Handbook of Oral Health

Handbook of Oral Health

Edited by Timothy Campbell

hayle
medical

New York

Hayle Medical,
750 Third Avenue, 9th Floor,
New York, NY 10017, USA

Visit us on the World Wide Web at:
www.haylemedical.com

ISBN: 978-1-63241-569-1

Cataloging-in-Publication Data

Handbook of oral health / edited by Timothy Campbell.
   p. cm.
Includes bibliographical references and index.
ISBN 978-1-63241-569-1
1. Mouth--Care and hygiene. 2. Oral medicine. 3. Dental care. 4. Dental public health.
5. Mouth--Diseases. 6. Dentistry. I. Campbell, Timothy.
RK60.7 .H36 2019
617.601--dc23

Table of Contents

Preface...IX

Chapter 1   **Molecular and clinical analyses of *Helicobacter pylori* colonization in inflamed dental pulp**..1
Ryota Nomura, Yuko Ogaya, Saaya Matayoshi, Yumiko Morita and
Kazuhiko Nakano

Chapter 2   **Evaluation of root resorption after comprehensive orthodontic treatment using cone beam computed tomography (CBCT)**...10
Yaqi Deng, Yannan Sun and Tianmin Xu

Chapter 3   **Perceptions and attitudes toward performing risk assessment for periodontal disease: a focus group exploration**..24
Thankam Thyvalikakath, Mei Song and Titus Schleyer

Chapter 4   **Dental caries and their association with socioeconomic characteristics, oral hygiene practices and eating habits among preschool children in Abu Dhabi, United Arab Emirates — the NOPLAS project**..34
Amal Elamin, Malin Garemo and Andrew Gardner

Chapter 5   **Shaping ability of protaper next compared with waveone in late-model three-dimensional printed teeth**...42
Zhi Cui, Zhao Wei, Minquan Du, Ping Yan and Han Jiang

Chapter 6   **Inequalities in oral health among adolescents in Gangneung**...........................50
Se-Hwan Jung, Myoung-Hee Kim and Jae-In Ryu

Chapter 7   **Parenting and oral health in an inner-city environment**...................................57
Shalini Nayee, Charlotte Klass, Gail Findlay and Jennifer E. Gallagher

Chapter 8   **Visual and radiographic caries detection: a tailored meta-analysis for two different settings**...67
Falk Schwendicke, Karim Elhennawy, Osama El Shahawy, Reham Maher,
Thais Gimenez, Fausto M. Mendes and Brian H. Willis

Chapter 9   **Are standardized caries risk assessment models effective in assessing actual caries status and future caries increment?**..76
Maria Grazia Cagetti, Giuliana Bontà, Fabio Cocco, Peter Lingstrom,
Laura Strohmenger and Guglielmo Campus

Chapter 10   **Children's dental fear and anxiety: exploring family related factors**................86
Lingli Wu and Xiaoli Gao

Chapter 11   **Glass hybrid restorations as an alternative for restoring hypomineralized molars in the ART model**...96
Juliana de Aguiar Grossi, Renata Nunes Cabral, Ana Paula Dias Ribeiro and
Soraya Coelho Leal

Chapter 12   **Panoramic radiographs and quantitative ultrasound of the radius and phalanx III to assess bone mineral status in postmenopausal women**....................103
Katarzyna Grocholewicz, Joanna Janiszewska-Olszowska,
Magda Aniko-Włodarczyk, Olga Preuss, Grzegorz Trybek, Ewa Sobolewska
and Mariusz Lipski

Chapter 13   **Perceived oral health and its association with symptoms of psychological distress, oral status and socio-demographic characteristics among elderly**....................111
Kari Elisabeth Dahl, Giovanna Calogiuri and Birgitta Jönsson

Chapter 14   **Rapid urease test (RUT) for evaluation of urease activity in oral bacteria in vitro and in supragingival dental plaque ex vivo**....................119
Gunnar Dahlén, Haidar Hassan, Susanne Blomqvist and Anette Carlén

Chapter 15   **Relations among obesity, family socioeconomic status, oral health behaviors and dental caries in adolescents: the 2010–2012 Korea National Health and nutrition examination survey**....................126
Jin Ah Kim, Hayon Michelle Choi, Yunhee Seo and Dae Ryong Kang

Chapter 16   **Lead exposure may affect gingival health in children**....................133
Borany Tort, Youn-Hee Choi, Eun-Kyong Kim, Yun-Sook Jung, Mina Ha,
Keun-Bae Song and Young-Eun Lee

Chapter 17   **Agony resulting from cultural practices of canine bud extraction among children under five years in selected slums of Makindye**....................140
Fiona Atim, Teddy Nagaddya, Florence Nakaggwa, Mary Gorrethy N-Mboowa,
Peter Kirabira and John Charles Okiria

Chapter 18   **The dental perspective on osteogenesis imperfecta in a Danish adult population**....................148
Kirstine Juhl Thuesen, Hans Gjørup, Jannie Dahl Hald, Malene Schmidt,
Torben Harsløf, Bente Langdahl and Dorte Haubek

Chapter 19   **Morphology of palatally displaced canines and adjacent teeth, a 3-D evaluation from cone-beam computed tomographic images**....................155
Rosalia Leonardi, Simone Muraglie, Salvatore Crimi, Marco Pirroni,
Giuseppe Musumeci and Rosario Perrotta

Chapter 20   **Can a brief psychological intervention improve oral health behaviour? A randomised controlled trial**....................164
U. Wide, J. Hagman, H. Werner and M. Hakeberg

Chapter 21   **The role of three interleukin 10 gene polymorphisms (− 1082 A > G, − 819 C > T, − 592 A > C) in the risk of chronic and aggressive periodontitis: a meta-analysis and trial sequential analysis**....................172
Hey Chiann Wong, Yuxuan Ooi, Shaju Jacob Pulikkotil and Cho Naing

Chapter 22   **Odontogenic ameloblast-associated protein (ODAM) in gingival crevicular fluid for site-specific diagnostic value of periodontitis**....................182
Hye-Kyung Lee, Soo Jin Kim, Young Ho Kim, Youngkyung Ko, Suk Ji and
Joo-Cheol Park

Chapter 23   **An assessment of strategies to control dental caries in Aboriginal children living in rural and remote communities** 190
Yvonne Dimitropoulos, Alexander Holden, Kylie Gwynne, Michelle Irving, Norma Binge and Anthony Blinkhorn

Chapter 24   **The Oral health status of children with autism Spectrum disorder in KwaZulu-Nata** 197
Magandhree Naidoo and Shenuka Singh

Chapter 25   **Factors associated with future dental care utilization among low-income smokers overdue for dental visits** 206
Paula R. Blasi, Chloe Krakauer, Melissa L. Anderson, Jennifer Nelson, Terry Bush, Sheryl L. Catz and Jennifer B. McClure

Chapter 26   **Assessment of the effect of the corticotomy-assisted orthodontic treatment on the maxillary periodontal tissue in patients with malocclusions with transverse maxillary deficiency** 218
Magdalena Sulewska, Ewa Duraj, Beata Bugała-Musiatowicz, Emilia Waszkiewicz-Sewastianik, Robert Milewski, Jan K. Pietruski, Eugeniusz Sajewicz and Małgorzata Pietruska

Chapter 27   **Oral health and health-related quality of life in HIV patients** 227
Vinicius da Costa Vieira, Liliane Lins, Viviane Almeida Sarmento, Eduardo Martins Netto and Carlos Brites

Chapter 28   **A new tooth brushing approach supported by an innovative hybrid toothbrush-compared reduction of dental plaque after a single use versus an oscillating-rotating powered toothbrush** 234
D. Klonowicz, M. Czerwinska, A. Sirvent and J-Ph. Gatignol

Chapter 29   **Evaluation of the relationship between maxillary posterior teeth and the maxillary sinus floor using cone-beam computed tomography** 242
Yechen Gu, Chao Sun, Daming Wu, Qingping Zhu, Diya Leng and Yang Zhou

Chapter 30   **Income and wealth as correlates of socioeconomic disparity in dentist visits among adults aged 20 years and over** 249
Alexander Kailembo, Carlos Quiñonez, Gabriela V. Lopez Mitnik, Jane A. Weintraub, Jennifer Stewart Williams, Raman Preet, Timothy Iafolla and Bruce A. Dye

Chapter 31   **What factors are associated with dental general anaesthetics for Australian children and what are the policy implications?** 259
John Rogers, Clare Delany, Clive Wright, Kaye Roberts-Thomson and Mike Morgan

Permissions

List of Contributors

Index

Preface

Every book is a source of knowledge and this one is no exception. The idea that led to the conceptualization of this book was the fact that the world is advancing rapidly; which makes it crucial to document the progress in every field. I am aware that a lot of data is already available, yet, there is a lot more to learn. Hence, I accepted the responsibility of editing this book and contributing my knowledge to the community.

Oral health is a branch of medicine concerned with teeth and other areas of the craniofacial complex including the temporomandibular joint and the supporting muscular, lymphatic, vascular, nervous and anatomical structures. Tooth decay is the most common disease occurring globally. Over 80% of cavities occur inside the fissures in teeth, which are not accessible by brushing. Teeth cleaning removes dental plaque and tartar and thus prevents cavities, gum disease, gingivitis and tooth decay. Professional cleaning involves scaling and polishing, debridement and fluoride treatment. Good oral hygiene is required for the prevention of tartar build-up and can be ensured with regular brushing and flossing. Dentures and retainers should also be cleaned regularly. A dentist or a dental surgeon specializes in the diagnosis, treatment and prevention of the conditions of the oral cavity. Complex procedures such as bone grafting, gingival grafts, invasive oral and maxillofacial surgical procedures, sinus lifts and implants, etc. are performed by a dental team comprising of the dentist, dental hygienists, dental therapists, dental technicians and dental assistants. This book contains some path-breaking studies in the field of oral health. It discusses the fundamentals as well as modern approaches of oral health and dentistry. It is a collective contribution of a renowned group of international experts.

While editing this book, I had multiple visions for it. Then I finally narrowed down to make every chapter a sole standing text explaining a particular topic, so that they can be used independently. However, the umbrella subject sinews them into a common theme. This makes the book a unique platform of knowledge.

I would like to give the major credit of this book to the experts from every corner of the world, who took the time to share their expertise with us. Also, I owe the completion of this book to the never-ending support of my family, who supported me throughout the project.

Editor

Molecular and clinical analyses of *Helicobacter pylori* colonization in inflamed dental pulp

Ryota Nomura*, Yuko Ogaya, Saaya Matayoshi, Yumiko Morita and Kazuhiko Nakano

Abstract

Background: Recently, dental pulp has been considered a possible source of infection of *Helicobacter pylori* (*H. pylori*) in children. We previously developed a novel PCR system for *H. pylori* detection with high specificity and sensitivity using primer sets constructed based on the complete genome information for 48 *H. pylori* strains. This PCR system showed high sensitivity with a detection limit of 1–10 cells when serial dilutions of *H. pylori* genomic DNA were used as templates. However, the detection limit was lower (10^2–10^3 cells) when *H. pylori* bacterial DNA was detected from inflamed pulp specimens. Thus, we further refined the system using a nested PCR method, which was much more sensitive than the previous single PCR method. In addition, we examined the distribution and virulence of *H. pylori* in inflamed pulp tissue.

Methods: Nested PCR system was constructed using primer sets designed from the complete genome information of 48 *H. pylori* strains. The detection limit of the nested PCR system was 1–10 cells using both *H. pylori* genomic DNA and bacterial DNA isolated from inflamed pulp specimens. Next, distribution of *H. pylori* was examined using 131 inflamed pulp specimens with the nested PCR system. In addition, association between the detection of *H. pylori* and clinical information regarding endodontic-infected teeth were investigated. Furthermore, adhesion property of *H. pylori* strains to human dental fibroblast cells was examined.

Results: *H. pylori* was present in 38.9% of inflamed pulp specimens using the nested PCR system. *H. pylori* was shown to be predominantly detected in primary teeth rather than permanent teeth. In addition, samplings of the inflamed pulp were performed twice from the same teeth at 1- or 2-week intervals, which revealed that *H. pylori* was detected in most specimens in both samplings. Furthermore, *H. pylori* strains showed adhesion property to human dental fibroblast cells.

Conclusion: Our results suggest that *H. pylori* colonizes inflamed pulp in approximately 40% of all cases through adhesion to human dental fibroblast cells.

Keywords: *Helicobacter pylori*, Inflamed pulp, Nested PCR method, Human dental fibroblast cells

Background

Helicobacter pylori is a Gram-negative microaerophilic bacterium found in the stomach that is responsible for gastric diseases [1]. Though details regarding its transmission and infection source remain unclear, the most likely route of infection is through the oral cavity [2]. To detect *H. pylori* in oral cavity specimens, molecular biological technique has been applied [3]. However, it is not easy to estimate the actual infection rate as *H. pylori* detected in the oral cavity has been reported to be 0–100% [4].

To overcome the difficulty of the detection of *H. pylori* in the oral specimens, we previously designed novel primer sets based on the information of the complete genome for 48 *H. pylori* strains in the database [5]. We searched genes including 16S rRNA, *vacA*, *cagA*, *glmM* (*ureC*), and *ureA* because these genes were used for *H. pylori* detection in published PCR methods with high

* Correspondence: rnomura@dent.osaka-u.ac.jp
Department of Pediatric Dentistry, Division of Oral Infection and Disease Control, Osaka University Graduate School of Dentistry, 1-8 Yamada-oka, Suita, Osaka 565-0871, Japan

frequency [6–10]. Among these genes, six sequences of at least 20 consecutive nucleotides conserved among all strains were found only in *ureA*, which were selected as primer sets for the detection. These primer sets produced amplicons for genomic DNA across *H. pylori* strains, but did not for *Helicobacter pullorum* and *Helicobacter felis* strains, the closest related species to *H. pylori*.

Most studies regarding *H. pylori* detection from oral specimens have focused on dental plaque or saliva specimens [11, 12]. A recent study showed that *H. pylori* was isolated from endodontic-infected root canals of primary teeth [13]. In addition, we detected *H. pylori* bacterial DNA in inflamed pulp specimens using our novel PCR method [5]. In the present study, we refined our system using a nested PCR method, which is much more sensitive than the previous single PCR method. The nested PCR method was then applied to investigate the actual *H. pylori* distribution in inflamed pulp specimens as well as correlations between the detection of *H. pylori* and clinical information regarding endodontic-infected teeth. Furthermore, the adhesion property of *H. pylori* strains to human dental fibroblast cells, which is considered an important virulence factor of *H. pylori* detected in inflamed pulp, was also investigated.

Method

Bacterial strains and growth condition

H. pylori reference strain 26,695 (ATCC 700392), J99 (ATCC 700824), ATCC 51932, and *H. pullorum* ATCC 51802 were purchased from Summit Pharmaceuticals International Corporation (Tokyo, Japan). *H. felis* ATCC 49179 was kindly provided by Professor Masakazu Kita (Department of Microbiology, Kyoto Prefectural University of Medicine, Kyoto, Japan). All strains were cultured by the method described previously using blood agar plates (Becton Dickinson, Franklin Lakes, NJ, USA) at 37 °C for 3 days [5]. Then, single colonies were selected, inoculated in 5 ml tryptic soy broth (Difco Laboratories, Detroit, MI, USA), and incubated at 37 °C for 3-5 days under microaerophilic conditions.

PCR system for *H. pylori* detection

H. pylori genomic DNA was extracted using a previously reported method for Gram-negative periodontitis-related bacteria [14]. We previously identified six sequences of at least 20 consecutive nucleotides in the *ureA* gene of 48 *H. pylori* strains registered in the GenBank database [5]. Based on these sequences, five primer sets (*ureA*-aF/aR, *ureA*-aF/bR, *ureA*-bF/aR, *ureA*-bF/bR, *ureA*-cF/cR) were constructed for PCR methods to detect *H. pylori* [5]. Among these primer sets, two primer sets for the first and second steps of the nested PCR method were selected as follows. First step PCR for *H. pylori* detection

was performed using primers *ureA*-aF (5′-ATG AAA CTC ACC CCA AAA GA-3′) and *ureA*-bR (5′-CCG AAA GTT TTT TCT CTG TCA AAG TCT A-3′); second step PCR was performed using primers *ureA*-bF (5′-AAA CGC AAA GAA AAA GGC ATT AA-3′) and *ureA*-aR (5′-TTC ACT TCA AAG AAA TGG AAG TGT GA-3′) (Fig. 1a). First step PCR was performed by amplifying 2 μl template genomic DNA extracted from cultured *H. pylori* strains or bacterial DNA extracted from dental pulp specimens in reactions of 20 μl total volume. Second step PCR was performed by amplifying 1 μl of the first PCR product used as a template in reactions of 20 μl total volume. Both PCR cycles of first and second steps of the nested PCR methods were performed as the single PCR method, described previously using TaKaRa Ex *Taq* polymerase (Takara Bio. Inc., Otsu, Japan) [5].

Specificity and sensitivity of the first and second step PCR systems

The specificity of primer sets for *H. pylori* detection was assessed using genomic DNA extracted from *H. pylori*, *H. pullorum*, and *H. felis*. The sensitivity of the PCR assays was determined using titrated cultures of *H. pylori* strain J99. The detection limits of the first step and second step PCR assays were determined using 10-fold serial dilutions of genomic DNA extracted from known numbers of bacterial cells. In addition, five inflamed pulp specimens were taken during root canal treatments. The total numbers of oral bacteria in these specimens were confirmed by plating serially diluted samples onto blood agar plates, which were anaerobically cultured at 37 °C for 4 days; specimens contained approximately 9×10^5–4×10^6 c.f.u. (mean 2.6×10^6 c.f.u.). Among these samples, two *H. pylori*-negative specimens were selected, which were confirmed using the nested PCR method described above. Two dental pulp specimens without bacterial infection were also collected during extraction of completely impacted wisdom teeth. Serial dilutions of known bacterial number of *H. pylori* were added to the inflamed and non-inflamed pulp specimens, followed by DNA extraction. Then, the detection limits of the first and second step PCR assays were determined using bacterial DNA as template.

Dental pulp specimens

This study was conducted in full adherence to the Declaration of Helsinki. The study protocol was approved by the Ethics Committee of Osaka University Graduate School of Dentistry (approval no. H23-E1-5). Prior to specimen collection, the subjects were informed of the study contents and written informed consent was obtained from all participants. When the participant was

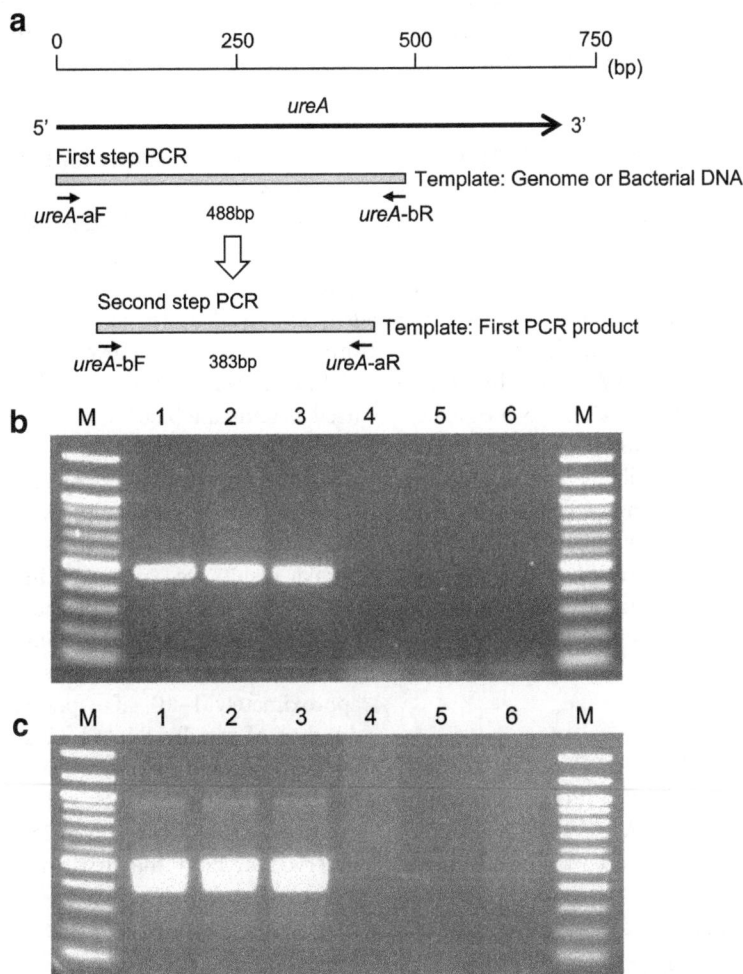

Fig. 1 Nested PCR method for *H. pylori* detection. **a** A schematic diagram of positions of the designed primers in this study. **b** Representative images showing the single PCR assay for *H. pylori* detection using *ureA*-aF and *ureA*-bR primer sets. **c** Representative images showing the nested PCR assay for *H. pylori* detection using *ureA*-aF and *ureA*-bR primer sets, followed by *ureA*-bF and *ureA*-aR primer sets. Lanes: 1, *H. pylori* 26,695; 2, J99; 3, ATCC 51932; 4, *H. pullorum* ATCC 51802; 5, *H. felis* ATCC 49179; 6, sterile water. M, molecular size marker (100 bp DNA ladder)

aged under 16, parental written informed consent was also obtained.

Inflamed pulp specimens were obtained from 131 subjects (age range: 1-19 years) who were treated at Osaka University Dental Hospital from February 2013 to February 2016. In our clinic, dental treatments including root canal treatments are performed children aged over 3 or 4 years. However, we performed the root canal treatments to the subjects with lower ages under restraint after the consent of the parents when the subjects have acute symptoms such as spontaneous pain or gingival abscess formation. The specimens were taken from patients who received root canal treatment under local anesthesia because of severe childhood caries ($n = 114$) or trauma ($n = 17$). The 101 and 30 specimens were obtained from primary and permanent teeth, respectively. Among 131 specimens, 36 were used in our previous study [5].

Inflamed pulp specimens taken from different teeth in the same patient were included among the 131 specimens and given a different specimen number.

Among 131 specimens, 20 specimens were taken additional sampling from the same teeth. All 20 specimens were collected from infected root canals with apical abscess formation. First samplings were performed in initial root canal treatments. When a gingival abscess formed, root canals were generally left unsealed and antibiotics were not applied during initial root canal treatments. Thus, second samplings were performed when the subjects visited the hospital for the second root canal treatment ($n = 20$). The detection frequencies of *H. pylori* between first and second samplings were compared.

The sampling method for dental pulp specimens was described previously [5]. The samples were stored on ice and immediately transported to our laboratory for testing. DNA extraction and nested PCR were performed as described above. To confirm that the amplified fragments in second step PCR were targeted species, ten positive bands were randomly selected and sequenced as described previously [15].

Adhesion to human dental pulp fibroblast cells (HDPFs)

The adhesion property of *H. pylori* strains to HDPFs was examined using a method described previously [16], with some modifications. Approximately 1×10^5 HDPFs were seeded in the tissue culture plates (Costar®, Corning Inc., Corning, NY, USA). The wells were washed with PBS and antibiotic-free medium was added, followed by the infection of 1×10^6 c.f.u. *H. pylori* in antibiotic-free medium. The medium was removed after 1.5 h of anaerobic incubation and infected cells were washed with PBS, and then added the sterile distilled water for disruption of the cells. Next, dilutions of cell lysates were plated onto blood agar plates and incubated at 37 °C for 3 days under microaerophilic conditions. The adhesion rates were calculated by the ratio of resuspended to infected cells. Data are shown as the mean ± standard deviation of triplicate experiments.

Statistical analyses

Statistical analyses were performed using the computational software package GraphPad Prism 6 (GraphPad Software Inc., La Jolla, CA, USA). Intergroup differences in each analysis were analyzed using Bonferroni's method after analysis of variance (ANOVA). A *P* value of less than 0.05 was considered to be statistically significant.

Results

Specificity and sensitivity for the first and second step PCR systems

The first and second step PCR primer sets produced amplicons consistent in size for genomic DNA of all *H. pylori* strains, but were not seen in *H. pullorum* and *H. felis* strains (Fig. 1b, c). The first and second step PCR primer sets showed a level of sensitivity at approximately 1–10 c.f.u. per reaction when *H. pylori* genomic DNA was used as template (Fig. 2a, b). However, the sensitivity of the first step PCR primer sets was decreased (10^2–10^3 c.f.u.) when the known number of serially diluted *H. pylori* was added to the infected pulp specimen, whereas the second PCR primer sets maintained a high sensitivity (Fig. 2c, d). Similar results were observed in both the first and second step PCR assays when another inflamed pulp specimen was used (data not shown). Furthermore, the sensitivities of the first and second step PCR primer sets were approximately 1–10 c.f.u. per reaction when the known number of serially diluted *H. pylori* was added to non-bacterial infected pulp specimens, though the bands in the first step PCR were weaker than those obtained from *H. pylori* genomic DNA (Fig. 2e, f). Similar results were observed in both the first and second step PCR assays

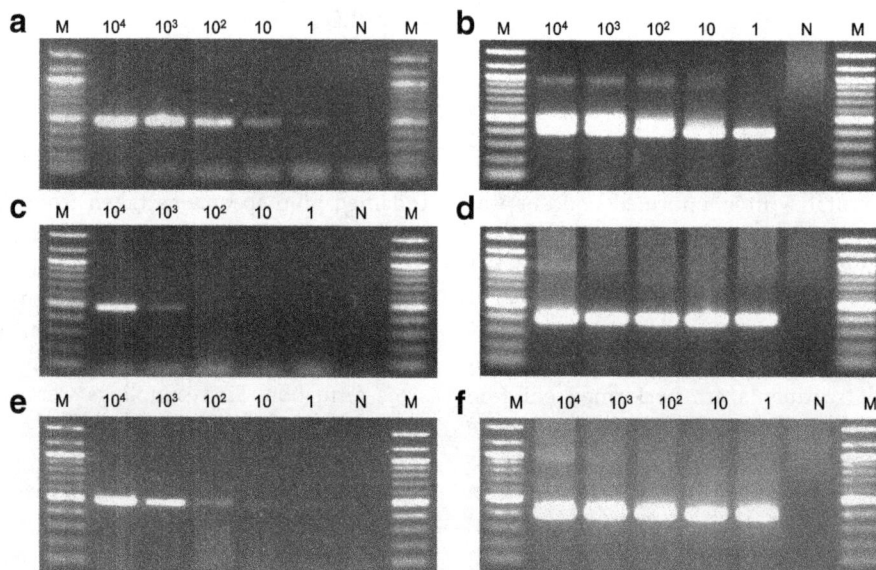

Fig. 2 Sensitivity of the single and nested PCR assays for *H. pylori* detection. Representative images showing the sensitivities of (**a**) single and (**b**) second step PCR assays for the detection of *H. pylori* J99 genomic DNA. Representative images showing the sensitivities of (**c**) single and (**d**) second step PCR assays for the detection of *H. pylori* bacterial DNA from inflamed pulp. Representative images showing the sensitivities of (**e**) single and (**f**) second step PCR assays for the detection of *H. pylori* bacterial DNA added to non-infected dental pulp. The *ureA*-aF and *ureA*-bR primer sets were used for the single PCR assay and *ureA*-bF and *ureA*-aR primer sets were used for the second step PCR assay. M, molecular size marker (100 bp DNA ladder)

when another non-infected pulp specimen was used (data not shown).

H. pylori Detection in inflamed pulp specimens

Figure 3a and b show representative results from the analyses of inflamed pulp specimens using the first and second PCR primer sets. *H. pylori* was detected in 4 of 131 (3.1%) root canal specimens in first step PCR, indicating that these samples contained more than 10^2–10^3 c.f.u. *H. pylori*. In second step PCR, 51 (38.9%) root canal specimens were *H. pylori*-positive, indicating that these samples contained more than 1–10 c.f.u. *H. pylori*. The nucleotide alignment of the fragment revealed that the second step PCR method could amplify the target sequence of *H. pylori*. The detection rate of *H. pylori* in second step PCR was significantly higher than that in first step PCR (***$P < 0.001$) (Fig. 3c). Additionally, there were no subjects in whom *H. pylori* was detected from all specimens taken from different teeth (Table 1). Among 20 specimens taken from the same teeth, 8 specimens were *H. pylori*-positive in the first sampling, 7 of which were *H. pylori*-positive in the second sampling (Fig. 3d). In addition, only 1 of 12 *H. pylori*-negative specimens showed positive results in the second sampling. There was no significant difference between the detection rate of *H. pylori* in specimens obtained from dental caries and that obtained from trauma (Fig. 3e). The detection rate of *H. pylori* in specimens obtained from primary teeth was higher than that obtained from permanent teeth, though there was no significant difference (Fig. 3f).

H. pylori Adhesion to HDPFs

All three tested *H. pylori* strains showed adhesion to HDPFs (Fig. 4a). Among these strains, 26,695 showed significantly higher adhesion rates than J99 (*$P < 0.05$). Confocal scanning laser microscopy demonstrated that *H. pylori* strain 26,695 clearly adhered to HDPFs (Fig. 4b).

Discussion

The reliable PCR system for the *H. pylori* detection in oral specimens requires high specificity and sensitivity levels since it is known that there are approximately 700 bacterial phylotypes found in the oral cavity [17]. To overcome difficulties in detecting *H. pylori* in the oral cavity, we previously designed novel primer sets using the complete genome information for 48 *H. pylori* strains registered in the GenBank database [5]. In that study, we found six sequences of at least 20 consecutive nucleotides conserved among all strains in the *ureA* gene. The *ureA* gene is known to encode the urease enzyme, which has been frequently used to develop PCR primers for *H. pylori* detection [7, 10, 18]. However, no

previous *ureA*-based primers were completely conserved among all strains registered in the database [5].

We previously constructed five primer sets (*ureA*-aF/aR, *ureA*-aF/bR, *ureA*-bF/aR, *ureA*-bF/bR, *ureA*-cF/cR) for the detection of *H. pylori* based on six sequences of at least 20 consecutive nucleotides [5]. These primer sets showed an appropriate level of sensitivity at approximately 1–10 c.f.u. per reaction for *H. pylori* genomic DNA. However, these primers sets revealed a sensitivity of approximately 10^2–10^3 cells for the detection of *H. pylori* DNA from inflamed pulp specimens. It has been reported that some PCR primers sets showed lower detection limits in *H. pylori* from gastric tissues or oral specimens compared with that from *H. pylori* genomic DNA [11]. In addition, we compared the sensitivities of detecting *H. pylori* from infected pulp specimens versus non-infected pulp specimens by adding a known number of serially diluted *H. pylori* to these specimens using the single PCR methods. The sensitivity in inflamed pulp specimens was much lower than that in non-infected pulp specimens, which indicated that numerous bacteria present at more than 10^6 c.f.u. in inflamed pulp may be the main cause for difficulty in detecting *H. pylori* in such specimens. Thus, we refined our system using a nested PCR method to improve the sensitivity for detection of *H. pylori* DNA from inflamed pulp tissue. Among the five primer sets beased on the *ureA* gene designed in our previous study, primer sets *ureA*-aF/bR and *ureA*-bF/aR were suitable for the nested PCR method.

Nested PCR is one of the most sensitive methods to detect a small number of bacteria from clinical specimens [19]. The specificity and sensitivity of target DNA amplification is estimated to be approximately 1000–10,000 times more sensitive than standard PCR [20]. Some researchers previously reported *H. pylori* detection using nested PCR methods [21]. However, complete genome information was unavailable when these nested PCR methods were reported. *H. pylori* 26,695 (ATCC 700392) is the first strain reported to identify the complete genome sequence in 1997, then only several complete genome sequences of *H. pylori* strains were reported until 10 years ago [22]. To our knowledge, this is the first study to propose a nested PCR method designed based on a large amount of genome information.

The detection rate of *H. pylori* from inflamed pulp specimens detected by single PCR with primer sets *ureA*-aF/*ureA*-bR were 3.0%, whereas that with primer set *ureA*-aF/*ureA*-aR was 15% [5]. However, the detection rate using primer set *ureA*-aF/*ureA*-aR was based on the results from only 40 specimens. Thus, the detection rate of the primer set *ureA*-aF/*ureA*-aR in 131 specimens was investigated in the present study, resulting in a detection rate of 5.3% (data not shown). Though the

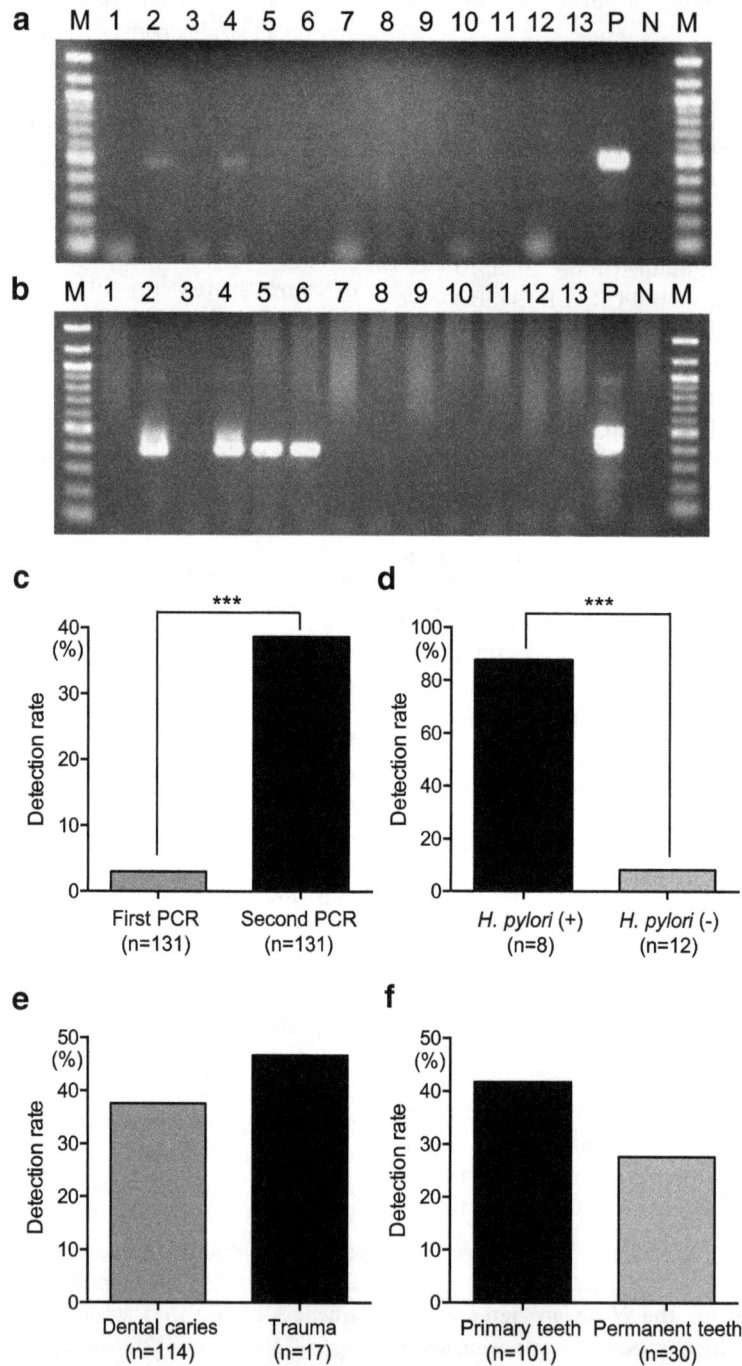

Fig. 3 Detection of *H. pylori* from inflamed pulp specimens using single and nested PCR assays. Representative results using inflamed pulp specimens with (**a**) single and (**b**) second step PCR. Lanes 1 through 13 are specimens collected from 13 different individuals; P, *H. pylori* strains 26,695 (positive control); N, sterile water. M, molecular size marker (100 bp DNA ladder). **c** Comparison of the detection rates of *H. pylori* from inflamed pulp specimens using single and second step PCR. **d** Detection rates of *H. pylori* in the second sampling from root canal specimens. The groups were categorized as *H. pylori*-positive or -negative in the first sampling. Comparison of the detection rates of *H. pylori* from specimens obtained from dental caries verses those from trauma (**e**) or in comparison between specimens obtained from primary teeth versus permanent teeth (**f**). Significant differences were determined using Bonferroni's method after ANOVA (***$P < 0.001$)

detection rate of *H. pylori* with primer set *ureA*-aF/*ureA*-aR was higher than that with primer set *ureA*-aF/*ureA*-bR, which may be because the primer set *ureA*-aF/*ureA*-aR was the most sensitive of all primer combinations [5], the detection limits of both primer sets were similar (approximately 1–10 cells using *H. pylori* genomic DNA). The

Table 1 Summary of *H. pylori* DNA detection of extirpated inflamed pulp specimens in the subjects who received root canal treatment several times

Subject	Dental caries extending pulp space (Age)				Detection Rate
1	ULA (2Y0M)	ULB (2Y1M)			0/2
	–	–			
2	URA (3Y9M)	URB (3Y9M)	ULA (3Y10M)		1/3
	+	–	–		
3	ULD (3Y10M)	URE (3Y11M)			0/2
	–	–			
4	LLC (4Y7M)	LRC (5Y5M)			1/2
	+	–			
5	LLE (5Y1M)	LLD (5Y3M)			0/2
	–	–			
6	URD (5Y2M)	LLE (5Y3M)			0/2
	–	–			
7	LLD (6Y0M)	LLE (7Y4M)			0/2
	–	–			
8	URD (6Y2M)	ULD (6Y4M)	URE (6Y5M)	LLE (6Y5M)	2/4
	+	+	–	–	
9	LLD (6Y11M)	LRE (7Y1M)			0/2
	–	–			
10	LRD (7Y4M)	URD (7Y5M)	LRD (7Y6M)		0/3
	–	–	–		
11	LLE (8Y1M)	URD (8Y2M)			0/2
	–	–			
12	LRE (7Y10M)	LRD (7Y10M)	LLE (7Y11M)	ULE (8Y0M)	2/4
	–	–	+	+	
13	LRD (8Y1M)	URD (10Y4M)			1/2
	+	–			
14	UL1 (9Y1M)	LL1 (10Y5M)			1/2
	–	+			
15	UR2 (11Y6M)	LR4 (11Y6M)	LR3 (11Y6M)	UL2 (11Y10M)	2/7
	+	–	–	–	
	UL5 (11Y10M)	UR5 (12Y1M)	UR4 (12Y1M)		
	–	+	–		
16	LL5 (14Y10M)	LL7 (14Y10M)			0/2
	–	–			

URE upper right primary second molar, *URD* upper right primary first molar, *URB* upper right primary lateral incisor, *URA* upper right primary central incisor, *ULA* upper left primary central incisor, *ULB* upper left primary lateral incisor, *ULD* upper left primary first molar, *ULE* upper left primary second molar, *LLE* lower left primary second molar, *LLD* lower left primary first molar, *LLC* lower left primary canine, *LRC* lower right primary canine, *LRD* lower right primary first molar, *LRE* lower right primary second molar, *UR5* upper left second premolar, *UR4* upper right first premolar, *UR2* upper right lateral incisor, *UL1* upper left central incisor, *UL2* upper left lateral incisor, *UL4* upper left first premolar, *UL5* I upper left second premolar, *LL7* lower left second molar, *LL5* lower left second premolar, *LL1* lower left central incisor, *LR3* lower right canine

single PCR method using primer set *ureA*-aF/*ureA*-aR is a simple and highly sensitive method; however, nested PCR is the most appropriate method for *H. pylori* detection because it showed highest sensitivity (1–10 cells) and detection rate (38.9%) in inflamed pulp specimens.

To determine the detailed distribution of *H. pylori* in inflamed pulp tissue, we analyzed the detection rate of *H. pylori* in 16 subjects who received root canal treatment in different teeth. In addition, *H. pylori* detection in 20 subjects with two samplings from the same tooth

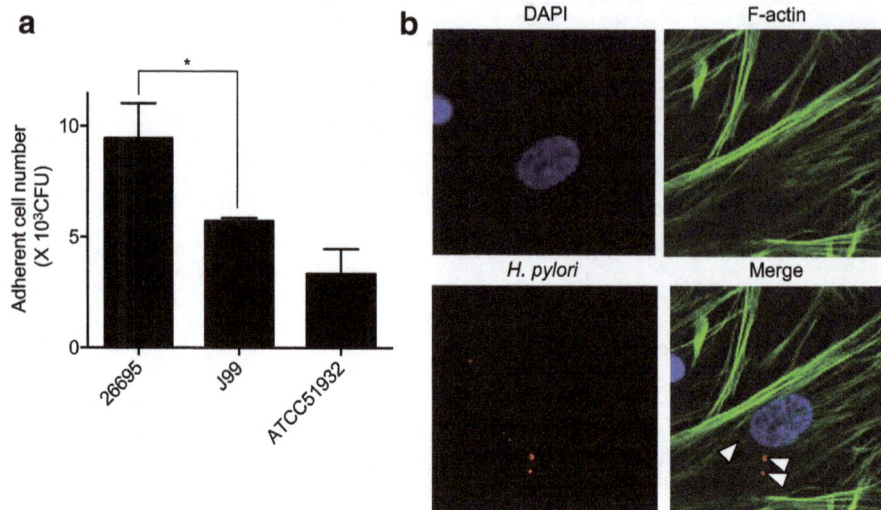

Fig. 4 Adhesion of *H. pylori* strains to human dental pulp fibroblast cells. **a** Adhesion rates were calculated based on the ratio of recovered to infected strains with an multiplicity of infection of 10. Significant differences were determined using Bonferroni's method after ANOVA (*$P < 0.05$). **b** Representative confocal scanning laser microscopic images of *H. pylori* strain 26,695 showing adhesion to human dental fibroblast cells following dual labeling. Nuclei are stained blue, bacterial cells adhering to HDPFs are stained red (arrows), and actin filaments are stained green

was performed. *H. pylori* was not detected from all inflamed pulp specimens in each individual, indicating that *H. pylori* was not widely distributed in teeth with infected root canals. However, most *H. pylori*-positive specimens were positive in the second sampling, suggesting that *H. pylori* was not transiently present but rather colonized the inflamed pulp tissue. Since the intervals between first and second samplings were approximately 1–2 weeks in most subjects, the precise colonization period of *H. pylori* in infected root canal remains unknown. Further studies should be performed to clarify this point. Comparison of the detection rates of *H. pylori* from specimens obtained from primary teeth versus permanent teeth revealed that higher detection rate of *H. pylori* was observed in specimens obtained from primary teeth. The result may be reasonable because *H. pylori* infections seem to be acquired in childhood [2].

Since *H. pylori* was not transiently present in infected root canal, we investigated the mechanism by which *H. pylori* colonizes pulp tissue by analyzing the adhesion property of *H. pylori* to HDPFs. Bacterial adhesion to host cells is considered an important virulence factor for many bacterial species [23]. For *H. pylori*, bacterial adhesion to gastric epithelium is a critical factor for *H. pylori* colonization [24]. However, there have been few reports focusing on *H. pylori* adhesion to cells obtained from oral origin, and, to our knowledge, this is the first study to investigate the adhesion properties of *H. pylori* to HDPFs. All three tested *H. pylori* strains showed adhesion to HDPFs, which is likely one of the reasons why *H. pylori* DNA was detected in inflamed pulp specimens. Among these strains, *cagA*-positive *H. pylori* strains

26,695 and J99 showed higher adhesion rates compared with *cagA*-negative *H. pylori* strain ATCC 51932. The *cagA* gene belongs to the *cag* pathogenicity island (PAI) [25]. The *cag* PAI contains several virulence genes, some of which were reported to be related to *H. pylori* adhesion to gastric epithelial cells [26, 27]. Though *cagA* is one of the possible genes related to *H. pylori* adhesion, various *H. pylori* adhesins have also been reported [28], and the adhesion mechanisms to HDPFs remain to be elucidated. Further studies should be performed to investigate bacterial adhesion induced by *H. pylori* virulence genes.

Conclusions

In summary, our nested PCR approach to detect *H. pylori* in inflamed pulp was constructed using two primers sets, both of which were designed based on conserved sequences in *H. pylori* strains. The nested PCR method showed a higher sensitivity than the single PCR method, which used only one primer set. In addition, *H. pylori* strains showed adhesion to HDPFs. These results clearly suggest that *H. pylori* may colonize dental pulp tissue.

Abbreviations
HDPFs: Human dental fibroblast cells; PBS: Phosphate-buffered saline

Acknowledgements
We thank Prof. Howard K. Kuramitsu, State University of New York at Buffalo, for editing the manuscript. We also thank Ms. Rewa Yanagisawa, WDB Co., Ltd., for technical support with molecular analyses.

Funding
This work was supported by JSPS KAKENHI Grant Number JP15H05049.

Authors' contributions
RN and KN designed the study, and experiments were performed by RN, YO, SM and YM. Data interpretation was performed RN and KN. RN wrote the paper under the supervision of KN. All authors read and approved the entire contents of the manuscript.

Competing interests
The authors declare that they have no competing interests.

References
1. Fennerty MB. *Helicobacter pylori*. Arch Intern Med. 1994;154:721–7.
2. Prasanthi CH, Prasanthi NL, Manikiran SS, Rama-Rao NN. Focus on current trends in the treatment of *Helicobacter pylori* infection: an update. Inter J Pharm Sci Rev Res. 2011;1:42–51.
3. Westblom TU, Bhatt BD. Diagnosis of *Helicobacter pylori* infection. Curr Topics Microbiol Immunol. 1999;241:215–35.
4. Silva DG, Tinoco EM, Rocha GA, Rocha AM, Guerra JB, Saraiva IE, Queiroz DM. *Helicobacter pylori* transiently in the mouth may participate in the transmission of infection. Mem Inst Oswaldo Cruz. 2010;105:657–60.
5. Ogaya Y, Nomura R, Watanabe Y, Nakano K. Detection of *Helicobacter pylori* DNA in inflamed dental pulp specimens from Japanese children and adolescents. J Med Microbiol. 2015;64:117–23.
6. Mapstone NP, Lynch DA, Lewis FA, Axon AT, Tompkins DS, Dixon MF, Quirke P. Identification of *Helicobacter pylori* DNA in the mouths and stomachs of patients with gastritis using PCR. J Clin Pathol. 1993;46:540–3.
7. Miyabayashi H, Furihata K, Shimizu T, Ueno I, Akamatsu T. Influence of oral *Helicobacter pylori* on the success of eradication therapy against gastric *Helicobacter pylori*. Helicobacter. 2000;5:30–7.
8. Wang J, Chi DS, Laffan JJ, Li C, Ferguson DA Jr, Litchfield P, Thomas E. Comparison of cytotoxin genotypes of *Helicobacter pylori* in stomach and saliva. Dig Dis Sci. 2002;47:1850–6.
9. Park CY, Kwak M, Gutierrez O, Graham DY, Yamaoka Y. Comparison of genotyping *Helicobacter pylori* directly from biopsy specimens and genotyping from bacterial cultures. J Clin Microbiol. 2003;41:3336–8.
10. Smith SI, Oyedeji KS, Arigbabu AO, Cantet F, Megraud F, Ojo OO, Uwaifo AO, Otegbayo JA, Ola SO, Coker AO. Comparison of three PCR methods for detection of *Helicobacter pylori* DNA and detection of *cagA* gene in gastric biopsy specimens. World J Gastroenterol. 2004;10:1958–60.
11. Sugimoto M, Wu JY, Abudayyeh S, Hoffman J, Brahem H, Al-Khatib K, Yamaoka Y, Graham DY. Unreliability of results of PCR detection of *Helicobacter pylori* in clinical or environmental samples. J Clin Microbiol. 2009;47:738–42.
12. Aksit Bıcak D, Akyuz S, Kıratlı B, Usta M, Urganci N, Alev B, Yarat A, Sahin F. The investigation of *Helicobacter pylori* in the dental biofilm and saliva samples of children with dyspeptic complaints. BMC Oral Health. 2017;17:67.
13. Hirsch C, Tegtmeyer N, Rohde M, Rowland M, Oyarzabal OA, Backert S. Live *Helicobacter pylori* in the root canal of endodontic-infected deciduous teeth. J Gastroenterol. 2012;47:936–40.
14. Amano A, Nakagawa I, Kataoka K, Morisaki I, Hamada S. Distribution of *Porphyromonas gingivalis* strains with *fimA* genotypes in periodontitis patients. J Clin Microbiol. 1999;37:1426–30.
15. Nakano K, Inaba H, Nomura R, Nemoto H, Takeda M, Yoshioka H, Matsue H, Takahashi T, Taniguchi K, et al. Detection of cariogenic *Streptococcus mutans* in extirpated heart valve and atheromatous plaque specimens. J Clin Microbiol. 2006;44:3313–7.
16. Nomura R, Ogaya Y, Nakano K. Contribution of the collagen-binding proteins of *Streptococcus mutans* to bacterial colonization of inflamed dental pulp. PLoS One. 2016;11:e0159613.
17. Robert J, Palmer JR. Composition and development of oral bacterial communities. Periodontol. 2013;64:20–39.
18. Peek RM Jr, Miller GG, Tham KT, Pérez-Pérez GI, Cover TL, Atherton JC, Dunn GD, Blaser MJ. Detection of *Helicobacter pylori* gene expression in human gastric mucosa. J Clin Microbiol. 1995;33:28–32.
19. Yamamoto Y. PCR in diagnosis of infection: detection of bacteria in cerebrospinal fluids. Clin Diagn Lab Immunol. 2002;9:508–14.
20. Takahashi T, Nakayama T, Tamura M, Ogawa K, Tsuda H, Morita A, Hara M, Togo M, Shiota H, et al. Nested polymerase chain reaction for assessing the clinical course of tuberculous meningitis. Neurology. 2005;64:1789–93.
21. Umeda M, Kobayashi H, Takeuchi Y, Hayashi J, Morotome-Hayashi Y, Yano K, Aoki A, Ohkusa T, Ishikawa I. High prevalence of *Helicobacter pylori* detected by PCR in the oral cavities of periodontitis patients. J Periodontol. 2003;74:129–34.
22. Oh JD, Kling-Bäckhed H, Giannakis M, Xu J, Fulton RS, Fulton LA, Cordum HS, Wang C, Elliott G, et al. The complete genome sequence of a chronic atrophic gastritis *Helicobacter pylori* strain: evolution during disease progression. Proc Natl Acad Sci U S A. 2006;103:9999–10004.
23. Ribet D, Cossart P. How bacterial pathogens colonize their hosts and invade deeper tissues. Microbes Infect. 2015;17:173–83.
24. Sheu BS, Yang HB, Yeh YC, Wu JJ. *Helicobacter pylori* colonization of the human gastric epithelium: a bug's first step is a novel target for us. J Gastroenterol Hepatol. 2010;25:26–32.
25. Jones KR, Whitmire JM, Merrell DS. A tale of two toxins: *Helicobacter Pylori* CagA and VacA modulate host pathways that impact disease. Front Microbiol. 2010;1:115.
26. Rieder G, Hatz RA, Moran AP, Walz A, Stolte M, Enders G. Role of adherence in interleukin-8 induction in *Helicobacter pylori*-associated gastritis. Infect Immun. 1997;65:3622–30.
27. Segal ED, Lange C, Covacci A, Tompkins LS, Falkow S. Induction of host signal transduction pathways by *Helicobacter pylori*. Proc Natl Acad Sci U S A. 1997;94:7595–9.
28. Ghosh P, Sarkar A, Ganguly M, Raghwan Alam J, De R, Mukhopadhyay AK. *Helicobacter pylori* strains harboring *babA2* from Indian sub population are associated with increased virulence in ex vivo study. Gut Pathog. 2016;8:1.

2

Evaluation of root resorption after comprehensive orthodontic treatment using cone beam computed tomography (CBCT)

Yaqi Deng, Yannan Sun and Tianmin Xu[*]

Abstract

Background: Orthodontic treatment can result in root resorption (RR). Traditional two-dimensional (2D) data exhibit magnification, deformation and positioning problems. Cone beam computed tomography (CBCT) contains more accurate three-dimensional (3D) information. This study identified and qualified the extent and location of root resorption using cone beam computed tomography (CBCT) after comprehensive orthodontic treatment.

Methods: Studies comparing the RR before and after comprehensive orthodontic treatment using CBCT were identified using electronic searches of databases, including Cochrane, PubMed, EMBASE, China National Knowledge Infrastructure (CNKI) and Web of Science, and manual searches in relevant journals and the reference lists of the included studies until Oct 25, 2017. The extraction of data and the risk of bias evaluation were conducted by two investigators independently. The methodological quality of the included studies was assessed using the methodological index for non-randomized studies (MINORS). Studies that reported the length and volume of teeth were used for quantitative analyses.

Results: Twelve studies were included in the meta-analysis. The length of all teeth after intervention was significantly shorter than that before treatment (MD = 0.80, 95% CI 0.56, 1.03, $P < 0.00001$). The sequence of RR from heaviest to lightest was maxillary lateral incisors, maxillary central incisors, mandibular anterior teeth, and maxillary canines. Studies were divided into two subgroups based on the use of tooth extraction. Root shortening after treatment was observed in both groups, and extraction caused more root resorption than was observed in the non-extraction group.

Conclusions: There were different degrees of root resorption after orthodontics, but it was clinically acceptable. Root resorption established in CBCT research was less serious and more accurate than that observed in the two-dimensional research. Current evidence suggests that root length and volume were reduced after orthodontic treatment. The order of the amount of RR was maxillary lateral incisors, maxillary central incisors and mandibular anterior teeth. Most of the articles were complicated by different confounding factors. Therefore, more high-quality clinical trials are needed to determine the risk factors of root resorption and optimal protocols for treatment and to draw more reliable conclusions.

Keywords: Root resorption, Cone beam computed tomography, Orthodontics, Meta-analysis

[*] Correspondence: tmxuortho@163.com
Department of Orthodontics, Peking University School and Hospital of
Stomatology, Beijing 100081, People's Republic of China

Background

External apical root resorption (EARR) is a reduction in root structure involving the apices, and it is a common phenomenon of orthodontic treatment in the modern world [1]. Most resorption is clinically insignificant, but severe root resorption threatens tooth longevity and causes tooth mobility or loss [2]. With improvements in orthodontic techniques and increased patient expectations, orthodontists need to be aware of EARR [3].

The prevalence of EARR is high, and the factors affecting it are complex and multiple, including internal and external factors. Internal factors are patient factors that include genetics, age at the start of treatment, gender, nutrition, root morphology, alveolar bone density, type of malocclusion, and so on [4–6]. External factors are primarily caused by orthodontic treatment, such as the type of appliance, treatment technique, continuous or intermittent force, force magnitude and direction, duration of the applied force, premolar extractions, tooth distance and root movement are risk factors for EARR [7–9]. The causes and mechanisms of resorption are not completely clear.

Different aspects of tooth resorption, including prevalence and degree, were investigated using conventional radiographs. Conventional radiographs include periapical film, panoramic radiograph, and lateral cephalometric images. Image distortion and magnification are common characteristics of panoramic radiography, also known as non-positioning radiographs, and this technique imprecisely measures cephalometric points [10, 11]. The disadvantages of this approach include confounded images caused by superimposed anatomic structures and a lack of right- and left-side information [12].

However, root resorption occurs 3-dimensionally, and 2D images cannot detect root resorption on lingual or buccal surfaces nor measure the volume of root loss. Therefore, quantification of treatment outcome using 2D images raised some criticism because of its reliability.

CBCT is an effective imaging method for the diagnosis of orthodontic root resorption using a 1: 1 ratio for reconstruction with no amplification error [13]. CBCT clearly shows the root structure, which results in more accurate qualitative judgment of orthodontic root resorption [14, 15]. CBCT images enhance cross-section research in three dimensions because the images may be observed at any angle using 3D reconstruction. Therefore, studies on RR using CBCT demonstrated improved accuracy and sensitivity in comparison with those using 2D data [16]. CBCT data contain equal image information of the right and left sides with no interference due to image overlap. Wang demonstrated that CBCT accurately measured tooth and root resorption volumes, and it was a more accurate and reliable 3D measuring

method for EARR investigation [17]. Another significant advantage of CBCT in root resorption studies is that it could be used in vivo, compared with Micro CT.

Weltman et al. [4] and Roscoe et al. [18] systematically reviewed root resorption associated with orthodontic treatment based on 2D images, but they did not do quantitative synthesis. There are no systematic reviews of root resorption associated with orthodontic treatment based on CBCT data, which is a more accurate and scientific method [19]. Therefore, it is necessary to integrate the data and conclusions of these trials. The purpose of this article is to report the results of a rigorous systematic review of the scientific literature relating to EARR in patients with fixed orthodontic appliances using the most accurate imaging information, CBCT.

Methods

This meta-analysis was performed in accordance with the guidelines of the Preferred Reporting Items for Systematic Reviews and Meta Analyses (PRISMA) checklist and PRISMA harm checklist items.

Types of studies

Study design: Randomized and non-randomized controlled trials, clinical trials, and prospective and retrospective reports were included. Longitudinal studies that observed root changes at different time points of treatment (before and after orthodontic treatment) were included. Self-controlled studies were included. Case reports, case series studies, descriptive studies, opinion articles and reviews were not included.

Types of participants

We included studies of orthodontic patients with no restrictions in the characteristics of occlusion, age or gender, and with available pre-and post-operative CBCT data. Patients with periodontitis were excluded. Pregnant patients and patients with systemic diseases, syndromes, pathologies, or history of root resorption were excluded.

Types of interventions

For comprehensive orthodontic treatment, patients in permanent dentition with fixed appliances, such as brackets and bands were included. Patients with different wire techniques and orthognathic surgery patients with pre-operative orthodontics with extraction treatment (bicuspid extraction on the upper and/or lower arch) or non-extraction were also included. Patients with local orthodontic treatment or stage treatment were excluded.

Types of outcome measures

Primary outcomes: Root resorption was evaluated using CBCT after orthodontic treatment. The primary outcomes were tooth/root length and tooth/root volume.

The PICOS format and null hypothesis are shown in Table 1.

Search methods for study identification

For the identification of studies to include or consider for this review, we developed detailed search strategies for each database searched. These strategies were based on the search strategy developed for MEDLINE but revised appropriately for each database. We searched the following databases: the CNKI database, the Cochrane Library, Web of Science, PubMed and EMBASE (to October 2017). We used no language or date restrictions in the searches of the electronic databases. The key words used to screen the databases are shown in Table 2. Citations of the remaining studies were examined to identify publications not located in the MEDLINE database. We contacted the authors of randomized controlled trials to identify any unpublished trials.

Data collection and analysis

Selection of studies The studies were screened, selected, and evaluated by two independent authors. Titles and abstracts were examined, and duplicate studies were eliminated. Full texts were obtained when the abstracts did not provide sufficient information. In the second phase of selection, eligibility criteria were used on the full articles. Any discrepancies in the inclusion of articles between reviewers were addressed via discussion until consensus was reached. Disagreements were resolved via discussion and consultation with a third author.

Data extraction and management Two independent authors (Deng and Sun) abstracted study data and evaluated data quality. Disagreements were adjudicated via consensus with a third reviewer (Xu). Data included study design (randomization procedure, blinding and

assessment endpoints) and patient characteristics (number, age, author, gender, indication, published years, and orthodontic site). When the data could not be culled from the article, we contacted the authors.

Methodological quality assessment

Two independent authors (Deng and Sun) assessed the quality of each study included in the meta-analysis using Methodological Index for Non-randomized Studies (MINORS). Evaluations were compared, and any inconsistencies between the review authors were discussed and resolved. For the self-controlled studies, the MINORS scores ranged from 9 to 15 out of a possible score of 16 (Table 3). There were no clear and consistent inclusion criteria for the included studies, but they were identified as moderate scientific evidence considering their prospective properties and the consecutive inclusion of participants.

Statistical analysis

Two authors independently screened the eligible studies, assessed the risk of bias in the trials and extracted data. The following outcomes of interest were recorded: tooth/root length and tooth/root volume. We calculated the mean differences (MD) with 95% confidence intervals (CI) for continuous data and risk ratios (RR) with 95% CI for dichotomous outcomes. Heterogeneity was tested using Cochrane's Q-test. $I^2 > 50\%$ was defined to indicate significant heterogeneity (I^2-value superior to 25, 50 and 75% corresponding to low, medium and high heterogeneity, respectively). Meta-analyses were performed using Review Manager 5.3 (Nordic Cochrane Centre, Copenhagen, Denmark). If the studies used similar participants and similar interventions, the fixed-effect model was used; if there was potential heterogeneity among studies, we preferred to use random-effects models. If sufficient data were available, we performed the following subgroup analyses: position of tooth; different intervention; extraction group and non-extraction group. If there were insufficient clinical trials for specific interventions or insufficient data for extraction, we qualitatively described the results. We then evaluated the influence of each subgroup on heterogeneity using forest plot analysis. Publication bias was assessed using funnel plot analysis.

Results
Description of studies
Search results

A total of 473 studies were obtained from the five databases. All abstracts were entered into the software Endnote (X8). The software screened for duplication, and 380 studies were retrieved. All the remaining studies were screened by the authors. A total of 206 abstracts

Table 1 PICOS format and null hypothesis

PICOS format	
Population	Patients with orthodontics
Intervention	Comprehensive orthodontics; not local orthodontics
Comparison	Before and after treatment
Outcome	Root resorption evaluated as tooth/root length and volume assessed using radiographic imaging CBCT
Null hypotheses	There is no difference in the incidence and severity of root resorption before and after comprehensive orthodontic treatment.

Table 2 Search results

Data base	Search strategy	Numbers
CNKI	Subject = root resorption AND Subject = orthodontic AND Subject = CBCT (accurate match)	103
Cochrane	Root resorption: ti, ab kw and Orthodontics: ti, ab, kw and cone beam computed tomography: ti, ab, kw	8
Web of Science	TS = ((root resorption) AND orthodontics AND (CBCT OR (Cone Beam Computed Tomography)))	34
PubMed	(Cone Beam Computed Tomography))) (root resorption) AND (root resorption) AND (orthodontics OR orthodontic) AND (CBCT OR (Cone Beam Computed Tomography))	132
EMBASE	'tooth disease' AND 'orthodontics' AND 'cone beam computed tomography' AND [1–1–1966]/sd NOT [30–9–2017]/sd AND [1966–2017]/py	178

were retrieved after excluding reviews, case reports, animal research and articles that did not conform to the research purpose. A total of 165 studies were excluded after full-text analysis for the following reasons: a. no results of CBCT examination; b. no assessment of root resorption; and c. local or stage treatment. Among 41 studies, 12 studies were analyzed quantitatively. The search results are presented in Table 2 and the flowchart of the literature search is presented in Fig. 1. Twelve studies were included in this review: Sun et al. [20]; Castro et al. [2]; Ahn et al. [13]; Wang et al. [21]; Wang et al. [22]; Qiao et al. [23]; Castro et al. [24]; Xu [25]; Wang et al. [26]; Oliveira et al. [27]; Ni et al. [28]; Zhang et al. [29].

Study characteristics

Study characteristics were summarized in Table 4.

Table 3 Methodological index for non-randomized studies (MINORS)

MINORS score Author	Year	1	2	3	4	5	6	7	8	Total
Sun et al.[20]	2012	green	green	green	green	yellow	green	green	red	13
Castro et al.[2]	2013	green	green	green	green	yellow	green	green	green	15
Ahn et al.[13]	2013	green	red	green	green	yellow	green	green	red	11
Wang et al.[21]	2013	green	green	green	green	yellow	yellow	green	yellow	13
Wang et al.[22]	2014	green	green	green	green	yellow	yellow	green	red	12
Qiao et al.[23]	2014	green	red	green	green	red	yellow	green	red	9
Castro et al.[24]	2015	green	green	green	green	yellow	yellow	green	red	12
Xu [25]	2015	green	yellow	green	green	yellow	yellow	green	red	11
Wang et al.[26]	2015	green	green	green	green	yellow	green	green	red	13
Oliveira et al.[27]	2016	green	red	green	green	red	green	green	green	12
Ni et al.[28]	2016	green	green	green	green	red	yellow	green	red	11
Zhang et al.[29]	2016	green	red	green	green	red	green	green	red	10

Items 1–12 represent: 1, a clearly stated aim; 2, inclusion of consecutive patients; 3, prospective collection of data; 4, endpoints appropriate to the aim of the study; 5, unbiased assessment of the study endpoint; 6, follow-up period appropriate to the aim of the study; and 7, loss to follow-up less than 5%; 8, prospective calculation of the study size. An item scored 0 means not mentioned, 1 means reported but inadequate, and 2 means reported and adequate. The total score was 16 for self-controlled studies. Use red for 0, yellow for 1 yellow and green for 2

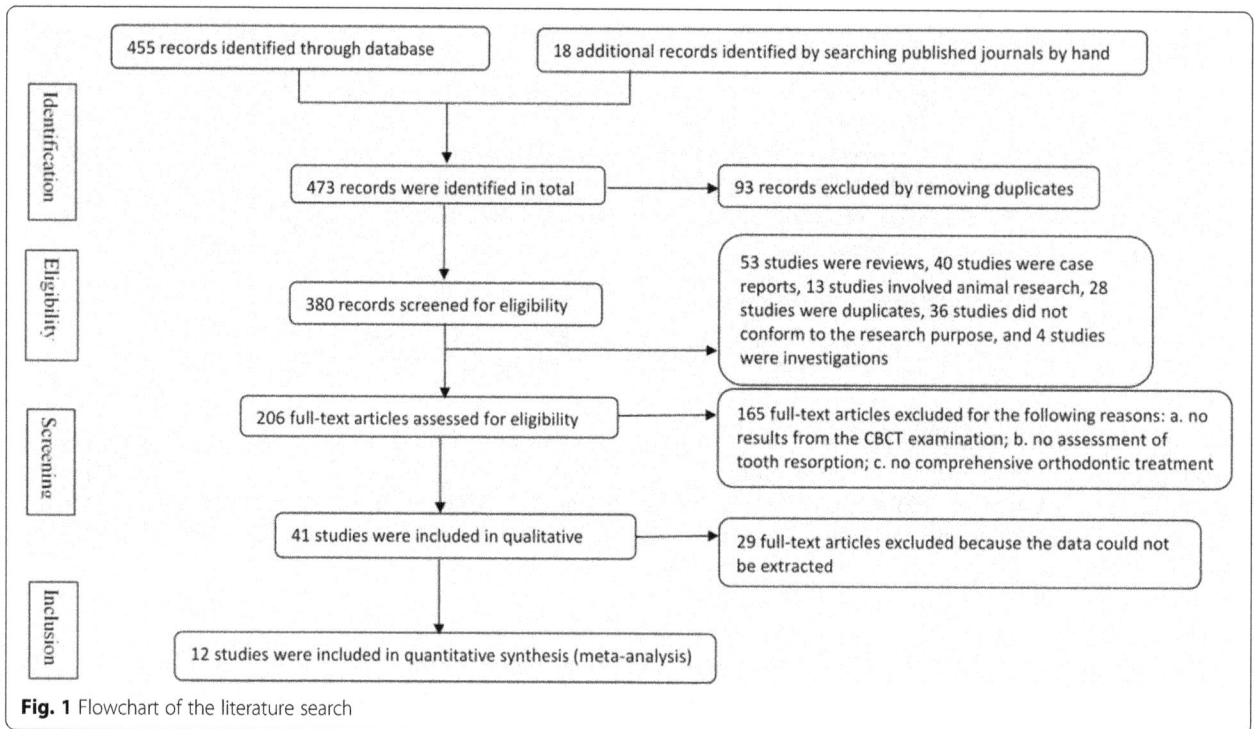

Fig. 1 Flowchart of the literature search

Characteristics of the participants A total of 247 participants were investigated and provided 1039 teeth in the 12 studies. The mean age of the participants ranged from 12.8 to 26.62 years, and both genders were included. Three studies [2, 24, 29] were based on teenagers, and the other studies included adults. Participants in four studies [20–22, 26] had skeletal malocclusion that was more serious than other studies, which may be the risk of root resorption.

Characteristics of the interventions All studies included comprehensive orthodontics, not local treatment, and the duration was between pre-treatment and post-treatment. Pre-operative decompensation of orthognathic surgery was also included. However, this type of intervention is different than normal treatment and may be one source of heterogeneity.

Characteristics of the outcomes Tooth length measurement method was primarily based on CBCT data. Tooth length was the distance from the apex to incisal edge or cusp. The volume index measurement method was performed using software for root reconstruction to calculate tooth volume before and after treatment. There was little methodological difference between the studies, and a low measurement bias could be considered.

Risk of bias in included studies The main bias was the implementation bias, which occurred in the process of

intervention. Multiple factors of root resorption were also interfering factors. Three articles [2, 20, 26] exhibited report bias.

Effects of interventions
Primary results
Tooth length—total teeth
Ten studies reported changes in tooth length using CBCT. Meta-analysis revealed medium heterogeneity (I^2 = 33%), and a random effect model was used. Post-treatment was comparable to pre-treatment (MD = 0.80, 95% CI 0.56, 1.03, $P < 0.00001$). The meta-analysis results are shown in Fig. 2. The funnel plot was more symmetrical, which indicates a small publication bias (Fig. 3). The source of heterogeneity may lie in the method of measurement. Ahn et al. and Wang et al.'s studies [13, 21, 22] measured the root length, which was the distance from the apex to the enamel dentin boundary, but other studies measured the tooth length as the distance from the cusp or incisal edge to apex.

Tooth length—maxillary central incisor
Seven studies reported changes of tooth length in maxillary central incisors using CBCT. Tooth length was significantly reduced after orthodontic treatment (MD = 0.84, 95% CI 0.56, 1.12, $P < 0.00001$). The meta-analysis results are shown in Fig. 4.

Table 4 Characteristics of the included studies

No.	Study	Participants	Outcomes	Evaluated teeth	Indications	Intervention	Duration
1	Sun et al. (2012) [20]	n = 17 (M10,F7;23.7y)	TV	(31,32,41,42)	Skeletal Class III	Pre-operative decompensation	7.6 m
2	Castro et al. (2013) [2]	n = 30 (M11,F19;13y)	TL	All teeth	Class I malocclusion with crowding	Straight-wire technique (Non-extraction)	22 m
3	Ahn et al. (2013) [13]	n = 37 (F37;26.62 ± 8.46y)	RL	Maxillary/Mandibular anterior teeth	Class I dentoalveolar protrusion	Straight-wire technique	1.8 ± 0.4 years
4	Wang et al. (2013) [21]	G1 n = 26 (M17,F9; 23.5 ± 3.2) G2 n = 30 (M14,F6; 24.8 ± 3.8)	RL	(31,32,41,42)	Surgical class III	Augmented corticotomy- assisted pre-surgical orthodontics Conventional procedures	Unclear
5	Wang et al. (2014) [22]	n = 8 (M5,F3;unclear)	RL	(31,32,41,42)	Severe Class III	Augmented corticotomy- assisted pre-surgical orthodontics	Unclear
6	Qiao et al. (2014) [23]	n = 10 (M4,F6;20.6 y)	TL	(11,12,13,21,22,23)	Extraction of 1st premolars	Straight-wire technique	12 m
7	Castro et al. (2015) [24]	G1 n = 6 (M2,F4;12.8 ± 1.8y) G2	TL	Posterior teeth with root-filled; Posterior teeth without root-filled	Permanent dentition Class I malocclusion with moderate dental crowding after RCT	Straight-wire technique	Unclear
8	Xu (2015) [25]	n = 18 (M8,F10;25y)	TL	(11,12,13,21,22,23)	Extraction of 1st premolars	Straight-wire technique	Unclear
9	Wang et al. (2015) [26]	n = 30 (M13,F17;22.32 ± 2.40y)	TV	(11,12,21,22,31,32, 41,42)	Skeletal Class III	Pre-operative decompensation	9.5 m
10	Oliveira et al. (2016) [27]	n = 11 (M5,F6;18-26y)	TL	(11,12,21,22)	Extraction of maxillary first premolars and retraction of maxillary incisors	Edgewise	Unclear
11	Ni et al. (2016) [28]	G1 n = 16 (M6,F10; 20.3 ± 3.2y) G2	TL	(11,12,13,21,22,23)	Moderate crowding in anterior teeth with root-filled; Moderate crowding in anterior teeth without root-filled	Straight-wire technique	18.3 ± 2.6 m
12	Zhang et al. (2016) [29]	n = 8 (M3,F5;13.25y)	TL;TV	(12,21)	Anterior cross-bite in earlypermanent dentition	Straight-wire technique	12 m

TL tooth length, RL root length, TV tooth volume, m month

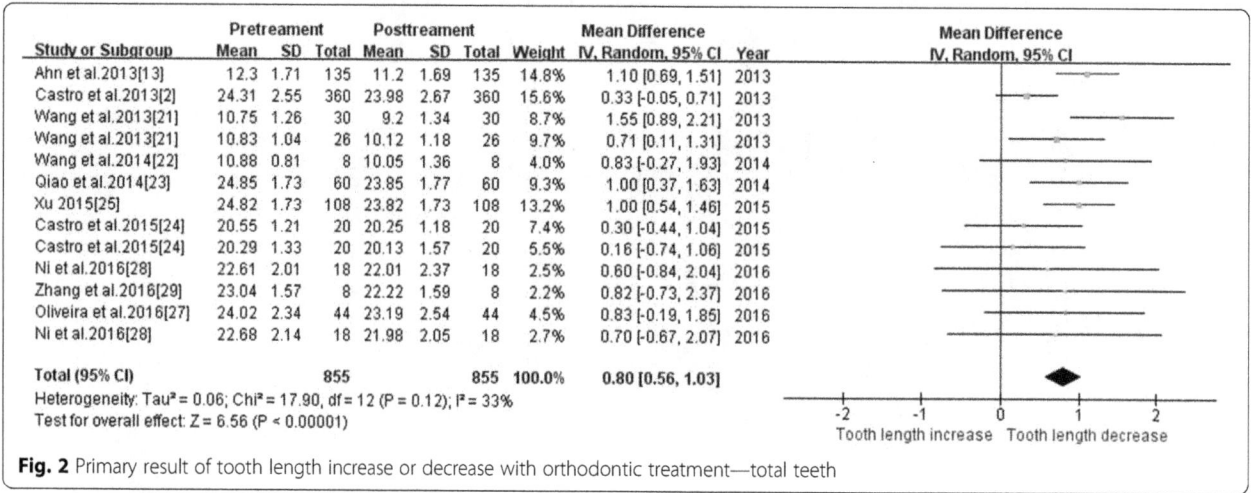

Study or Subgroup	Pretreatment Mean	SD	Total	Posttreatment Mean	SD	Total	Weight	Mean Difference IV, Random, 95% CI	Year
Ahn et al.2013[13]	12.3	1.71	135	11.2	1.69	135	14.8%	1.10 [0.69, 1.51]	2013
Castro et al.2013[2]	24.31	2.55	360	23.98	2.67	360	15.6%	0.33 [-0.05, 0.71]	2013
Wang et al.2013[21]	10.75	1.26	30	9.2	1.34	30	8.7%	1.55 [0.89, 2.21]	2013
Wang et al.2013[21]	10.83	1.04	26	10.12	1.18	26	9.7%	0.71 [0.11, 1.31]	2013
Wang et al.2014[22]	10.88	0.81	8	10.05	1.36	8	4.0%	0.83 [-0.27, 1.93]	2014
Qiao et al.2014[23]	24.85	1.73	60	23.85	1.77	60	9.3%	1.00 [0.37, 1.63]	2014
Xu 2015[25]	24.82	1.73	108	23.82	1.73	108	13.2%	1.00 [0.54, 1.46]	2015
Castro et al.2015[24]	20.55	1.21	20	20.25	1.18	20	7.4%	0.30 [-0.44, 1.04]	2015
Castro et al.2015[24]	20.29	1.33	20	20.13	1.57	20	5.5%	0.16 [-0.74, 1.06]	2015
Ni et al.2016[28]	22.61	2.01	18	22.01	2.37	18	2.5%	0.60 [-0.84, 2.04]	2016
Zhang et al.2016[29]	23.04	1.57	8	22.22	1.59	8	2.2%	0.82 [-0.73, 2.37]	2016
Oliveira et al.2016[27]	24.02	2.34	44	23.19	2.54	44	4.5%	0.83 [-0.19, 1.85]	2016
Ni et al.2016[28]	22.68	2.14	18	21.98	2.05	18	2.7%	0.70 [-0.67, 2.07]	2016
Total (95% CI)			855			855	100.0%	0.80 [0.56, 1.03]	

Heterogeneity: Tau² = 0.06; Chi² = 17.90, df = 12 (P = 0.12); I² = 33%
Test for overall effect: Z = 6.56 (P < 0.00001)

Fig. 2 Primary result of tooth length increase or decrease with orthodontic treatment—total teeth

Tooth length—maxillary lateral incisor

Six studies reported changes of tooth length in maxillary lateral incisors using CBCT. Tooth length of maxillary lateral incisors was significantly reduced after treatment (MD = 0.90, 95% CI 0.58, 1.22, $P < 0.00001$). The meta-analysis results are shown in Fig. 5.

Tooth length—maxillary canine

Five studies reported changes in maxillary canine. Meta-analysis revealed low heterogeneity (I^2 = 19%), and a fixed-effect model was used. The tooth length was significantly shorter after treatment (MD = 0.68, 95% CI 0.37, 1.00, $P < 0.00001$). The meta-analysis results are shown in Fig. 6.

Tooth length— mandibular anterior teeth

Three studies reported changes of tooth length in mandibular anterior teeth using CBCT. Meta-analysis revealed high heterogeneity (I^2 = 63%), and a random-effect model was used. Sensitivity tests were performed after the removal of different study groups in Wang et al. [21], and the heterogeneity was reduced to 0%. Post-treatment was comparable to pre-treatment (MD = 0.53 95% CI 0.16, 0.90, $P < 0.00001$). The meta-analysis results are shown in Figs. 7 and 8.

Tooth length—tooth extraction & non-tooth extraction

The study was divided into two subgroups, tooth extraction and non-extraction, based on the orthodontic

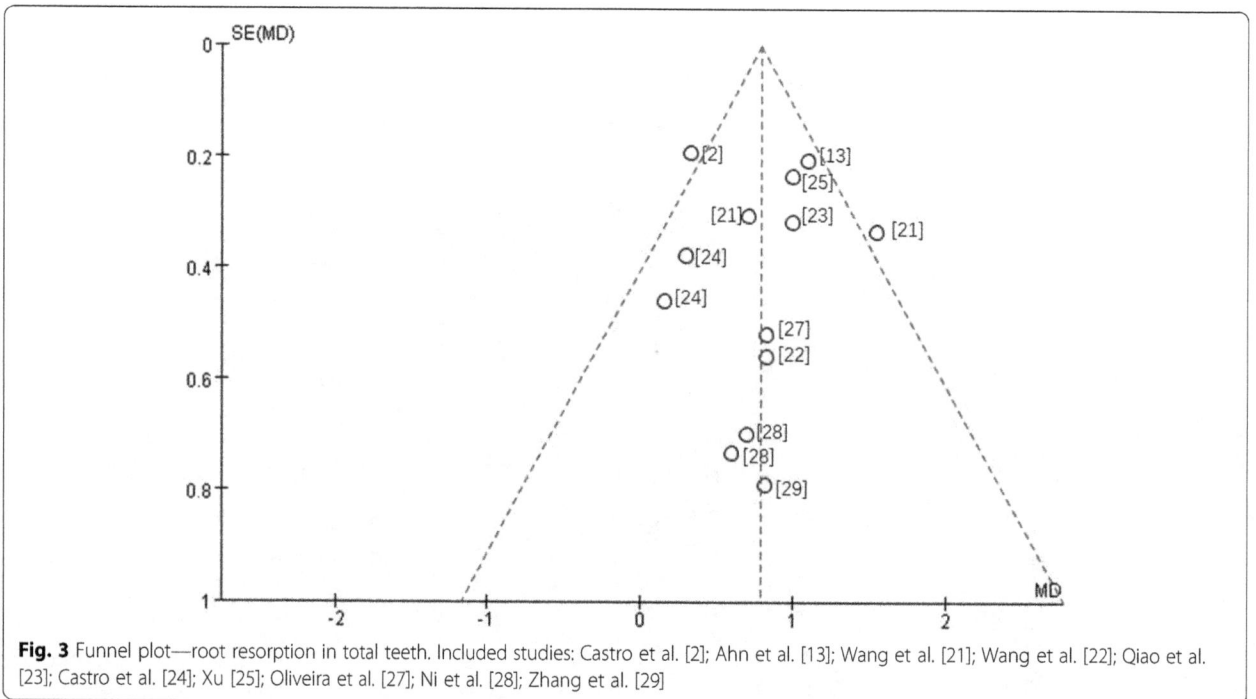

Fig. 3 Funnel plot—root resorption in total teeth. Included studies: Castro et al. [2]; Ahn et al. [13]; Wang et al. [21]; Wang et al. [22]; Qiao et al. [23]; Castro et al. [24]; Xu [25]; Oliveira et al. [27]; Ni et al. [28]; Zhang et al. [29]

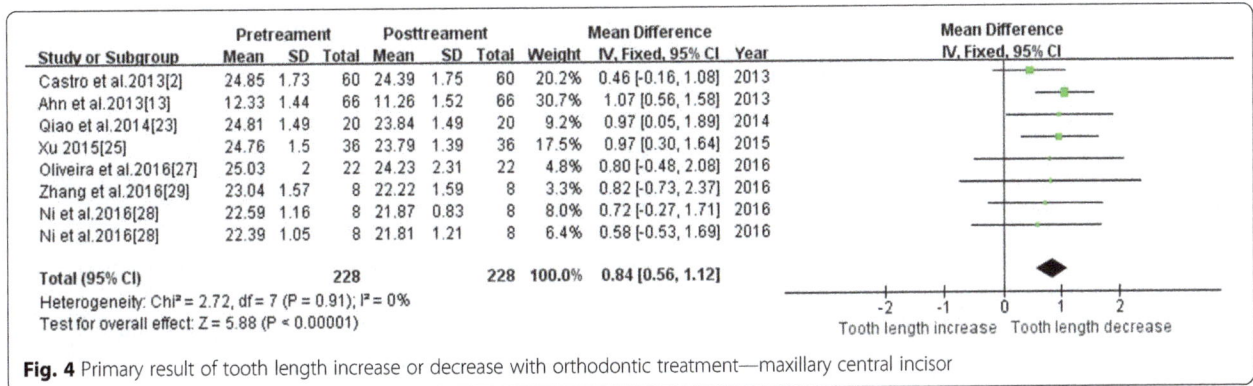

Study or Subgroup	Pretreament Mean	SD	Total	Posttreatment Mean	SD	Total	Weight	Mean Difference IV, Fixed, 95% CI	Year
Castro et al.2013[2]	24.85	1.73	60	24.39	1.75	60	20.2%	0.46 [-0.16, 1.08]	2013
Ahn et al.2013[13]	12.33	1.44	66	11.26	1.52	66	30.7%	1.07 [0.56, 1.58]	2013
Qiao et al.2014[23]	24.81	1.49	20	23.84	1.49	20	9.2%	0.97 [0.05, 1.89]	2014
Xu 2015[25]	24.76	1.5	36	23.79	1.39	36	17.5%	0.97 [0.30, 1.64]	2015
Oliveira et al.2016[27]	25.03	2	22	24.23	2.31	22	4.8%	0.80 [-0.48, 2.08]	2016
Zhang et al.2016[29]	23.04	1.57	8	22.22	1.59	8	3.3%	0.82 [-0.73, 2.37]	2016
Ni et al.2016[28]	22.59	1.16	8	21.87	0.83	8	8.0%	0.72 [-0.27, 1.71]	2016
Ni et al.2016[28]	22.39	1.05	8	21.81	1.21	8	6.4%	0.58 [-0.53, 1.69]	2016
Total (95% CI)			228			228	100.0%	0.84 [0.56, 1.12]	

Heterogeneity: Chi² = 2.72, df = 7 (P = 0.91); I² = 0%
Test for overall effect: Z = 5.88 (P < 0.00001)

Fig. 4 Primary result of tooth length increase or decrease with orthodontic treatment—maxillary central incisor

approach. The following heterogeneity test results were demonstrated: $p = 0.96$ and 0.12, I^2 was 0 and 40%, respectively; the two subgroups combined together $p = 0.18$, I^2 was 28%. Subgroup analysis demonstrated $CHI^2 = 1.10$, $P = 0.29$, and subgroup differences were not statistically significant. Therefore, we speculated whether extraction or not was less affected to heterogeneity. The heterogeneity source in the non-extraction group arose from control group in Wang et al. [21]. The overall effect value ($Z = 7.10$, $P < 0.00001$) suggests that the effect of extraction treatment on tooth length was statistically significant. The total effect of the tooth extraction group was 1.03 [0.77, 1.30], and the total effect value of the non-extractive group was 0.77[0.37, 1.18]. Tooth extraction may have caused more root resorption. The meta-analysis results are shown in Fig. 9.

Tooth length—different interventions
The study was divided into three subgroups, straight wire, augmented corticotomy-assisted presurgical orthodontics and edgewise technique, based on the orthodontic technique. Subgroup analysis demonstrated that subgroup differences were not statistically significant. Therefore, we speculated different intervention of heterogeneity was less affected. The total effect of the straight wire group was 0.8 [0.52, 1.08], the total effect value of the augmented corticotomy-assisted presurgical orthodontics group was 0.74[0.21, 1.27] and the total

effect of the edgewise group was 0.83[– 0.19, 1.85]. The augmented corticotomy-assisted presurgical orthodontics may cause less root resorption. The meta-analysis results are shown in Fig. 10.

Root volume
Three studies reported changes in root volume using CBCT. The results of meta-analysis revealed that the root volume before and after orthodontic treatment was significantly different (MD = 23.12, 95% CI 17.88, 28.36 $P < 0.00001$). The root volume was significantly reduced after treatment. The meta-analysis results are shown in Fig. 11.

Discussion
Summary of main results
Evidence suggests that orthodontic treatment causes an increased incidence and severity of apical root resorption. Tooth length and root volume were reduced after orthodontic intervention.

Overall completeness and applicability of evidence
Numerous CBCT studies investigated root resorption before and after orthodontic treatment, but quantitative data of the extraction were only available in 12 articles for a meta-analysis. We chose two major indicators, tooth/root length and root volume, to reflect root resorption. Other indicators that reflect changes were not

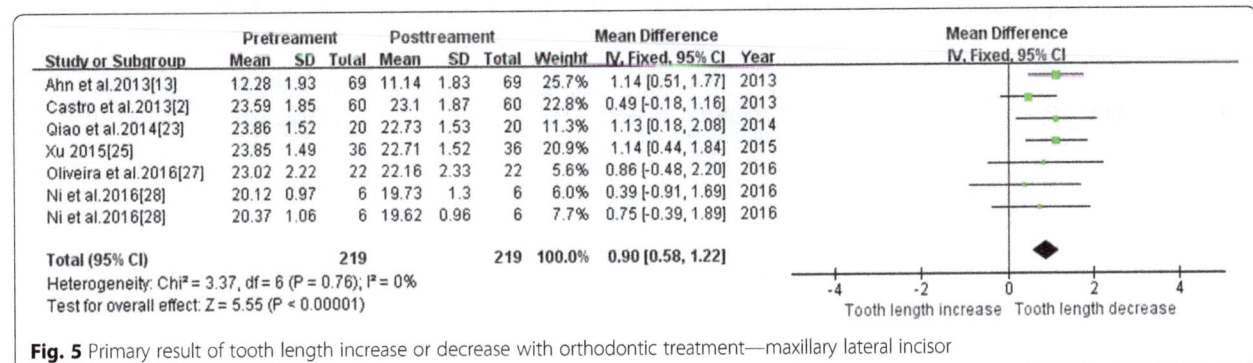

Study or Subgroup	Pretreament Mean	SD	Total	Posttreatment Mean	SD	Total	Weight	Mean Difference IV, Fixed, 95% CI	Year
Ahn et al.2013[13]	12.28	1.93	69	11.14	1.83	69	25.7%	1.14 [0.51, 1.77]	2013
Castro et al.2013[2]	23.59	1.85	60	23.1	1.87	60	22.8%	0.49 [-0.18, 1.16]	2013
Qiao et al.2014[23]	23.86	1.52	20	22.73	1.53	20	11.3%	1.13 [0.18, 2.08]	2014
Xu 2015[25]	23.85	1.49	36	22.71	1.52	36	20.9%	1.14 [0.44, 1.84]	2015
Oliveira et al.2016[27]	23.02	2.22	22	22.16	2.33	22	5.6%	0.86 [-0.48, 2.20]	2016
Ni et al.2016[28]	20.12	0.97	6	19.73	1.3	6	6.0%	0.39 [-0.91, 1.69]	2016
Ni et al.2016[28]	20.37	1.06	6	19.62	0.96	6	7.7%	0.75 [-0.39, 1.89]	2016
Total (95% CI)			219			219	100.0%	0.90 [0.58, 1.22]	

Heterogeneity: Chi² = 3.37, df = 6 (P = 0.76); I² = 0%
Test for overall effect: Z = 5.55 (P < 0.00001)

Fig. 5 Primary result of tooth length increase or decrease with orthodontic treatment—maxillary lateral incisor

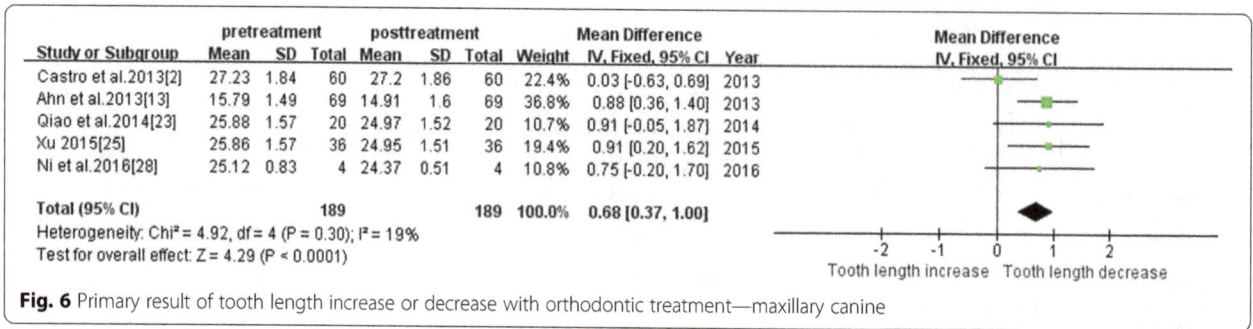

Study or Subgroup	pretreatment			posttreatment			Weight	Mean Difference IV, Fixed, 95% CI	Year	Mean Difference IV, Fixed, 95% CI
	Mean	SD	Total	Mean	SD	Total				
Castro et al.2013[2]	27.23	1.84	60	27.2	1.86	60	22.4%	0.03 [-0.63, 0.69]	2013	
Ahn et al.2013[13]	15.79	1.49	69	14.91	1.6	69	36.8%	0.88 [0.36, 1.40]	2013	
Qiao et al.2014[23]	25.88	1.57	20	24.97	1.52	20	10.7%	0.91 [-0.05, 1.87]	2014	
Xu 2015[25]	25.86	1.57	36	24.95	1.51	36	19.4%	0.91 [0.20, 1.62]	2015	
Ni et al.2016[28]	25.12	0.83	4	24.37	0.51	4	10.8%	0.75 [-0.20, 1.70]	2016	
Total (95% CI)			189			189	100.0%	0.68 [0.37, 1.00]		

Heterogeneity: Chi² = 4.92, df = 4 (P = 0.30); I² = 19%
Test for overall effect: Z = 4.29 (P < 0.0001)

Tooth length increase   Tooth length decrease

Fig. 6 Primary result of tooth length increase or decrease with orthodontic treatment—maxillary canine

included, and numerical integration and meta-analysis were not performed. Quantitative analysis of other indicators may be performed using numerical analyses to improve the data on this issue.

Quality of the evidence
Twelve articles were included in this meta-analysis, and all of the studies were non-randomized controlled trials. Randomized controls cannot be used because it is ethically impossible to perform CBCT screenings in patients who have not undergone orthodontic treatment. All studies were self-controlled, which reflects the impact of intervention on these patients more accurately. All patients were diagnosed and measured using CBCT, which excluded the shortcomings of magnification and distortion in 2D image data. All data sources were evaluated more accurately and reproducibly by CBCT, which is the most accurate method of obtaining data in vivo. Methodological evaluation scores from 9 to 15, and 4 studies received scores that were above or equal to 13, which were considered as high quality. One study was below 10 and was considered low quality. The remaining studies were of medium quality. The overall quality of the selected literature was good. There were 3 prospective trials, and the remaining trials were retrospective experiments. Prospective experimental evidence will provide more adequate data.

Potential biases in the review process
The different orthodontic technologies, such as straight wire and edge wise, and corticotomy, incompleteness of some of the reports and lack of quality control in some

trials may have contributed to bias in study assessments. We made every attempt to limit bias in the review process by ensuring a comprehensive search for potentially eligible studies. Time limitations prevented the search of additional databases and sources, which may have identified additional published and unpublished studies. There may also be publication bias because of the lack of publication of negative results. We strictly controlled the inclusion of exclusion criteria. There were only two prospective experiments, while others were retrospective studies. There may be biases in sample selection and dropout. The sample size of all studies was relatively small, and only one of the studies calculated the sample size [27].

The age distribution did not completely cover the age of patients with orthodontic treatment, but it covered the span of treatment for most patients. However, there were few samples for adolescent studies, and many patients of orthodontic treatment are adolescents in clinical practice. Therefore, whether the conclusions of this meta-analysis are well suited for adolescent samples must be further studied.

Primary outcome tooth length

Tooth position Total tooth root length was reduced after orthodontic treatment, and the included studies exhibited a small publication bias. The effect value indicated that the maxillary lateral incisors were the most absorbed, followed by the maxillary central incisors, mandibular anterior teeth and upper canines. Nanekrungsan et al. [8] found that the maxillary lateral incisors

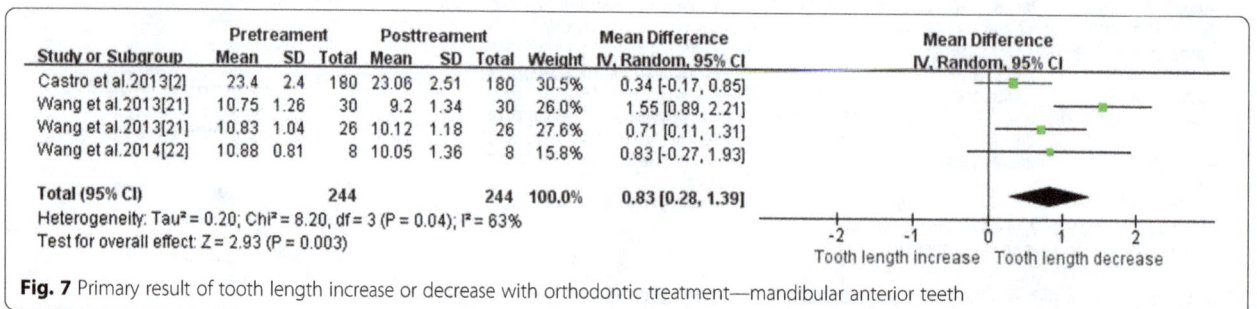

Study or Subgroup	Pretreament			Posttreament			Weight	Mean Difference IV, Random, 95% CI	Mean Difference IV, Random, 95% CI
	Mean	SD	Total	Mean	SD	Total			
Castro et al.2013[2]	23.4	2.4	180	23.06	2.51	180	30.5%	0.34 [-0.17, 0.85]	
Wang et al.2013[21]	10.75	1.26	30	9.2	1.34	30	26.0%	1.55 [0.89, 2.21]	
Wang et al.2013[21]	10.83	1.04	26	10.12	1.18	26	27.6%	0.71 [0.11, 1.31]	
Wang et al.2014[22]	10.88	0.81	8	10.05	1.36	8	15.8%	0.83 [-0.27, 1.93]	
Total (95% CI)			244			244	100.0%	0.83 [0.28, 1.39]	

Heterogeneity: Tau² = 0.20; Chi² = 8.20, df = 3 (P = 0.04); I² = 63%
Test for overall effect: Z = 2.93 (P = 0.003)

Tooth length increase   Tooth length decrease

Fig. 7 Primary result of tooth length increase or decrease with orthodontic treatment—mandibular anterior teeth

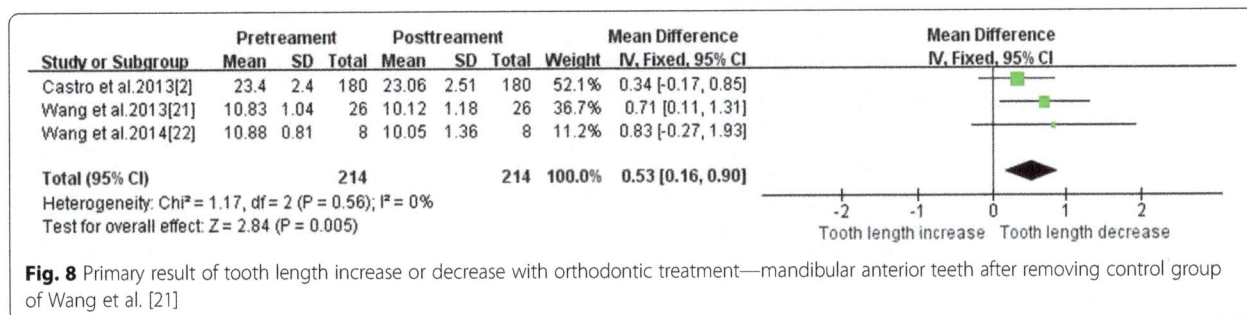

Study or Subgroup	Pretreatment Mean	SD	Total	Posttreament Mean	SD	Total	Weight	Mean Difference IV, Fixed, 95% CI
Castro et al.2013[2]	23.4	2.4	180	23.06	2.51	180	52.1%	0.34 [-0.17, 0.85]
Wang et al.2013[21]	10.83	1.04	26	10.12	1.18	26	36.7%	0.71 [0.11, 1.31]
Wang et al.2014[22]	10.88	0.81	8	10.05	1.36	8	11.2%	0.83 [-0.27, 1.93]
Total (95% CI)			214			214	100.0%	0.53 [0.16, 0.90]

Heterogeneity: Chi² = 1.17, df = 2 (P = 0.56); I² = 0%
Test for overall effect: Z = 2.84 (P = 0.005)

Fig. 8 Primary result of tooth length increase or decrease with orthodontic treatment—mandibular anterior teeth after removing control group of Wang et al. [21]

were primarily reduced after treatment. Yu et al. [30] found that the maxillary lateral incisors exhibited greater resorption than maxillary central incisors and canines using CBCT. Kennedy et al. [31] also found that the maxillary lateral incisors were more prone to root resorption than the central incisors. Pejicic et al. [32] found that lateral incisors were primarily affected, and mean values ranged from 0.5 mm to 3 mm, which is consistent with the conclusions of our study. Previous 2D studies [3, 33, 34] found that maxillary central incisors were the most affected teeth. Sameshima et al. [11] demonstrated that the absorption order was the upper central incisors, the upper lateral incisors, the lower central incisors, and the lower lateral incisors. Jung et al. [35] found that the maxillary central incisors were the most resorbed, with 27% undergoing greater than 1 mm of root resorption. Inaccuracies caused by the magnification and overlap of 2D data, the different types of patient malocclusion, or the different treatment methods may explain the differences in absorption of the anterior teeth.

A meta-analysis of Segal et al. [36] was based on 2D data and demonstrated a strong correlation between root resorption and apical displacement. The mean resorption of upper central incisors was 1.421 ± 0.448 mm, which was slightly higher than the present study (MD = 0.84,CI[0.56,1.12]). Two-dimensional data may over-estimated root resorption.

The present meta-analysis revealed that the root resorption of the upper central incisors and upper lateral incisors were similar, and it was difficult to determine which tooth was the most affected. The sample of 3D studies was quite small. Therefore, larger 3D sample sizes and more clinical trial evidence are required to supplement and confirm these conclusions.

The heterogeneity of root resorption of the mandibular anterior teeth was high partially because two studies measured the root length and other studies measured tooth length. Removal of the data from control group of Wang et al. [21] reduced the heterogeneity to zero, which suggested that this data was the source of heterogeneity. This group was pre-operative orthodontic of

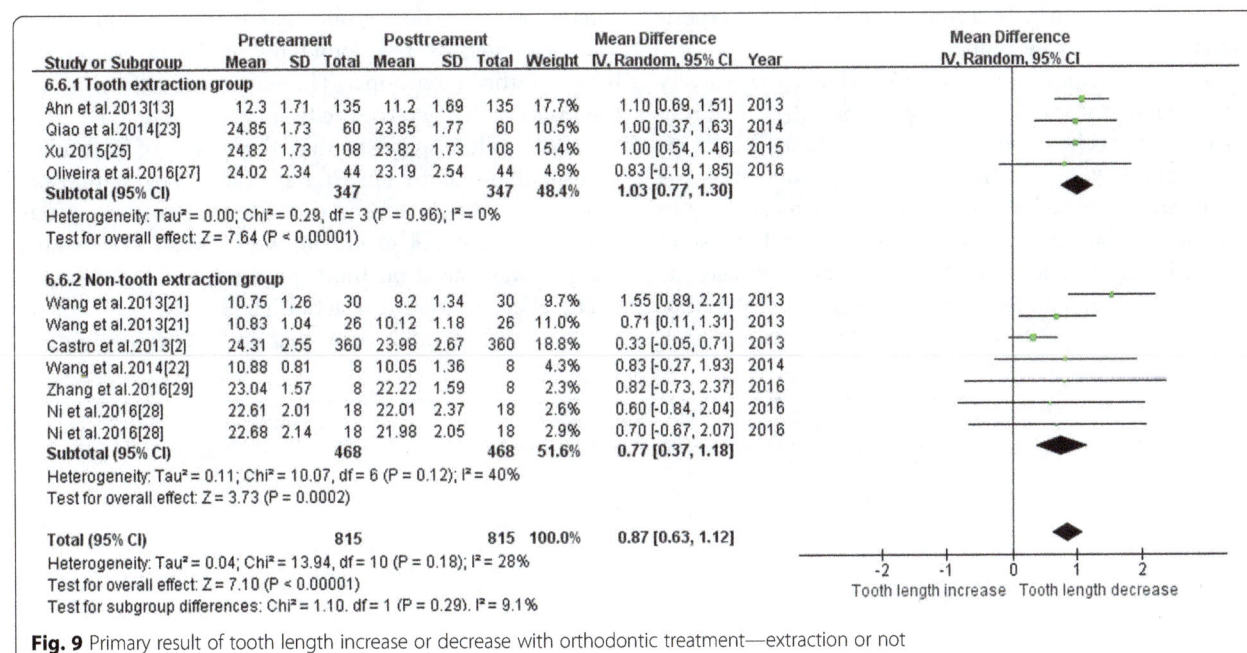

Fig. 9 Primary result of tooth length increase or decrease with orthodontic treatment—extraction or not

Study or Subgroup	pretreatment Mean	SD	Total	posttreatment Mean	SD	Total	Weight	Mean Difference IV, Random, 95% CI	Year
7.1.1 Straight wire technique									
Ahn et al.2013[13]	12.3	1.71	135	11.2	1.69	135	14.8%	1.10 [0.69, 1.51]	2013
Wang et al.2013[21]	10.75	1.26	30	9.2	1.34	30	8.2%	1.55 [0.89, 2.21]	2013
Castro et al.2013[2]	24.31	2.55	360	23.98	2.67	360	15.6%	0.33 [-0.05, 0.71]	2013
Qiao et al.2014[23]	24.85	1.73	60	23.85	1.77	60	8.8%	1.00 [0.37, 1.63]	2014
Xu 2015[25]	24.82	1.73	108	23.82	1.73	108	12.9%	1.00 [0.54, 1.46]	2015
Castro et al.2015[24]	20.55	1.21	20	20.25	1.18	20	6.9%	0.30 [-0.44, 1.04]	2015
Castro et al.2015[24]	20.29	1.33	20	20.13	1.57	20	5.1%	0.16 [-0.74, 1.06]	2015
Ni et al.2016[28]	22.68	2.14	18	21.98	2.05	18	2.4%	0.70 [-0.67, 2.07]	2016
Ni et al.2016[28]	22.61	2.01	18	22.01	2.37	18	2.2%	0.60 [-0.84, 2.04]	2016
Zhang et al.2016[29]	23.04	1.57	8	22.22	1.59	8	1.9%	0.82 [-0.73, 2.37]	2016
Oliveira et al.2016[27]	24.02	2.34	44	23.19	2.54	44	4.1%	0.83 [-0.19, 1.85]	2016
Subtotal (95% CI)			821			821	83.0%	0.80 [0.52, 1.08]	
Heterogeneity: Tau² = 0.09; Chi² = 17.82, df = 10 (P = 0.06); I² = 44%									
Test for overall effect: Z = 5.57 (P < 0.00001)									
7.1.2 Augmented corticotomy-assisted presurgical orthodontics									
Wang et al.2013[21]	10.83	1.04	26	10.12	1.18	26	9.3%	0.71 [0.11, 1.31]	2013
Wang et al.2014[22]	10.88	0.81	8	10.05	1.36	8	3.6%	0.83 [-0.27, 1.93]	2014
Subtotal (95% CI)			34			34	12.9%	0.74 [0.21, 1.27]	
Heterogeneity: Tau² = 0.00; Chi² = 0.04, df = 1 (P = 0.85); I² = 0%									
Test for overall effect: Z = 2.73 (P = 0.006)									
7.1.3 Edgewise technique									
Oliveira et al.2016[27]	24.02	2.34	44	23.19	2.54	44	4.1%	0.83 [-0.19, 1.85]	2016
Subtotal (95% CI)			44			44	4.1%	0.83 [-0.19, 1.85]	
Heterogeneity: Not applicable									
Test for overall effect: Z = 1.59 (P = 0.11)									
Total (95% CI)			899			899	100.0%	0.80 [0.57, 1.02]	
Heterogeneity: Tau² = 0.05; Chi² = 17.91, df = 13 (P = 0.16); I² = 27%									
Test for overall effect: Z = 7.00 (P < 0.00001)									
Test for subgroup differences: Chi² = 0.05, df = 2 (P = 0.98). I² = 0%									

Tooth length increase — Tooth length decrease (scale: −2, −1, 0, 1, 2)

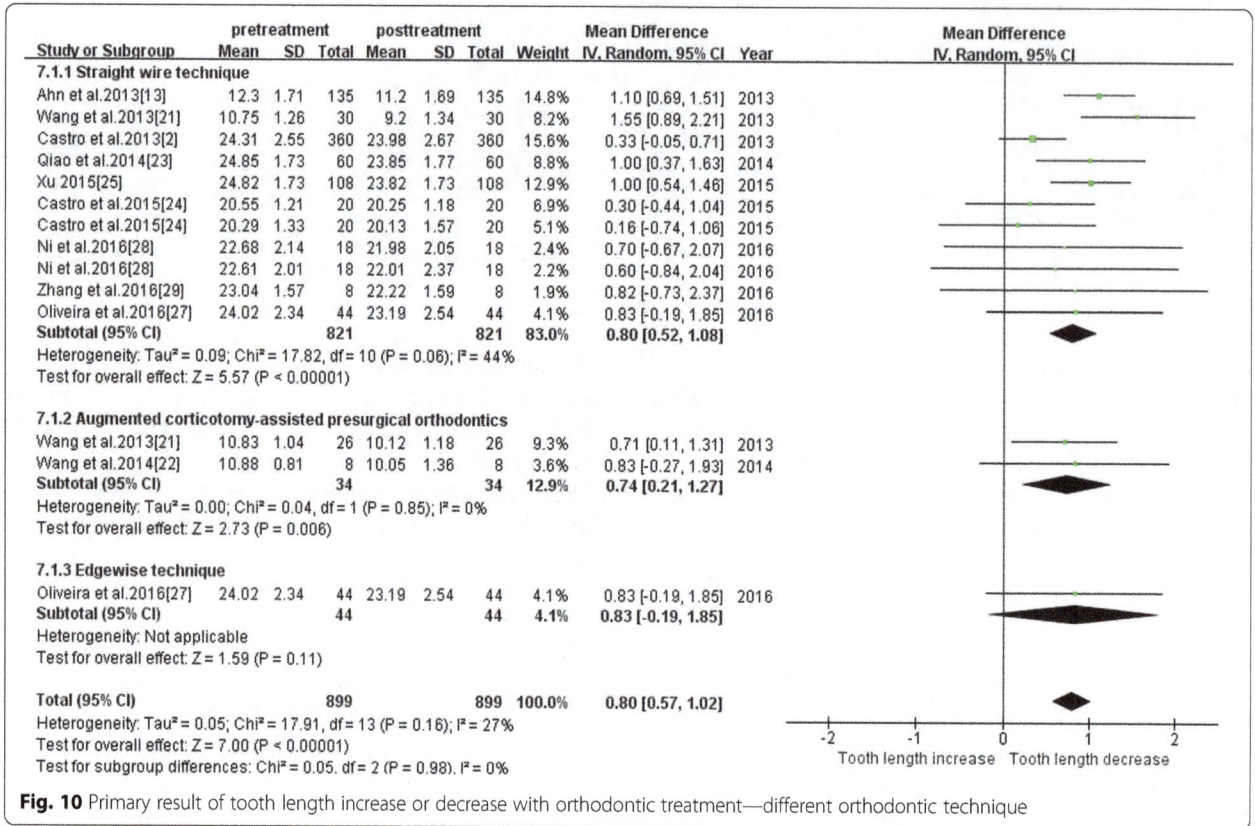

Fig. 10 Primary result of tooth length increase or decrease with orthodontic treatment—different orthodontic technique

orthognathic surgery patients, which resulted in greater root resorption (1.55 ± 0.66 mm). Experimental group was also pre-operatively compensated, but corticotomy was added. A previous study demonstrated that corticotomy reduced the duration of treatment and resulted in lower root resorption compared to traditional methods. Therefore, the value of experimental group may be reduced.

The key of orthodontics prior to orthognathic surgery lies in the anterior teeth for compensation [37]. The root much more easily touches the alveolar bone, which increases the risk of root resorption [38]. Some scholars confirmed that maxillary root resorption is most likely to occur in the patients with bony malocclusion because of the maximum distance of tooth movement, especially the incisors [39, 40]. Therefore, the data suggest that orthopedic orthodontic treatment of skeletal malocclusion using simple orthodontics will cause more root resorption, regardless of cortical osteotomy intervention.

Extraction vs non-extraction There is controversy about root resorption following extraction and non-extraction methods. The present study was divided into two subgroups: extraction group and non-extraction group. The heterogeneity test found no significant difference between the subgroups. Therefore, the effect of extraction on the heterogeneity is speculative. The overall effect value suggests that the effect of extraction treatment on tooth length was statistically significant. The heterogeneity source of the non-extraction group arose from control group in Wang et al. [21], whose analysis was based on tooth position.

The effect of tooth extraction (1.03 ± 0.27) on root resorption was greater than that in the non-extraction

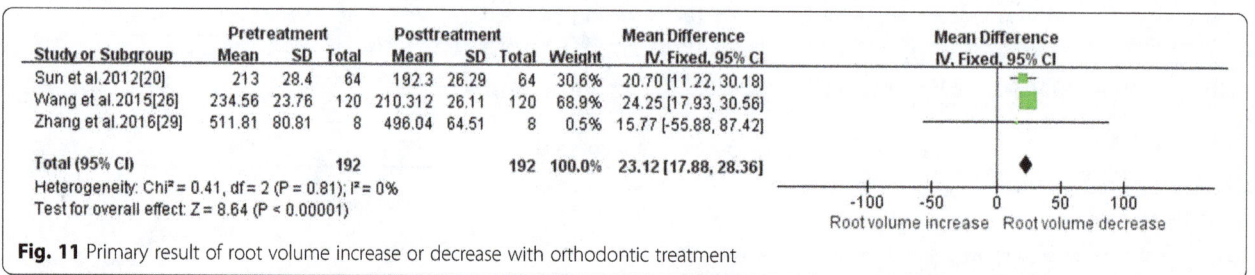

Study or Subgroup	Pretreatment Mean	SD	Total	Posttreatment Mean	SD	Total	Weight	Mean Difference IV, Fixed, 95% CI
Sun et al.2012[20]	213	28.4	64	192.3	26.29	64	30.6%	20.70 [11.22, 30.18]
Wang et al.2015[26]	234.56	23.76	120	210.312	26.11	120	68.9%	24.25 [17.93, 30.56]
Zhang et al.2016[29]	511.81	80.81	8	496.04	64.51	8	0.5%	15.77 [-55.88, 87.42]
Total (95% CI)			192			192	100.0%	23.12 [17.88, 28.36]
Heterogeneity: Chi² = 0.41, df = 2 (P = 0.81); I² = 0%								
Test for overall effect: Z = 8.64 (P < 0.00001)								

Root volume increase — Root volume decrease (scale: −100, −50, 0, 50, 100)

Fig. 11 Primary result of root volume increase or decrease with orthodontic treatment

group (0.77 ± 0.40). Baumrind et al. [41] found no association between tooth extraction and root resorption in a 2D study, which is consistent with the Kaley et al. [42] study. However, Sameshima et al. [11] found that removal of four first premolar teeth resulted in more root resorption than removal of two maxillary premolar teeth or no removal. The incidence of EARR was 3.72 times higher in patients who received extractions than patients without extraction [43]. Sun et al. [44] further confirmed that tooth extraction compared to non-extraction treatment caused more root resorption, which is consistent with the conclusions of the present meta-analysis. Jung et al. [35] found that maxillary central incisors resorption was 0.6 ± 0.67 mm in the non-extraction group and 0.98 ± 0.82 mm in the extraction group. The mean values are close to the present meta-analysis, but the standard deviation was smaller in our meta-analysis than in his study. In conclusion, the extraction group exhibited greater RR than the non-extraction group. The three-dimensional data were more accurate, and the root resorption that occurred in clinical treatment was not as serious as expected.

Different interventions According to the subgroup analysis of the intervention methods, the intervention was not considered as the main source of heterogeneity in this study. According to the effect value from largest to smallest of root resorption was edgewise, straight wire and augmented corticotomy-assisted presurgical orthodontics. However, there was only one study of edgewise, so more clinical studies were needed for the comparison between edgewise and other orthodontic techniques. The corticotomy group had a slightly lower root resorption than the straight wire group, suggesting that corticotomy may also reduce tooth root resorption in addition to accelerating tooth movement [45].

Primary outcome tooth volume
Root resorption is not just a two-dimensional change in length, it actually occurs in three dimensions, including on the buccal-lingual and mesial-distal sides. Therefore, the volume index is more realistic than the length index, which reflects the root resorption accurately. All three studies [20, 26, 29] focused on the maxillary and mandibular incisors and were consistent with no heterogeneity in the length index.

Factors affecting root resorption

Treatment duration Clinical studies demonstrated that a long course of treatment may cause more serious root resorption [41, 46–48]. Therefore, clinical orthodontists should avoid prolonged orthodontic treatment. However, if the patient has had root resorption or root resorption

prior to treatment, orthodontic treatment will increase the degree and speed of root resorption, which causes severe root resorption [46]. However, some studies reported no correlation between treatment duration and apical root loss [34, 49].One possible reason is that patients prolonged the treatment because of untimely referral. The limited periods of activation during the prolonged referral period in a lighter force system may also explain this difference. Harry et al. [50] suggested that the stress duration is the more serious reason than the magnitude of force. Segal et al.'s meta-analysis based on 2D data demonstrated a strong correlation between root resorption and duration [36].

Treatment duration is a risk factor of root resorption, but it is also correlated with it. We included data before and after comprehensive orthodontic treatment rather than topical or stage treatment to exclude changes in tooth length that occurred only after months of adduction or depression. Normal orthodontic treatment of a general course is 2–3 years, and stage data may not reflect the complete response to an entire treatment. The present study included before and after treatment data, which reduced the bias to some extent. These results provide the best available evidence for clinical decisions to minimize the risk and severity of apical root resorption. Therefore, clinicians should be very careful when moving anterior teeth over a long distance and a long time.

Limitations

1. There were many confounding factors, such as tooth movement distance, magnitude of force, alveolar shape and technique. There was no regression analysis of age, gender or other risk factors. Original studies did not meet consistent inclusion and exclusion criteria and provided limited information about age and could not be compared quantitatively. We hope that more unified reference planes and measurement methods may be used in future quantitative analyses.
2. Only non-randomized controlled trials (self-controlled trials) were included because of the lack of a large number of related RCT experiments due to limited conditions.
3. Most of the included trials (9 papers) resulted in changes in the length of the tooth, and root resorption was a three-dimensional change, not only in two dimensions. However, only three studies included volume changes.
4. Most of the research focused on the upper and lower anterior teeth, and root resorption of the upper and lower posterior teeth was less studied. Therefore, total dentition root resorption severity and impact factors require further experiments to verify.

Clinical significance

It is necessary to inform patients of the risk of root resorption prior to orthodontic treatment. Significant shortening of the root length will lead to inappropriate crown-root ratios and adjacency to the periodontal tissue. Apical resorption greater than 3 mm is equivalent to 1 mm of bone loss, which will accelerate the periodontal disease process. The treatment program must be re-evaluated if serious root resorption is found. Future experiments should be based on a reasonable sample size and the implementation of the entire orthodontic process to ensure the effect value.

The above meta-analysis demonstrated that the average value of root resorption was approximately 1 mm, and the upper limit did not exceed 2 mm. Sharpe's grading standards indicated that the first grade was slightly blunt (1–2 mm) [51]. The results were grade 1. Malmgren's rating standard indicates that level 1 is irregular root contour and level 2 is root resorption apically amounting to less than 2 mm (minor resorption) [40]. The most serious case did not exceed 2 degrees, and it was a mild absorption.

Conclusions

The following conclusions are drawn based on the existing research:

1. Evidence suggests that orthodontic treatment increased the incidence and severity of apical root resorption. Tooth length and root volume were reduced after orthodontic intervention, but these changes were in a clinically acceptable range.
2. Different tooth positions exhibited different degrees of absorption, and the sequence of RR from heaviest to lightest was maxillary lateral incisors, maxillary central incisors, mandibular anterior teeth, and maxillary canines.
3. Tooth extraction may result in more root resorption than non-extraction.
4. Most of the patients measured using CBCT exhibited root resorption within the clinically acceptable range. The RR value of CBCT was lower than the 2D data.

However, more methods are needed to provide more reliable evidence for clinical trials based on CBCT data. Experimental studies on treatment, the distance and angle of tooth movement, and correction techniques may provide more clinical guidance for orthodontic treatment of RR reduction.

Abbreviations

2D: Two-dimensional; 3D: Three-dimensional; CBCT: Cone beam computed tomography; CNKI: China National Knowledge Infrastructure; EARR: External apical root resorption; m: Month; MINORS: Methodological index for non-randomized studies; PRISMA: Preferred Reporting Items for Systematic Reviews and Meta Analyses; RL: Root length; RR: Root resorption; TL: Tooth length; TV: Tooth volume

Authors' contributions

YD and YS were responsible for study selection, quality assessment, data extraction and data synthesis. YD drafted the manuscript. TX participated in the research design and revision of the manuscript. All authors read and approved the final manuscript.

Competing interests

The authors declare that they have no competing interests.

References

1. Killiany DM. Root resorption caused by orthodontic treatment: an evidence-based review of literature. Semin Orthod. 1999;5:128–33.
2. Castro IO, Alencar AH, Valladaresneto J, Estrela C. Apical root resorption due to orthodontic treatment detected by cone beam computed tomography. Angle Orthod. 2013;83:196–203.
3. Jiang RP, Mcdonald JP, Fu MK. Root resorption before and after orthodontic treatment: a clinical study of contributory factors. Eur J Orthod. 2010;32:693–7.
4. Weltman B, Vig KW, Fields HW, Shanker S, Kaizar EE. Root resorption associated with orthodontic tooth movement: a systematic review. Am J Orthod Dentofac Orthop. 2010;137:462–76.
5. Martins DR, Tibola D, Janson G, Maria FR. Effects of intrusion combined with anterior retraction on apical root resorption. Eur J Orthod. 2012;34:170–5.
6. Picanço GV, de Freitas KM, Cançado RH, Valarelli FP, Picanço PR, Feijão CP. Predisposing factors to severe external root resorption associated to orthodontic treatment. Dental Press J Orthod. 2013;18:110–20.
7. Acar A, Canyürek U, Kocaaga M, Erverdi N. Continuous vs. discontinuous force application and root resorption. Angle Orthod. 1999;69:159–63.
8. Nanekrungsan K, Patanaporn V, Janhom A, Korwanich N. External apical root resorption in maxillary incisors in orthodontic patients: associated factors and radiographic evaluation. Imaging Sci Dent. 2012;42:147–54.
9. Parker RJ, Harris EF. Directions of orthodontic tooth movements associated with external apical root resorption of the maxillary central incisor. Am J Orthod Dentofac Orthop. 1998;114:677–83.
10. Peck JL, Sameshima GT, Miller A, Worth P, Hatcher DC. Mesiodistal root angulation using panoramic and cone beam CT. Angle Orthod. 2007;77:206–13.
11. Sameshima GT, Asgarifar KO. Assessment of root resorption and root shape: periapical vs panoramic films. Angle Orthod. 2001;71:185–9.
12. Baumrind S, Miller D, Molthen R. The reliability of head film measurements. 3 Tracing superimposition. Am J Orthod. 1976;70:617–44.
13. Ahn HW, Moon SC, Baek SH. Morphometric evaluation of changes in the alveolar bone and roots of the maxillary anterior teeth before and after en masse retraction using cone-beam computed tomography. Angle Orthod. 2013;83:212–21.
14. Dudic A, Giannopoulou C, Leuzinger M, Kiliaridis S. Detection of apical root resorption after orthodontic treatment by using panoramic radiography and cone-beam computed tomography of super-high resolution. Am J Orthod Dentofac Orthop. 2009;135:434–7.
15. Durack C, Patel S, Davies J, Wilson R, Mannocci F. Diagnostic accuracy of small volume cone beam computed tomography and intraoral periapical radiography for the detection of simulated external inflammatory root resorption. Int Endod J. 2011;44:136–47.
16. Estrela C, Bueno MR, Leles CR, Azevedo B, Azevedo JR. Accuracy of cone beam computed tomography and panoramic and periapical radiography for detection of apical periodontitis. J Endod. 2008;34:273–9.
17. Wang Y, He S, Guo Y, Wang S, Chen S. Accuracy of volumetric measurement of simulated root resorption lacunas based on cone beam computed tomography. Orthod Craniofac Res. 2013;16:169–76.
18. Roscoe MG, Meira JB, Cattaneo PM. Association of orthodontic force system and root resorption: a systematic review. Am J Orthod Dentofac Orthop. 2015;147:610–26.

19. Liedke GS, Da SH, Da SH, Dutra V, de Figueiredo JA. Influence of voxel size in the diagnostic ability of cone beam tomography to evaluate simulated external root resorption. J Endod. 2009;35:233–5.

20. Sun BY, Wang L, Deng RX, Ding Y. Comparative evaluation of root resorption in mandibular incisors following the treatment of adults with skeletal class III. Prog Mod Biomed. 2012;12:1098–100.

21. Wang B, Shen G, Fang B, Yu H, Wu Y. Augmented corticotomy-assisted presurgical orthodontics of class III malocclusions: a cephalometric and cone-beam computed tomography study. J Craniofac Surg. 2013;24:1886–90.

22. Wang B, Shen G, Fang B, Yu H, Wu Y, Sun L. Augmented corticotomy-assisted surgical orthodontics decompensates lower incisors in class III malocclusion patients. J Oral Maxillofac Surg. 2014;72:596–602.

23. Qiao YQ, Zhu FJ, Cui SX. Study of CBCT for root resorption of the anterior teeth of maxillary during adult orthodontic treatment. Med Innov China. 2014;11:006–9.

24. Castro I, Valladares-Neto J, Estrela C. Contribution of cone beam computed tomography to the detection of apical root resorption after orthodontic treatment in root-filled and vital teeth. Angle Orthod. 2015;85:771–6.

25. Xu SD. Explore the evaluation of adult orthodontic treatment of root resorption with CBCT. Gen J Stomatol. 2015;2:98–9.

26. Wang F, Wang JG, Zhang XZ. Examining incisor root resorption using CBCT after orthodontic treatment for adults with skeletal class III malocclusion. Tianjin Med J. 2015;43:390–3.

27. Oliveira TM, Claudino LV, Mattos CT, Sant'Anna EF. Maxillary dentoalveolar assessment following retraction of maxillary incisors: a preliminary study. Dental Press J Orthod. 2016;21:82–9.

28. Ni M, Lei Y, Chen WJ, Wu GR. Cone beam computed tomography study on the apical root resorption after orthodontic treatment in root-filled teeth. Stomatologie. 2016;36:233–6.

29. Zhang RF, Wang HM, Bai YX, Li S. Effects of orthodontic force on upper central incisor's developing roots. Beijing J Stomatol. 2016;24:335–7.

30. Yu JH, Shu KW, Tsai MT, Hsu JT, Chang HW, Tung KL. A cone-beam computed tomography study of orthodontic apical root resorption. J Dent Sci. 2013;8:74–9.

31. Kennedy DB, Joondeph DR, Osterberg SK, Little RM. The effect of extraction and orthodontic treatment on dentoalveolar support. Am J Orthod. 1983;84:183–90.

32. Pejicic A, Bertl M, Čelar A. Extent and prognosis of apical root resorption due to orthodontic treatment. Int J Stomat Occ Med. 2012;5:147–54.

33. Ousehal L, Lazrak L, Essmaali FE, Ngom PI. Apical root resorption in patients wearing orthodontic appliances. Odontostomatol Trop. 2012;35:12–8.

34. Makedonas D, Lund H, Hansen K. Root resorption diagnosed with cone beam computed tomography after 6 months and at the end of orthodontic treatment with fixed appliances. Angle Orthod. 2013;83:389–93.

35. Jung YH, Cho BH. External root resorption after orthodontic treatment: a study of contributing factors. Imaging Sci Dent. 2011;41:17–21.

36. Segal GR, Schiffman PH, Tuncay OC. Meta analysis of the treatment-related factors of external apical root resorption. Orthod Craniofac Res. 2004;7:71–8.

37. Worms FW, Isaacson RJ, Speidel TM. Surgical orthodontic treatment planning: profile analysis and mandibular surgery. Angle Orthod. 1976;46:1–25.

38. Vardimon A, Oren E, Ben-Bassat Y. Cortical bone remodeling/tooth movement ratio during maxillary incisor retraction with tip versus torque movements. Am J Orthod Dentofac Orthop. 1998;114:520–9.

39. Horiuchi A, Hotokezaka H, Kobayashi K. Correlation between cortical plate proximity and apical root resorption. Am J Orthod Dentofac Orthop. 1998; 114:311–8.

40. Levander E, Malmgren O. Evaluation of the risk of root resorption during orthodontic treatment: a study of upper incisors. Eur J Orthod. 1988;10:30–8.

41. Baumrind S, Korn EL, Boyd RL. Apical root resorption in orthodontically treated adults. Am J Orthod Dentofac Orthop. 1996;110:311–20.

42. Kaley J, Phillips C. Factors related to root resorption in edgewise practice. Angle Orthod. 1991;61:125–32.

43. Mcnab S, Battistutta D, Taverne A, Symons AL. External apical root resorption following orthodontic treatment. Angle Orthod. 2000;70:227–32.

44. Sun J, Wu YY, Wei D, Li W. Study of effect of different premolar extraction models on the incisor root resorption using panoramic radiography and cone beam computed tomography. Stomatologie. 2014;34:608–10.

45. Faedda GL, Baldessarini RJ. Treatment-emergent mania in pediatric bipolar disorder: a retrospective case review. J Affect Disord. 2004;82:149–58.

46. Brezniak N, Wasserstein A. Root resorption after orthodontic treatment: part 1. Literature review. Am J Orthod Dentofac Orthop. 1993;103:138–46.

47. Mohandesan H, Ravanmehr H, Valaei N. A radiographic analysis of external apical root resorption of maxillary incisors during active orthodontic treatment. Eur J Orthod. 2007;29:134–9.

48. Brin I, Tulloch JF, Koroluk L, Philips C. External apical root resorption in class II malocclusion: a retrospective review of 1- versus 2-phase treatment. Am J Orthod Dentofac Orthop. 2003;124:151–6.

49. Jiang F, Chen J, Kula K, Gu H, Du Y, Eckert G. Root resorptions associated with canine retraction treatment. Am J Orthod Dentofac Orthop. 2017;152:348–54.

50. Harry MR, Sims MR. Root resorption in bicuspid intrusion. A scanning electron microscope study. Angle Orthod. 1982;52:235–58.

51. Sharpe W, Reed B, Subtelny JD, Polson A. Orthodontic relapse, apical root resorption, and crestal alveolar bone levels. Am J Orthod Dentofac Orthop. 1987;91:252–8.

3

Perceptions and attitudes toward performing risk assessment for periodontal disease: a focus group exploration

Thankam Thyvalikakath[1]* ⓘ, Mei Song[2] and Titus Schleyer[3]

Abstract

Background: Currently, many risk assessment tools are available for clinicians to assess a patient's periodontal disease risk. Numerous studies demonstrate the potential of these tools to promote preventive management and reduce morbidity due to periodontal disease. Despite these promising results, solo and small group dental practices, where most people receive care, have not adopted risk assessment tools widely, primarily due to lack of studies in these settings. The objective of this study was to explore the knowledge, attitudes, and beliefs of dental providers in these settings toward risk-based care through focus groups.

Methods: We conducted six focus group sessions with 52 dentists and dental hygienists practicing in solo and small group practices in Pittsburgh, PA and New York City (NYC), NY. An experienced moderator and a note-taker conducted the six sessions, each including 8–10 participants and lasting approximately 90 min. All sessions were audio-recorded and transcribed verbatim. Two researchers coded the focus group transcripts. Using a thematic analysis approach, they reviewed the coding results to identify important themes and selected representative excerpts that best described each theme.

Results: Providers strongly believed identifying risk factors could predict periodontal disease and use this information to change their patients' behavior. A successful risk assessment tool could assist them in educating and changing their patient's behaviors to adopt a healthy lifestyle, thus enabling them to play a major role in their patients' overall health. However, to achieve this goal, it is essential to educate all dental providers and not just dentists on performing risk assessment and translating the results into actionable recommendations for patients. According to study participants, the research community has focused more on translating research findings into a risk assessment tool, and less on how clinicians would use these tools during patient encounters and if it affects a patients' risk or outcome.

Conclusions: Dental practitioners were open to performing risk assessment as routine care and playing a bigger role in their patients' overall health. Recommendations to overcome major barriers included educating dental providers at all levels, conducting more research about their adoption and use in real-world settings and developing appropriate reimbursement models.

Keywords: Risk assessment, Risk assessment tool, Risk factors, Periodontal disease, Electronic health records, Electronic dental records, Dental informatics, Biomedical informatics

* Correspondence: tpt@iu.edu
[1]Dental Informatics Core, Department of Cariology, Operative Dentistry & Dental Public Health, Indiana University School of Dentistry, Research Scientist, Center for Biomedical Informatics, Regenstrief Institute, Inc, 1050 Wishard Boulevard, R2206, Indianapolis, IN 46202, USA
Full list of author information is available at the end of the article

Background

Periodontal disease is a significant oral health problem induced by dental-plaque bacteria and host-mediated inflammation of the gums. It is the sixth most prevalent chronic condition in the world [1–3] and accounts for approximately 46% of adult periodontitis and 9% of severe periodontal disease in the US [1, 4]. Mounting evidence also suggests a potential association of periodontal disease with systemic diseases such as diabetes, cardiovascular disease, cancer and stroke [1, 5, 6]. Furthermore, poor oral health and tooth loss can negatively affect a person's self-esteem and overall quality of life [1, 7]. With adults retaining their teeth much longer, oral health remains an important component of their overall health [7]. Unfortunately, many at-risk patients are not identified at the time of routine dental examination. They appear to be in good periodontal health despite the fact they may have underlying risk factors that increase their probability of periodontal disease in the future [8–10].

Until recently, clinicians and researchers considered all people equally susceptible to periodontal disease as most adults suffered from the disease with age [6, 10, 11]. In contrast, it is now a fact that susceptibility to and severity of periodontal disease varies among adults [5]. Many studies have significantly expanded our understanding of the etiology and pathogenesis of periodontal disease. Research has identified many risks and risk-modifying factors [5, 6, 12, 13]. As a result, professional dental associations and dental schools emphasize risk assessment and preventive management for periodontal disease. This approach requires clinicians to perform a thorough patient examination and integrate findings into an accurate and valid assessment of a patient's current disease status and future disease risk [14].

Currently, many risk assessment tools are available for clinicians to assess a patient's periodontal disease risk [11, 15–21]. Most tools leverage the information clinicians routinely collect or patients self-report and compute a risk or disease score based on the risk factors. This score is then used to recommend an appropriate treatment plan for the respective patient. A systematic review of these tools indicated their ability to identify subjects with a different probability of periodontitis progression and/or tooth loss in various populations. Other studies demonstrated clinicians' high agreement with the periodontal diagnosis made by a risk assessment tool [18], their positive attitude towards using such tools [20] and improved patient care outcome and practice productivity [20, 22].

Despite these promising results, solo and small group dental practices, where most people receive care, have not adopted risk assessment tools widely, primarily due to lack of studies focusing on risk assessment in these

settings [20]. For instance, limited research has investigated dental practitioners' perception of risk assessment and incorporation of risk assessment into their daily practice. In addition, while risk assessment may inform patient care, it is not clear how a particular patient may benefit from treatment based on risk assessment [11, 23]. Also, lessons learned in large organizational settings may not be generalizable to small practice settings due to differences in patient characteristics and approaches to providing care [24].

In this study, we explored the views and attitudes of dental practitioners in solo and small-group practices towards a risk-based care approach through focus groups. We also assessed their perceived barriers and facilitators towards using risk assessment tools. Focus groups are an established method to explore the issues affecting novel interventions in clinical practice [25]. The informal and unstructured nature of focus groups helped in elucidating user needs and attitudes and identified significant barriers and opportunities for a risk-based care. Leveraging this knowledge can help better understand the needs of dental practitioners as well as inform the design of future risk assessment tools to improve patient care.

Methods

Participant recruitment

We recruited a purposive sample of 52 dental practitioners from Pittsburgh, Pennsylvania (PA), and New York City, New York (NY) and conducted six focus group sessions. In Pittsburgh, we conducted two sessions with dentists and hygienists practicing in urban and suburban areas respectively. In New York City, we conducted one session each with dentists and hygienists. We selected this sample with the intention to explore potential similarities and differences in the research topic between urban and suburban practitioners in academic versus nonacademic settings.

Participants were recruited through local dental study clubs, hygienist associations, University of Pittsburgh School of Dental Medicine part-time faculty list and the Practitioner Engaged in Applied Research & Learning (PEARL) practice-based research network of New York University. These organizations sent an initial email invitation to their members that contained a brief study description, inclusion criteria and an honorarium offer upon complete participation. They also sent a reminder message 2 weeks later. We contacted interested clinicians and confirmed they met the following inclusion criteria: be in active practice (> 30 h/week of clinical activity), graduated from a US-based educational program and be fluent in English.

Script development

A five-member panel of two dentists, one hygienist and two researchers with qualitative research expertise developed the focus group script. They developed questions geared towards exploring important issues associated with the adoption of a risk-based care for periodontal disease. The questions included dentists' main focus in the first patient examination; their definition and perception of a risk-based care; current periodontal risk assessment practices; and opinions on the benefits and drawbacks of applying a risk-based approach. We also designed questions to identify major professional, social, cultural, workflow and technical issues that facilitate or hinder the implementation of a risk-based care approach. Additional file 1: Appendix A presents the script used in the focus group sessions. To facilitate the discussion, we used the Previser Risk calculator (PRC) (PreViser Corp., Mount Vernon, WA) [9, 26] as an example to help participants think about risk assessment.

Focus group sessions

An experienced moderator and a note-taker conducted the six sessions, each including 8–10 participants and lasting approximately 90 min (See Additional file 1: Appendix A). After a short warm-up period, the moderator started the discussion, guiding the questions with the script and a handout of the sample risk assessment tool interface of Previser Risk calculator (PRC) (PreViser Corp., Mount Vernon, WA) [9, 26] when necessary. At the end of each session, participants filled out an exit survey on their practice experience, type of practice, patient population, periodontal charting tools (Additional file 2: Appendix B). The sessions were audio-recorded and transcribed verbatim by professional transcriptionists.

Coding and data analysis

One informatics researcher (Thankam Paul Thyvalikakath (TPT)), and a qualitative researcher (Mei Song (MS)) coded the focus group transcripts, using the qualitative data analysis software NVivo 10 (QSR International, Australia). They first coded one transcript independently with open coding (the process of selecting and naming categories, and identifying commonalities of the data). They reviewed the codes and discussed any disagreements to reach consensus. Through open coding, they identified a set of higher-level codes to guide subsequent coding. Afterward, they annotated and coded all transcripts using the higher-level codes and subcodes accordingly. Using a thematic analysis method [27], through constant comparison, the two researchers reviewed the coding results, discussed agreements and resolved discrepancies to identify important themes. They then selected representative excerpts that best described each theme to prepare the study results.

Results

A total of 27 dentists and 25 hygienists participated in the focus group sessions. The dentist group consisted of 16 male and 11 female participants, and the hygienist group consisted of all female participants. Tables 1 and 2 describe the demographics and patient characteristics of these participants. Our analysis focused on dental practitioners' perceptions of a risk-based dental care, the ways

Table 1 Characteristics of Focus Group Participants (n = 52)

Characteristics	Number	Percent
Gender		
Male	16	(30.8)
Female	36	(69.2)
Position		
Dentist	27	(51.9)
Hygienist	25	(48.1)
Type of Practice[a]		
Solo practice	26	(50.0)
Group practice	14	(26.9)
Community clinic/public health	2	(3.8)
Hospital	3	(5.8)
Other: VA, academic	7	(13.5)
Clinical Experience		
1–10 years	8	(15.4)
11–20 years	10	(19.2)
21–25 years	11	(21.2)
> 25 years	23	(44.2)
Frequency of performing periodontal examination		
Once or more each 6 months	21	(40.4)
At least once a year	24	(46.2)
At least once every 2 years	3	(5.8)
< once every 2 years	1	(1.9)
Never	2	(3.8)
Missing	1	(1.9)
Frequency of referral to periodontist		
0–24%	28	
25–49%	6	
50–74%	7	
75% or more	7	
Worked for a periodontist	3	
Use of Patient Chart[a]		
Paper chart only	15	(28.8)
Computer chart only	8	(15.4)
Both paper and computer chart	20	(38.5)
Unclear	9	(17.3)

[a]Four participants worked at more than one practices, only data applicable to their primary work is counted

Table 2 Characteristics of patients treated by the focus group participants (n = 52)

Patient population[a]	Number	Percent
Mainly White patients	27	(51.9)
Mainly African American patients	16	(30.8)
Both White and African American patients	1	(1.9)
Other: Hispanics, Asians	8	(15.4)
Percentage of patients with public insurance		
0–10%	31	(63.46)
More than 10%	4	(7.69)
More than 20%	6	(11.54)
More than 50%	2	(3.86)
Majority of patients are in public programs	9	(17.31)
Number of patients treated with periodontal disease/week		
0–9 patients	32	(61.5)
10–19	11	(21.15)
20–49	8	(15.38)
50 or more	1	(1.92)

[a]Four participants worked at more than one practices, only data applicable to their primary work is counted

they performed risk assessment, the benefits of and barriers to performing risk assessment and suggested strategies to overcome barriers. Major themes that emerged from the discussion are described below.

Perceptions of a risk-based care approach

When asked how they defined a risk-based dental care, the majority of providers interpreted it as conducting a certain type of risk assessment for patients. Most commonly, it involved identifying all possible risk factors and assessing their impact on a patient's oral health. These factors included pre-existing dental problems such as periodontal diseases; medical conditions such as heart diseases, diabetes, high blood pressure; smoking and alcohol drinking; diet habits; and oral hygiene. One hygienist said, *"It's host resistance. It's smoking. It's health. It's medical condition. It's psychological condition. They're all risk factors that you have to either ask or assess with your intuition and kind of put that all together and how individually all those things affect this one person."*

Providers viewed risk assessment not only on how it affects patients' ongoing problems but also from the perspective of preventive management. They believed identifying risk factors could predict clinical manifestation of some dental diseases and could use this information to motivate patients for behavior change. One dentist commented, *"From a preventive dentistry standpoint, prevent the progression of the initiation of any kind of dental disease and injury. We do have a lot of patients who are very active and the children come in with a tremendous*

amount of injuries. We look to see if we can assess what their behaviors are to make sure or at least decrease the possibility of any type of dental disease or pathology, or even injury."

Interestingly, a small number of providers (two dentists and two hygienists) perceived risk assessment as evaluating the impact on treatment outcomes. They tried to assess how well a patient would be successful with the proposed treatment given his risk factors. For instance, one dentist said he modified a patient's treatment based on caries risk assessment: conservative treatment with remineralization in some cases but more aggressive in others. Another dentist described a different scenario, *"If you have somebody that's 25 years old, and every tooth in their mouth is severely decayed, chances are you being real successful with this patient are somewhat limited, whereas if somebody comes in at 25 and they need one or two small fillings, you can show them why, they can correct their behavior, and they're gonna be good the rest of their life."*

For the two hygienists, they seemed to focus on patients' financial conditions, rather than personal risk factors. For patients who could afford any treatment needed, the risk level for a bad outcome would be low; for those who had no access to care other than free care services, their risk level would be high. Therefore, *"risk-based assessment can mean a lot of different things depending on your setting,"* as one hygienist concluded.

Current practice of risk-based care

For most study participants, risk assessment was not an intentional and purposeful task they performed for a new patient; instead, they integrated it into the comprehensive examination. Typically, information gathered from the patient brought certain risk factors to the dentist's attention, such as having diabetes or smoking. During the oral status evaluation, especially the periodontal examination, clinical signs or symptoms triggered the dentist to probe more on potential risk factors. However, dentists did not consider the periodontal evaluation as a form of risk assessment. One dentist noted, *"I don't call it risk assessment; it's my periodontal exam. I'm doing the attachment levels, the pocket depths, those types of things. First I do a little mini-screening to see do they need a comprehensive perio exam. If yes, we open that record up and do that."*

While most dentists used numbers, such as pocket depth and bleeding index, in the periodontal evaluation, they relied mostly on personal knowledge, expertise and practice experience to assess a patient's oral health and risk factors. With no formal or systematic tools, dentists evaluated risk factors mentally and subjectively. As a dentist summarized, *"Frankly we don't use tools...all we do is you know, like intuitive finding. You look at the patient, and you get some bells off in your head... I know my knowledge base, I see some signs and symptoms, and then I kind of move on to another thing."*

A handful of dentists, however, performed risk assessment more systematically, using tools varying from forms to algorithms and software. Two dentists used the American Dental Association's (ADA) caries risk assessment form and one used caries management by risk assessment form (CAMBRA). One office developed an internal form to assess and assign patients to different risk categories. Another office used a system called Structure Chart, a voice-activated application with a built-in risk assessment function that allows hygienists to record various index, plot periodontal data over time, send updated charting and forms to dentists and deliver a summary report to patients with recommendations. The risk levels, as a hygienist commented, *"were easy to understand and it prompts them to ask questions about their own health, which is good, 'cause I think it's more meaningful when it comes from them."* As a very helpful tool for patient education, this system was well received by hygienists in the office.

Benefits of performing risk assessment in dental care
To encourage discussion among study participants, we showed them a sample of the risk assessment tool and asked what benefits they perceived it would have on dental care. Thus, the benefits presented here include what they experienced in their practices as well as the perception of a risk assessment tool they may not have used personally.

Risk assessment helps dentists practice preventive dentistry
Some dentists felt assessing risk would allow them to identify individual risk factors and categorize patients based on their risk levels for dental diseases. Documentation of this information served as a reminder to dentists during future visits to monitor specific symptoms for preventive care. One dentist in Pittsburgh said it helped him *"set up a checklist so that there is something that I tend to look on occasion; it's there to remind me to take a good look at that."* This approach is helpful to prevent dental problems from happening or diagnosing a problem at an early stage so that *"it will be intercepted and treated early, thus earlier treatment, simpler treatment."*

Risk-based care helps dental providers play a bigger role in patients' health
Providers believed that risk-based dental care could identify not only risk factors for oral diseases but also those affecting a patient's overall health. As such, assessing risk would help raise the awareness of the oral-systemic connection in the dental community.

Subsequently, being mindful of this connection would motivate them to play a bigger role in patients' health, so that they are *"not just saving teeth and keeping gums healthy, what we do also have an impact on the health of their heart, pancreas, and lungs. It's really about taking responsibility as a practitioner."* Taking greater responsibility would also motivate dental practitioners to take a more holistic view of patient health and integrate dental care into medical care. *"It's a valuable thing to have us as dentists included in the overall health improvement of a patient, and oral health being part of it,"* commented a New York dentist.

Risk assessment helps educate patients and dental students
Participants unanimously agreed that a big value of risk-based care is to help them better educate and communicate with patients, especially with the assistance of well-designed and validated risk assessment tools. We provided a sample risk assessment results of the tool that included number scales, charts, graphs and color-coded results. Many participants felt such a tool would be helpful to patients in multiple ways. With the information presented as a summary report, patients can review their results in a concise and easy to understand format. The actionable recommendations are especially valuable to patients who can *"leave with something where they can look at what happened at that visit and know what to do for the future so that they have a plan in their hand."*

Study participants also considered the tool valuable for educating dental students. It may be debatable to use one numerical score to summarize a patient's risk level, but from an academic standpoint, some participants believed it could be a useful guideline to learn risk assessment *"especially for the younger dentist going in, first-year or second-year dental students."* Others shared this view, but considered the tool *"too repetitive"* and less useful for more experienced dentists as they *"may not even need the tool to evaluate (risks) quicker or more concisely."*

Risk-based care helps boost the business of dental practices
In addition to clinical care and education, providers suggested risk-based care has the potential to improve the business side of dentistry. Specifically, performing risk assessment and educating patients would likely improve patients' satisfaction and acceptance with treatment and increase revenue over time. Being able to categorize patients based on risk level would potentially save hygienists' time by avoiding unnecessary work for low-risk patients. As one dentist said, *"If you could subcategorize those perio patients, you could save man-hours in time and submitting to insurance forms. These would all be benefits."* Other providers proposed a less mentioned benefit from a liability standpoint. A few

dentists expressed concern that sometimes patients suspected being gouged when receiving more treatment. If dentists "*had some solid numbers documented in the records,*" they would have some proof in hand so the patient "*would have no way out.*"

Barriers to performing risk assessment in dental care

Providers agreed that performing risk assessment would be useful to improving patient care; however, they identified five barriers that deterred this practice in dental offices. These encompassed various aspects of dental practice, from the nature of performing risk assessment, acceptance by providers, to patients' reaction and financial considerations.

Risk assessment tools lack scientific validation

The most reported barrier concerned the quality of risk assessment tools. Though several tools are available on the market, providers were concerned about the science behind them and the accuracy and validity of the risk assessment. For instance, commenting on the sample tool, one dentist said, "*If there were valid science behind it, it would be a very useful tool. I think one of the issues or problems with this particular risk assessment calculator and other ones is that there isn't enough medicine behind it.*"

To be considered valid, providers wanted to see well designed studies that evaluated these tools and results published in good scientific journals. More importantly, they would be more convinced of the tool's usefulness if studies could show performing risk assessment "*is a corollary to the success of treatment outcome.*" For periodontal disease, they wanted to see if treatment based on risk assessment would produce positive results, as a dentist asked, "*for the severe category patients, when we do aggressive periodontal therapy and surgery and adjunctive chemotherapeutic perio treatment, do we get positive or negative results?*"

Risk assessment is time-consuming and under-reimbursed

As risk assessment involves identifying multiple factors, a comprehensive assessment could be a challenging task. Gathering and documenting all information would require dentists to spend extra time that many could not afford in a regular 30–40 min appointment. To exacerbate the problem, they felt the format and content of risk assessment tools were not very user-friendly. Many preferred to "*just go through a few slides or a few drop down boxes to get the results,*" so if they had to "*answer two or three pages just to get a quantitative number, it's not worth it, quite honestly,*" as one dentist said. With extra time spent, providers expected reimbursement for performing a risk assessment. Thus a lack of it posed an important barrier to them. One dentist commented, "*It does sound crass, but time is money...Dentistry is my livelihood, not my hobby. So if I get a questionnaire that's gonna take me an hour to fill out, and the insurance company reimburses me $15.00?*"

Implementing risk assessment programs can be costly

While providers showed interest in risk assessment, they were cautious about adding another technology-based tool in the office when some offices do not even have a computer in every operatory. The cost of purchasing and implementing a tool came to their mind immediately, as one dentist posed these questions, "*How much does this cost me? How much training or man-hours is it gonna take to implement this?*" A hygienist added the potential cost of printing out the summary report generated by a tool. "*We know that taking this would be the best tool, but cost-effectiveness is an issue when you're handing someone two or three pages of anything, because haven't we all just really been aggravated by the cost of ink?*"

Some dentists are resistant to change their practice routine

A few participants reported that some dentists practiced with a relatively fixed mindset and were reluctant to embrace changes in dentistry, be it using an electronic dental record or practicing risk assessment. They are slow to embrace new technologies and new ways of practice. A dentist offered his observation, "*There are many older people that haven't jumped on the bandwagon 'cause of the comfort zone of what they're doing and how they're generating their money. They're making their income, so why change that? Why upset that apple cart?*"

Changing patient health behaviors is difficult and challenging

For risk-based care to produce the best results, patients need to accept it. However, providers often encountered patients who do not value preventive care. These patients come to a dentist to fix existing problems, not to prevent future diseases. Dentists found it extremely difficult to motivate them to change oral health habits. One dentist shared a conversation with a young patient who smoked since a very early age, "*When I told a young fellow, 'You have quite a tobacco pouch here. You really need to stop this. You're 19 years old.' I got back, 'Grandma gave me my first chew at four years old. What's the matter? You're telling me my grandma doesn't know what's going on?*" Two hygienists experienced similar frustration when trying to refer people to get the periodontal treatment desperately needed, but to no avail, "*It's been my feeling all along that the people we recommend to go to a periodontal office never go. We can look back on their chart forever. They're not going.*"

Performing risk assessment results in unintended consequences

In addition to the above barriers, providers identified several unintended consequences of performing risk assessment that further discouraged them. One potential drawback is that doing risk assessment requires entering much information into the computer, which consequently reduces the face time with patients. As a result, the dental provider-patient relationship may suffer. Another unintended result could be the misuse of risk assessment results by insurance companies to refuse coverage for treatment. Providers were concerned that insurance companies would challenge the treatment recommended by a tool that may not fit their rules. The third potential outcome is some patients may be shocked and turned off by a high-risk score generated by a risk assessment tool. Dentists worried that these patients could lose hope and stop trying to improve their oral health altogether.

Facilitators for performing risk-based care

According to study participants, the primary factor for adopting a risk-based care was to educate all stakeholders involved in patient care. Other facilitators included making risk assessment a standard practice and risk assessment tools universally accepted; providing monetary incentives to providers and having access to well-designed and scientifically validated risk assessment tools. We describe them briefly in this section:

Promoting risk assessment to all stakeholders in the dental care

Providers believed that education is the key to the adoption of risk-based care. It is especially important to start the education in dental school so *"students will come out of school wanting to do risk assessment as they learned."* Then they should teach risk assessment to support staff, such as hygienists and dental assistants. Dentists emphasized the need to teach students not only the meaning of risk assessment but also how to interpret numeric results in a meaningful way. As one dentist suggested, *"A number is just a number. But how do you make it relevant to you as a practitioner? How do you make it relevant to the patient? So there comes education again."* The third piece of the education is patients. Providers hoped to educate patients more on the oral-systemic connections to better understand their risk profile. With education, they expected patients to *"speak the same language, and hopefully, gets a little bit more motivated (about their health)."*

Making risk assessment standard and universally acceptable

Providers believed it is imperative that risk assessment is made a standard of care to enable its wide adoption.

They expected the endorsement by dental associations to play an important role. For example, to adopt a periodontal risk assessment tool, a dentist suggested, *"if you got the American Academy of Periodontology on board and endorsed it, the ADA would jump on board. And just like PSR (Periodontal Screening and Recording) scores, it would become universally acceptable."* Once a standard of care, more people will accept the idea and become an adopter. Providers also proposed the additional value of using universally acceptable risk assessment tools for patient care. For instance, when a patient switches a dental office, the new dentist will understand his risk history and profile instantly if the two dentists use the same tool. This universal approach will ease care coordination between different providers.

Providing monetary incentives to dental practitioners

As previously described, a major barrier to performing risk assessment was a lack of reimbursement for dentists. Given the pressing time constraints of the current practice environment, providers, especially dentists, were clear that the ability to generate more revenue would be a big facilitator for risk assessment. One dentist said, *"This may sound callous, but overall, the bulk of dentists who practice dentistry as a business look at the business of dentistry different than the practice of dentistry. We like the new remote control whose 50 buttons does the magic thing, but if it isn't gonna make me money, I'm not going to be quick to jump on the bandwagon."*

Having access to well-designed, scientifically validated and easy to use risk assessment tools

When all other favorable factors are in place, access to well-designed, clinically based and scientifically validated tools becomes the deciding factor for providers to take up risk assessment. Throughout the discussion, they proposed numerous suggestions for designing an ideal tool. As we will address the details of the requirements in a separate article, we provide a concise summary of their opinions here.

According to them, a risk assessment tool should include multiple features and functions, the most important being that it must consider all relevant factors to calculate the risk score. They suggested adding factors, such as patients' oral pH, personal life and even emotional status such as *"are they going through a divorce? Is their stress level higher than normal?"* In addition, the tool should emphasize factors linking dental to medical conditions; track patient changes over time; connect other risk assessment tools, such as caries assessment; and provide personalized recommendations to patients. A valid risk assessment tool needs to assign the right weights to different risk factors to calculate an accurate and personalized risk score. After development, the tool should be tested in well-designed scientific studies. When delivering patient results, they expected the summary report to be concise and tailored to each patient, with better data visualization, clearer, and color-coded scales and written in easy to understand grade-level language. For optimal adoption, this tool also *"needs to be incorporated, not in a stand-alone program, but into a computer program that the office is using"* in the workflow, as one hygienist commented.

Discussion

This study performed a progressive exploration of general dentists' and hygienists' perceptions and attitudes regarding a risk-based care approach for periodontal disease. A major finding of this study is the dental providers' strong emphasis that a successful risk assessment tool would assist them in educating and changing their patient's behavior to adopt healthy lifestyle behaviors. They expressed risk assessment played a major role in practicing preventive dentistry and enabling patients to have better outcomes. The study participants also highlighted that performing risk assessment could enable them to play a bigger role in their patients' overall health. To achieve this goal, it is essential to educate all dental providers and not just dentists on performing risk assessment. It is equally important to teach them to interpret and translate the results into actionable recommendations for patients.

We did not detect significant differences between dentists and hygienists in their perceptions and attitudes toward risk-based care. Both groups viewed risk assessment as identifying all possible risk factors and assessing their impact on a patient's oral health. They also agreed on the various benefits of and barriers to performing risk assessment. However, sometimes they focused on different aspects of risk assessment. For example, dentists focused on treatment outcome when assessing a patient's risk level while some hygienists looked more at his/her ability to pay for treatment. On the benefits of risk assessment, dentists focused more on performing preventive dentistry and playing a bigger role in patients' overall health while hygienists focused on educating patients about oral disease and the connection to medical conditions. It is important to note that these differences mainly stem from the respective clinical roles dentists and hygienists play in the office.

Our study also identified key factors to be addressed to make risk assessment part of routine dental care and to promote preventive management. In this section, we propose directions for future research in this field. We hope these suggestions can leverage practitioners' positive attitudes and address their concerns to promote preventive management of periodontal disease through risk assessment. It is important to note that medicine also

faces the same challenges of adopting risk assessment tools observed in dentistry [28–32]. Since dentistry is yet to adopt a risk-based treatment approach widely, it has the advantage of implementing risk assessment tools that are designed based on dental practitioners' and patients' needs.

Developing standardized and reproducible measures to assess risk for periodontal disease

Currently, dental practitioners mostly rely on their expert knowledge and practice experience to evaluate patients' risk for periodontal disease. In most cases, they consider this intuitive evaluation sufficient but do admit that acquisition of the skill may require years of experience and learning, especially for new dental school graduates. Thus, it is important for clinicians to assess an individual's periodontal disease risk and status in objective and standardized ways. Future work should focus on developing standardized and reproducible measures for periodontal risk assessment. Over time, such approaches can provide valuable data to conduct comparative effectiveness research that will lay the foundation for evidence-based dentistry.

Evaluating risk assessment tools to improve process and patient outcomes

In this study, a major barrier to the adoption of current tools is the lack of scientific evaluation. Admittedly, developing a good decision support tool is a difficult endeavor; however, study participants feel that the research community has overemphasized on translating research findings into a risk assessment tool, not on evaluating if and how it can reduce a patient's risk. We need more research to validate the risk assessment results in clinical settings to answer critical questions, such as how clinicians interpret the risk scores, how they use the results to make treatment decisions, how they educate patients and promote shared decision-making, and ultimately how risk assessment tools improve treatment processes and patient outcomes.

Exploring new models of payment to perform risk assessment

Both dentists and hygienists are highly concerned about the current reimbursement model that limits them from performing risk assessment and preventive management. This concern clearly shows that developing scientifically valid and easy to use tools alone are insufficient for clinicians to perform risk assessment. It is critical that the dental profession and researchers explore new models of payment to incentivize providers to conduct risk assessment and transition to a preventive model that will reduce dental diseases and dental care costs.

Developing innovative and integrative approach to collect patient information

Study participants reported the extra time needed to gather and record information as a notable barrier. We need to develop more innovative approaches to reuse existing data from various sources and improve the user-interface of clinical systems. With the huge amount of data available electronically in the electronic dental record (EDR), electronic health record (EHR), and other sources, how to reuse them more efficiently and effectively remains an important research question. We envision that data collection may use an integrative approach, for instance, by combining patient self-reported general health and lifestyle data collected before visits, dental data collected during patient visits, and medical data automatically imported from other sources before or after visits.

Designing smart tools to help patients track, monitor and change behaviors

A perfect tool may help providers to predict and prevent oral diseases, but it may not guarantee to change patients' health behaviors. In addition to incorporating an educational component in the risk assessment results, simple-to-use tools such as smartphone apps could be developed to motivate patients to monitor and improve their oral health behaviors.

Promoting an integrated care and prevention approach

Dentists in the study embraced the idea of playing a role like primary care physicians. As some medical conditions manifest first in the oral cavity, dental practitioners are in a unique position to identify them earlier than physicians. Moreover, oral diseases share many of the same risk factors with medical conditions such as cardiovascular disease, diabetes, respiratory disease and cancer; thus promoting an integrated care and prevention approach is crucial to improving patient outcomes, population health and reducing per capita costs of healthcare. While it is still debatable if dentists should perform certain screening procedures and claim reimbursement, their openness to a bigger role may play a significant part in raising patients' awareness of oral-systemic connection and facilitating care coordination for their general health. As indicated in the study, participating in patients' overall health brings providers more career satisfaction than financial gains.

Limitations

A major limitation of this study is that we recruited a convenience sample of dentists and hygienists from Pittsburgh and New York City. In the selection process, we purposefully sampled dental practitioners from metro vs. suburban areas to explore potential differences among them on the research questions. However, with Pittsburgh and NYC being densely populated metropolitan areas, the point of views of these providers may not reflect views of providers in other parts of the country, especially those in rural areas or working with specific patient populations. Therefore, the results may not be generalizable to all dental practitioners. To generalize our results, we plan to administer a nation-wide survey of dentists and hygienists based on the themes that emerged from this study. Secondly, participation inequality existed in the focus group sessions. In certain sessions, a few active participants contributed more to the discussion on using risk assessment tools. However, this should not be a serious concern since each participant had a different experience in using these tools. We were more interested in identifying what experience they had in risk assessment and less in who had that experience. Finally, opinions on the research questions may change as the tools become more readily available. It will be helpful to conduct a similar study to compare the results.

Conclusions

Most dentists and hygienists in the study defined risk-based care as identifying all possible risk factors and assessing the impact on patients' oral diseases. Dental practitioners were open to performing risk assessment as a routine care practice and playing a bigger role in patients' overall health. But the extra time needed and lack of reimbursement, the difficulty to change provider and patient behaviors, and the limited availability of scientifically validated tools all posed as roadblocks. To overcome these barriers, dental community should work towards the following: educate providers about risk-based care at all levels; promote risk assessment as standard of care; develop innovative and integrative methods to collect patient data; conduct scientific research to validate risk assessment tools and study their adoption and use in real-world settings; and build simple and easy to use electronic tools to motivate changes in oral health behavior.

Abbreviations

ADA: American dental association; CAMBRA: Caries management by risk assessment; EDR: Electronic dental record; EHR: Electronic health record; MS: Mei Song; NY: New York; NYC: New York City; PA: Pennsylvania; PEARL: Practitioner engaged in applied Research & Learning; PRC: Previser risk calculator; PSR: Periodontal screening and recording; TPT: Thankam Paul Thyvalikakath; WA: Washington

Acknowledgements

We gratefully acknowledge the study participants. We acknowledge Late Dr. Frederick Curro and Ms. Ashley Gill and the PEARL Network at the New York University for assistance with recruiting New York City (NYC) dentists and hygienists and conducting the focus group sessions in NYC. We acknowledge Dr. Gerardo Maupome and Ms. Merry Jo Thoele for reviewing the focus group questions and Ms. Jane Thomas for moderating the sessions. We also thank Mr. Michael Dziabiak for his assistance with conducting the study and Mr. Andres Rodriguez for his assistance with formatting the manuscript. This project was partially supported by the Clem MacDonald chair account and the Lilly Endowment Inc. Physician Scientist Initiative.

Funding
This study was funded in part by the grant 5K08DE018957 from the National Institute for Dental and Craniofacial Research, a component of NIH. The funding agency did not have any role in the design of the study and collection, analysis, and interpretation of data and in writing the manuscript.

Authors' contributions
TPT conceptualized the study, drafted focus group questions, recruited participants, collected data, analyzed the results, wrote, and finalized the manuscript. MS assisted with conceptualizing the study, drafting the focus group questions, analyzing study results and writing the manuscript. She also finalized the manuscript. TS guided conceptualizing the study and data analysis. He also reviewed and finalized the manuscript. All authors read and approved the final version of the manuscript.

Authors' information
TPT is a dentist and biomedical informatics researcher. Her experiences and knowledge include learning end-users' decision-making process using user-centered design and cognitive engineering methods, developing, implementing and evaluating clinical decision support systems and leveraging electronic health records data for clinical research and quality improvement purposes. MS expertise is in conducting qualitative studies to understand the needs of the end-users of a particular intervention and in applying thematic analysis. TS is a dentist and senior biomedical informatics researcher. His experiences and knowledge include applying user-centered design methods to investigate users' workflow and developing, implementing and evaluating clinical decision support systems.

Competing interests
The authors declare that they have no competing interests.

Author details
[1]Dental Informatics Core, Department of Cariology, Operative Dentistry & Dental Public Health, Indiana University School of Dentistry, Research Scientist, Center for Biomedical Informatics, Regenstrief Institute, Inc, 1050 Wishard Boulevard, R2206, Indianapolis, IN 46202, USA. [2]Microbicide Trials Network, Magee-Womens Research Institute, 204 Craft Avenue, Pittsburgh, PA 15213, USA. [3]Center for Biomedical Informatics, Regenstrief Institute, Inc. Indiana University School of Medicine, 1101 West Tenth Street, Indianapolis, IN 46202, USA.

References
1. Eke PI, Wei L, Thornton-Evans GO, Borrell LN, Borgnakke WS, Dye B, et al. Risk indicators for periodontitis in US adults: NHANES 2009 to 2012. J Periodontol. 2016;87:1174–85.
2. Eke PI, Dye BA, Wei L, Slade GD, Thornton-Evans GO, Borgnakke WS, et al. Update on prevalence of periodontitis in adults in the United States: NHANES 2009 to 2012. J Periodontol. 2015;86:611–22.
3. CDC. Gum Disease Information [Internet]. 2014 [cited 2017 Aug 14]. Available from: https://www.perio.org/consumer/gum-disease.htm
4. Hujoel P, Zina L, Cunha-Cruz J, López R. Specific infections as the etiology of destructive periodontal disease: a systematic review. Eur J Oral Sci. 2013;121:2–6.
5. Bouchard P, Carra MC, Boillot A, Mora F, Rangé H. Risk factors in periodontology: a conceptual framework. J Clin Periodontol. 2017;44:125–31.
6. Genco RJ, Borgnakke WS. Risk factors for periodontal disease. Periodontol 2000. 2013;62:59–94.
7. Buset SL, Walter C, Friedmann A, Weiger R, Borgnakke WS, Zitzmann NU. Are periodontal diseases really silent? A systematic review of their effect on quality of life. J Clin Periodontol. 2016;43:333–44.
8. Kye W, Davidson R, Martin J, Engebretson S. Current status of periodontal risk assessment. J Evid Based Dent Pract. 2012;12:2–11.
9. Page RC, Krall EA, Martin J, Mancl L, Garcia RI. Validity and accuracy of a risk calculator in predicting periodontal disease. J Am Dent Assoc. 2002;133:569–76.
10. Douglass CW. Risk assessment and management of periodontal disease. J Am Dent Assoc. 2006;137(Suppl):27S–32S.
11. Lang NP, Suvan JE, Tonetti MS. Risk factor assessment tools for the prevention of periodontitis progression a systematic review. J Clin Periodontol. 2015;42:S59–70.
12. Van Dyke TE, Sheilesh D. Risk factors for periodontitis. J Int Acad Periodontol. 2005;7:3–7.
13. AlJehani YA. Risk factors of periodontal disease: review of the literature. Int J Dent. 2014;2014:1–9.
14. Tonetti MS, Eickholz P, Loos BG, Papapanou P, van der Velden U, Armitage G, et al. Principles in prevention of periodontal diseases. J Clin Periodontol. 2015;42:S5–11.
15. Trombelli L, Farina R, Ferrari S, Pasetti P, Calura G. Comparison between two methods for periodontal risk assessment. Minerva Stomatol. 2009;58:277–87.
16. Lang NP, Tonetti MS. Periodontal risk assessment (PRA) for patients in supportive periodontal therapy (SPT). Oral Health Prev Dent. 2003;1:7–16.
17. Page RC, Martin JA, Loeb CF. The oral health information suite (OHIS): its use in the management of periodontal disease. J Dent Educ. 2005;69:509–20.
18. Mullins JM, Even JB, White JM. Periodontal management by risk assessment: a pragmatic approach. J Evid Based Dent Pract. 2016;16(Suppl):91–8.
19. Garcia RI, Compton R, Dietrich T. Risk assessment and periodontal prevention in primary care. Periodontol 2000. 2016;71:10–21.
20. Mertz E, Bolarinwa O, Wides C, Gregorich S, Simmons K, Vaderhobli R, et al. Provider attitudes toward the implementation of clinical decision support tools in dental practice. J Evid Based Dent Pract. 2015;15:152–63.
21. Chandra RV. Evaluation of a novel periodontal risk assessment model in patients presenting for dental care. Oral Health Prev Dent. 2007;5:39–48.
22. Busby M, Chapple E, Matthews R, Chapple ILC. Practitioner evaluation of a novel online integrated oral health and risk assessment tool: a practice pilot. Br Dent J. 2013;215:115–20.
23. Asimakopoulou K, Newton JT, Daly B, Kutzer Y, Ide M. The effects of providing periodontal disease risk information on psychological outcomes - a randomized controlled trial. J Clin Periodontol. 2015;42:350–5.
24. Brocklehurst PR, Ashley JR, Tickle M. Patient assessment in general dental practice – risk assessment or clinical monitoring? BDJ. 2011;210:351–4.
25. Sofaer S. Qualitative research methods. Int J Qual Heal Care. 2002;14:329–36.
26. Martin JA, Page RC, Loeb CF, Levi PA. Tooth loss in 776 treated periodontal patients. J Periodontol. 2010;81:244–50.
27. Braun V, Clarke V. Using thematic analysis in psychology. Qual Res Psychol. 2006;3:77–101.
28. Cresswell K, Majeed A, Bates DW, Sheikh A. Computerised decision support systems for healthcare professionals: an interpretative review. Inform Prim Care. 2012;20:115–28.
29. Sittig DF, Wright A, Osheroff JA, Middleton B, Teich JM, Ash JS, et al. Grand challenges in clinical decision support. J Biomed Inform. 2008;41:387–92.
30. Légaré F, Ratté S, Gravel K, Graham ID. Barriers and facilitators to implementing shared decision-making in clinical practice: update of a systematic review of health professionals' perceptions. Patient Educ Couns. 2008;73:526–35.
31. Carter-Harris L, Gould MK. Multilevel barriers to the successful implementation of lung cancer screening: why does it have to be so hard? Ann Am Thorac Soc. 2017;14:1261–5.
32. Bates DW, Kuperman GJ, Wang S, Gandhi T, Kittler A, Volk L, et al. Ten commandments for effective clinical decision support: making the practice of evidence-based medicine a reality. J Am Med Inform Assoc. 2003;10:523–30.

4

Dental caries and their association with socioeconomic characteristics, oral hygiene practices and eating habits among preschool children in Abu Dhabi, United Arab Emirates — the NOPLAS project

Amal Elamin[1]* ⓘ, Malin Garemo[1] and Andrew Gardner[2]

Abstract

Background: Dental caries are a global public health problem and influence the overall health of children. The risk factors for caries include biological, socio-behavioral and environmental factors. This cross-sectional study assessed dental caries and their associations with socioeconomic factors, oral hygiene practices and eating habits among Emirati and non-Emirati children in Abu Dhabi, United Arab Emirates (UAE).

Methods: The stratified sample comprised children aged 18 months to 4 years recruited from 7 nurseries. The World Health Organization (WHO) decayed, missing and filled teeth index (dmft) was used to analyze the dental status of the children. Parents completed a questionnaire regarding demographics, food consumption and oral habits. The study was approved by the Research Ethics Committee at Zayed University, UAE (ZU15_029_F).

Results: A total of 186 children with a mean age of 2.46 years, of which 46.2% were Emirati, participated. Overall, 41% of the children had dental caries. The mean dmft±SD was 1.70 ± 2.81 with a mean ± SD decayed component (dt) of 1.68 ± 2.80 and mean ± SD filled component (ft) of 0.02 ± 0.19. Emirati children showed higher mean dmft, Plaque Index and Significant Carries Index values than non-Emirati children ($P < 0.000$). Low maternal education, rural nursery location, infrequent tooth-brushing, frequent consumption of high-sugar food items and Emirati nationality were factors significantly associated with dental caries.

Conclusions: In this study, 4 out of 10 nursery children were found to have dental caries. Sociodemographic factors, dietary and oral health habits were associated with dental caries. Effective oral health interventions tailored to improve eating habits and the dental screening of children in this age group are imperative to mitigate these concerns.

Keywords: Dental caries, Oral hygiene practices, High sugar intake, United Arab Emirates, Preschool children, Socio-economic status, Socio cultural factors, Nurseries

* Correspondence: Amal.Elamin@zu.ac.ae
[1]Department of Health Sciences, College of Natural and Health Sciences, Zayed University, P.O. Box 144534, Abu-Dhabi, United Arab Emirates
Full list of author information is available at the end of the article

Background

Good oral health status at a young age is of the utmost importance for children's development, overall health and well-being [1]. Epidemiological studies have revealed that dental caries are the most prevalent chronic disease worldwide in the pediatric community and represent a costly burden to health care services [2, 3]. There is ample evidence supporting the fact that the caries status of young, permanent dentition is closely related to the status of the primary dentition, indicating the importance of understanding the risk factors for caries in the early years of life [4, 5].

Dental caries are a multifactorial disease, with many risk factors contributing to their initiation and progression. The risk factors can be categorized as biological, environmental or socio-behavioral [1]. In preschoolers, high consumption of sucrose, sweet drinks, high sugar intake between meals, and frequent snacking have all been associated with dental caries [6, 7]. Additionally, the quality of a child's oral hygiene practices and the parents' ability to withhold cariogenic snacks are also factors associated with dental caries [1, 8]. Some studies have found an association between tooth-brushing and lower caries prevalence, although the findings are inconsistent [7, 9, 10]. Moreover, socioeconomic factors such as income, education level and family size impact disease prevalence [11–14]. In developing countries, children from urban areas experience a higher prevalence of dental caries, in contrast to industrialized countries, where the highest caries rates have been observed among deprived social groups and ethnic minorities [2, 15].

The global prevalence of childhood caries varies widely, with the lowest prevalence reported in some Western countries, such as Sweden, Italy and the USA [16]. Conversely, a higher prevalence has been reported in the Middle East, where many countries are still undergoing economic transition and the health care system is still developing [6, 7, 10, 17–20]. Despite the fact that oral health care is free for United Arab Emirates (UAE) nationals, a high prevalence of dental caries (range: 74.1–83%) among 4- to 5-year-olds and a high decayed, missing and filled teeth index (dmft) (range: 3.07–10.9) have been reported in different areas of the UAE [6, 7, 17]. A study conducted in Abu Dhabi in 1998 found a high prevalence of dental caries in children aged 2, 4 and 5 years, but to date, very limited data are available on the dental status of toddlers and preschoolers, indicating a clear knowledge gap [21].

The aim of this cross-sectional study was to assess dental caries and their association with socioeconomic factors, oral hygiene practices and eating habits among Emirati and non-Emirati nursery children aged 18 months to 4 years living in Abu Dhabi, UAE.

Methods

Subjects and study design

The data for this cross-sectional study were collected in 2015/2016. The target population was nursery children between 18 months and 4 years of age residing in the capital district of Abu Dhabi. A stratified random sampling design was used where clusters consisted of nurseries stratified geographically across urban, suburban and rural areas. The three strata were proportional to the number of nurseries in each geographical area. Seven nurseries participated, representing the three strata. Access to the parents of the children in the target age group was achieved through face-to-face interaction during pickup and drop offs using bilingual study investigators. Parents were provided with oral and written information about the study prior to them being asked to consent to their child taking part. Data were collected through oral examination and a structured questionnaire. This study is part of a project titled 'Nutrition, Oral Health, Physical Development, Lifestyle, Anthropometry and Socioeconomic Status' (NOPLAS).

Questionnaire

Consenting parents completed a self-administered structured questionnaire in either English or Arabic (see Additional file 1). The questionnaire collected information about socio-economic background (e.g., maternal and paternal education levels, self-rated financial status) and oral hygiene and dental health practices (e.g., details about tooth-brushing, dental visits, past dental history). The questionnaire also asked about eating habits using a 42-item Food Frequency Questionnaire (FFQ) covering all food groups, including 9 high-sugar food items (flavored milk, cakes, biscuits, fruit juices, syrups and cordials, soft drinks, ice cream, chocolate, and sweets). The FFQ contained five response choices: 'more than 1 time/day', '6–7 times/week', '3–5 times/week', '1–2 times/week', and 'fewer than 1 time/ week or never'. The mean intake frequency of the nine sugary foods was used to assess the associations between the dental indices and sugary food consumption. Similarly, the mean intake frequency for the other 33 food categories was used as a measure of non-sugary food intake.

Oral examination

Prior to the field study, the intra-examiner reliability was measured by repeated examinations performed on children to assess the intra-examiner agreement of caries status and dental plaque, using Cohen's Kappa statistics. Others have suggested an acceptable intra-examiner agreement of $\kappa > 0.61$–0.93 for caries [22, 23]. In this study a $\kappa > 0.93$ was used as an acceptable intra examiner reliability for caries. The results indicated a complete intra examiner reliability for caries yielding $\kappa = 1.0$, while for plaque, κ was calculated as 0.924. The participating children were examined by one trained dentist experienced in working with children under field conditions. The children were examined at the nurseries in the presence of a familiar adult, such as a nurse or teacher, and their nursery friends. To reduce anxiety, the dentist explained to the child what would be done prior to the examination. The World Health Organization (WHO) caries-scoring index for primary dentition, the dmft, was used to describe the dental caries status of each child [24]. Plaque was recorded using the Plaque Index (PI) [25]. Each intra-oral clinical examination was performed with the child seated in a conventional school chair facing a window with sunlight access under standard conventional light with the dentist wearing a headlight. The examination was carried out using a sterilized, disposable set consisting of an illuminated mouth mirror (Denlite, Welch Allyn Ltd., Navan, Co Meath, Ireland) and a blunt ball-ended probe (Diagnostic Probe, Hu-Freidy Dental, Chicago, Illinois, USA) with an end diameter of 0.5 mm. The dentist recorded the findings for each child on a scoring sheet. The assessments were performed only on cooperative and happy children, regardless of parental approval, to ensure the wellbeing of the children.

Ethical consideration

This study was performed in agreement with the Ministry of Social Affairs, UAE. The study received full ethical approval from the Research Ethics Committee at Zayed University, UAE (ZU15_029_F) and complied with the Declaration of Helsinki Ethical Principles for Medical Research. Permissions and approvals were obtained from nursery management. Prior to participation, the parents were provided with detailed information about the study in Arabic and English. Written consent was obtained for each participant.

Statistical analysis

The statistical software package SPSS version 24.0 was used for all statistical analyses (IBM Corp., Armonk, NY, UAS 2016). The mean dmft score was used to calculate the Significant Carries Index (SIC) as described by Bratthall [26]. Dental caries, mean dmft and SIC were used to determine the extent of dental caries, and the association of other variables with these indices was evaluated using t-tests, Pearson correlations or non-parametric tests, including chi-square tests as appropriate. A P-value ≤ 0.05 was considered statistically significant.

Results

A total of 186 children (40.9% girls), with a mean age of 2.46 years, participated in the study (Fig. 1). Parents reported their children to be healthy, with no health conditions known to affect oral health status. One-third of the children (34.4%) were enrolled in nurseries located

in urban areas, 36.6% in nurseries located in suburban areas and 29.0% in nurseries located in rural areas. Half of the children (54.3%) were > 36 months old, 11.3% were between 18 and 24 months old, and the remaining children (34.4%) were between 25 and 36 months old. The sample had a heterogeneous background, and children were categorized into Emirati children (46.2%) and non-Emirati children (53.8%) based on their nationality, as reported by their parents. The non-Emirati group was comprised of Western, Eastern Mediterranean and Southeast Asian children. The population residing in rural areas is mainly Emirati; thus, the nursery located in this area had mainly Emirati children enrolled, whereas the other locations hosted children of mixed nationalities. There were significant differences in the parents' education level, as 75.4% of Emirati fathers had a university degree compared to 95.3% of non-Emirati fathers ($P<0.01$), and the corresponding values for mothers were 63.9% vs. 91.1%, respectively ($P<0.01$). None of the families considered themselves poor, and 98.6% rated their economic status as middle income, and 1.4% rated themselves as wealthy. A loss analysis revealed that considerably more Emirati families did not return the questionnaire compared to non-Emirati families (34.1% vs. 3.2%, respectively, $P<0.001$).

Each nursery was visited at least three times for the oral examination, resulting in 74.7% of the children undertaking the dental assessment, with the remaining children refusing the examination or being absent on all three visits (Fig. 1). Overall, 41% of children had dental caries. Decayed teeth (98.7%) contributed the most to the dmft scores. The mean $\pm$ SD dmft was 1.70 ± 2.81 with a mean $\pm$ SD decayed component (dt) of 1.68 ± 2.80 and a mean $\pm$ SD filled component (ft) of 0.02 ± 0.19. There were no missing teeth due to caries (mt). No significant difference was found in the mean dmft between boys and girls, but as shown in Table 1, the Emirati children had considerably more decayed teeth (dt) and higher dmft than the non-Emirati children ($P<0.000$). Furthermore, the Emirati children had a significantly higher mean dmft when residing in rural areas than those in urban or suburban areas ($P=0.03$).

Figure 2 shows the distribution of dmft scores in the four dental quadrants. Dental caries occurred most frequently in the maxillary teeth and in the posterior teeth of both jaws.

Figure 3 illustrates the prevalence of dental caries by nationality and age group. Caries were present in children below 24 months of age, and the prevalence increased with age with significant differences between nationalities in children > 36 months old ($P=0.001$). Table 2 shows the SIC results divided by nationality, gender, nursery location and age group. The PI was considerably higher among Emirati children than non-Emirati

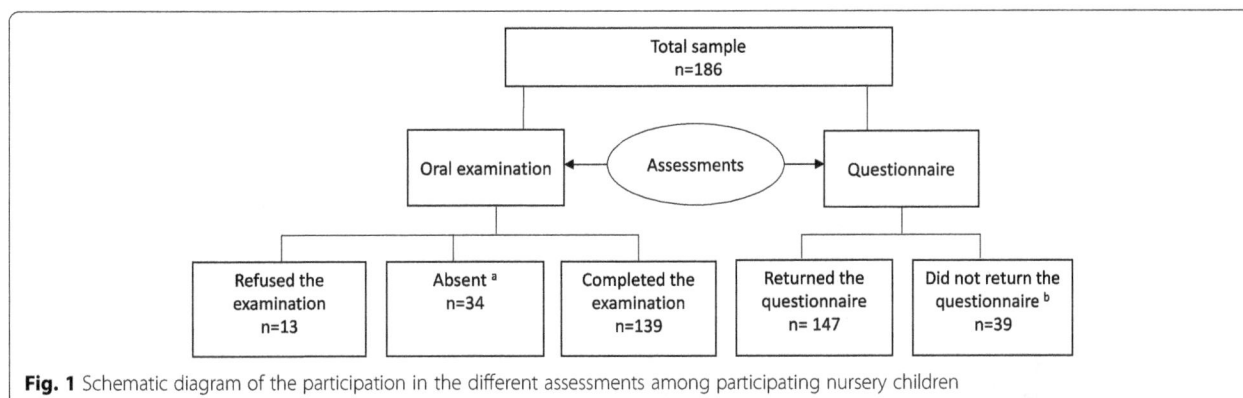

Fig. 1 Schematic diagram of the participation in the different assessments among participating nursery children

children, 1.8 ± 1.0 vs. 0.9 ± 1.0 ($P < 0.000$), with no differences by gender or age.

A majority of the children (75.3%) brushed their teeth at least one time per day, while the remaining children (24.7%) brushed their teeth irregularly or never. There were considerably fewer Emirati children who brushed their teeth daily than non-Emirati children (57.9% vs. 86.5% respectively, $P < 0.000$). Analysis of tooth-brushing habits showed that 52.9% of the children brushed their teeth together with an adult; in 44.3% of these cases, the brushing was done by an adult, and in 2.9% of the cases, the children brushed their teeth by themselves. A vast majority (95.6%) used a regular toothbrush with only 4.6% using an electric toothbrush. More than a quarter of the children (27.9%) had, according to their parents, visited a dentist. Regular checkups were the main reason for the dental visits, with the secondary reason being dental trauma or fissure sealant application. Ten children (6.8%), all Emirati children, reported current dental complaints due to toothache, speech difficulties or habit-related malocclusions. When parents were asked about their perception of their child's dental health, 91.5% of parents rated the dental health of their child as very good or satisfactory, whereas 7.5% perceived it as dissatisfactory. Emirati parents had a lower perception of their child's dental health and dental appearance than non-Emirati parents ($P = 0.009$ and $P = 0.01$, respectively). Table 3 shows the associations between dental caries and univariate socioeconomic variables. Maternal education and parents' perceptions about their child's dental status were independent variables significantly associated with the mean dmft and SIC values.

The frequency of consumption of high-sugar food items is shown in Table 4. The intake of sugary foods was positively associated with the dmft ($r = 0.37$, $P < 0.001$). Children who had had caries (dmft> 0) consumed high-sugar food items more frequently than those who were caries free ($P = 0.003$). Children included in the SIC also consumed high-sugar food items more frequently than those who were not ($P = 0.003$).

Discussion

Dental health is associated with speech development, eating ability, and overall health in young children [27]. Many caries prediction models have implicated caries in primary dentition as a strong predictor of future caries in permanent dentition [4]. In this stratified sample of children attending nurseries in Abu Dhabi, the prevalence of dental caries was found to be 41%. The univariate analysis revealed that Emirati nationality, low maternal education, rural geographic location of the nursery, and frequent consumption of high-sugar food items were associated with caries in this study population.

The overall mean dmft of 1.7 was lower than that of recent findings by Kowash demonstrating a mean dmft of 10.9 in children below 5 years of age in the Eastern Region of the UAE [6]. While the overall caries status was 41, 64.7% of the Emirati children > 3 years had caries which is on par with regional studies showing that 68–89% of 3- to 5-year-old children were affected by

Table 1 Mean decayed teeth (dt), filled teeth (ft) and dmft scores divided by nationality among nursery children

	Total (n)	Decayed (dt)		Filled (ft)		dmft score[b]	
		n (%)	Mean (SD)	n (%)	Mean (SD)	n (%)	Mean (SD)
All children	139	57 (41.0)	1.70 (2.8)	2 (1.4)	0.02 (0.1)	57 (41.0)	1.68 (2.8)
Emirati children	63[a]	35 (55.6)	2.57 (3.2)	1 (1.6)	0.03 (0.2)	35 (55.6)	2.60 (3.2)
Non-Emirati children	63[a]	16 (25.4)	0.75 (1.8)	0 (0)	0 (0)	16 (25.4)	0.75 (1.8)

Abbreviations: dmft decayed, missing and filled teeth index, *dt* decayed teeth, *ft* filled teeth
[a]Thirteen children out of the total of 139 children did not report nationality
[b]No children had missing teeth due to dental caries

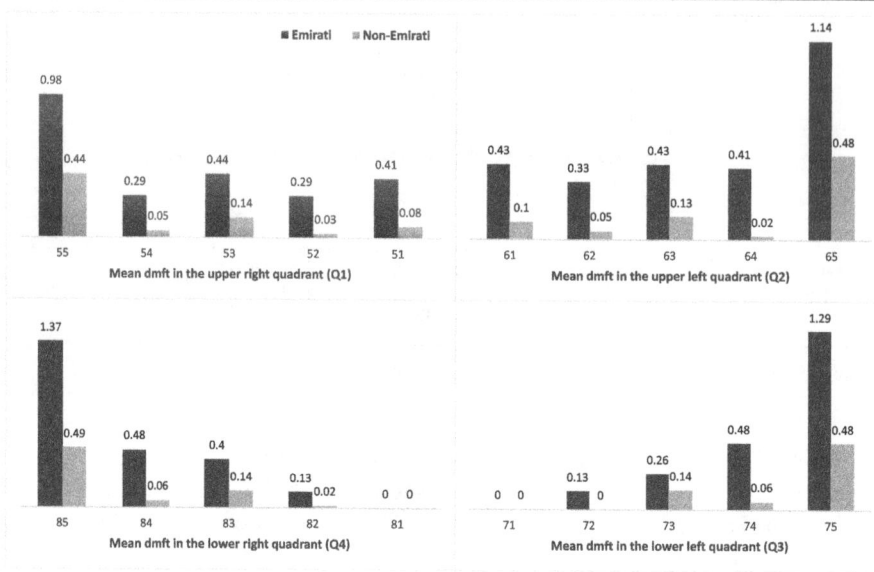

Fig. 2 The distribution of the dmft in the four dental quadrants among nursery children

caries [6, 7, 10, 17–20, 28]. The SIC was calculated for one third of the population with the highest caries scores to focus on the group with the most severe caries status [26]. The SIC was found to be almost three times as high as the mean dmft, and while it is always higher, the large difference between the two indices is concerning. A positive association between the dmft index and PI was also found, which is consistent with some studies, whereas others did not find such an association [29, 30].

Culture influences norms of oral health practices, recognition of illness and health care-seeking practices [31]. Although Gulf Cooperation Council countries, including the UAE, have undergone economic transition, it has been suggested that these countries still share some aspects of developing countries such as poor health profiles and low

health literacy rates [32]. While caries were found in both nationality groups, all indices (dmft, SIC and PI) in the univariate analyses were significantly higher in Emirati children, as was the consumption of high-sugar food items. Although high sugar intake has been associated with caries in many other studies, it is startling to find a strong association at such a young age, confirming a habit of frequent intake of discretionary calories [33, 34]. One could hypothesize that these findings could be attributed to sociocultural factors, as Emirati families seem to share a practice of frequently including high-sugar food items in their children's diet. Prediction models exploring specific determinants of dental caries, and potential confounders are essential to fully understand the etiology of dental caries in this population.

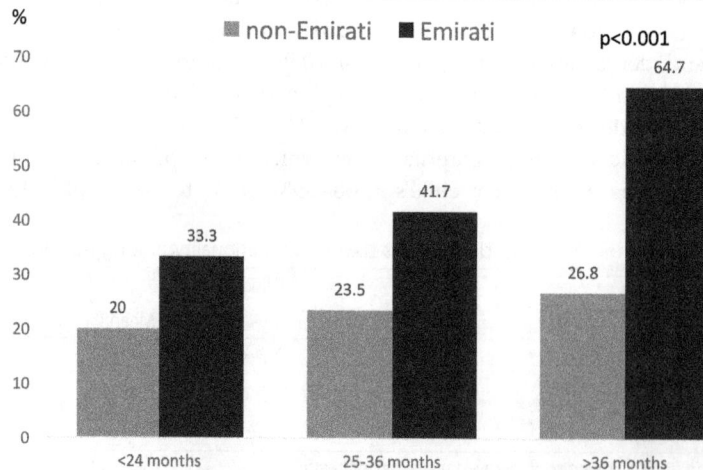

Fig. 3 Dental prevalence caries in nursery children divided by age-group and nationality

Table 2 Association between Significant Caries Index (SIC) and sample variables among nursery children

	SIC			x^2	P-value
	n	%	Mean dmft (SD)		
Nationality				17.29	0.000
Emirati	32	50.8	5.0 (3.0)		
Non-Emirati	10	15.9	4.1 (3.0)		
Gender				2.069	0.15
Boys	32	38.6	4.7 (2.5)		
Girls	15	24.8	5.1 (3.7)		
Nursery				21.677	0.000
Urban	6	12	3.2 (1.2)		
Suburban	19	36.5	4.9 (3.3)		
Rural	22	59.5	5.1 (2.9)		
Age group				3.59	0.166
18–24 months	2	25	3.5 (0.7)		
25–36 months	9	21.4	4.7 (3.6)		
> 36 months	32	37.6	4.9 (3.0)		

Abbreviations: SIC Significant Caries Index, *dmft* decayed, missing and filled teeth index, *SD* standard deviation

Dental status was also related to the level of urbanization and the age of the participants. Children in rural area experienced more caries and had more visible plaque than children in other geographical locations, which is consistent with studies conducted elsewhere [35, 36]. Dental caries were found in children below the age of 2, comparable to studies in Nigeria and Thailand that reported caries in children as young as 12 months of age [37, 38]. In this study, the dmft increased with age

indicating the cumulative effect consistent with findings in other studies [39]. The rate of caries in non-Emirati children increased from 20% in children below 2 years of age to 26.8% in children above 3 years of age and the rate of caries in Emirati children almost doubled from 33.3 to 64.7% in the corresponding age groups.

A substantial body of literature has documented an inverse association between socioeconomic status and the of dental caries [14, 29, 40, 41]. Analysis of socioeconomic variables in this study revealed that the mother's level of education was strongly associated with dental caries. However, this inverse association between education level and dental caries was not observed in relation to the father's education, suggesting the importance of improving health education primarily in mothers [14, 40]. Consistent with previous reports from the region, a toothbrush was the most common brushing aid among children [42, 43]. Tooth-brushing is considered a relatively affordable method of reducing the risk of dental caries mainly via the exposure to fluoride from toothpaste concurrently with mechanical cleansing [44]. In other studies, brushing at least twice daily has been associated with reduced caries occurrence, a finding that could not be confirmed in this study [45]. Despite the fact that oral health services are free for the Emirati population and health insurance is compulsory for non-Emiratis, the utilization of dental services was relatively low in both groups, consistent with other studies conducted in the region [43]. Thus further studies need to focus on understanding how the utilization of dental services can be improved.

This study was conducted in nurseries, i.e., an educational setting under field conditions, which may have strengthened the study design because it is well

Table 3 Associations between dental caries and univariate socioeconomic variables among nursery children in Abu Dhabi. N = 147

Independent variable	Groups	%	Mean dmft (SD)	P-value[a]	Mean SIC (SD)	P-value[b]
Father's education level	High school or below	12.6	2.9 (3.6)	0.062	5.3 (3.3)	0.065
	University degree	87.4	1.2 (2.5)		4.6 (3.2)	
Mother's education level	High school or below	20.8	3.2 (3.7)	0.000	5.4 (3.40)	0.001
	University degree	79.2	0.9 (2.2)		4.5 (3.0)	
Self-rated financial status	Lower middle income	2.2	2.5 (3.5)		5.0 (–)	0.775
	Middle income	62.6	1.6 (3.0)	0.651	5.4 (0.6)	
	Higher middle income	33.8	1.1 (2.1)		3.9 (2.2)	
	Wealthy	1.4	–		–	
Parents' perception of their child's dental status	Very good	41.5	1.0 (1.8)	0.000	3.9 (2.10)	0.000
	Satisfactory	51.0	1.1 (2.3)		4.5 (2.9)	
	Dissatisfactory	6.8	6.9 (4.1)		6.9 (4.1)	
	Very dissatisfactory	0.7	–		0 (0)	

Abbreviations: dmft decayed, missing and filled teeth index, *SIC* significant caries index, *SD* standard deviation
[a]The significance of the dmft scores as measured by the Mann-Whitney U test or Kruskal-Wallis test as appropriate
[b]the significance of SIC scores as measured by Pearson chi-square or Fisher's exact tests as appropriate

Table 4 Consumption of high-sugar food items based on the FFQ divided by nationality

Food category	Emirati children (N = 58)			Non-Emirati children (N = 89)			P-value
	> 6 times/w (%)	1–5 times/w (%)	< 1 time/w (%)	> 6 times/w (%)	1–5 times/w (%)	< 1 time/w (%)	χ^2 2 df
Flavored milk	31.6	42.1	26.3	14.3	21.4	64.3	0.000
Muffins/donuts or similar	25.9	65.5	8.6	9.3	43.0	47.7	0.000
Biscuits/cookies and similar	25.9	58.6	15.5	19.8	54.7	25.6	0.316
Juices	67.3	29.1	3.6	36.8	46.0	17.2	0.001
Syrups/fruit punches/fruit squash	10.5	28.1	61.4	2.4	8.3	89.3	0.000
Soft drinks	3.7	25.9	70.4	1.2	7.1	91.7	0.005
Ice cream	7.1	48.2	44.6	1.1	49.4	49.4	0.159
Chocolates	33.9	51.8	14.3	1.2	62.8	36.0	0.000
Candy/sweets (not chocolates)	23.2	51.8	25.0	4.7	32.6	62.8	0.000

Abbreviations: FFQ Food Frequency Questionnaire

recognized that hospital-based studies have higher selection bias and subjects are less representative of the general population [46]. Furthermore, the stratified sampling allowed the inclusion of children from areas of differing degrees of urbanization. However, there are some limitation to studies conducted in educational institutes. Unless preschool education is mandatory such studies have no access to subjects who do not attend nurseries. As preschool education is not mandatory in the UAE, the study results cannot be generalized to this segment of the population. As recommended by other researchers, efforts were made to maximize the participation rate by receiving the full support of the nursery administration, the dissemination of electronic and printed invitations, including bilingual investigators and establishing face-to-face contact with parents during regular drop off/pickup times [47]. Repeated visits to the nurseries was also a strategy used to optimize participation. An unexpected challenge related to recruitment was the difficulty accessing parents, unlike what has been reported in other child health studies [47]. In most cultures, parents drop off and pick up their children from nurseries. However, in the UAE, a culture of bringing the children to nurseries by household helpers (e.g., maids and drivers) or by bus was found to be a major limiting factor in accessing large numbers of families, hence the sample size was impacted and a variation in the participation rate was found, as shown in the loss analysis. Accordingly, the sample size can be considered a limitation of this study, suggesting that the results need to be interpreted with caution. The lack of mandatory dental checkups in this age group poses a challenge for accessing large, unbiased groups of children. An alternative strategy could be to recruit children through household visits, which would not necessarily be more efficient for recruitment as it is labor-intensive and costly.

Conclusions

In conclusion, 4 out of 10 nursery children in this study with a mean age of 2.46 years had dental caries. Lower maternal education, rural nursery location, infrequent tooth-brushing, Emirati nationality and frequent consumption of high-sugar food items were all factors associated with dental caries. The findings that Emirati children consumed significantly more sugar compared to non-Emirati children and had more dental caries may imply the need for targeted interventions. The findings of this study need to be supported by longitudinal, population-based studies. Health education for parents of young children should be considered to improve eating habits. In addition, introducing mandatory dental checkups, starting in toddlers, could be a proactive strategy to screen, prevent and intervene early.

Abbreviations

CI: Confidence interval; dmft: Decayed, missing and filled teeth index; dt: Decayed teeth; FFQ: Food frequency questionnaire; ft.: Filled teeth; mt: Missing teeth; SD: standard deviation; SIC: Significant caries index; UAE: United Arab Emirates

Acknowledgements

We would like to thank The Ministry of Social Affairs, Abu Dhabi and the nurseries' management and staff for supporting the NOPLAS project. Furthermore, we would like to acknowledge the children and their parents for participating. We would also like to thank Noor Al-Edawi for conducting the dental examinations and Farah, Nahed, Shajiya, Dhuha, Shaima, Maitha and Edward for their support in data collection and data entry. Finally, we would like to thank Zayed University for the financial support.

Funding

This research project (titled NOPLAS: Nutrition, Oral Health, Physical Development, Lifestyle, Anthropometric and Socioeconomic Status of Preschool Children in Abu Dhabi) received funding from the Research Incentive Fund (R16055) at Zayed University, UAE. The funding body had no role in the design of the study and collection, analysis, and interpretation of data and in writing the manuscript.

Authors' contributions

AE and MG contributed to the design of the study, data collection, data analysis and writing of the manuscript. AG contributed to the data analysis and writing of the manuscript. All the authors read and approved the final manuscript.

Competing interests

The authors declare that they have no competing interests.

Author details

[1]Department of Health Sciences, College of Natural and Health Sciences, Zayed University, P.O. Box 144534, Abu-Dhabi, United Arab Emirates. [2]School of Molecular Sciences, University of Western Australia, Crawley, Perth, WA 6009, Australia.

References

1. Selwitz RH, Ismail AI, Pitts NB. Dental caries. Lancet. 2007;369:51–9.
2. Edelstein BL. The dental caries pandemic and disparities problem. BMC Oral Health. 2006;6(Suppl 1):S2.
3. Petersen PE, Bourgeois D, Ogawa H, Estupinan-Day S, Ndiaye C. The global burden of oral diseases and risks to oral health. Bull World Health Organ. 2005;83:661–9.
4. Li Y, Wang W. Predicting caries in permanent teeth from caries in primary teeth: an eight-year cohort study. J Dent Res. 2002;81:561–6.
5. Vadiakas G. Case definition, aetiology and risk assessment of early childhood caries (ECC): a revisited review. Eur Arch Paediatr Dent. 2008;9:114–25.
6. Kowash MB. Severity of early childhood caries in preschool children attending Al-Ain dental Centre, United Arab Emirates. Eur Arch Paediatr Dent. 2015;16:319–24.
7. Kowash MB, Alkhabuli JO, Dafaalla SA, Shah A, Khamis AH. Early childhood caries and associated risk factors among preschool children in Ras Al-Khaimah, United Arab Emirates. Eur Arch Paediatr Dent. 2017;18:97–103.
8. Hong CH, Bagramian RA, Hashim Nainar SM, Straffon LH, Shen L, Hsu CY. High caries prevalence and risk factors among young preschool children in an urban community with water fluoridation. Int J Paediatr Dent. 2014;24:32–42.
9. Elidrissi SM, Naidoo S. Prevalence of dental caries and toothbrushing habits among preschool children in Khartoum state, Sudan. Int Dent J. 2016;66:215–20.
10. Chedid NR, Bourgeois D, Kaloustian H, Baba NZ, Pilipili C. Caries prevalence and caries risk in a sample of Lebanese preschool children. Odontostomatol Trop. 2011;34:31–45.
11. Farsi N, Merdad L, Mirdad S. Caries risk assessment in preschool children in Saudi Arabia. Oral Health Prev Dent. 2013;11:271–80.
12. Sankeshwari RM, Ankola AV, Tangade PS, Hebbal MI. Association of socio-economic status and dietary habits with early childhood caries among 3- to 5-year-old children of Belgaum city. Eur Arch Paediatr Dent. 2013;14:147–53.
13. Congiu G, Campus G, Luglie PF. Early childhood caries (ECC) prevalence and background factors: a review. Oral health Prev Dent. 2014;12:71–6.
14. Tanaka K, Miyake Y, Sasaki S, Hirota Y. Socioeconomic status and risk of dental caries in Japanese preschool children: the Osaka maternal and child health study. J Public Health Dent. 2013;73:217–23.
15. Hooley M, Skouteris H, Boganin C, Satur J, Kilpatrick N. Parental influence and the development of dental caries in children aged 0-6 years: a systematic review of the literature. J Dent. 2012;40:873–85.
16. Anil S, Anand PS. Early childhood caries: prevalence, risk factors, and prevention. Front Pediatr. 2017;5:157.
17. El-Nadeef MA, Hassab H, Al-Hosani E. National survey of the oral health of 5-year-old children in the United Arab Emirates. East Mediterr Health J. 2010;16:51–5.
18. Alkhtib A, Ghanim A, Temple-Smith M, Messer LB, Pirotta M, Morgan M. Prevalence of early childhood caries and enamel defects in four and five-year old Qatari preschool children. BMC Oral Health. 2016;16:73.
19. Al-Mutawa SA, Shyama M, Al-Duwairi Y, Soparkar P. Dental caries experience of Kuwaiti kindergarten schoolchildren. Community Dent Health. 2010;27:213–7.
20. Qadri G, Nourallah A, Splieth CH. Early childhood caries and feeding practices in kindergarten children. Quintessence Int. 2012;43:503–10.
21. Al-Hosani E, Rugg-Gunn A. Combination of low parental educational attainment and high parental income related to high caries experience in pre-school children in Abu Dhabi. Community Dent Oral Epidemiol. 1998;26:31–6.
22. Cleaton-Jones P, Hargreaves JA, Fatti LP, Chandler HD, Grossman ES. Dental caries diagnosis calibration for clinical field surveys. Caries Res. 1989;23:195–9.
23. Bolin AK, Bolin A, Koch G. Children's dental health in Europe: caries experience of 5- and 12-year-old children from eight EU countries. Int J Paediatr Dent. 1996;6:155–62.
24. World Health Organization. Oral health survey: basic methods. 5th ed. Geneva: World Health Organization; 2013.
25. Loe H. The gingival index, the plaque index and the retention index systems. J Periodontol. 1967;38(Suppl):610–6.
26. Bratthall D. Introducing the significant caries index together with a proposal for a new global oral health goal for 12-year-olds. Int Dent J. 2000;50:378–84.
27. Bagramian RA, Garcia-Godoy F, Volpe AR. The global increase in dental caries. A pending public health crisis. Am J Dent. 2009;22:3–8.
28. Dashash M, Blinkhorn A. The dental health of 5 year-old children living in Damascus, Syria. Community Dent Health. 2012;29:209–13.
29. King NM, Wu II, Tsai JS. Caries prevalence and distribution, and oral health habits of zero- to four-year-old children in Macau, China. J Dent Child (Chic). 2003;70:243–9.
30. Oliveira LB, Sheiham A, Bonecker M. Exploring the association of dental caries with social factors and nutritional status in Brazilian preschool children. Eur J Oral Sci. 2008;116:37–43.
31. Kelesidis N. A racial comparison of sociocultural factors and oral health perceptions. J Dent Hyg. 2014;88:173–82.
32. Alkhamis A, Hassan A, Cosgrove P. Financing healthcare in Gulf cooperation council countries: a focus on Saudi Arabia. Int J Health Plann Manag. 2014; 29:e64–82.
33. Colak H, Dulgergil CT, Dalli M, Hamidi MM. Early childhood caries update: a review of causes, diagnoses, and treatments. J Nat Sci Biol Med. 2013;4:29–38.
34. Zukanovic A. Caries risk assessment models in caries prediction. Acta Med Acad. 2013;42:198–208.
35. Smith L, Blinkhorn A, Moir R, Brown N, Blinkhorn F. An assessment of dental caries among young aboriginal children in new South Wales, Australia: a cross-sectional study. BMC Public Health. 2015;15:1314.
36. Kaminska A, Szalewski L, Batkowska J, Wallner J, Wallner E, Szabelska A, Borowicz J. The dependence of dental caries on oral hygiene habits in preschool children from urban and rural areas in Poland. Ann Agric Environ Med. 2016;23:660–5.
37. Vachirarojpisan T, Shinada K, Kawaguchi Y, Laungwechakan P, Somkote T, Detsomboonrat P. Early childhood caries in children aged 6-19 months. Community Dent Oral Epidemiol. 2004;32:133–42.
38. World Health Organization. WHO Expert Consultation on Public Health Intervention against Early Childhood Caries: report of a meeting, Bangkok, Thailand 26–28 January 2016. Geneva: World Health Organization; 2017. (WHO/NMH/PND/17.1)
39. Mwakayoka H, Masalu JR, Namakuka Kikwilu E. Dental Caries and Associated Factors in Children Aged 2–4 Years Old in Mbeya City, Tanzania. J Dent (Shiraz). 2017;18:104–11.
40. Al-Meedani LA, Al-Dlaigan YH. Prevalence of dental caries and associated social risk factors among preschool children in Riyadh, Saudi. Pak J Med Sci. 2016;32:452–6.
41. Sayegh A, Dini EL, Holt RD, Bedi R. Oral health, sociodemographic factors, dietary and oral hygiene practices in Jordanian children. J Dent. 2005;33:379–88.
42. Al-Darwish MS. Oral health knowledge, behaviour and practices among school children in Qatar. Dent Res J (Isfahan). 2016;13:342–53.
43. Al-Ansari JM, Al-Jairan LY, Gillespie GM. Dietary habits of the primary to secondary school population and implications for oral health. J Allied Health. 2006;35:75–80.
44. Polk DE, Geng M, Levy S, Koerber A, Flay BR. Frequency of daily tooth brushing: predictors of change in 9- to 11-year old US children. Community Dent Health. 2014;31:136–40.
45. Gibson S, Williams S. Dental caries in pre-school children: associations with social class, toothbrushing habit and consumption of sugars and sugar-containing foods. Further analysis of data from the National Diet and nutrition survey of children aged 1.5-4.5 years. Caries Res. 1999;33:101–13.
46. Ness KK, Leisenring W, Goodman P, Kawashima T, Mertens AC, Oeffinger KC, Armstrong GT, Robison LL. Assessment of selection bias in clinic-based populations of childhood cancer survivors: a report from the childhood cancer survivor study. Pediatr Blood Cancer. 2009;52:379–86.
47. Claudio L, Stingone JA. Improving sampling and response rates in children's health research through participatory methods. J Sch Health. 2008;78:445–51.

5

Shaping ability of protaper next compared with waveone in late-model three-dimensional printed teeth

Zhi Cui[1], Zhao Wei[2], Minquan Du[3], Ping Yan[1*] and Han Jiang[1*]

Abstract

Background: Comparison of the shaping ability of advanced nickel-titanium (Ni-Ti) instruments is of great interest to the field of endodontics. However, the models used to study canal preparation still lack uniformity, relevance to reality and complexity. The aim of this study was thus to compare the shaping abilities of the ProTaper Next (PN) and WaveOne (WO) Ni-Ti instruments in three-dimensional (3D)-printed teeth, which may overcome the present defects of most real teeth and model teeth including 3D S-shaped canals.

Methods: Six teeth and their corresponding 3D-printed replicas were prepared using the same kind of Ni-Ti instrument. The pre- and post-preparation volumes, surface areas and transportation of the canals were measured to compare the teeth with their replicas. Twenty 3D-printed teeth with S-shaped canals were used to support the preparation study. The S-shaped canals were then scanned to measure their volumes and surface areas. Next, the two kinds of instruments were used to prepare the 3D-printed canals ($n = 10$ per group). The volume and surface area of the canals, the transportation along the two curvatures and the percentage of unprepared surface area were measured. Micro-CT and VGstudio2.2 (VG2.2) software were used to perform scans and collect data throughout the research. The paired-samples T test and Kruskal-Wallis H test were used for statistical analysis.

Results: There was no significant difference between the real canals and the printed ones post-preparation ($P > .05$). The printed S-shaped root canals had a unified shape, with a small standard deviation and range. The WO group had higher mean values for the volume and superficial area measurements compared with the PN group ($P < .05$). No differences in the untouched areas were found between the two systems ($P > .05$). PN caused less transportation at the apical curve than WO did ($P < .05$).

Conclusions: In conclusion, 3D-printed teeth are suitable for the study of Ni-Ti rotary instruments. Furthermore, the PN rotary system caused less transportation at the apical curve than the WO system did in complicated root canal procedures.

Keywords: Printed resin teeth, Three-dimensional S-shaped root canal, ProTaper next, WaveOne, Micro-computed tomography imaging

* Correspondence: WB000275@whu.edu.cn; jianghan@whu.edu.cn
[1]The State Key Laboratory Breeding Base of Basic Science of Stomatology (Hubei-MOST) & Key Laboratory of Oral Biomedicine Ministry of Education, School & Hospital of Stomatology, Wuhan University, Luoyu Road, Wuhan City 237, China
Full list of author information is available at the end of the article

Background

Shaping and cleaning root canals are essential parts of endodontic chemo-mechanical disinfection. Many experiments have focused on comparing the shaping abilities of nickel-titanium (Ni-Ti) instruments in extracted teeth and simulated root canals [1]. However, use of the former teeth cannot ensure uniformity [2], and the latter lack relevance to reality as well as complex morphology [3].

Three-dimensional (3D) printing is a novel technology that can change manufacturing methods. Combined with stomatological approaches, various appliances have been 3D-printed in the dental field, such as drill guides for dental implants; physical models for prosthodontics, orthodontics and surgery; and craniomaxillofacial and orthopaedic implants [4]. In a recent study, 3D-printed teeth were also introduced into preparation research [5, 6].

The ProTaper Next (PN; Dentsply Maillefer, Ballaigues, Switzerland) and WaveOne (WO; Dentsply Maillefer) systems are based on innovative metallurgy in which manufacturers introduce M-Wire alloy to improve the fatigue life and flexibility of the files. ProTaper Next is the successor of ProTaper Universal and has superior torque and speed. The off-centred rectangular cross-section gives the file a snake-like "swaggering" movement [7], which can generate an enlarged space for debris removal. WO is a single-file system, and combined with the balanced force technique, the file can turn a shorter angular distance. This motion reduces the file stress and plastic deformation [8].

Although these Ni-Ti instruments are advanced and popular in clinical treatment, few studies have researched which file system is more suitable for the treatment of complex root canals. In the present study, the shaping abilities of PN and WO were compared in 3D-printed teeth which contained unified 3D S-shaped root canals. The null hypothesis was that there would be no difference between the two Ni-Ti instruments in terms of the analysed parameters.

Methods

Selection and characterization of teeth

Extracted permanent molars and maxillary premolars with mature apices and no previous root canal therapy were selected from a pool of extracted teeth. Radiographic images of each tooth were acquired in the buccolingual and mesiodistal orientations. Based on the results, three maxillary first premolars and three mandibular first molars, with two narrow root canals (30–40°), were selected for the analysis [9]. Micro-CT (Scanco Medical, Bassersdorf, Switzerland), which outputs images in TIFF format and has a resolution of 30 μm, was used to scan these teeth. VGstudio Max version 2.2 (VG2.2) software (Volume Graphics, Heidelberg, Germany) was then used to manage the TIFF images into a 3D construction and to output data in STL format.

Resin tooth creation using 3D printing technology

The machine, ProJet 3500 HDMax (3D Systems, South Carolina, America), used for 3D printing has a precision of 16 μm and can be used with two materials [4]. The printer use UV-curable plastic, VisiJet M3 Crystal (3D Systems, South Carolina, America), and support material, VisiJet S300 (3D Systems, South Carolina, America), which allow for hands-free, melt-away removal without damaging the delicate structures. Every tooth was created in duplicate, such that there were six experimental pairs, including twelve pairs of root canals.

Root canal instruments

Both of the real and duplicate tooth were instrumented using a new suite of PN with permanent rotation at 300 rpm and 3 Ncm. All instruments were operated with an X-Smart Plus endodontic motor (Dentsply Maillefer). A #10 K-file (Dentsply Maillefer) was used to dredge the root canals and measure the working length, which was defined as 1 mm shorter than the distance from the reference plane to the point where the file tip was visible under the visual field of a microscope (Leica M320 F12, Germany). The PN X1 (size 17, .04 taper) and, X2 (size 25, .06 taper) were selected as the appropriate files because of the size of the root canals. The preparation processes were as follows:

1. X1 was moved in the apical direction using a 33 mm mm in-and-out motion and with light apical pressure. Sufficient irrigation was conducted after three or four motions. This process was repeated until the working length was completed.
2. X2 was used to complete the work using the same method.

Micro-CT scanning and VG2.2 analysis

The VG2.2 was used to calculate the volume and surface area of each root canal by measuring the region of interest. Before preparation, the printed teeth were scanned by micro-CT, and the surface area and volume were measured using VG2.2. The post-preparation parameters were then determined using the same method. VG2.2 could overlap pre- and post-preparation samples through the best-matching function and determine the geometric centres by measuring the points on the border of the sections automatically. The transportation value of the canals was defined as the distance between the approximate centres of the fixed sections of the pre- and post-preparation root canals [10]. A dipstick was then used to help to measure the transportation at four sections, respectively located 1 mm, 3 mm, 5 mm, and 9 mm from the apex.

Comparing shaping abilities of Ni-Ti instruments

A mandibular first molar was chosen to conform to antecedent methods and standards. This tooth had a complex distal root canal that contained two curves with different dimensions and positions. Utilizing the model tooth, twenty resin teeth were printed and used to measure the volume and surface area. The replicas were then separated into two groups ($n = 10$). The resin teeth in the PN group were prepared as previously described. The WO group was instrumented using a reciprocating working motion of 170° counterclockwise and 50° clockwise with a primary file (size 25, 0.08 taper). All the preparation operations were completed by a sole endodontist who was experienced in these techniques and who had been sufficiently trained using both true and printed teeth. Every resin tooth had its own suit of instruments. The preparation process for the WO system was as follows:

1. A single file was used to approximately shape the coronal two-thirds of the canal length with a progressive up-and-down movement with no more than three or four repetitions.
2. The canal was irrigated with copious distilled water.
3. The file was applied to the whole length using the same process. During the process, only a small amount of force was required.

The transportation and the proportion of the unshaped surface area were detected in the two curves of the S-shaped canal (the cervical half and the apical half). The un-instrumented surface area was measured by counting the number of static voxels in the non-overlapping area [11]. All of the results were obtained using VG2.2.

Statistical analysis

The statistical analysis was performed with SPSS (IBM SPSS Statistics 21; SPSS Inc., Chicago, IL). The different parameters of the twelve pairs of root canals were analysed using the paired-samples T test or the Wilcoxon signed-rank test. The uniformity of the twenty printed canals was then assessed based on the standard deviation, maximum and minimum. Other multiple comparisons of the shaping abilities of the two instrument groups were analysed using the independent-samples T test or the Mann-Whitney U test. The statistical significance level was set at $P < .05$.

Results

Comparison of real root canals and 3D-printed canals

Figure 1 shows one pair of the six pairs of real teeth and their 3D-printed counterparts. Before preparation, the volume and surface area of the real canals were not

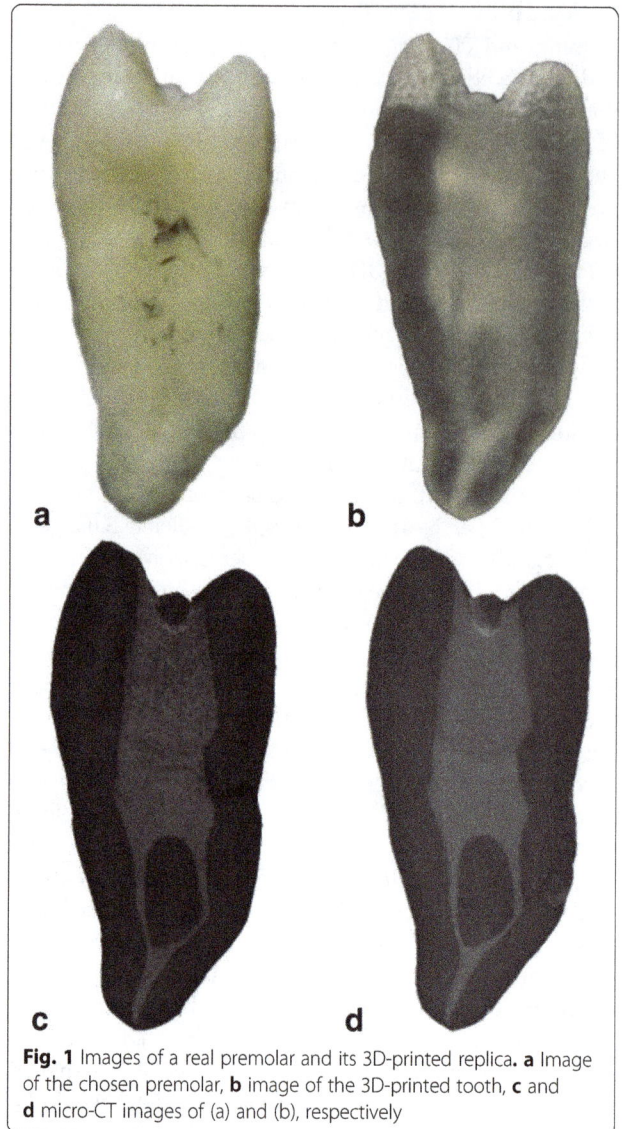

Fig. 1 Images of a real premolar and its 3D-printed replica. **a** Image of the chosen premolar, **b** image of the 3D-printed tooth, **c** and **d** micro-CT images of (a) and (b), respectively

significantly different from those of the printed canals ($P > .05$) (Table 1). In addition, similarly, after preparation, the volumes and surface areas of the true canals and duplicates were not significantly different ($P > .05$) (Table 1). There was no significant difference in the transportation of the real root canals and the duplicate canals in any of the four sections ($P > .05$) (Table 2). Overlapping images of the root canals of the chosen pair of teeth are shown in Fig. 2.

Twenty 3D-printed root canals

Different views of the construction of the S-shaped root canal can be seen in Fig. 3. The mean volume of the original simulated root canals was $1.92 \pm .03$ mm^3, with a minimum value of 1.87 mm^3 and a maximum value of 1.95 mm^3. The mean surface area of the pre-prepared root canals was $19.00 \pm .13$ mm^2. Here, 19.26 mm^2 and

Table 1 Volumes and surface areas of real and 3D-printed canals pre- and post-preparation ($n = 12$)

Group	Volume before preparation (mm³)	Volume after preparation (mm³)	Surface area before preparation (mm²)	Surface area after preparation (mm²)
	Mean ± SD	Mean ± SD	Mean ± SD	Mean ± SD
Real teeth	2.82 ± .74	2.94 ± .75	19.61 ± 3.65	20.51 ± 3.58
3D-printed teeth	2.78 ± .73	2.97 ± .77	19.57 ± 3.60	20.59 ± 3.24
P value	.289[b]	.064[a]	.387[b]	.494[a]

[a]Paired-samples T test ($P < .05$)
[b]Wilcoxon signed-rank test ($P < .05$)

18.81 mm² were the minimum and maximum values, respectively.

Volume and surface area in two groups
The volume and surface area values in the WO group were greater than the values in the PN group ($P < .05$) (Table 3).

Percentage of unshaped area in two groups
Based on the data shown in Table 4, both groups had remaining unshaped areas in the apical and coronal halves. Notably, there was more untouched area in the coronal half compared with the apical half. However, for the untouched proportion of the two halves of the canals, there was no difference between the groups ($P > .05$).

Transportation in two groups
The mean transportation in the PN group at the apical curve was less than that at the cervical curve. A similar result was obtained in the WO group (Table 5). WO caused more transportation at the apical curve than PN did ($P < .05$); however, there was no difference between the two groups at the cervical curve ($P > .05$).

Discussion
The use of 3D-printed teeth in this type of comparative study, which assessed the shaping abilities of two Ni-Ti instrument systems, is a novel application of this powerful technology. In previous studies, researchers used extracted teeth to more accurately simulate clinical conditions [7, 10, 12–18]. However, real teeth have unique root canal systems, interfering with the uniformity of experiments [19]. Collection of the appropriate

Table 2 Transportation in four sections of real and printed canals after preparation ($n = 12$)

Group	1 mm from apex (mm)	3 mm from apex (mm)	5 mm from apex (mm)	9 mm from apex (mm)
	Mean ± SD	Mean ± SD	Mean ± SD	Mean ± SD
Real teeth	.047 ± .037	.053 ± .042	.052 ± .052	.013 ± .014
3D-printed teeth	.053 ± .042	.06 ± .053	.056 ± .056	.014 ± .016
P value	.084[b]	.058[b]		.655[b]

[b]Wilcoxon signed-rank test ($P < .05$)

human teeth for in vitro examination and measurement of the curvature parameters for classification also make the experiments much more complicated. Other studies have used resin blocks [4, 20–25], but the physical properties of resin include greater hardness than for dentin [26]. Additionally, the simulated constructions do not reflect the diversity of real root canal morphology [27]. The frequency of instrument failure and the duration of the procedure using such simulated teeth are also not generalizable to clinical situations [28].

In the present study, duplicate teeth were successfully 3D printed based on scanning and digital reconstruction. No differences were found in the post-preparation volume, surface area or transportation between the 3D-printed teeth and the real teeth. This finding suggests that 3D-printed teeth could be suitable for comparing the shaping abilities of different Ni-Ti instruments. One of the advantages of 3D-printed teeth is that they can provide the uniformity and relevance to reality. Thus, the data from this research may be applicable to real-life clinical operations. The volumes of the true canals and duplicates were not significantly different after the preparation, however, the p-value ($p = 0.064$) is close to the significativity. The posibility is that the material of printed tooth need more similar of physical properties and bio-performances with natural dentin.

Earlier studies on the morphology of root canals have indicated that nearly all canals have two curvatures [29]. Other studies have demonstrated that an S-shaped root canal increases the difficulty of preparation and the risk of instrument fracture [20]. Compared with previous experimental root canals with single [7, 12, 15–18, 23, 30] or two-dimensional S-shaped [20, 21, 23, 24, 26] curvatures, printed teeth with a stereo S-shaped root canal can simulate the clinical conditions and challenges of preparing such a canal. With the progress of 3D printing technology, our hope is that computer design technology will be able to adjust the degree, radius, location and other shape details of curvatures to satisfy different study criteria.

Utilizing 3D-printed teeth, the shaping abilities of two NiTi instruments were compared. In contrast to the results of earlier research with extracted teeth [12, 13], the WO primary file removed more dentin and yielded a

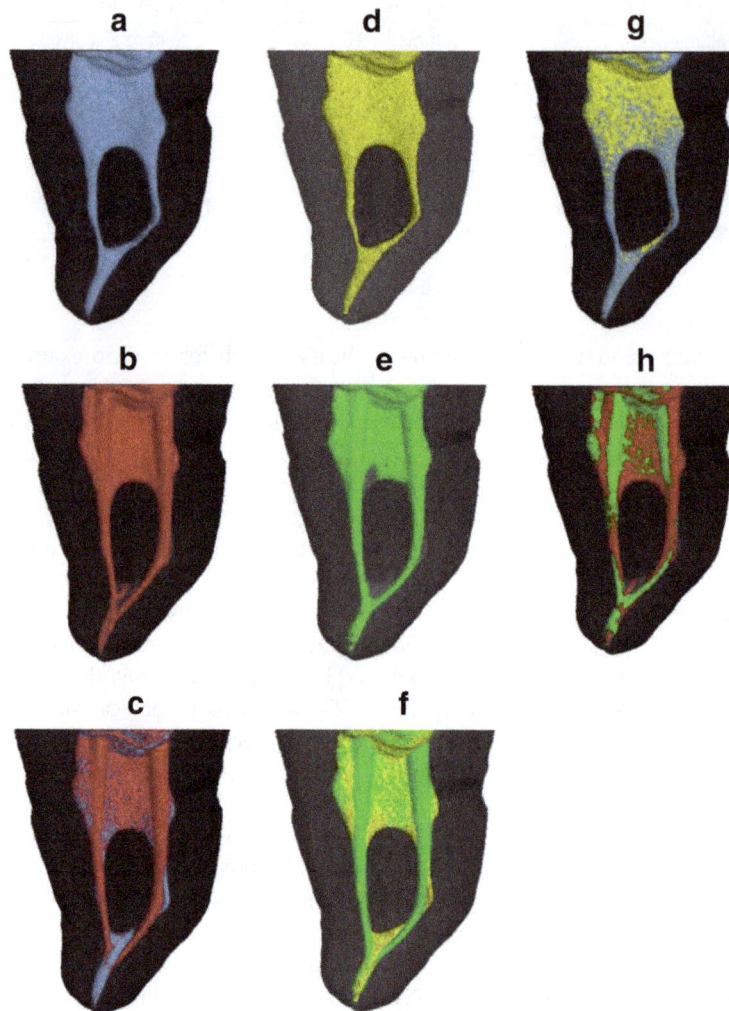

Fig. 2 Images comparing the original premolar to a 3D-printed replica tooth. (**a**) (**b**) (**c**) Images of the root canal of a premolar, showing the pre-preparation canals in blue and the post-preparation areas in red. (**c**) The untouched areas are presented after overlapping (**a**) and (**b**). Pre-preparation, post-preparation and overlapping root canal images for the 3D-printed tooth are shown in yellow (**d**), green (**e**), and (**f**), respectively. (**g**) and (**h**) show overlapping canal images for the real premolar and the 3D-printed tooth before and after preparation, respectively

larger post-preparation surface area than the PN X2 did. In previous studies, although the degree and radius of the original curvature of true teeth were considered when allocating the teeth into groups, the volume and surface area of the canals were not sufficient to differentiate the teeth. Differences in canal morphology may affect canal preparation, and positive results may be influenced by discrepancies between canal shapes [31, 32]. The two indexes thus cannot be measured in resin blocks using a two-dimensional method.

In the current study, both groups exhibited a greater unshaped area in the cervical curvature region than in the apical region. This result was similar to that of a study by Cabanilas using WO and other instruments [33]. The finding may be due to the fact that the root canals had a capacious oval part in the coronal half and a conspicuous constriction in the apical half. This consideration implies that the selection of the appropriate primary file should be based on the integral root shape of the tooth in question. The remaining smear layers require sufficient chemical irrigation [34].

Both instrument groups cause more transportation in the coronal curves and less in the apical ones. This finding is corroborated by the results of previous experiments [14, 15, 21], which revealed a decreased tendency towards transportation from the cervical part to the apical part. The reason for this result may be that a longer diameter for the file predisposes it to resist deformation forces and straighten the coronal part. We observed the same phenomenon as that described in the results of Zhao's study [12]: the WO system produced more transportation at the apical curvature than the PN system

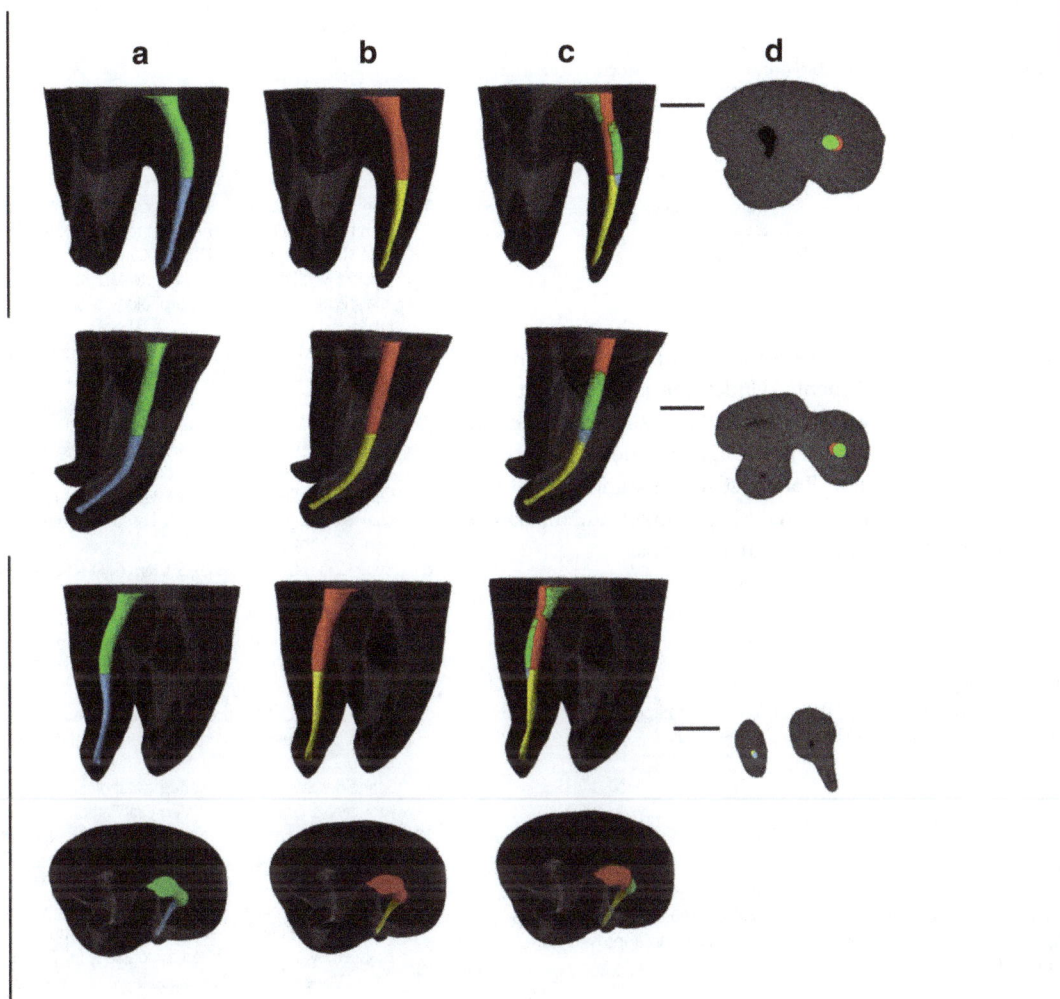

Fig. 3 The different directions of the overlapping images of the S-shaped root canals. The coronal curvatures of the pre- and post-preparation canals are shown in green and red, respectively. The pre- and post-preparation apical regions are shown in blue and yellow, respectively. Column **a** shows images of the prepared root canals, and images of the post-preparation canals are shown in column **b**. In column **c**, the untouched areas are presented after overlapping the images in the **a** and **b** columns. Finally, column **d** shows the sections of the overlapping canals

did. The PN X1 (size 17, 0.04 taper) plays a key role in the preliminary enlargement of the apical part of the canal, which reduces the degree of curvature and the pressure on the main file [35]. For the WO system, the relatively larger taper of the primary file increases the degree of transportation [7, 36, 37]. However, Davut's study [13] indicated that the two instrument systems produce similar levels of transportation in the apical half of curved canals. The various software programs and methods that are used for measurement affect the accuracy of studies, and the transportation data vary considerably between the available published studies. The widely accepted measurement method should therefore be further discussed and researched.

Table 3 Volumes and surface areas of post-preparation simulated canals ($n = 10$)

Instrument	Volume (mm³)		Surface area (mm²)	
	Mean ± SD	Min-Max	Mean ± SD	Min-Max
ProTaper Next	3.21 ± .04	3.16–3.27	21.22 ± .77	20.24–22.70
WaveOne	3.37 ± .06	3.24–3.46	22.67 ± .61	21.89–23.63
P value	<.001[d]		<.001[c]	

[c]Independent-samples T test (P < .05)
[d]Mann-Whitney U test (P < .05)

Table 4 Percentages of unprepared areas in the apical and coronal halves of canals ($n = 10$)

Instrument	Unprepared apical area (%)		Unprepared coronal area (%)	
	Mean ± SD	Min-Max	Mean ± SD	Min-Max
ProTaper Next	11.03 ± .96	10.11–12.8	55.70 ± 1.25	53.26–57.19
WaveOne	12.06 ± 1.21	9.25–13.10	55.53 ± 1.01	53.48–57.24
P value	.683[c]		.684[c]	

[c]Independent-samples T test (P < .05)

Table 5 Transportation at the apical and coronal curvatures ($n = 10$)

Instrument	Apical curvature (mm)		Coronal curvature (mm)	
	Mean ± SD	Min-Max	Mean ± SD	Min-Max
ProTaper Next	0.14 ± .03 0.19	0.09–0.20	0.41 ± .04 0.43	0.37–0.50
WaveOne	±.05	0.11–0.27	±.06	0.35–0.50
P value	.014[c]		.404[c]	

[c]Independent-samples T test ($P < .05$)

Conclusions

Here, 3D-printed teeth were found to be suitable for the study of Ni-Ti instruments. Under the study conditions, the null hypothesis was rejected. PN had superior function in reducing transportation in the apical potion of the complex root canal system. Both instruments adhered to the original simulated root canal shape, however, unshaped areas still existed in the root canal systems.

Abbreviations
3D: three-dimensional; Ni-Ti: Nickel-titanium; PN: Protaper next; VG2.2: VGstudio2.2; WO: Waveone

Authors' contributions
Conceived and designed the experiments: PY, HJ. Performed the experiments: ZC, ZW. Analysed the data: HJ, ZC, MD, ZW. Wrote the paper: ZC, MD, PY, HJ. All authors of this study have read and approved our manuscript, and this is the case.

Author information
Zhi Cui, Ping Yan (corresponding author), Han Jiang (corresponding author): The State Key Laboratory Breeding Base of Basic Science of Stomatology (Hubei-MOST) & Key Laboratory of Oral Biomedicine Ministry of Education, School & Hospital of Stomatology, Wuhan University, Luoyu Road 237, Wuhan City, China. Zhao Wei: Department of Dentistry, Second Hospital of Baoding, 338 Dongfeng West Road, Baoding, China. Minquan Du: Department of Prevention, School and Hospital of Stomatology, Wuhan University, 237 Luoyu Road, Wuhan, China.

Competing interests
The authors declare that they have no competing interests.

Author details
[1]The State Key Laboratory Breeding Base of Basic Science of Stomatology (Hubei-MOST) & Key Laboratory of Oral Biomedicine Ministry of Education, School & Hospital of Stomatology, Wuhan University, Luoyu Road, Wuhan City 237, China. [2]Department of Dentistry, Second Hospital of Baoding, 338 Dongfeng West Road, Baoding, China. [3]Department of Prevention Dentistry,

School and Hospital of Stomatology, Wuhan University, 237 Luoyu Road, Wuhan, China.

References
1. Ahn SY, Kim HC, Kim E. Kinematic effects of nickel-titanium instruments with reciprocating or continuous rotation motion: a systematic review of in vitro studies. J Endod. 2016;42:1009–17.
2. Versiani MA, Pécora JD, Sousa-Neto MD. Microcomputed tomography analysis of the root canal morphology of single-rooted mandibular canines. Int Endod J. 2013;46:800–7.
3. Hülsmann M, Gressmann G, Schäfers F. A comparative study of root canal preparation using FlexMaster and HERO 642 rotary NiTi instruments. Int Endod J. 2003;36:358–66.
4. Dawood A, Marti Marti B, Sauret-Jackson V, Darwood A. 3D printing in dentistry. Br Dent J. 2015;219:521–9.
5. Ordinola-Zapata R, Bramante CM, Duarte MA, Cavenago BC, Jaramillo D, Versiani MA. Shaping ability of Reciproc and TF adaptive systems in severely curved canals of rapid microCT-based prototyping molar replicas. J Appl Oral Sci. 2014;22:509–15.
6. Byun C, Kim C, Cho S, Baek SH, Kim G, Kim SG, et al. Endodontic treatment of an anomalous anterior tooth with the aid of a 3-dimensional printed physical tooth model. J Endod. 2015;41:961–5.
7. Saber SE, Nagy MM, Schäfer E. Comparative evaluation of the shaping ability of ProTaper next, iRaCe and Hyflex CM rotaty NiTi files in severely curved root canals. Int Endod J. 2014;48:131–6.
8. Wan J, Rasimick BJ, Musikant BL, Deutsch AS. A comparison of cyclic fatigue resistance in reciprocating and rotary nickel-titanium instruments. Aust Endod J. 2011;37:122–7.
9. Schneider SW. A comparison of canal preparations in straight and curved root canals. Oral Surg Oral Med Oral Pathol. 1971;32:271–5.
10. Özer SY. Comparison of root canal transportation induced by three rotary systems with noncutting tips using computed tomography. Oral Surg Oral Med Oral Pathol Oral Radiol Endod. 2011;111:244–50.
11. Stern S, Patel S, Foschi F, Sherriff M, Mannocci F. Changes in centering and shaping ability using three nickel-titanium instrumentation techniques analysed by micro-computed tomography (μCT). Int Endod J. 2012;45:514–23.
12. Zhao D, Shen Y, Peng B, Haapasalo M. Root canal preparation of mandibular molars with 3 nickel-titanium rotary instruments: a micro-computed tomographic study. J Endod. 2014;40(11):1860–4.
13. Capar ID, Ertas H, Ok E, Arslan H, Ertas ET. Comparative study of different novel nickel-titanium rotary Systems for Root Canal Preparation in severely curved root canals. J Endod. 2014;40(6):852–6.
14. Deepak J, Ashish M, Fatil N, Kadam N, Yadav V, Jagdale H. Shaping ability of 5(th) generation Ni-Ti rotary Systems for Root Canal Preparation in curved root canals using CBCT: an in vitro study. J Int Oral Health. 2015;7:57–61.
15. Elnaghy AM, Elsaka SE. Evaluation of root canal transportation, centering ratio, and remaining dentin thickness associated with ProTaper next instruments with and without glide path. J Endod. 2014;40:2053–6.
16. Celikten B, Uzuntas CF, Kursun S, Orhan AI, Tufenkci P, Orhan K, et al. Comparative evaluation of shaping ability of two nickel-titanium rotary systems using cone beam computed tomography. BMC Oral Health. 2015;15:32.
17. Peters OA, Peters CI, Schönenberger K, Barbakow F. ProTaper rotary root canal preparation: effects of canal anatomy on final shape analysed by micro CT. Int Endod J. 2003;36:86–92.
18. Dhingra A, Ruhal N, Miglani A. Evaluation of single file systems Reciproc, Oneshape, and WaveOne using cone beam computed tomography -an in vitro study. J Clin Diagn Res. 2015;9:ZC30–4.
19. Adnan AH, Mazen IT, Elias MF. Methodologies used in quality assessment of root canal preparation techniques: review of the literature. J of Taibah University Med Sci. 2015;10:123–31.
20. Stavileci M, Hoxha V, Görduysus Ö, Tatar I, Laperre K, Hostens J, et al. Effects of preparation techniques on root canal shaping assessed by micro-computed tomography. Med Sci Monit Basic Res. 2013;19:163–8.
21. Al-Sudani D, Grande NM, Plotino G, Pompa G, Di Carlo S, Testarelli L, et al. Cyclic fatigue of nickel-titanium rotary instruments in a double (S-shaped) simulated curvature. J Endod. 2012;38:987–9.

22. Ba-Hattab R, Pröhl AK, Lang H, Pahncke D. Comparison of the shaping ability of GT® series X, twisted files and AlphaKite rotary nickel-titanium systems in simulated canals. BMC Oral Health. 2013;13:72.

23. Wu H, Peng C, Bai Y, Hu X, Wang L, Li C. Shaping ability of ProTaper universal, WaveOne and ProTaper next in simulated L-shaped and S-shaped root canals. BMC Oral Health. 2015;15:27.

24. Yoo YS, Cho YB. A comparison of the shaping ability of reciprocating NiTi instruments in simulated curved canals. Restor Dent Endod. 2012;37:220–7.

25. Wei Z, Cui Z, Yan P, Jiang H. A comparison of the shaping ability of three nickel-titanium rotary instruments: a micro-computed tomography study via a contrast radiopaque technique in vitro. BMC Oral Health. 2017;17:39.

26. Ceyhanli KT, Kamaci A, Taner M, Erdilek N, Celik D. Shaping ability of two M-wire and two traditional nickel-titanium instrumentation systems in S-shaped resin canals. Niger J Clin Pract. 2015;18:713–7.

27. Paqué F, Musch U, Hülsmann M. Comparison of root canal preparation using RaCe and pro taper rotary Ni-Ti instruments. Int Endod J. 2005;38:8–16.

28. Peters OA. Current challenges and concepts in the preparation of root canal systems: a review. J Endod. 2004;30:559–71.

29. Hülsmann M, Peters OA, Dummer PM. Mechanical preparation of root canals: shaping goals, techniques and means. Endod Top. 2005;10:30–76.

30. Willershausen B, Kasaj A, Rőhrig B, et al. Radiographic investigation of frequency and location of root canal curvatures in human mandibular anterior incisors in vitro. J Endod. 2008;34:152–6.

31. Giannastasio D, Rosa RA, Peres BU, Barreto MS, Dotto GN, Kuga MC, et al. Wizard CD plus and ProTaper universal: analysis of apical transportation using new software. J Appl Oral Sci. 2013;21:468–74.

32. Peters OA, Laib A, Gohring TN, Barbakow F. Changes in root canal geometry after preparation assessed by high-resolution computed tomography. J Endod. 2001;27:1–6.

33. De-Deus G. Research that matters - root canal filling and leakage studies. Int Endod J. 2012;45:1063–4.

34. Haapasalo M, Shen Y, Qian W, Gao Y. Irrigation in endodontics. Dent Clin N Am. 2010;54:291–312.

35. Cabanillas C, Monterde M, Pallarés A, Aranda S, Montes R. Assessment using AutoCAD software of the preparation of dentin walls in root canals produced by 4 different endodontic instrument systems. Int J Dent. 2015; 2015:517203.

36. Patiño PV, Biedma BM, Liébana CR, Cantatore G, Bahillo JG. The influence of a manual glide path on the separation rate of NiTi rotary instruments. J Endod. 2005;31:11–6.

37. Marzouk AM, Ghoneim AG. Computed tomographic evaluation of canal shape instrumented by different kinematics rotary nickel-titanium systems. J Endod. 2013;39:906–9.

6

Inequalities in oral health among adolescents in Gangneung, South Korea

Se-Hwan Jung[1], Myoung-Hee Kim[2] and Jae-In Ryu[3*] ⓘ

Abstract

Background: This study aims to evaluate inequality in oral health among adolescents and to explain the mechanisms of such inequalities in Gangneung, South Korea.

Methods: One thousand two hundred sixty-seven students in their first year from four vocational and three general schools participated in the baseline survey of 2011, and 84.7% of them were surveyed again in 2013. Oral examinations by the same dentist and a self-administered questionnaire were repeated during both waves. Outcome measure for oral health was the existence of untreated dental caries (DT). As socioeconomic position (SEP) indicators, school type (general vs. vocational), father's and mother's education, perceived economic status, and Family Affluence Scale (FAS) were measured. Variables measuring oral health related behaviours included tooth brushing frequency, frequency of eating snacks and drinking sodas, smoking, and annual visits to dental clinics. Chi-square tests and panel logistic regression were adopted to examine the associations between dental caries and SEP indicators by STATA version 15.1.

Results: Having a less educated father and attending a vocational school were significant predictors for untreated caries after controlling for SEP indicators. However, students from general schools, higher SEP by father's education, perceived economic status, or FAS, or having non-smoking experience or annual visits to dental clinics were more likely to stay caries-free.

Conclusions: There were socioeconomic inequalities in oral health on an adolescent panel. Given that oral health status during adolescents can persist throughout the course of a person's life, intervention to tackle such inequalities and school environments are required.

Keywords: Adolescent health, Schools, Socioeconomic factors

Background

Various studies have recognized that there are socioeconomic inequalities in health [1–3] and oral health [4, 5]. A gap exists across all levels of socioeconomic groups, especially between the highest and the lowest ones. Furthermore, such inequalities are observed throughout the course of a person's life, from childhood to adulthood and into old age [6–9]. However, there are differing opinions for the existence of health inequality in a specific life stage: adolescence.

West [10, 11] suggested that adolescents exhibit dissimilar health inequality patterns when compared to other age groups because this group can be "characterised by the absence or disappearance of class variation." To the contrary, others have claimed that findings on health equality among adolescents are the result of inappropriate measurements for socioeconomic position (SEP) indicators [12, 13]. These studies argued that commonly used SEP indicators, including education, occupation, and income levels, are not appropriate for adolescents. For example, there was a significant health gap in adolescents when using alternative SEP indicators such as the Family Affluence Scale (FAS) [14] and perceived socioeconomic status [15]. Subsequent to these debates, studies in different settings have attempted to verify both positions but a consensus stills has not been reached [16–18].

Recently, there have been several longitudinal studies dealing with inequality in adolescent oral health by SEP indicators. A life-course research in cohort of New Zealand children concluded that there was an effect from childhood SEP [19]. A study from Sweden showed

* Correspondence: jaeinryu@khu.ac.kr
[3]Department of Preventive and Social Dentistry, College of Dentistry, Kyung Hee University, 26 Kyungheedae-ro, Dongdaemun-gu, Seoul 02447, South Korea
Full list of author information is available at the end of the article

that there is limited effect from SEP only after considering the previous experience of caries [20]. Polk et al. [21] and Newacheck [22] also reported that there was an SEP gradient in caries experiences in the U.S. Another longitudinal study from Iowa cohort revealed that there is a gap by SEP, especially maternal educational levels [23]. However, Curtis, using the same cohort data from Iowa Fluoride Study (IFS), recently argued that 'the role of SES in caries may not be as important as previously thought'. Meanwhile, another group of scholars have focused on school characteristics as an alternative to traditional SEP indicators [24–27] or influential effectors for behaviour, especially in S. Korea [28, 29], to determine health inequalities in adolescents. Others have reported that the residential area was a socioeconomic predictor of oral health inequality among adolescents [30, 31].

In terms of oral health, adolescence is of special importance because permanent dentition is complete and parental supervision of oral health behaviours weakens. Indeed, dental caries is a unique health condition aggravating during the schooling period. On the other hand, as they are amenable by health education and highly receptive to public health programs, interventions may be effective and the effects may be long lasting.

This study aims to evaluate inequality in oral health among adolescents by various SEP indicators and to explain the mechanisms of such inequalities in Gangneung, a city in South Korea.

Methods

Study participants

The aim of this panel study was to explore inequality in untreated caries among adolescents. The city of Gangneung has eleven high schools; two in rural areas and nine in urban areas [32]. By the school types, there were six general schools, four vocational schools, and one art school. The aim of the general schools is to support students' academic development and entry into college. By contrast, the aim of the vocational schools is to prepare students to enter the workforce directly after graduation. The one art school in this study was excluded due to its unique characteristics. First, the schools were categorized by its location as an urban or rural area. There was only one general and one vocational school in the rural area, so both of them were included. Among the other eight schools in the urban area, three vocational schools and two general schools were selected as study samples. Because they have fewer students than the general schools, all of the vocational schools were included. Two general schools were randomly selected by their close proximity to sampled vocational schools. Only first year students, 15-yr-old, were invited to participate in consideration of the follow-up survey after two years. All of the students were sixteen

years old because middle school education is mandatory in South Korea, so the freshman in high school were all the same age. The research team sent the consent forms for oral examinations and surveys to students' parents or guardians with a brief introduction. Only students who returned completed consent forms from their parents or guardians were included in the study. Among 1371 students, ninety-seven declined to participate, and seven were excluded due to incomplete answers on the questionnaires. Finally, 1267 students were enrolled into the panel.

The Institutional Review Board in Gangneung-Wonju National University Dental Hospital reviewed and approved this study (GWNUDH IRB-2011-1-3). The Gangneung Health Centre and the Gangneung Office of Education with their district offices also consented to the study and supported the administrative process.

Study variables and measurement

Outcome measure for oral health was the untreated dental caries according to the Korean National Oral Health Survey (KNOHS) standard [33], which follows the guideline established by the WHO methods for oral health survey [34]. The untreated dental caries "D" component, which includes carious teeth, filled teeth with recurrent decay, teeth with only the root left, defective filling with caries, temporary filling, and teeth with a filled tooth surfaces but with other surface decayed.

The examinations were conducted in a classroom of the surveyed schools using their table and chairs with a lightweight portable examination light. The plane mouth mirrors, periodontal probes that conform to WHO specifications, and several pairs of tweezers were supplied for the survey. The same dentist who was trained according to the Korean National Oral Health Survey (KNOHS) confirmed the students' oral status twice in three years. To have reliable intra-examiner reliability, the dentist examined 20 students before the main study. He re-examined them one week later for calibration, and the kappa consistency was 0.91, good agreement [35]. The status transition in dental caries between 2011 and 2013 were classified as follows: 1) no to no (remained caries-free); 2) yes to no (received treatment); 3) no to yes (developed new dental caries); and 4) yes to yes (remained untreated caries).

Self-administered questionnaire surveys were administered, and items were derived from the Korean Youth Risk Behaviour Web-based Survey (KYRBWS) [36, 37] and from the guidelines in "Delivering better oral health: an evidence-based toolkit for prevention" [38]. As SEP indicators, school type (general vs. vocational), father's and mother's education level, perceived economic status, and FAS were measured. Father's and mother's education level was categorized into two groups; high school graduation or below vs. college graduation or above. The perceived economic status were re-categorised as high (high, high-middle, and middle) vs. low (middle-low and low). The FAS score was calculated by summing up dummy variables to represent the ownership of a family car, private bedroom for the student, computers, and the number of family vacations in the past year. FAS scores range from zero to nine, and students with scores larger than five were defined as 'high' and the others as 'low' group. Variable to measure oral health related behaviours included tooth brushing frequency ('twice or more a day' vs. 'less than twice a day'), frequency of snacks and drinking sodas ('less than once a day' vs. 'once or more a day'), smoking ('no' vs. 'yes'), and annual visits of dental clinics at least once a year ('yes' or 'no').

Statistical analysis

Annual prevalence of untreated caries (decayed teeth; 'D rate') and proportion of status transition in dental caries over the follow-up was examined according to various SEP indicators and oral health related behaviours by chi-square tests. In order to identify independent effects of SEP variables and contributions of covariates to oral health status with considering panel design, unconditional panel logistic regression models were estimated. Data analysis was carried out using STATA version 15.1 statistical software package (StataCorp, Texas).

Results

The characteristics of the study participants are displayed in the Table 1. At the baseline survey of 2011, the participation rate was 92.4%, and a total of 1267 students participated. The follow-up rate was 84.7% in 2013 with the drop of 194 students. Attrition was more common in vocational schools (27.3%) than general schools (7.4%). However, this did not present significant changes

in the distribution of gender and SEP indicators of the sample between waves (Additional file 1: Table S1).

At both waves, the students who were from vocational schools, less educated fathers, and 'low' groups of perceived economic status and FAS were more likely to have untreated dental caries. As for oral health behaviours, tooth brushing and annual visits were inversely associated with D rates. Smoking was strongly associated with D rates in both waves (Table 2).

The odds ratios (ORs) for untreated caries were estimated after adjusting for SEP indicators only in Model 1, and SEP indicators and oral health related behaviours covariates together in Model 2 (Table 3). As for D rates, fathers' education and school type remained significant after controlling for other SEP indicators. Even after incorporating health behaviour variables in the models, they still showed significant effects with attenuation.

The status transition in dental caries over the follow-up is shown in Table 4. Students from general schools, in higher SEP measured by father's education, perceived economic status, or FAS, drinking soda less than a day, without smoking experience, and to have annual visits to dental clinics were more likely to stay caries-free ($p < 0.01$).

Discussion

Our analysis of the adolescent panel in Gangneung, South Korea, verified the existence of significant differences in untreated dental caries by school type and father's education, and in caries experience by gender and father's education. Oral health-related behaviours attenuated but did not explain away such effects.

Differences in oral health by school type can be attributed to the fact that schools are a place where youths form a unique culture. Here, they begin to be independent from their family, spending most of the day with their peers. In a society where college graduation is the

Table 1 The characteristics of study participants by school type in Gangneung

School location	School type	Sampled population N	Respondents in baseline 2011 (1st grade, 15-yr-old) N	Gender		Respondents in follow-up 2013 (3rd grade, 17-yr-old) N
				Boys N (%)	Girls N (%)	
Total		1371	1267	690(54.5)	577(45.5)	1073
Rural						
School A	General	93	88	41(46.6)	47(53.4)	71
School B	Vocational	155	133	48(36.1)	85(63.9)	99
Urban						
School C	General	341	335	335(100.0)		314
School D	General	360	343		343(100.0)	324
School E	Vocational	296	242	242(100.0)		168
School F	Vocational	58	58	24(41.4)	34(58.6)	45
School G	Vocational	68	68		68(100.0)	52

Table 2 Numbers and percentages of adolescents who have untreated dental caries (D rate) by survey year in Gangneung

D rate	2011 (1st grade, 15-yr-old) N = 1267		2013 (3rd grade, 17-yr-old) N = 1073	
Total	217(17.1)		153(14.3)	
Gender				
Girls	92(15.9)		62(12.2)	
Boys	125(18.1)		91(16.1)	
School type				
General	94(12.3)	***	70(9.9)	***
Vocational	123(24.6)		83(22.8)	
Father's education				
College or above	50(10.5)	***	33(7.7)	***
High school or below	137(19.8)		98(17.0)	
Mother's education				
College or above	46(13.3)		31(10.3)	
High school or below	143(17.6)		101(14.4)	
Perceived economic status				
High	145(15.6)	*	99(12.6)	**
Low	72(21.4)		54(19.2)	
FAS				
High	171(15.6)	***	115(12.5)	***
Low	46(27.4)		38(26.0)	
Frequency of tooth-brushing				
≥2	182(16.2)	*	137(14.0)	
< 2	35(24.5)		16(17.4)	
Frequency of eating snacks				
< 1	71(15.7)		118(13.4)	*
≥1	131(17.3)		35(18.9)	
Frequency of drinking soda				
< 1	99(15.1)		134(13.6)	
≥1	95(18.6)		19(21.1)	
Smoking experience				
No	124(13.8)	***	91(12.0)	**
Yes	93(25.3)		62(19.6)	
Annual visits to dental clinic				
Yes	84(14.6)	*	55(10.7)	**
No	133(19.2)		98(17.6)	

*p < 0.05, **p < 0.01, ***p < 0.001

Table 3 Adjusted odds ratio and 95% confidence intervals estimated from unconditional panel logistic regression models for D rate among adolescents in Gangneung (N = 2003)

D rate	Model 1†		Model 2‡	
Gender				
Girls (vs. boys)	0.65(0.39–1.06)		0.71(0.41–1.23)	
School type				
Vocational (vs. general)	3.10(1.79–5.35)	***	2.68(1.46–4.92)	**
Father's education				
High school (vs. college)	2.15(1.15–4.01)	*	2.04(1.05–3.98)	*
Mother's education				
High school (vs. college)	0.92(0.48–1.76)		0.86(0.43–1.73)	
Perceived economic status				
Low (vs. high)	1.03(0.62–1.71)		1.05(0.61–1.81)	
FAS				
Low (vs. high)	1.82(0.95–3.49)		1.80(0.88–3.64)	
Frequency of tooth-brushing				
< 2 (vs. N ≥ 2)			1.42(0.72–2.83)	
Frequency of eating snacks				
≥1 (vs. N < 1)			1.64(1.00–2.70)	
Frequency of drinking soda				
≥1 (vs. N < 1)			1.13(0.66–1.95)	
Smoking experience				
Yes (vs. no)			1.72(1.02–2.92)	*
Annual visits to dental clinic				
No (vs. yes)			1.91(1.22–3.01)	**

† Model 1: adjusted for gender, school type, father's education, mother's education, subjective economic status, and FAS
‡ Model 2: adjusted for gender, school type, father's education, mother's education, subjective economic status, FAS, frequency of tooth brushing, eating snacks, and drinking soda, smoking, and annual visits to dental clinics
*p < 0.05, **p < 0.01, ***p < 0.001. - mean VIF (=1.37) < 10

in assault, harassment, and adolescent prostitution [39]. Another Korean study found that even after controlling for individual-level SEP indicators and psychological stress, students in vocational schools engaged more in risky behaviours, for example smoking and drinking, and less in health-promoting behaviours, such as tooth brushing [40, 41].

There was no significant difference by gender in untreated dental caries. It is contrary to the findings in the 2012 Korean National Oral Health Survey, which showed higher prevalence of decayed teeth among girls by 10.6% [42]. Martinez-Mier and Zandona [43] argued that caries is multifactorial disease attributable to diverse factors, including genetic and hormonal factors as well as cultural influences, behavioural, and dietary practices. Kawamura and colleagues attributed the better oral health of girls to more frequent tooth brushing and their desires to possess healthy teeth [44]. It was suggested that their concern for good oral health motivates them

norm, vocational schools could be a symbolic representation of social disadvantages, which are related to poor health and undesirable health behaviours. There was a report that male and female students in Korean vocational schools are more likely to engage in nonconformant behaviours, including smoking, alcohol consumption, unexcused absences, running away from home, and sexual relationships, as well as to be involved

Table 4 Condition transition for untreated caries over the two-year follow-up in Gangneung adolescent at 2013 (N = 1073)

	Caries status change (from 2011 to 2013)				
	No → No[a]	Yes → No[b]	No → Yes[c]	Yes → Yes[d]	
Total	834 (77.7)	86 (8.1)	61 (5.7)	92 (8.6)	
Gender					
Girls	397 (78.3)	48 (9.5)	25 (4.9)	37 (7.3)	
Boys	437 (77.2)	38 (6.7)	36 (6.4)	55 (9.7)	
School type					***
General	585 (82.5)	54 (7.6)	37 (5.2)	33 (4.7)	
Vocational	249 (68.4)	32 (8.8)	24 (6.6)	59 (16.2)	
Father's education					***
College or above	361 (84.5)	33 (7.7)	23 (5.4)	10 (2.3)	
High school or below	432 (74.9)	47 (8.2)	34 (5.9)	64 (11.1)	
Mother's education					
College or above	244 (81.1)	26 (8.6)	18 (6.0)	13 (4.3)	
High school or below	545 (77.8)	55 (7.9)	38 (5.4)	63 (9.0)	
Perceived economic status					**
High	621 (78.8)	68 (8.6)	47 (6.0)	52 (6.6)	
Low	209 (74.4)	18 (6.4)	14 (5.0)	40 (14.2)	
FAS					***
High	732 (79.2)	77 (8.3)	52 (5.6)	63 (6.8)	
Low	100 (68.5)	8 (5.5)	9 (6.6)	29 (19.9)	
Frequency of tooth-brushing					
≥2	764 (77.9)	80 (8.2)	53 (5.4)	84 (8.6)	
< 2	70 (76.1)	6 (6.5)	8 (8.7)	8 (8.7)	
Frequency of eating snacks					
< 1	699 (79.1)	67 (7.6)	47 (5.3)	71 (8.0)	
≥1	131 (70.8)	19 (10.3)	14 (7.6)	21 (11.4)	
Frequency of drinking soda					**
< 1	777 (79.0)	72 (7.3)	53 (5.4)	81 (8.2)	
≥1	57 (63.3)	14 (15.6)	8 (8.9)	11 (12.2)	
Smoking experience					***
No	611 (80.8)	54 (7.1)	42 (5.6)	49 (6.5)	
Yes	223 (70.4)	32 (10.1)	19 (6.0)	43 (13.6)	
Annual visits to dental clinic					**
Yes	410 (79.5)	51 (9.9)	18 (3.5)	37 (7.2)	
No	424 (76.1)	35 (6.3)	43 (7.7)	55 (9.9)	

[a]No → No as remaining caries-free, [b]Yes → No as being treated with fillings, [c]No → Yes as developing dental caries, and [d]Yes → Yes as remaining untreated caries
**p < 0.01, ***p < 0.001

to visit dental clinics for treatment more often than males. Indeed, we found that students who visited dental clinics more regularly had a reduced likelihood of having untreated caries; adolescents who visited the dental clinic more regularly to receive treatment had less untreated caries.

It is noteworthy that father's education but not mother's education was a strong predictor of oral health

in Korean adolescents. This is contrary to the report that mothers play an important role in the child development of oral health [45]. First, the cut-off level of mother's education might be inappropriate to capture the differences; in fact, only 30% of students in the panel had mothers who had graduated college, which means that the 'low' education group consisted of heterogeneous individuals, resulting in non-differential misclassification.

Second, although parents' education level is associated with health literacy and awareness and thereby children's behaviours and service utilisation [46], parental influence wanes during transitional developmental periods [47]. Children have a desire to be similar with their friends, and such desires become stronger in older adolescents [48]. Therefore, mother's education might have little impact on the oral health and behaviours of adolescents in this panel. Along the same line, in our study, father's education as surrogate marker of household material conditions might be a better indicator of cultural and behavioural resources than mother's education. In Korea, fathers are generally family breadwinners, and there is a clear correlation between fathers' education and family economic status. As a mid-sized semi-urban city, Gangneung provides less job opportunities. In this context, father's education could surpass other SEP indicators in representing household socioeconomic conditions.

The oral health behaviours of the study panel improved during the follow-up. For instance, the prevalence of eating less snacks went from under 37.5% at baseline to 82.7% at the second wave. Students exhibiting healthier behaviours increased dramatically in terms of oral health; they brushed teeth more and consumed less snacks and soda. All of this generally contributes to better oral health [49–51], and indeed D rates with untreated caries in our panel declined over time.

This study has some limitations. First, although differential sample attrition between general and vocational schools did not bring out differences in the distribution of socioeconomic factors among students, we cannot be sure that there was no systematic difference in oral health-related behaviours between participants and dropouts. Second, we could not fully explain why the strong effect of father's education persisted even after controlling for oral health-related behaviours. Third, because the panel was composed of high-school students only, it was hard to conduct follow-ups after their graduation. In order to examine long-term effects of oral health and related behaviours in adolescents, it would thus be necessary to expand the panel range to primary school students as they begin to formulate health behaviours.

Conclusion

We found socioeconomic inequalities in oral health based on an adolescent panel from Gangneung. Given that poor oral health and undesirable oral health-related behaviours during the adolescent period could last throughout a person's lifetime [52], there should be an immediate intervention to tackle such inequalities and school environments.

Acknowledgements

This research was supported by Basic Science Research Program through the National Research Foundation of Korea (NRF) funded by the Ministry of Education (2011-0011208). The authors thank to the Gangneung Health Centre and the Gangneung Office of Education for supporting the administrative process.

Authors' contributions

All authors contributed extensively to the work presented in this paper. SH has made substantial contributions to conception and design, acquisition of data, and interpretation of data; JI has been involved in analysis and interpretation of data and drafting the manuscript; MH has been revising it critically for important intellectual content; and All authors have given final approval of the version to be published. Each author have participated sufficiently in the work to take public responsibility for appropriate portions of the content and agreed to be accountable for all aspects of the work in ensuring that questions related to the accuracy or integrity of any part of the work are appropriately investigated and resolved.

Competing interests

The authors declare that they have no competing interests.

Author details

[1]Department of Preventive Dentistry, College of Dentistry, Gangneung-Wonju University, 120 Gangneungdaehag-ro, Gangneung City, Gangwon Province 25457, South Korea. [2]Center for Health Equity Research, People's Health Institute, 36 Sadangro 13-gil, 2nd floor, Dongjak-gu, Seoul 07004, South Korea. [3]Department of Preventive and Social Dentistry, College of Dentistry, Kyung Hee University, 26 Kyungheedae-ro, Dongdaemun-gu, Seoul 02447, South Korea.

References

1. Townsend P, Davidson N. Inequalities in health: the black report. Harmondsworth: Penguin; 1982.
2. Whitehead M. The health divide: inequalities in health in the 1980s. London: Health Education Authority; 1987.
3. Marmot MG, Wilkinson RG. Social determinants of health. 2nd ed. Oxford; New York: Oxford University Press; 2006.
4. Marmot M, Bell R. Social determinants and dental health. Adv Dent Res. 2011;23(2):201–6.
5. Gilbert GH, Duncan RP, Shelton BJ. Social determinants of tooth loss. Health Serv Res. 2003;38(6 Pt 2):1843–62.
6. Galobardes B, Lynch JW, Davey Smith G. Childhood socioeconomic circumstances and cause-specific mortality in adulthood: systematic review and interpretation. Epidemiol Rev. 2004;26:7–21.
7. Ben-Shlomo Y, Kuh D. A life course approach to chronic disease epidemiology: conceptual models, empirical challenges and interdisciplinary perspectives. Int J Epidemiol. 2002;31(2):285–93.
8. Smith GD. Life-course approaches to inequalities in adult chronic disease risk. Proc Nutr Soc. 2007;66(2):216–36.
9. Smith GD, Hart C, Blane D, Hole D. Adverse socioeconomic conditions in childhood and cause specific adult mortality: prospective observational study. BMJ. 1998;316(7145):1631–5.
10. West P. Health inequalities in the early years: is there equalisation in youth? Soc Sci Med. 1997;44(6):833–58.
11. West P, Sweeting H. Evidence on equalisation in health in youth from the west of Scotland. Soc Sci Med. 2004;59(1):13–27.
12. Currie CE, Elton RA, Todd J, Platt S. Indicators of socioeconomic status for adolescents: the WHO health behaviour in school-aged children survey. Health Educ Res. 1997;12(3):385–97.

13. Piko BF, Fitzpatrick KM. Socioeconomic status, psychosocial health and health behaviours among Hungarian adolescents. Eur J Pub Health. 2007;17(4):353–60.

14. Currie C, Molcho M, Boyce W, Holstein B, Torsheim T, Richter M. Researching health inequalities in adolescents: the development of the health behaviour in school-aged children (HBSC) family affluence scale. Soc Sci Med. 2008; 66(6):1429–36.

15. Goodman E, Adler NE, Kawachi I, Frazier AL, Huang B, Colditz GA. Adolescents' perceptions of social status: development and evaluation of a new indicator. Pediatrics. 2001;108(2):E31.

16. Goodman E. The role of socioeconomic status gradients in explaining differences in US adolescents' health. Am J Public Health. 1999;89(10):1522–8.

17. Siahpush M, Singh GK. A multivariate analysis of the association between social class of origin and current social class with self-rated general health and psychological health among 16-year-old Australians. Aust NZ J Med. 2000;30(6):653–9.

18. Vuille JC, Schenkel M. Social equalization in the health of youth. The role of the school. Eur J Pub Health. 2001;11(3):287–93.

19. Poulton R, Caspi A, Milne BJ, Thomson WM, Taylor A, Sears MR, Moffitt TE. Association between children's experience of socioeconomic disadvantage and adult health: a life-course study. Lancet. 2002;360(9346):1640–5.

20. Kallestal C, Wall S. Socio-economic effect on caries. Incidence data among Swedish 12-14-year-olds. Community Dent Oral Epidemiol. 2002;30(2):108–14.

21. Polk DE, Weyant RJ, Manz MC. Socioeconomic factors in adolescents' oral health: are they mediated by oral hygiene behaviors or preventive interventions? Community Dent Oral Epidemiol. 2010;38(1):1–9.

22. Newacheck PW, Hung YY, Park MJ, Brindis CD, Irwin CE Jr. Disparities in adolescent health and health care: does socioeconomic status matter? Health Serv Res. 2003;38(5):1235–52.

23. Warren JJ, Van Buren JM, Levy SM, Marshall TA, Cavanaugh JE, Curtis AM, Kolker JL, Weber-Gasparoni K. Dental caries clusters among adolescents. Community Dent Oral Epidemiol. 2017;45(6):538–44.

24. Fruhstorfer BH, Mousoulis C, Uthman OA, Robertson W. Socio-economic status and overweight or obesity among school-age children in sub-Saharan Africa - a systematic review. Clin Obes. 2016;6(1):19–32.

25. Martins-Oliveira JG, Jorge KO, Ferreira RC, Ferreira EF, Vale MP, Zarzar PM. Risk of alcohol dependence: prevalence, related problems and socioeconomic factors. Cien Saude Colet. 2016;21(1):17–26.

26. Nabe-Nielsen K, Krolner R, Mortensen LH, Jorgensen MB, Diderichsen F. Health promotion in primary and secondary schools in Denmark: time trends and associations with schools' and students' characteristics. BMC Public Health. 2015;15:93.

27. Henkel D, Zemlin U. Social inequality and substance use and problematic gambling among adolescents and young adults: a review of epidemiological surveys in Germany. Curr Drug Abuse Rev. 2016;9(1):26–48.

28. Heo J, Oh J, Subramanian SV, Kawachi I. Household and school-level influences on smoking behavior among Korean adolescents: a multilevel analysis. PLoS One. 2014;9(6):e98683.

29. Kim H, Kim EK, Choi ES, Kim YJ, Lee HJ, Kim JJ, Jang HS, Shim KS, Jeon SN, Kang YH, et al. The determinants of adolescent smoking by gender and type of school in Korea. J Prev Med Public Health. 2006;39(5):379–88.

30. Mathur MR, Tsakos G, Millett C, Arora M, Watt R. Socioeconomic inequalities in dental caries and their determinants in adolescents in New Delhi, India. BMJ Open. 2014;4(12):e006391.

31. Mathur MR, Tsakos G, Parmar P, Millett CJ, Watt RG. Socioeconomic inequalities and determinants of oral hygiene status among urban Indian adolescents. Community Dent Oral Epidemiol. 2016;44(3):248–54.

32. Gangneung City. The statistical yearbook of Gangneung city. Gangneung: Gangneung City; 2012.

33. Ministry of Health and Welfare. Korean National Oral Health Survey 2010. Seoul: Ministry of Health and Welfare; 2010.

34. World Health Organization. Oral health surveys : basic methods. 5th ed. Geneva: World Health Organization; 2013.

35. Bowling A. Sample size and sampling for quantitative research. In: Research methods in health: investigating health and health services. 2nd ed. Buckingham; Philadelphia: Open University Press; 2002. p. 165–92.

36. Korea Centers for Disease Control and Prevention Reliability and validity of Korean youth risk behavior web-based survey questionnaire. Seoul: Korea centers for disease control and Prevention; 2009.

37. Korea Centers for Disease Control and Prevention The statistics of Korean youth risk behavior web-based survey 2011. Seoul: Ministry of Education, Ministry of Health and Welfare, Korea centers for disease control and Prevention; 2012.

38. Public Health England. Delivering better oral health: An evidence-based toolkit for prevention. 3rd ed. London: Department of Health, National Health Service, The British Association for the Study of Community Dentistry; 2014.

39. Kim DS. Experience of parent-related negative life events, mental health, and delinquent behavior among Korean adolescents. J Prev Med Public Health. 2007;40(3):218–26.

40. Jung SH, Tsakos G, Sheiham A, Ryu JI, Watt RG. Socio-economic status and oral health-related behaviours in Korean adolescents. Soc Sci Med. 2010; 70(11):1780–8.

41. Kim SI, Lee HR, Ma DS, Park DY, Jung SH. The differences of oral health-related behaviors by type of school among high school students in Gangneung city. J Korean Acad Oral Health. 2012;36(4):309–14.

42. Ministry of Health and Welfare. Ministry of Health and Welfare statistical year book 2012. Seoul: Ministry of Health and Welfare; 2012.

43. Martinez-Mier EA, Zandona AF. The impact of gender on caries prevalence and risk assessment. Dent Clin N Am. 2013;57(2):301–15.

44. Kawamura M, Takase N, Sasahara H, Okada M. Teenagers' oral health attitudes and behavior in Japan: comparison by sex and age group. J Oral Sci. 2008; 50(2):167–74.

45. Murakami K, Kondo N, Ohkubo T, Hashimoto H. The effect of fathers' and mothers' educational level on adult oral health in Japan. Community Dent Oral Epidemiol. 2016;44(3):283–91.

46. Mejia GC, Ha DH. Dental caries trends in Australian school children. Aust Dent J. 2011;56(2):227–30.

47. Hall-Scullin E, Goldthorpe J, Milsom K, Tickle M. A qualitative study of the views of adolescents on their caries risk and prevention behaviours. BMC oral health. 2015;15(1):141.

48. Stokes E, Ashcroft A, Platt MJ. Determining Liverpool adolescents' beliefs and attitudes in relation to oral health. Health education research. 2006; 21(2):192–205.

49. Harris NO, García-Godoy F, Nathe CN. Primary preventive dentistry, 8th edn. Boston: Pearson; 2014.

50. Daly B, Watt R, Batchelor P, Treasure E. Essential dental public health. Oxford; New York: Oxford University Press; 2002.

51. Pine CM. Community oral health. Oxford; Boston: Wright; 1997.

52. Due P, Krolner R, Rasmussen M, Andersen A, Trab Damsgaard M, Graham H, Holstein BE. Pathways and mechanisms in adolescence contribute to adult health inequalities. Scand J Public Health. 2011;39(6 Suppl):62–78.

7

Parenting and oral health in an inner-city environment: a qualitative pilot study

Shalini Nayee[1], Charlotte Klass[1], Gail Findlay[2] and Jennifer E. Gallagher[1*] ⓘ

Abstract

Background: Preventable oral diseases such as dental caries remain common in the United Kingdom. Clustering of poor health is observed within deprived communities, such as inner-city areas, where elevated levels of dental need are associated with lower uptake of dental care. Successful oral health promotion (OHP) initiatives are contingent upon effective community engagement. The aim of this pilot study was to engage with families with young children to explore community views on oral health and dental care and thus tailor OHP initiatives more effectively to their needs.

Methods: Qualitative research, involving individual interviews and triad focus groups with parents/caregivers, was conducted in a south London inner-city community as part of a 'Well London' programme initiative.

Results: Seventeen parents/caregivers participated in this pilot study. Parents/caregivers described a spectrum of oral health behaviours based on their social history, past dental experiences and cultural influences. All parents described a clear desire to create healthy lives for their children; however, two broad groups were apparent, termed 'Oral Health Prioritisers' and 'Oral Health Non-prioritisers'. The former reported regularly accessing dental care for their children, believing that oral health contributes to systemic health. Non-prioritisers, however, preferentially used key services considered most beneficial to their child's wellbeing. Dental services were considered a low priority for this group, where oral health was synonymous with absence of pain. Participants in both groups favoured OHP initiatives involving a range of health and social care services, with schools at the epicentre of programmes. First-time parents were proposed as an important group requiring support in future OHP initiatives with evidence suggesting that first-born children may have delayed presentation to a dentist.

Conclusions: The findings suggest that this inner-city community may contain sub-groups with contrasting perspectives on oral health and oral health behaviours; nevertheless, there was support for a systems approach to oral health promotion initiatives involving a range of health and social care services, including a critcal role for schools, and actively connecting with first-time parents. The findings provide the basis for further research.

Keywords: Oral health promotion, Parenting, Oral health, Access to dental care

Background

Parents living in deprived, inner city environments face an array of challenges to establish and maintain healthy lifestyles for their families. Common risk factors for chronic oral and systemic disease, such as poor diet, obesity and lack of exercise, disproportionately impact upon deprived families [1], due to clustering of multiple risk factors within such communities [2]. These effects are further exacerbated within inner city areas due to

the convergence of multiple factors including mobile populations, weak social networks [3], financial insecurity and lack of engagement with preventive health services [4], resulting in worse systemic and oral health compared with more affluent communities.

Lambeth, a densely populated inner London borough with high levels of deprivation, faces a spectrum of dental and general health challenges, exemplified by lower life expectancy for its residents than in London and England overall [5]. Oral disease is common, with approximately 10% of 3-year old [6], and 24% of 5-year old children [7], found to have at least one untreated carious

* Correspondence: jenny.gallagher@kcl.ac.uk
[1]King's College London Dental Institute, Population and Patient Health Division, Denmark Hill, London SE5 9RS, UK
Full list of author information is available at the end of the article

tooth. Nevertheless the objective 'need' for oral care does not translate to perceived need for oral care amongst its residents, with dental attendance rates persistently lower than London and national averages, particularly amongst children [8]. Recent data show that 41% of Lambeth children did not access any NHS dental services over a two-year period [8], with this figure, encompassing all parts of Lambeth, masking substantially worse access rates within northern localities of the borough. Amongst adult residents the situation appears worse with 49% of adults not accessing any NHS dental services over a two-year period [8], suggesting a prevailing culture of irregular dental attendance, albeit that some may possibly choose to access services privately. The dichotomy between high levels of dental disease but persistently low uptake of dental services suggests there is a poor 'fit' between the community and local dental services [9].

Low uptake of primary care dental services leads to more advanced presentation of dental disease, with provisional data showing that dental caries is the most common primary diagnosis amongst young children in England requiring admission to hospital [10]. Moreover, children from deprived communities are over-represented in such admissions, such that they are twice as likely to require hospital admission for dental care as children from the most affluent communities [11].

Increased uptake of dental services represents a fundamental step in improving oral health within this community, and similar communities, not only giving local residents exposure to evidence-based preventive care and advice [12], but also contributing to improved oral health awareness, which can be sustained in the community for future generations. Recent oral health statistics for 3-year old children showing high caries experience amongst this cohort [6], also highlight the critical importance of early access to dental care, with childhood oral disease an important predictor of future oral disease.

Oral health and uptake of dental services can be improved significantly through appropriate oral health promotion (OHP) initiatives [13]. Moreover, targeting of these initiatives towards families with young children provides a pragmatic way to improve both current and future oral health outcomes, with this child-centric approach mirroring recent recommendations for transforming public health in London [14]. OHP initiatives are deemed successful if they provide sustained improvement in health outcomes, with the onus on local communities to facilitate this effort. Ensuring that OHP initiatives can be sustained by local communities requires detailed community consultation during planning and development, as parental knowledge, attitudes and beliefs may differ widely from those of dentists and service planners/commissioners [15]. Community engagement is also critical for improving health equity,

acting to improve social cohesion, foster mutual responsibility and empower the local community [1].

The aim of this qualitative study was to investigate how parents/caregivers with young children perceive oral health; to understand the key factors and beliefs that have shaped these perceptions of oral health; and to understand how these perceptions affect oral health behaviours, including uptake of dental care. These findings will be used to provide insight into how OHP initiatives can be formulated to improve oral health within this community, and similar communities.

This study was nested within the wider public health 'Well London' programme which involves community engagement and is based on a development framework for communities and local organisations to work together to improve health, wellbeing and reduce inequalities [16]. A three-year Well London (Phase 2) initiative was focussed in the neighbourhood where the parents/care giver respondents in this study were residents [17], to inform specific dental aspects of the programme.

Methods

This study involved a dual method qualitative approach, encompassing individual semi-structured interviews and triad focus groups of up to three participants [18], to consult with parents/caregivers of young children. Hereafter, parents/caregivers will be referred to as parents to enhance the flow of the paper.

Parents (aged 18 years and over) living in a North Lambeth estate, or its proximity, were invited to participate in this pilot study through recruitment via local community events, children's centres and schools. Research ethics approval was sought and obtained from King's College London Research Ethics Committee (BDM/13/14-29); this included consent to publish participants' data.

Verbal and written informed consent was obtained from all parents agreeing to take part in the Additional file 1. Parents were also invited to complete an information sheet, providing the researchers with basic demographic information. Participants were assigned to individual interviews or triad focus groups based on their personal preference. Triad focus groups provided parents with an opportunity to interact with one another other and explore novel themes that emerged from these interactions, but on a sufficiently small scale that more personal or sensitive topics could be discussed. Individual interviews provided parents with a preference for one-to-one conversations with an opportunity to share their views with researchers.

Interviews and focus groups were conducted by two female researchers (SN and CK). Interview/focus group venues were selected based on ease for informants, with use of local community centres and children's centres.

Topics for discussion during interviews/focus group were outlined in a pre-determined topic guide, informed by the Additional file 2. These included to: perceptions of oral health; oral health knowledge and behaviours; barriers to oral care; and oral health promotion initiatives to improve oral health and increase uptake of dental care.

Focus groups lasted up to 35 min and interviews from 30 to 65 min. Interviews/focus groups were arranged until saturation was reached: in total 17 parents were consulted in this study, through a combination of eight individual interviews and four triad interviews.

Data analysis

All data were transcribed and analysed using the 'framework' method by Ritchie and Lewis, 2003 [18]. This iterative process entailed listening to audio recordings and reading transcripts obtained from the first six interviews/focus groups. These initial interviews/focus groups were coded, from which initial categories were identified by three researchers (SN, CK and JEG). Categories and themes were used to construct an initial analytical framework, to which relevant codified sections of interviews/focus groups were added by a single researcher (SN). Subsequent interviews/focus groups were analysed, and the analytical framework modified to reflect additional emergent themes, followed by creation of a summary framework matrix. Finally, data interpretation was performed to distil the content and meaning of the data into underlying theoretical principles, with construction of typologies to broadly define and explain the differing views within the sample population.

Results

Approximately 80 parents were provided with a summary of the study, half of whom declined to receive any further information, most commonly citing lack of time due to work commitments. It was also apparent that a small sub-group of parents had challenging personal circumstances that rendered their lives too chaotic to consider participating in this study. Amongst the 40 parents who did voice initial interest in participation, approximately 20 parents were lost due to the requirement for parents to spend at least 24 h considering their potential participation before being contacted again by researchers, in line with ethics committee stipulations. Eight parents participated in individual interviews and nine in triad interviews/small focus groups.

Participant demographics

Interviews/focus groups were performed until a representative sample was obtained, and saturation was reached with respect to the views and ideas expressed by informants. In total 17 individuals participated in this research, comprising 15 mothers, one father and one grandmother. Available demographic information for all informants is summarised in Table 1. Approximately 50% of the study informants were first generation migrant parents who had not been raised in the UK. In presenting the findings, parents will be denoted with the abbreviation 'P' and the grandparent with 'GP', females as [F] and the male informant as [M].

A community with divergent perspectives of oral health

In common with many inner-city environments, the population of this South London community is characterised by the diversity of its residents, with respect to ethnicity, socio-economic status and cultural background. This diversity is reflected in the study sample and the spectrum of attitudes, views and beliefs that were encountered throughout this study. At either end of this spectrum were two distinct views of oral health and patterns of oral health behaviours (Fig. 1). 'Oral Health Prioritisers' were motivated by the underlying

Table 1 Demographic details of informants participating in individual interviews and triad focus groups

Gender	Number
Females	16
Males	1
Age group	
25–34	9
35–44	6
45–54	1
55–64	1
Relationship to children	
Parent	16
Grandparent	1
Ethnicity	
White British	3
Black (Unspecified)	6
Black (African)	5
Black (British)	1
North African	1
South American	1
Residence	
Within the estate	6
In close proximity to estate	11
Number of children	
1	5
2	9
3	1
4	1
5	1

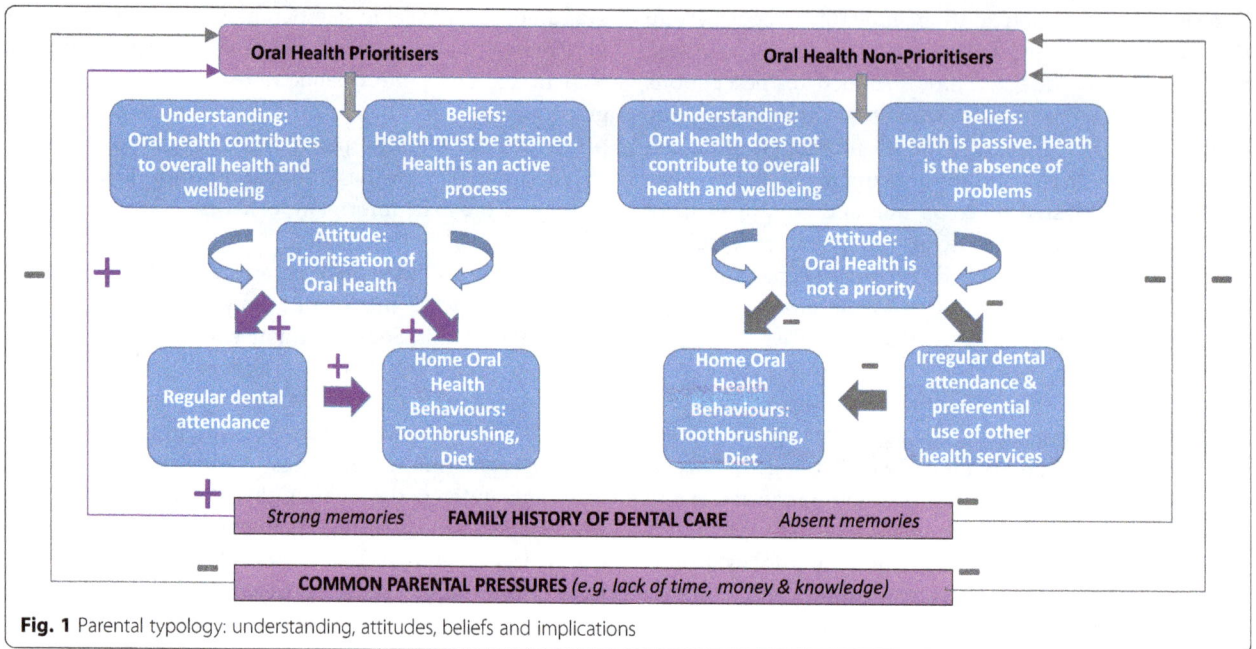

Fig. 1 Parental typology: understanding, attitudes, beliefs and implications

belief that oral health forms an integral component of a child's overall health and wellbeing, attained through specific habits, routines and behaviours, as summarised by one mother:

> *[It's] The food you eat, the drinks you drink and the way you brush your teeth* (P12[F], 9.422)

In contrast, 'Oral Health Non-prioritisers' considered oral health to be unrelated to a child's overall health and wellbeing, believing oral health to be synonymous with lack of symptoms, notably pain. These views were exemplified by one respondent who had lived in the community for 10 years and had not taken their children to a dentist:

> *I just think the dentist is a bit ... [low priority] ... to be honest with you I don't know where the dentist is* (P2[M], 2.072)

Oral Health Prioritisers were often critical of Oral Health Non-prioritisers, attributing their behaviour to lack of care for their children, or even laziness. One grandmother suggested that dental anxiety may contribute to the irregular dental attendance of Oral Health Non-prioritisers, although she did not feel this excused their behaviour:

> *It's probably not a case of not wanting to take them, maybe the parents were scared of the dentist themselves...or they were working and could not take them to the dentist, but I am sure there could have been a way that parents could take time out to take the child to the dentist* (GP[F], 8.290)

Selective engagement with health services

Parental perceptions of oral health made an important contribution to use and knowledge of local dental services, with contrasting dental attendance patterns between Oral Health Non-prioritisers and Oral Health Prioritisers. The effects of lower overall health literacy and health awareness amongst Oral Health Non-prioritisers, compared with Oral Health Prioritisers, were evident with respect to dental attendance. There was lack of awareness of professional preventive dental care amongst Oral Health Non-prioritisers, with some parents never having been to the dentist, or only having visited the dentist for the first time during adulthood. There was a common assumption that dental services in London are predominantly private, acting to reinforce the belief that dental care is a non-essential health service, which should only be accessed for specific problems. Oral Health Non-prioritisers described dental visits in the context of being 'forced' to go and discussed costs of dental care in terms of 'fear':

> *...most of them are private. So... you are scared* (P2[M], 2.102)

One mother, who had never been to the dentist, considered private care to be a major obstacle to seeking dental care, even when in pain:

> *...if I don't have enough money to go to the private dentists, that means even if I'm in pain I prefer taking paracetamol* (P16[F], 12.309)

Some Oral Health Non-prioritisers also cited the practicalities of accessing dental care as a substantial barrier to accessing dental care. One mother, aware of her family's entitlement to free dental care and of the notion of attending the dentist for a 'check-up', had only taken one of her five children to the dentist:

It's important to go to the check-up, but I never go...
I'm busy that's why. (P11[F], 7.258-7.260)

In theory, these barriers (with the exception of cost) could be applicable to all preventive health services within the community. Nevertheless, all Oral Health Non-prioritisers in this study described voluntarily engaging with community baby clinics and children's centres for preventive care and advice. It was apparent that Oral Health Non-prioritisers restricted their engagement to a limited number of key health services they considered most beneficial to their children's health. The perceived irrelevance of oral health to overall health/wellbeing rendered dental care a low priority service.

The importance of underlying belief systems is underscored by the fact that the majority of Oral Health Prioritisers interviewed described a range of barriers to accessing dental care. These included: concern about the costs of NHS care; being advised that routine NHS care was only available privately; lack of space in dental practices for children's buggies; suboptimal communication from members of the dental team; adverse treatment outcomes; and difficulty obtaining appointments during school holidays. Despite these barriers to care, Oral Health Prioritisers described patterns of regular dental attendance for their families, suggesting that beliefs regarding the importance of oral health were a critical determinant of dental attendance.

The power of history
Investigation of parents' perceptions of oral health and oral health behaviours highlighted the critical influence of past experiences. It was apparent that parents considered their own childhood experiences to be a key driver of their current behaviours. Many Oral Health Prioritisers attributed their good oral health behaviours to repeating and copying the actions of their own parents, as described by one mother:

... every six months we went... all of us went to the
dentist and we always brushed our teeth morning and
night and that's the way it was... So that's what I do
with my daughter. (P14[F], L10.116 - 10.118)

Oral Health Prioritisers raised in the UK recounted enjoying dental appointments during childhood, recalling the excitement of leaving school to visit the dentist,

although there were also negative memories such as having treatment under 'gas and air' which inevitably meant that they would have had teeth removed under general anaesthetic or sedation. Some Oral Health Prioritiser migrant parents reported adapting their childhood routines to their new environment and resources, as described by one mother raised in West Africa. She had implemented a strict routine of regular dental visits and twice-daily supervised toothbrushing regime for her children, attributing her current fastidiousness to her own childhood experiences:

...I encourage [children] to clean their teeth, which
sometimes is not easy...I said to [son], you are so lucky,
you've got toothbrush, you've got toothpaste...I can
remember... we go overnight, after they've cooked with
the wood, in the morning the ash is cold and that's
what they will give you to go and scrub your teeth,
and you scrub your teeth until they are squeaky clean.
(P7[F], L4.014-4.018)

Repetition and copying of childhood experiences was also observed amongst Oral Health Non-prioritisers, with none of these parents reporting a history of regular dental attendance during their own childhoods. Indeed, amongst many parents there was a complete absence of childhood memories of home oral care or dental attendance, whether positive or negative. Lack of positive oral health behaviours during their own childhoods reassured some Oral Health Non-prioritisers that their current behaviours would not be detrimental to their child's health. Other parents felt that changing some elements of their own childhood experiences would be sufficient. One mother with a childhood history of irregular dental attendance summarised her feelings by saying:

... I guess, to be honest, I don't see [visiting the dentist]
as a priority now. As long as I know that I'm doing
what needs to be done in terms of brushing ... Yeah, it's
not really much of a priority (P15[F], L11.097)

The need for OHP initiatives
All informants, whether Oral Health Prioritisers or Oral Health Non-prioritisers, demonstrated limitations in their oral health knowledge. In fact, an inverse relationship between parents' self-perceived oral health knowledge and objective knowledge was evident. For example, many parents described limitations in their knowledge about toothbrushing, yet provided detailed descriptions of their family's twice-daily brushing regimens. In contrast, the majority of parents reported confidence in their dietary knowledge yet probing of dietary practices revealed large gaps in knowledge, with descriptions consistent with children consuming diets with high cariogenic

potential. Many parents found it challenging to restrict sugar, making reference to others, particularly grandparents and family friends, providing sweets; teachers using sweets to reward pupils; or children simply having a 'sweet-tooth'. Moreover, some parents demonstrated confusion about the role of sugar, as described by one parent:

> *Well sugar is not good, but kids need sugar to grow* (P2[M], L2.055)

Consumption of fruit juices was prevalent amongst the majority of families in this study, with fruit juices perceived as preferable to carbonated drinks, as described by one Oral Health Prioritiser mother:

> *What they need to do is open more juice bar things or even in schools, have a little juice bar, say try this, try this, you can give out samples, let the kids decide what they like.* (P1[F], L1.206)

Discussion about dental visits also revealed that although the children of some informants had no caries experience, others across the spectrum of behaviours, knowledge and beliefs, from Oral Health Prioritisers to Oral Health Non-prioritisers, made reference to their children requiring fillings or other operative dental treatment.

The importance of connecting – Making a difference

All participating parents acknowledged that OHP initiatives would be of most benefit if they adopted a systems approach, encompassing a range of health and social care services. The power of such an approach (both formal and informal) was apparent through the stories of parents who had transitioned from being an Oral Health Non-prioritiser to an Oral Health Prioritiser. For example, one migrant mother was hospitalised when she initially arrived in the UK, bringing her into contact with social workers. Their assistance facilitated engagement with primary care health services, and some two decades later, she attributed her health awareness and positive health behaviours to this early support. Another mother with a history of symptomatic dental attendance recalled a passing comment from her General Medical Practitioners (GMP) regarding registering her two-year old daughter with the dentist:

> *I think the GP told me to... and they registered her, and they said we need to go to have the first appointment so that's why I went. (P10[F], 6.122)*

After this initial appointment with the dentist, the family developed a routine of regular dental appointments, demonstrating the utility of informal OHP for increasing uptake of dental care and fostering positive oral health behaviours.

Lack of oral health literacy amongst first-time parents

Whilst parents in the community had diverse views on specific OHP initiatives, there was clear sentiment on who should be targeted by OHP initiatives, namely first-time parents. Many informants described the overwhelming nature of being a first-time parent, with lack of information forcing parents to rely on instincts and 'common-sense'. The majority were unsure about the correct age to start brushing their children's teeth, or when the first dental visit should be made. As a consequence, parents reported that first-born children often had their first dental visit much later than younger siblings.

Parents felt that dietary advice was more readily available for first-time parents, with health visitors and children's centres being an important source of information. Parents with minimal contact with dentists were often reliant on health visitors and GMPs for oral health information, although the extent and standard of information provided was variable, as described by one young mother:

> *... I don't think there was a discussion [with the health visitor] about the dentist...because he was quite young then...in my mind anyway, you don't really think he needs to start going to the dentist when he's a baby, so yeah, that was it, it was more about brushing and how many times to brush and that kind of thing* (P15, L11.006)

How to support first-time parents

Preference for a systems approach encompassing GMPs, health visitors, children's centres, baby clinics and pharmacies was common amongst parents. Notably, there was little mention of desire for increased support from dentists themselves. This was particularly evident amongst parents who had little engagement with dental professionals and services. Many parents welcomed the idea of increased written information in the form of posters and leaflets, with distribution in antenatal classes, baby clinics/immunisation centres and children's centres. Parents also favoured OHP delivered in group settings in baby clinics and children's centres, enabling them to establish support networks with other parents, and perceiving this approach to be less intimidating than information delivered via health visitors in their own homes.

A critical role for schools

Parents suggested a wide range of OHP initiatives they felt would benefit their community, and similar communities, and a summary of views is provided in Table 2. Participants were keen for schools to be at the epicentre of

Table 2 Summary of parental views on different OHP initiatives

OHP initiative	Level of parental support High = Majority support Medium = Support for initiative, with caveats Low = Lack of overall support	Summary of parental views
Improving oral health		
Fluoride Varnish Schemes	High	• Lack of awareness of fluoride varnish amongst the majority of parents • Most parents supported idea after initiative summarised • Parents keen for implementation via schools rather than in the community.
School-based toothbrushing clubs	Medium	• Most parents felt initiative would help busy parents • Concerns about infection control amongst parents with highest levels of health awareness • Some concerns about potential for disruption on lessons. • Many parents reported more problems with toothbrushing at weekends (due to loss of normal routine) than during school-days
School dental education sessions	Medium	• Likely to have an impact as children more receptive to information delivered by external speakers (e.g. dentists, dental nurses/hygienists, dental students) than their parents • Sessions must be interactive to engage pupils • Sessions will only have a transient effect if parents are not sufficiently involved
Dental education sessions for parents	Medium	• Parents are always keen for information that may benefit that child's health and wellbeing • Lack of time to attend during working-hours • Community drop-in sessions suggested, but may not attract many parents
Healthy eating initiatives in schools	High	• Concern about unhealthy school dinners and use of sweets/chocolates to reward pupils • Initiative does not target fast-food outlets in close proximity to local schools
Increasing uptake of dental care		
School-based dental screening	High	• The only method of ensuring all children are seen by a dentist • UK-raised parents who recalled dental screening in their childhoods very supportive of reintroduction
Distribution of dental passports	High	• Simple but effective method, as frames dental visits in a positive way • Distribution through schools is easiest method
Text message reminders	High	• Would encourage preventive dental care • Should come via schools, as many already operate a text messaging service

community-wide OHP initiatives, with readily available access to all school-age children, and minimal disruption for busy parents. School dental screening was popular, and considered by many the most equitable method of increasing uptake of dental care, for others, as summarised by one grandmother on behalf of the community:

Because some children just didn't go to the dentist. And somebody needed to help those children whose mums couldn't be bothered to get off their bottoms and take their child to the dentist (GP1, 8.288)

Initiatives to increase exposure to fluoride via toothbrushing and fluoride varnish schemes were broadly

supported, although there were contrasting views on the practicalities of toothbrushing schemes, particularly in relation to infection control:

...because they are taught to be so independent in school it freaks me out a bit that my son would pick up someone else's toothbrush and use it (P6 [F], L3.102)

It is a good idea. Everybody's got their own toothbrushes ... let's say they're doing PE... everybody's got their PE kit, everybody knows their PE kit. So it's the same, everybody's got their toothbrush, everybody knows their toothbrush, so that is a good idea (P7[F], L4.118)

Overall, many parents felt that additional support from schools was critical to supplement their personal efforts to implement positive oral and general health behaviours, due to the considerable pressures of family life, common in this and similar communities, as described by one mother:

...we have got enough as mothers to, you know, deal with at home. And you know you can be mum, you can be dad, you know, you are the referee, so it's nice that, you know, school do back up what you are saying at home (P6[F], L3.043)

Discussion

This pilot study has identified two distinct groups of parents within this inner-city community. One group (termed Oral Health Prioritisers) considered oral health to be attainable through a combination of diet, oral hygiene and regular dental attendance, whilst the other (termed Oral Health Non-prioritisers) considered oral health to be synonymous with an absence of symptoms and reported irregular patterns of dental attendance.

Lack of familiarity with preventive dental care has previously been reported amongst migrant mothers in Australia [19], and this present study reflects this finding to an extent. Some first-generation migrant parents participating in focus groups were surprised to learn they could take their children to a dentist for preventive care as well as interventive treatment. Similarly amongst some non-migrant parents there was no awareness of professionally delivered preventive care. On the other hand, some first-generation migrant parents reported having implemented strict oral care regimens for their children, with respect to diet, oral hygiene and dental attendance. Clearly, factors beyond migration patterns have shaped the two distinct perspectives of oral health observed in this study.

Within this community, the decisive factor appeared to be whether parents believed oral health to be a component of their child's overall health and wellbeing. All parents described a clear desire to create healthy lives for their children, and for Oral Health Prioritisers' oral health was perceived to be a component of systemic health. In contrast, Oral Health Non-prioritisers considered oral health to be entirely distinct from overall health and wellbeing and accorded little priority to oral health. Oral Health Non-prioritisers were willing to engage with preventive services relating to systemic health (via children's centres and baby clinics) but rarely, if ever, reported engaged with local dental services.

The beliefs and actions of these two groups of parents were reportedly shaped by past events, especially childhood experiences. It has been observed that negative experiences of dental care during childhood may manifest during adulthood, through parents delaying dental treatment for themselves and their children [20]. In our study, a striking absence of any memories relating to childhood dental visits was observed amongst Oral Health Non-prioritisers. In contrast, Oral Health Prioritisers had strong memories of childhood dental appointments, and whilst primarily positive, some were negative. Crucially, all parents reporting a history of regular dental attendance during childhood were Oral Health Prioritisers. This finding underlines the importance of parenting skills and encouraging early access to dental care for families, as childhood dental attendance patterns strongly shape attendance patterns during adulthood [21].

Both groups of parents identified additional barriers to dental attendance that have previously been documented in the literature [22]. These included time, cost, dental anxiety, concerns about availability of NHS care and poor communication from the dental team. Notably, language was not identified as a particular barrier to accessing dental care, although this may reflect the study methodology, as some parents with weaker English language skills were reluctant to participate in focus groups/interviews. This study has also highlighted the importance of community consultation for understanding local barriers, which may otherwise remain undiscovered. Within this community, there were specific concerns regarding the visibility of local practices, their size and the difficulties of taking pushchairs/buggies into these facilities.

The potential for some parents to 'transition' from being a Non-prioritiser to an Oral Health Prioritiser is an interesting finding in this pilot. Supporting a positive transition is critical to increase uptake of dental care and improve oral health and requires further exploration. Equally important, is the observation that no parents reported the converse; however, given the small numbers involved, caution should be exercised. The discovery of two distinct groups of parents within this community suggests that whilst it may be possible to direct some initiatives towards the whole community, most likely through schools and the wider health and social care systems, tailored initiatives will also be needed for those who don't prioritise dental care. Particularly as OHP initiatives in dental practices will have little scope to reach Oral Health Non-prioritisers who rarely access dental services; first-born children may have delayed presentation to the dentist compared with younger siblings; and, parents will not have access to school initiatives until their firstborn is around 5 years of age.

In this context, the potential benefits of a systems approach are suggested by these findings, harnessing the influence of children's centres, schools, GMPs and other health professionals to signpost dental services and embed

OHP initiatives within the community. This approach is in accordance with current national and international health promotion programmes. Positive early experience is recognised as vital to ensure children are ready to learn, ready for school and have good life chances [23], and it is vitally important to make an overt link to dental services in support of socially deprived families.

This group of parents considered schools as significant resource for supporting oral health, an approach for which there is much support. The World Health Organisation (WHO) has identified schools as a critical setting for health promotion, enabling targeting of not only students, but the wider community of staff and parents [24]. Their Global School Health Initiative promotes the concept of 'Health Promoting Schools', with oral health promotion a key aspect of this initiative due to the high global burden of preventable dental disease, and shared risk factors for oral and systemic disease [24]. Moreover, national programmes within the UK such as ChildSmile in Scotland [25], and Designed to Smile in Wales [26], have demonstrated the feasibility and efficacy of OHP programmes that combine community initiatives with nursery and school-based programmes. This systems approach may have the added benefit of protecting individual services from excessive additional workloads, as areas of deprivation often exhibit an inverse care law, where there is a mismatch between the high needs for healthcare and supply of healthcare [27]. Residents in the most deprived communities are more likely to have multiple co-morbidities and psychosocial problems [27], resulting in complex health needs that may be best managed with multidisciplinary input.

One final consideration with respect to designing OHP initiatives is the possibility of additional sub-groups within this community that were not reached within this study. A plausible extension of the typologies defined in this study would be a third group of parents who appear to neglect both oral and systemic health, so-called 'Health Non-prioritisers'. The current findings should therefore be tested on larger samples across a range of inner-city culturally diverse settings to gain deeper understanding of parents' views and supportive action. The methods used in this study may have created an inherent bias, whereby parents who pay little heed to health and wellbeing do not use services where study recruitment was undertaken, have little interest in engaging with health researchers or participating in community consultation, or, have lives that are too chaotic to find time to participate in an interview or focus group when approached through schools. This group of parents undoubtedly represents those most in need of support via OHP initiatives and it would seem likely that a systems approach could assist with reaching this group of families.

Limitations and strengths of study

This study presents the findings of interviews and focus groups with 17 parents in an inner city South London community. Whilst this is a relatively small sample size, it exceeds the acceptable size for hard to reach groups [28], and robust qualitative research [29]. Whilst there were informants from the main ethnic groups on the estate, younger parents, aged 16–24 years, did not participate despite efforts to recruit these individuals; younger parents may have specific views and beliefs that are not represented in this study. The lack of male participants is also acknowledged, although it is noted that the vast majority of primary caregivers encountered by the researchers in this community were female. Whilst parents with limited English language skills were invited to participate in this study, it is accepted that parents with the most limited English language skills may also have been deterred from participating in this research due to its qualitative nature. Future research should enable interviews to be undertaken in their mother tongue or via a translator, either of which has resource implications.

Research exploring oral health in inner city communities tends to focus on specific ethnic or cultural groups; this study provides insight on review of the attitudes and beliefs shaping participant's oral health behaviours, and as such, many of the findings may be applicable to other diverse inner-city communities. Whilst these results provide insight to the perceptions and beliefs of those interviewed, further research is required to test and develop these findings to provide more generalisable insights. Future studies, exploring such issues, should gain ethical consent to interview parents when they are approached, and found to be willing and interested to participate, rather than arranging appointments to do so. These parents should of course be able to withdraw their data within an agreed time frame if they change their minds, without giving a reason.

Conclusion

In conclusion, the evidence from this pilot study suggests that sub-groups within this inner-city area may place different emphases on oral health. None-the-less, participating parents favour a systems approach to OHP initiatives, involving a range of health and social care services, including a critcal role for schools, and actively connecting with first-time parents. These approaches may assist in reaching families who rarely engage with dental services and enable specific OHP initiatives to be delivered within this community. The findings provide the basis for further research.

Acknowledgements
The authors would like to recognise the support given by participating parents, primary schools and children centres and the work of Chris Hadfield, Well London Phase 2 Project Co-ordinator for this Vauxhall Gardens scheme.

Funding
The Vauxhall Gardens Well London initiative was funded from Big Lottery Funding through the London Mayoral Office, the University of East London and Lambeth Local Authority, all of which were represented on the Steering Group for the Vauxhall Gardens Project, supporting its conduct, funding and overseeing the practical actions arising from this community engagement. The following researchers were funded by their respective organisations King's College London (JEG), King's College Hospital NHS Foundation Trust (SN) and London Health Education England/Public Health England (CK) for their contribution to the research. GF received dual funding from University of East London and the Big Lottery.
In summary, Big Lottery Funding therefore directly supported GF's contribution to the research from design of the study, interpretation of data, redrafting of the manuscript and the additional costs of the fieldwork through KCL (refreshments and transcription). KCL and the NHS therefore largely supported the design of the study and collection, analysis, and interpretation of data and in writing the manuscript.

Authors' contributions
JEG and CK designed this study; GF who leads the evaluation of Well London initiatives, provided advice and support on this nested oral health study within the wider programme of research and interpretation of the data; SN and CK performed fieldwork; SN, CK and JEG analysed the data and produced the initial draft of the manuscript. All authors (JEG, CK, SN, GF) have contributed to redrafting of the manuscript, have approved the final version and are accountable for this work.

Authors' information
Shalini Nayee is a former Dental Core Trainee and researcher on this project. Charlotte Klass is a former specialty trainee in Dental Public Health and honorary researcher. Professor Findlay, the Well London Lead overall and for this project is Director of Health Improvement at the Institute for Health and Human Development, University of East London. Professor Jenny Gallagher, the dental and local operational lead for this Well London Phase 2 project, is Newland-Pedley Professor of Oral Health Strategy, Honorary Consultant in Dental Public Health and Dean for International Affairs.

Competing interests
Both academic departments (UEL and KCL) have received funding for Well London initiatives. Staff at UEL conceived the Well London initiative, bid for resources and were involved in running and evaluating the programmes across London (GF). JEG at KCLDI received Big Lottery funding via Lambeth LA to run the Vauxhall Gardens Phase II initiative and support this exploratory fieldwork.

Author details
[1]King's College London Dental Institute, Population and Patient Health Division, Denmark Hill, London SE5 9RS, UK. [2]Institute for Health and Human Development, University of East London Stratford Campus, Water Lane, London E12 4LZ, UK.

References
1. Marmot M, Allen J, Bell R, Bloomer E, Goldblatt P. WHO European review of social determinants of health and the health divide. Lancet. 2012;380(9846):1011–29. (1474-547X (Electronic)). https://doi.org/10.1016/S0140-6736(12)61228-8.
2. Poortinga W. The prevalence and clustering of four major lifestyle risk factors in an English adult population. Prev Med. 2007;44(2):124–8. (0091-7435 (Print))
3. Cattell V. Poor people, poor places, and poor health: the mediating role of social networks and social capital. Soc Sci Med. 2001;52(10):1501–16. (0277-9536 (Print))
4. Hanson CL, Allin LJ, Ellis JG, Dodd-Reynolds CJ. An evaluation of the efficacy of the exercise on referral scheme in Northumberland, UK: association with physical activity and predictors of engagement. A naturalistic observation study. BMJ Open. 2013; https://doi.org/10.1136/bmjopen-2013-002849.
5. Greater London Authority. London Borough Profiles. 2013. https://bmjopen.bmj.com/content/bmjopen/3/8/e002849.full.pdf.
6. Public Health England. Oral health survey of three-year-old children 2013. A report on the prevalence and severity of dental decay; 2014. http://www.nwph.net/dentalhealth/survey-results%203(12_13).aspx.
7. Public Health England. National Dental Epidemiology Programme for England: oral health survey of five-year-old children 2012. A report on the prevalence and severity of dental decay; 2013. http://www.nwph.net/dentalhealth/survey-results5.aspx?id=1.
8. NHS Dental Statistics for England 2012-2013. http://www.hscic.gov.uk/catalogue/PUB10871.
9. Penchansky R, Thomas JW. The concept of access: definition and relationship to consumer satisfaction. Med Care. 1981;19(2):127–40. (0025-7079 (Print))
10. The Royal College of Surgeons of England. Report on the State of Children's Oral Health. Faculty of Dental Surgery. 2015. In. https://www.rcseng.ac.uk/library-and-publications/rcs-publications/docs/report-childrens-oral-health/.
11. Moles DR, Ashley P. Hospital admissions for dental care in children: England 1997-2006. Br Dent J. 2009;206(7):E14. (1476-5373 (Electronic))
12. England PH. Delivering better oral health: an evidence-based toolkit for prevention. Third ed; 2014.
13. Passalacqua A, Reeves AO, Newton T, Hughes R, Dunne S, Donaldson N, Wilson N. An assessment of oral health promotion programmes in the United Kingdom. Eur J Dent Educ. 2012;16(1):e19–26. (1600-0579 (Electronic))
14. Better Health for London. https://www.london.gov.uk/sites/default/files/better_health_for_london.pdff.
15. Scambler S, Klass C, Wright D, Gallagher JE. Insights into the oral health beliefs and practices of mothers from a north London Orthodox Jewish community. BMC Oral Health. 2010;10:14. (1472-6831 (Electronic))
16. Well London: communities working together for a healthier city. http://www.welllondon.org.uk/.
17. Vauxhall Gardens Estate (Phase 2 Programme). http://www.welllondon.org.uk/1111/lambeth-vauxhall-gardens-estate.html.
18. Gale NK, Heath G, Cameron E, Rashid S, Redwood S. Using the framework method for the analysis of qualitative data in multi-disciplinary health research. BMC Med Res Methodol. 2013;18:13–117. (1471-2288 (Electronic))
19. Riggs E, Gussy M, Gibbs L, van Gemert C, Waters E, Kilpatrick N. Hard to reach communities or hard to access services? Migrant mothers' experiences of dental services. Aust Dent J. 2014;59(2):201–7. (1834-7819 (Electronic))
20. Smith PA, Freeman R. Remembering and repeating childhood dental treatment experiences: parents, their children, and barriers to dental care. Int J Paediatr Dent. 2010;20(1):50–8. (1365-263X (Electronic))
21. Listl S. Inequalities in dental attendance throughout the life-course. J Dent Res. 2012;91(7 Suppl):91S–7S. (1544-0591 (Electronic))
22. Hill KB, Chadwick B, Freeman R, O'Sullivan I, Murray JJ. Adult Dental Health Survey 2009: relationships between dental attendance patterns, oral health behaviour and the current barriers to dental care. Br Dent J. 2013;(1):214, 25–32. (1476-5373 (Electronic))
23. Public Health England. Health matters: giving every child the best start in life. 5th ed. London: PHE; 2016.
24. Jurgensen N, Petersen PE. Promoting oral health of children through schools–results from a WHO global survey 2012. Community Dent Health. 2013;30(4):204–18. (0265-539X (Print))
25. Macpherson LM, Ball GE, King P, Chalmers K, Gnich W. Childsmile: the child oral health improvement programme in Scotland. Prim Dent J. 2015;4(4):33–7. (2050-1684 (Print))
26. Howells L. Designed to smile–tackling caries in young children in Wales. Prim Dent J. 2015;4(4):20–1. (2050-1684 (Print)). http://www.designedtosmile.org/
27. Mercer SW, Watt GC. The inverse care law: clinical primary care encounters in deprived and affluent areas of Scotland. Ann Fam Med. 2007;5(6):503–10. (1544-1717 (Electronic))
28. Baker SE, Edwards R, Doidge M. How many qualitative interviews is enough?: Expert voices and early career reflections on sampling and cases in qualitative research. 2012.

8

Visual and radiographic caries detection: a tailored meta-analysis for two different settings, Egypt and Germany

Falk Schwendicke[1*], Karim Elhennawy[1], Osama El Shahawy[2,3], Reham Maher[2,3], Thais Gimenez[4], Fausto M. Mendes[4] and Brian H. Willis[5]

Abstract

Background: Diagnostic meta-analyses on caries detection methods should assist practitioners in their daily practice. However, conventional meta-analysis estimates may be inapplicable due to differences in test conduct, applied thresholds and assessed population between settings. Our aim was to demonstrate the impact of tailored meta-analysis of visual and radiographic caries detection to different settings using setting-specific routine data.

Methods: Published systematic reviews and meta-analyses on the accuracy of visual and radiographic caries detection were used. In two settings (a private practice in Germany and a public health clinic in Egypt), routine data of a total of 100 (n = 50/practice) consecutive 12–14 year-olds were collected. Test-positive rates of visual and radiographic detection for initial and advanced carious lesions on occlusal or proximal surfaces of molars were used to tailor meta-analyses. If prevalence data were available, these were also used for tailoring.

Results: From the original reviews, 210 and 100 heterogeneous studies on visual and radiographic caries detection were included in our meta-analyses. For radiographic detection, sensitivity and specificity estimates derived from conventional and tailored meta-analysis were similar. For visual detection of advanced occlusal carious lesions, the conventional meta-analysis yielded a sensitivity and specificity (95% CI) of 64.6% (57–71) and 90.9% (88–93), whereas the tailored estimates for Egypt were 75.1% (70–81) and 84.9% (82–89), respectively, and 43.7% (37–51) and 96.5% (95–97) for Germany, respectively.

Conclusion: Conventional test accuracy meta-analyses may yield aggregate estimates which are inapplicable to specific settings. Routine data may be used to produce a meta-analysis estimate which is tailored to the setting and thereby improving its applicability.

Keywords: Caries detection, Decision making, Diagnostic accuracy studies, Evidence-based dentistry, Medical informatics

Background

To detect carious lesions, dentists can use a number of methods, namely visual or visual-tactile detection, radiography, or further methods employing, for example, laser-fluorescence or near-infrared light. The accuracy of the methods is measured in terms of their sensitivity and specificity. The more sensitive methods allow the detection of early lesions, which facilitates non- or

micro-invasive treatment [1, 2], but they can also lead to over-detection and overtreatment. The risks of over- and under-detection further depend on the chosen cut-off for a positive result and how the test is conducted [3–6] – does one practitioner look or search more intently for lesions than another for instance?

Theoretically, the sensitivity and specificity, and hence risks of over- and under-detection, may be determined by a Diagnostic Accuracy Study (DAS). However, DAS may vary significantly in how visual or radiographic assessment is applied, the threshold for a positive result and the type of target disorder being investigated. The

* Correspondence: falk.schwendicke@charite.de
[1]Department of Operative and Preventive Dentistry, Charité –
Universitätsmedizin Berlin, Aßmannshauser Str. 4-6, 14197 Berlin, Germany
Full list of author information is available at the end of the article

test positive rate (the proportion of those who tested positive in all those tested) captures some of these features.

Moreover, DAS are often performed on different populations (many DAS on caries are performed in vitro), with different prevalence rates and patient case-mixes. This is well recognized and is sometimes described as 'spectrum bias' or more accurately 'spectrum effects' and is known to affect test performances [7]. Diagnostic meta-analysis aims to accommodate this heterogeneity [8], and provides estimates for the average sensitivity, specificity and positive or negative likelihood ratios [3, 6].

However, an average estimate may be unrepresentative of an individual dental practitioner who may use a different threshold, execute the test differently and see a population of patients which is quite different from that represented by the average sensitivity and specificity [3, 6, 9].

In response to this challenge, tailored meta-analysis (TMA) has been developed [10, 11]. Essentially the method combines routine data collected from the setting with the research data from DAS. In particular, routine data can often be collected to estimate the test positive rate and, in some cases, the prevalence. The novel aspect of the method lies in the exploitation of logical relations between the test positive rate, prevalence, sensitivity and specificity. Thus, if the first two are known it allows us to deduce the ranges of values for the sensitivity and specificity, and these may be used to tailor the selection of studies to the setting of interest for meta-analysis. Importantly, when the sensitivity and specificity for a detection method is tailored to the setting of interest this affects the positive and negative predictive values for the test in the setting, which may ultimately affect treatment decisions.

The present study used TMA to estimate the accuracy of visual and radiographic caries detection in two very different settings, Germany and Egypt. As an example, we used a population of 12- to 14-year olds, with caries detection on proximal and occlusal surfaces of permanent molars. We aimed at providing specific accuracy estimates for the two settings, hypothesizing that tailored accuracies differ between settings and from those yielded by conventional meta-analysis.

Methods
Study design
Conventional diagnostic meta-analyses synthesize all available data on a specific detection method. In contrast, TMA synthesizes only those data applying to a specific setting and/or particular examiners, for example with regards to test positive rate or prevalence. The present study performed TMA using three different data sources: (1) Two published systematic reviews and meta-analyses of DASs on visual and radiographic caries

detection; (2) Routine data from a private practice in Germany and a public health clinic in Egypt were collected to estimate the respective test-positive rates; (3) Prevalence data for visually detected occlusal carious lesions were collected for both settings.

These are now discussed below.

Systematic reviews
Details on the systematic review processes have been described elsewhere [3, 6]. Briefly, two reviewers searched PubMed, Embase and Cochrane Central for studies reporting accuracy data on visual [3] or radiographic detection of carious lesions [6]. The included studies reported a reference test (often histological assessment, but also other reference standards like invasive opening of the presumed lesion) to measure the performance of the index test (visual or radiographic detection). Both in vitro (the majority of studies) and clinical studies were included.

For our study, only those studies which reported sufficient data to estimate the sensitivity and specificity of the method for the proximal and/or occlusal surfaces of permanent teeth were considered. We extracted true positive, true negative, false positive and false negative numbers for each study. Data were separately extracted for studies on

1. radiographic or visual caries detection
2. detection of occlusal or proximal surfaces
3. initial and advanced lesions or only advanced lesions

Note that the definition of initial and advanced lesions was not standardized; most studies regarded cavitated lesions or those clinically and/or radiographically extended in dentin as advanced, which left non-cavitated lesions or those confined to enamel as being initial. Such dichotomization is useful, as the threshold of cavitation or dentin involvement is often used to decide between non-invasive (non-operative) and invasive (operative, restorative) treatment.

Overall, eight different subsets of data were extracted (data on visual caries detection on proximal surfaces were later discarded, as accessibility of these surfaces varied widely). As not all of the studies reported on each subset, the number of included studies varied considerably between subsets. The data used for each subset may be found in the Additional file 1.

Routine data collection
For the present study, routine data were defined as data routinely collected on a population of patients without specific scientific purpose. Routine data thus carry the advantage that they will be available from a large range

of settings, (for example claims data) and capture real-life practice. Routine data collection was approved by the local ethics committees (Charité ethics EA2 137/14; Cairo university ethics 16/7/3), and only anonymized aggregated data were used for statistical evaluation.

Over 6 months, routine examination data were collected on 50 consecutive patients aged 12–14 years old attending for a regular dental examination in each of the settings. This age was chosen, as the data were available to estimate the test positive rate and prevalence for 12-year olds in both Germany and Egypt. Patients not falling into this age band or where their data were not fully available (for example due to non-compliance with the diagnostic process) were excluded.

The data were collected by two examiners, one in each setting, and each having more than 15 years of experience in dental practice as well as experience in visual and radiographic lesion detection and evaluation.

The private practice in Germany served approximately 3000 regularly attending patients and was situated in a mid-sized town in rural Northern Germany. Regular epidemiologic surveys indicate comparatively high caries experience in this area [12, 13]. The university clinic in Egypt served approximately 250 patients per day and was situated in Giza, metropolitan region of Cairo.

Visual caries detection on molars was performed using ICDAS criteria [14], with ICDAS scores 1 and 2 being recorded as "initial lesions" and scores 3–6 as "advanced lesions". Tooth cleaning was not routinely performed prior to the assessment, but calculus and plaque were removed if considered to be needed by the dentist. A standard dental mirror (of different manufacturers both within and between practices), a straight-ended dental probe and a 3-in-1 air/water syringe in standard dental chairs (Germany: Dentorest, Ritter, Biberach, Germany; Egypt: Belmont clesta, Takara Belmont, Tokyo, Japan) were used, with teeth being dried during examination. Cotton rolls were not regularly used during examination.

Data on visual detection were recorded only for occlusal surfaces, as visual accessibility of proximal surfaces in this age group varied greatly between patients due to different eruption status of teeth. For sealed teeth, detection was performed as far as the sealant allowed; in most cases, the surface was deemed not assessable. Restored occlusal surfaces were excluded as well. If more than one lesion was detected per occlusal surface, the worst score was recorded.

Radiographic bitewing caries detection was performed for both occlusal and proximal surfaces. In Germany, analogue Kodak Insight films (Eastman Kodak, Rochester, NY, USA) were used. Films were exposed for 0.08 s at 70kVp and 7 mA, and developed in a Dürr Dental XR 24 processing machine (Dürr, Bietigheim-Bissingen, Germany). In Egypt, Kodak Intraoral E-speed films were

exposed for 0.12 s at 70kVp and 7 mA, and manually developed. Films were used in various bitewing holders (this varied across but also within settings, given this being routine application). A scoring system describing lesions in outer and inner enamel (E1, E2) and outer, middle and inner dentin (D1–3) was used. Surfaces not assessable (due to radiographic projection, or restorations or orthodontic bands present) were excluded, as were third molars. Scores were rescored into initial (E1, E2) and advanced lesions (D1-D3). Data on detection of non-occlusal and non-proximal detection were not included.

Thus, for each of the tests (visual inspection or radiography) routine data from each of the two settings were used to describe the number of lesions (initial or advanced) as a proportion of the total number of assessed (occlusal or proximal) surfaces. This enabled an interval estimate for each of the respective test positive rates.

Estimation of the prevalence

For the two settings, we estimated the prevalence rates of visually detected initial and advanced, as well as only advanced occlusal carious lesions. For Germany, data from a city of similar size location and socioeconomic structure and a similar population of rather high risk children were used [15]. We assumed 73% of the reported lesions to be located occlusally [16]. Assuming eight occlusal molar surfaces being present and deducing the reported number of restorations (again assuming 73% being located occlusally) resulted in a tooth-level prevalence of 45% for initial and advanced, and 22% for only advanced lesions, respectively. Note that the assumption of all occlusal lesions being located on molars is a simplification and might lead to some distortion. For Egypt, data on caries experience from Cairo, the metropolis region Giza belongs to, were available [17], with 65% of reported initial and advanced lesions being situated on occlusal surfaces. Again, we assumed the lesions to be distributed among eight occlusal surfaces, which resulted in a tooth-level prevalence of 12.9% for all (initial and advanced) and 8.1% for only advanced lesions, respectively.

Statistical analysis

Willis and Hyde [10, 11] have previously demonstrated that if the test positive rate is known this constrains the region of values that the sensitivity and specificity take in receiver operating characteristic (ROC) space. This region is constrained further if the prevalence is also known. Thus, an *applicable region* for the test sensitivity and specificity may be derived based on the test positive rate and prevalence. In essence, it represents the feasible set of (sensitivity, specificity) pairs for the test given the information we have collected on the test positive rate and prevalence. Furthermore since the test positive rate and prevalence vary with the test (visual or radiography), target disorder (all lesions or only advanced lesions) and setting (Germany and Egypt) the applicable region is particular to the respective combination of these.

After deriving the applicable region, each study is compared with this region by first deriving the maximum likelihood estimate (MLE) for the sensitivity and specificity subject to it being constrained to lie in the applicable region [10, 11]. This is then compared with the observed sensitivity and specificity and low probability studies ($p < 0.025$) are excluded. The resulting tailored set of studies is then aggregated using a bivariate random effects model to derive estimates for the sensitivity and specificity [18] - this is the TMA estimate.

The test positive rate ranges used to derive the applicable region in the TMA corresponded to the 99% confidence intervals derived from the routine data collected from each of the settings. The ranges used for the prevalence rates were based on a plausible interval that contained the point prevalence estimates derived for the setting (Table 1).

There is no reliable statistical method for estimating the level of heterogeneity when using bivariate measures (sensitivity, specificity). However, the ROC plot provides a visual representation of the dispersion of studies which is indicative of the level of heterogeneity.

Results

From the original reviews [3, 6], 210 studies on visual caries detection and 100 studies on radiographic caries detection were included in our meta-analyses (see Additional file 1). Inspection of the ROC plots for the conventional meta-analyses demonstrates widespread dispersion of studies, suggesting that heterogeneity is present in all the analyses as expected. Figures 1 and 2 illustrate this for the radiographic detection of occlusal lesions and the visual detection of advanced occlusal lesions.

From the routine data interval estimates for the test positive rate and prevalence were calculated (Table 1) and these were used to derive an applicable region [10, 11] for each of the tests in Egypt and Germany. This is illustrated for the radiographic detection of occlusal lesions and the visual detection of advanced occlusal lesions in Figs. 1 and 2.

In Fig. 1 the applicable regions for Egypt and Germany are close and overlap in large areas of the ROC space, whereas in Fig. 2 they occupy discrete regions. Thus, the visual detection of advance occlusal lesions in Egypt is likely to have sensitivity and specificity which is in a completely different region of ROC space from that of Germany. Furthermore, from Fig. 2 the conventional point estimate (all studies included) lies between the applicable regions for both Egypt and Germany and is significantly different from the tailored estimate for Germany.

The location of the applicable region in ROC space affects the number of studies included in the tailored meta-analyses and in general, tailoring to the setting reduces the number of studies applicable (Table 2). Thus for the visual detection of all occlusal lesions out of the 67 studies included in the original meta-analysis only 51 studies were applicable to Egypt and only 12 studies were applicable to Germany. This can have profound effects on the estimates for the sensitivity and specificity which are plausible for these two settings.

Table 3 illustrates the effects tailoring has on the likelihood ratios for the test. The most marked differences occur with the visual detection of occlusal lesions. In contrast, radiographic detection is broadly consistent across both settings (Egypt and Germany) and in line with the average estimates when all studies are included.

The positive and negative predictive values (PPV, NPV) for the tests are given in Tables 4 and 5 using the point prevalence estimates for the settings where available. Again the differences between Egypt and Germany are large for visual detection and are driven by the differences in the prevalence and likelihood ratios. A PPV

Table 1 Test positive rate and prevalence rates used in tailored meta-analysis

	Egypt				Germany			
	Test positive rate		Prevalence		Test positive rate		Prevalence	
	Lower limit	Upper limit	Lower limit	Upper limit	Lower limit	Upper limit	Lower limit	Upper limit
Visual detection								
advanced occlusal	0.20	0.33	0.01	0.15	0.05	0.26	0.15	0.30
all occlusal	0.30	0.44	0.05	0.20	0.13	0.28	0.35	0.55
Radiographic detection								
advanced occlusal	0.14	0.26	0.09	0.29	0.06	0.18	0.01	0.21
all occlusal	0.14	0.26	0.09	0.29	0.06	0.19	0.01	0.21
advanced proximal	0.02	0.07			0.03	0.08		
all proximal	0.03	0.08			0.07	0.14		

The lower and upper limits for the test positive rates are 99% confidence interval limits derived from the routine data. The lower and upper limits for the prevalence rates are plausible limits based on a priori point estimates

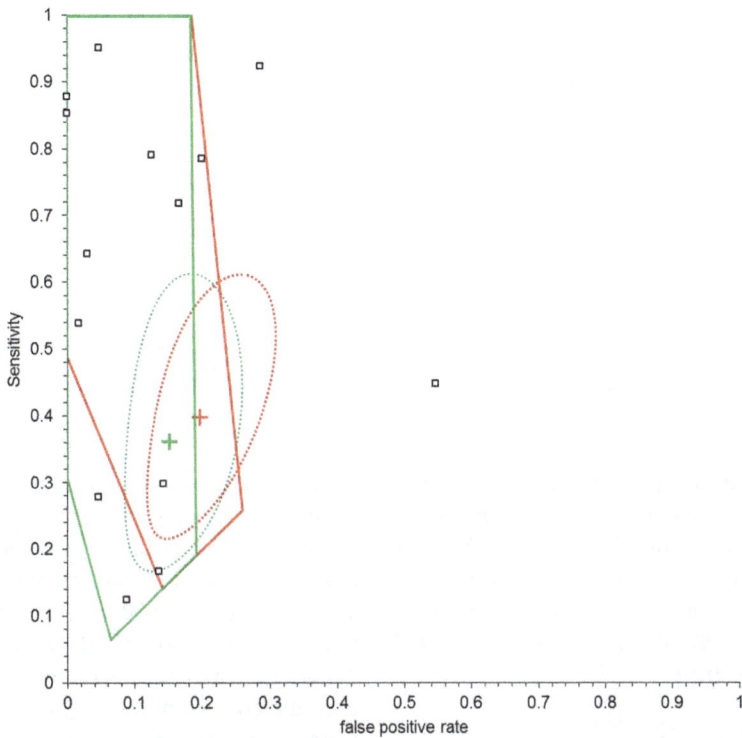

Fig. 1 Comparison of tailored meta-analyses for the radiographic detection of all occlusal lesions for Egypt (red) and Germany (green). Also given are the summary estimates (cross) with the associated 95% confidence ellipses

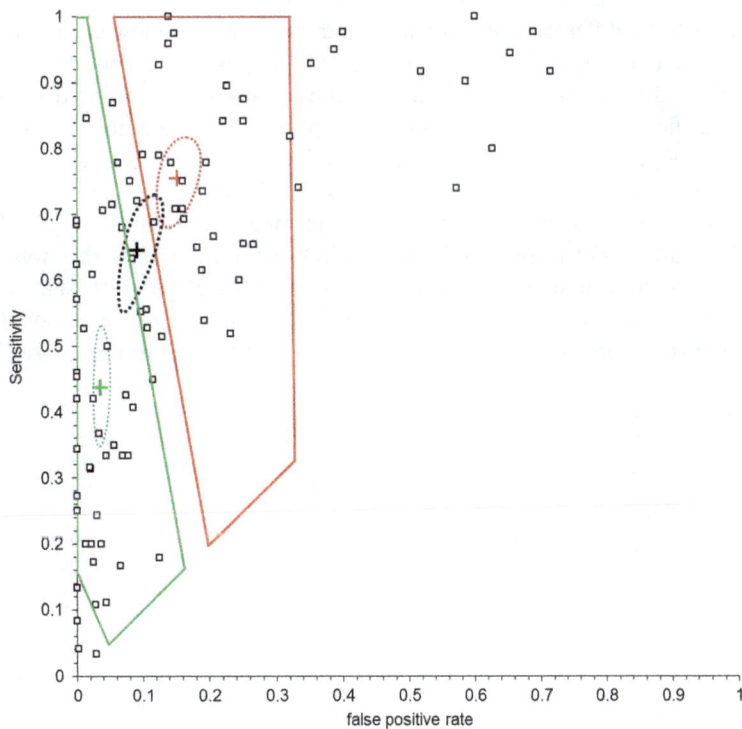

Fig. 2 Comparison of tailored meta-analyses for the visual detection of advanced occlusal lesions for Egypt (red), Germany (green) and the conventional meta-analysis (black). Also given are the summary estimates (cross) with the associated 95% confidence ellipses

Table 2 Mean (95% CI) sensitivity and specificity for all studies, tailored to Egypt and tailored to Germany

	ALL			Egypt			Germany		
	n	Sensitivity	Specificity	n	Sensitivity	Specificity	n	Sensitivity	Specificity
Visual detection									
advanced occlusal	94	64.6% (57–71)	90.9% (88–93)	55	75.1% (70–81)	84.9% (82–89)	50	43.7% (37–51)	96.5% (95–97)
all occlusal	67	85.5% (81–89)	75.3% (70–80)	51	85.8% (82–89)	77.0% (73–81)	12	49.1% (40–58)	91.2% (88–94)
Radiographic detection									
advanced occlusal	44	52.3% (44–60)	89.3% (86–92)	38	54.2% (47–61)	89.1% (86–92)	36	50.8% (43–59)	91.4% (88–94)
all occlusal	14	38.6% (25–54)	77.8% (70–84)	11	39.7% (25–56)	80.4% (72–87)	9	36.0% (20–56)	84.8% (77–90)
advanced proximal	22	44.4% (38–51)	95.5% (94–97)	22	44.4% (38–51)	95.5% (94–97)	22	44.4% (38–51)	95.5% (94–97)
all proximal	38	43.2% (36–51)	90.0% (87–92)	31	40.2% (32–48)	92.5% (91–94)	34	40.5% (33–48)	91.7% (90–93)

n = number of studies

of 82% for visual detection of all occlusal lesions in the German setting suggests it should be used for ruling in occlusal lesions when the test is positive, whilst in Egypt the same test performs with a PPV of 36%. In contrast, a negative test result is more useful to clinicians in Egypt (NPV = 97%) compared with an NPV of 69% in the German setting.

Discussion

When identifying carious lesions, general dental practitioners are faced with a specific patient population, where the prevalence rates of different lesions (and stages) are not always represented by those obtained from individual studies. Moreover, each practitioner will apply methods differently, yielding different test positive rates in the hands of different dentists. As a result, the PPV and/or NPV from a DAS are possibly very different from those found in a specific practice. The resulting over- and under-detection have implications both on a clinical and a public health level [4, 5].

When deciding if and how to apply a caries detection method, dentists should be cautious not to solely rely on the aggregate estimates from conventional diagnostic test meta-analyses particularly if there is widespread heterogeneity, as the implicit assumption of 'one-size fits all' may be untenable. The heterogeneity [19] stemming from factors like study design, test execution, threshold and patient spectrum can be generally described. However, it is difficult to determine which factors are responsible for the result of heterogeneity between DAS, and these cannot be addressed by conventional meta-analysis. Tailored meta-analysis circumvents this by using information directly from the setting of interest to determine which sub-group of studies are likely to reflect the performance in that setting.

We used tailored meta-analysis to assess whether the summary estimate of all DAS included in conventional meta-analysis is accurate in a setting such as Germany or Egypt. Including setting-specific test positive rates and prevalence allowed us to tailor our diagnostic meta-analysis. We showed that for visual detection of occlusal lesions the tailored meta-analysis estimates for Egypt and Germany do not coincide whereas for radiographic detection they do. This may have a number of reasons. First, test conduct may differ, starting from who performed the examinations (both visual and radiographically) and how exactly this was done. Obviously, these aspects will not be 100% standardized even under controlled settings, and it is impossible to standardize them across settings in routine care. Tailoring meta-analysis

Table 3 Mean (95% CI) Positive and Negative Likelihood Ratios (LR) for all studies, tailored to Egypt and tailored to Germany

	ALL			Egypt			Germany		
	n	Positive LR	Negative LR	n	Positive LR	Negative LR	n	Positive LR	Negative LR
Visual detection									
advanced occlusal	94	7.09 (5.6–8.9)	0.39 (0.3–0.5)	55	5.0 (4.3–5.8)	0.29 (0.2–0.4)	50	12.5 (9.2–16.9)	0.58 (0.5–0.7)
all occlusal	67	3.46 (2.8–4.3)	0.19 (0.15–0.25)	51	3.73 (3.1–4.4)	0.18 (0.14–0.24)	12	5.56 (3.7–8.5)	0.56 (0.46–0.68)
Radiographic detection									
advanced occlusal	44	4.90 (3.7–6.5)	0.53 (0.46–0.62)	38	5.96 (3.7–6.6)	0.51 (0.44–0.60)	36	5.87 (4.3–8.0)	0.54 (0.46–0.63)
all occlusal	14	1.74 (1.3–2.4)	0.79 (0.65–0.96)	11	2.02 (1.4–2.9)	0.75 (0.60–0.94)	9	2.36 (1.4–4.1)	0.76 (0.58–0.99)
advanced proximal	22	9.82 (7.3–13.3)	0.58 (0.52–0.65)	22	9.82 (7.3–13.3)	0.58 (0.52–0.65)	22	9.82 (7.3–13.3)	0.58 (0.52–0.65)
all proximal	38	4.30 (3.4–5.5)	0.63 (0.56–0.72)	31	5.34 (4.2–6.8)	0.65 (0.57–0.74)	34	4.89 (3.9–6.2)	0.65 (0.57–0.73)

Table 4 Positive Predictive Values (PPV) of different tests for Egypt and Germany where prevalence rates are available

	Egypt			Germany		
	Prevalence	Positive LR	PPV	Prevalence	Positive LR	PPV
Visual detection						
advanced occlusal	8.1%	5.00	30.6%	22.0%	12.5	77.9%
all occlusal	12.9%	3.73	35.6%	45.0%	5.56	82.0%
Radiographic detection						
advanced occlusal	19.0%	5.96	58.3%	10.0%	5.87	39.5%
all occlusal	19.0%	2.02	32.1%	11.0%	2.36	22.6%

can be useful here to yield setting-specific estimates which are more applicable under the specific circumstances. Second, prevalence rates differed, as described, reflecting different health conditions and risk factors (diet, availability of fluoride, oral hygiene), but also test positive rates. For example, we only evaluated accessible surfaces, which usually meant for occlusal surfaces, unsealed ones. In Germany, unsealed surfaces are found mainly in patients with irregular utilization of dental services; these patients usually also show high caries risk [12]. Low risk patients usually attend the dentist regularly; the majority of occlusal surfaces in these surfaces are sealed for preventive reasons [12]. The resulting high test positive rate for caries lesions in the available surfaces is a result of this; consequently, visual detection had high specificity and PPV, but relatively low NPV. Hence, on occlusal surfaces, dentists in this specific German setting can expect positive detections of caries on occlusal surfaces to be true, and treat accordingly. Negative detections, in contrast, may be false; an additional (more sensitive) diagnostic measure could be applied additionally to increase the NPV. In contrast, in Egypt the tooth level prevalence of occlusal lesions was very low, resulting in low specificity and low PPV of visual detection. Hence, positive detections should be regarded with caution and an additional test for verifying the positive test result should be considered prior to applying (invasive) treatments.

In contrast, for radiographic assessments, tailored meta-analysis did not yield significantly different findings

for both settings or compared to conventional meta-analysis. This may have a number of reasons, too. First, we did not tailor for prevalence of proximal lesions; this was, as no epidemiologic data for both settings was available. Hence, our estimates for radiographic detection are not as tailored as those for visual detection. Second, prevalence rates may indeed be similar in both settings (something we don't know) for proximal lesions. Third, it can be assumed that interpreting radiographs is -to some degree- more objective than visual assessment; the impact of test conduct may be lower for radiographic than for visual detection. Fourth, heterogeneity was generally lower for DSA on radiographic detection; the impact of tailoring will automatically be lower under such circumstances. Last, the number of studies included in this meta-analysis was lower; confidence intervals for any accuracy estimates were wider due to lower statistical power and differences between settings less likely to be detected.

Limitations
The main driver of tailored meta-analysis is the interval estimate for the test positive rate which determines the size of the applicable region. The interval estimate for the prevalence helps refine the applicable region further. Thus the estimates may be subject to selection bias. This was mitigated by sampling consecutive patients although it is still possible that an unrepresentative sample was selected.

Table 5 Negative Predictive Values (NPV) of different tests for Egypt and Germany where prevalence rates are available

	Egypt			Germany		
	Prevalence	Negative LR	NPV	Prevalence	Negative LR	NPV
Visual detection						
advanced occlusal	8.1%	0.29	97.5%	22.0%	0.58	85.9%
all occlusal	12.9%	0.18	97.4%	45.0%	0.56	68.6%
Radiographic detection	19.0%	0.51	89.3%	10.0%	0.54	94.3%
advanced occlusal	19.0%	0.75	85.0%	11.0%	0.76	91.4%
all occlusal	8.1%	0.29	97.5%	22.0%	0.58	85.9%

Only certain surfaces on molars were assessed as both visual occlusal and radiographic proximal assessment are useful detection methods here. In practice, dentists would assess other teeth and surfaces, too. This may affect the prevalence rates reported in this study.

Many of the primary studies were conducted in vitro and showed high risk of bias, often due to unrealistically high prevalence of lesions and potential spectrum bias. However, when there are multiple sources of heterogeneity the individual contributions of the different sources of heterogeneity are unlikely to be determined. In such an instance, tailored meta-analysis may afford the advantage of being probabilistic rather than deterministic in its study selection.

Some surfaces were not accessible for inspection due to teeth not being fully erupted, teeth overlapping on radiographs, presence of sealants or presence of restorations. The presence of a restoration indicates a previous lesion on the surface and omitting such cases from the data could potentially lead to the test positive rate being underestimated. However, there were only a few such cases and their effect on our estimates is likely to be limited.

Recommendations

Diagnostic accuracy studies should be scrutinized for their applicability to different settings, and a critical risk of bias assessment with a focus on setting-specific prevalence and patient spectrum should be performed. A systematic assessment of the risk of bias may be made using tools such as QUADAS-2 [20] prior to the study conduct to allow a higher internal validity.

It is clear from this analysis and others [10, 11] that the summary estimates yielded from conventional meta-analysis of diagnostic accuracy studies have the potential to be inapplicable in particular clinical settings and tailored meta-analysis potentially overcomes this. Although at presence it remains the reserve of statisticians, a user-friendly package in which medical practitioners could readily implement it in the clinical setting would widen the access of the technique.

One of the difficulties for systematic reviewers is the inadequate reporting of data in the primary studies. The STARD statement, which provides standards on reporting of primary diagnostic studies, aimed to address this [21]. Although any improvements in reporting remain largely the responsibility of primary research investigators, journals have a role in facilitating this process and ensuring the STARD statement is fully observed in published diagnostic test accuracy studies.

Although tailored meta-analysis produces estimates which are plausible, their validity is yet to be established. Recently there have been developments in the evaluation of the validity of meta-analysis estimates [22]. Potentially such methods could be used to investigate the validity of tailored meta-analysis findings, but at present this an area for future research.

Existing or newly developed guidelines on caries detection methods should include not only generic, but tailored accuracy estimates, where possible, before deciding to recommend or refute the application of a detection method. Routinely collected data (which is increasingly available) might be useful for such tailoring. In the long term, tailoring might be performed using routine data via practice software, with generated outputs assisting practitioners in individualized decision-making.

Conclusions

Conventional test accuracy meta-analyses may yield aggregate estimates which are inapplicable to specific settings due to the failure of the summary estimate to capture the variation in test performance across different settings. However, routine data collected from the setting of interest may be combined with secondary research to modify this estimate to produce an estimate which is tailored to the setting. This estimate is more likely to be representative of the test accuracy within the setting of interest. Test accuracy meta-analyses should be scrutinized for their applicability to different settings and tailoring may eventually be useful for individualized decision-making.

Abbreviations

DAS: Diagnostic accuracy study; ICDAS: International Caries Detection and Assessment System; MLE: Maximum likelihood estimate; NPV: Negative predictive value; PPV: Positive predictive value; ROC: Receiver Operating Characteristics; TMA: Tailored Meta-Analysis

Funding

BHW is in receipt of an Medical Research Council Clinician Scientist's award (MR/N007999/1). The funding body had no role in the design of the study and collection, analysis, and interpretation of data and in writing the manuscript.

Authors' contributions

FS and BW developed the study, analyzed and interpreted the data. FS collected data and wrote the manuscript. KE, OES, RM collected data, interpreted the findings and provided feedback to the manuscript. TG and FMM provided data, interpreted the findings and provided feedback to the manuscript. All authors read and approved the final manuscript.

Consent for publication

The routine data use was granted by the Charité ethics (EA2 137/14) and the Cairo university ethics (16/7/3). No separate informed consent procedure for publication was needed, mainly only aggregate data are published.

Competing interests

The authors declare that they have no competing interests.

Author details
[1]Department of Operative and Preventive Dentistry, Charité – Universitätsmedizin Berlin, Aßmannshauser Str. 4-6, 14197 Berlin, Germany. [2]Department of Pediatric Dentistry, Cairo University, Giza, Egypt. [3]Department of Pediatric Dentistry, Cairo University, 11 el Saraya Street, Manial, Cairo, Egypt. [4]Department of Pediatric Dentistry, School of Dentistry, University of São Paulo, Av. Lineu Prestes, São Paulo 2227, Brazil. [5]Institute of Applied Health Research, University of Birmingham, Edgbaston, Birmingham B15 2TT, UK.

References
1. Baelum V, Heidmann J, Nyvad B. Dental caries paradigms in diagnosis and diagnostic research. Eur J Oral Sci. 2006;114(4):263–77.
2. Baelum V, Hintze H, Wenzel A, Danielsen B, Nyvad B. Implications of caries diagnostic strategies for clinical management decisions. Community Dent Oral Epidemiol. 2012;40(3):257–66.
3. Gimenez T, Piovesan C, Braga MM, Raggio DP, Deery C, Ricketts DN, Ekstrand KR, Mendes FM. Visual inspection for caries detection: a systematic review and meta-analysis. J Dent Res. 2015;94(7):895–904.
4. Schwendicke F, Paris S, Stolpe M. Detection and treatment of proximal caries lesions: milieu-specific cost–effectiveness analysis. J Dent. 2015; 43(6):647–55.
5. Schwendicke F, Stolpe M, Meyer-Lueckel H, Paris S. Detecting and treating occlusal caries lesions: a cost-effectiveness analysis. J Dent Res. 2015;94(2):272–80.
6. Schwendicke F, Tzschoppe M, Paris S. Radiographic caries detection: a systematic review and meta-analysis. J Dent. 2015;43(8):924–33.
7. Willis BH. Spectrum bias–why clinicians need to be cautious when applying diagnostic test studies. Fam Pract. 2008;25(5):390–6.
8. Willis BH, Quigley M. Uptake of newer methodological developments and the deployment of meta-analysis in diagnostic test research: a systematic review. BMC Med Res Methodol. 2011;11(1):1–8.
9. Mendes FM, Novaes TF, Matos R, Bittar DG, Piovesan C, Gimenez T, Imparato JC, Raggio DP, Braga MM. Radiographic and laser fluorescence methods have no benefits for detecting caries in primary teeth. Caries Res. 2012;46(6):536–43.
10. Willis BH, Hyde CJ. Estimating a test's accuracy using tailored meta-analysis—how setting-specific data may aid study selection. J Clin Epidemiol. 2014;67(5):538–46.
11. Willis BH, Hyde CJ. What is the test's accuracy in my practice population? Tailored meta-analysis provides a plausible estimate. J Clin Epidemiol. 2015;68(8):847–54.
12. Micheelis W, Schiffner U. Vierte Deutsche Mundgesundheits-Studie (DMS IV). In: IDZ Materialreihe. Edited by Institut der Deutschen Zahnärzte, vol. 31. Deutscher Ärzteverlag, Cologne; 2006.
13. DAJ. Epidemiologische Begleituntersuchungen zur Gruppenprophylaxe 2000. In: Gutachten aus den Bundesländern bzw Landesteilen Deutsche Arbeitsgemeinschaft für Jugendzahnpflege; 2001.
14. Ismail AI, Sohn W, Tellez M, Amaya A, Sen A, Hasson H, Pitts NB. The international caries detection and assessment system (ICDAS): an integrated system for measuring dental caries. Community Dent Oral Epidemiol. 2007; 35(3):170–8.
15. Pieper K, Weber K, Margraf-Stiksrud J, Heinzel-Gutenbrunner M, Stein S, Jablonski-Momeni A. Evaluation of a preventive program aiming at children with increased caries risk using ICDAS II criteria. Clin Oral Investig. 2013; 17(9):2049–55.
16. Jablonski-Momeni A, Winter J, Petrakakis P, Schmidt-Schäfer S. Caries prevalence (ICDAS) in 12-year-olds from low caries prevalence areas and association with independent variables. Int J Paediatr Dent. 2013;24(2):90–7.
17. Mobarak EH, Shabayek MM, Mulder J, Reda AH, Frencken JE. Caries experience of Egyptian adolescents: does the atraumatic restorative treatment approach offer a solution? Med Princ Pract. 2011;20(6):545–9.
18. Chu H, Cole SR. Bivariate meta-analysis of sensitivity and specificity with sparse data: a generalized linear mixed model approach. J Clin Epidemiol. 2006;59(12):1331–2. author reply 1332-1333
19. Whiting P, Rutjes AW, Reitsma JB, Glas AS, Bossuyt PM, Kleijnen J. Sources of variation and bias in studies of diagnostic accuracy: a systematic review. Ann Intern Med. 2004;140(3):189–202.
20. Whiting PF, Rutjes AW, Westwood ME, Mallett S, Deeks JJ, Reitsma JB, Leeflang MM, Sterne JA, Bossuyt PM, QUADAS-2 Group. QUADAS-2: a revised tool for the quality assessment of diagnostic accuracy studies. Ann Intern Med. 2011;155(8):529–36.
21. Bossuyt PM, Reitsma JB, Bruns DE, Gatsonis CA, Glasziou PP, Irwig LM, Moher D, Rennie D, de Vet HC, Lijmer JG, Standards for Reporting of Diagnostic Accuracy. The STARD statement for reporting studies of diagnostic accuracy: explanation and elaboration. Ann Intern Med. 2003; 138(1):W1–12.
22. Willis BH, Riley RD. Measuring the statistical validity of summary meta-analysis and meta-regression results for use in clinical practice. Stat Med. 2017;36(21):3283–301.

Are standardized caries risk assessment models effective in assessing actual caries status and future caries increment?

Maria Grazia Cagetti[1,2]* (iD), Giuliana Bontà[1], Fabio Cocco[2,3], Peter Lingstrom[4], Laura Strohmenger[1,2] and Guglielmo Campus[2,3]

Abstract

Background: Assessing caries risk is an essential element in the planning of preventive and therapeutic strategies. Different caries risk assessment (CRA) models have been proposed for the identification of individuals running a risk of future caries. This systematic review was designed to evaluate whether standardized caries risk assessment (CRA) models are able to evaluate the risk according to the actual caries status and/or the future caries increment.

Methods: Randomized clinical trials, cross-sectional studies, cohort studies, comparative studies, validation studies and evaluation studies, reporting caries risk assessment using standardized models (Cariogram, CAMBRA, PreViser, NUS-CRA and CAT) in patients of any age related to caries data recorded by DMFT/S or ICDAS indices, were included. PubMed, Scopus and Embase were searched from 2000 to 2016. A search string was developed. All the papers meeting the inclusion criteria were subjected to a quality assessment.

Results: One thousand three-undred ninety-two papers were identified and 32 were included. In all but one, the Cariogram was used both as sole model or in conjunction with other models. All the papers on children ($n = 16$) and adults ($n = 12$) found a statistically significant association between the risk levels and the actual caries status and/or the future caries increment. Nineteen papers, all using the Cariogram except one, were classified as being of good quality. Three of four papers comprising children and adults found a positive association. For seven of the included papers, Cariogram sensibility and specificity were calculated; sensibility ranged from low (41.0) to fairly low (75.0), while specificity was higher, ranging from 65.8 to 88.0. Wide 95% confidence intervals for both parameters were found, indicating that the reliability of the model differed in different caries risk levels.

Conclusions: The scientific evidence relating to standardized CRA models is still limited; even if Cariogram was tested in children and adults in few studies of good quality, no sufficient evidence is available to affirm the method is effective in caries assessment and prediction. New options of diagnosis, prognosis and therapy are now available to dentists but the validity of standardized CRA models still remains limited.

Keywords: Dental caries, Dental caries susceptibility, Dental health surveys, Risk assessment, Review

* Correspondence: maria.cagetti@unimi.it
[1]Department of Biomedical, Surgical and Dental Sciences, University of Milan, Via Beldiletto 1, 20142 Milan, Italy
[2]WHO Collaboration Centre for Epidemiology and Community Dentistry, Via Beldiletto 1, 20142 Milan, Italy
Full list of author information is available at the end of the article

Background

Different caries risk assessment (CRA) models have been proposed for the identification of individuals running a risk of future caries [1–7].

Caries is a multifactorial disease resulting from a series of events occurring in a chain that lasts for years where clinical, microbiological, behavioral and social factors are involved in the process. In view of its multifactorial nature, a multivariate approach is necessary [8]. The scientific basis for caries risk assessment, prevention and treatment on an individual patient basis requires incessant development, specification and continuing validation [9]. Scientific evidence proving CRA methods' validity is limited [3]. Past caries experience is regarded as the single most powerful caries predictor in all age groups [4–7, 10]. Different measures of past caries experience are often included in analytical models of multi-risk studies. Nevertheless, there are consequences of including past caries experience measures for both prediction and multi-risk models since this parameter will hide the effects of weaker indicators of high risk individuals or of other caries risk-factors [11].

Caries risk assessment still has great potential to enhance patient care as it is the corner stone of a minimal invasive care plan, allowing the determination of the appropriate non-invasive as well as invasive interventions and recall strategies [12], but still today, a great need to standardize study design, outcome measures and reporting of data in studies on CRA is required [13].

Standardized models including different combinations of risk and protective factors (Table 1) have been developed from the 2000s onwards to predict caries; they can be summarized in two main categories, those using an algorithm with a software program and those using standardized questionnaires (self-submitted and/or through an interview). Moreover, CRA methods could be used as an effective health-education tool to change the attitudes and behaviors of patients/parents/caregivers towards good oral hygiene and dietary habits maintenance [14].

Nowadays, no systematic reviews are available on the performances of standardized models. Recent reviews have attempted to assess the validity of different caries risk assessment models/factors [3, 10, 13]. Two reviews combined single clinical parameters and standardized

Table 1 Different factors included in each standardized Caries Risk Model

	Software programs			American Dental Association models		
Factors	NUS-CRA 11 factors	Cariogram 9 factors	PreViser 11 factors	ADA 11 factors	CAMBRA 14 factors	CAT 12 factors
Socio-demographic						
Age	X		X			
Ethnicity	X					
Family socioeconomic status	X			X	X	X
Behavioural						
Infant feeding history	X				X	
Diet	X	X	X	X	X	X
Fluoride	X	X	X	X	X	X
Dental attendance			X	X	X	X
Clinical						
Oral hygiene	X	X	X	X	X	X
Past caries	X	X	X	X	X	X
White spot lesions				X	X	X
Enamel defects						X
Dental appliance			X	X	X	X
Systemic health	X	X	X	X	X	X
Medication				X	X	
Salivary and microbiological						
Saliva flow rate		X	X	X	X	X
Saliva buffering capacity		X				
Mutans streptococci	X	X	X		X	X
Lactobacilli	X	X	X		X	

NusCra National University of Singapore Caries Risk Assessment, *CAMBRA* Caries Management By Risk Assessment, *ADA* caries risk assessment by American Dental Association, *CAT* America Academy of Pediatric Dentistry's Caries Assessment Tool

caries risk assessment models [3, 13]. The only exter-
nally validated model was the Cariogram [13]; the accuracy of the standardized model was found to be limited
in pre-school children, based on two papers [15, 16].
The search literature contained a time frame from 1966
to 2006 with a refresh in 2011, so the most recent papers
were not included in the review. Otherwise, Tellez et al.
[3] aimed to appraise the evidence in caries prediction of
two standardized CRA models, Cariogram, and Caries
Management by Risk Assessment (CAMBRA), and two
guidelines of the American Dental Association (ADA)
and the American Academy of Pediatric Dentistry
(AAPD), taking into account six longitudinal studies. In
this review, the literature search was also stopped in
2011. Senneby et al. [13] evaluated the association
between previous caries experience, microbiological
tests, buffering capacity, salivary flow rate, oral hygiene,
dietary habits, socio-demographic variables and the future caries lesion development. The evidence was considered of low quality and was lacking in regards to the
studied methods. The literature search was stopped in
January 2015.

Starting from these premises, this review aimed to
evaluate the current literature on standardized CRA
models, verifying whether the risk level measured using
different tools is associated with the actual caries status
and/or the future caries increment.

Methods
This systematic review was conducted and reported following the Preferred Reporting Items for Systematic Reviews and Meta-analyses (PRISMA Statement) checklist.

Protocol and registration
The review method and planning were registered at
Prospero (PROSPERO 2016:CRD42016038590).

Eligibility criteria
Randomized controlled trial (RCT), cross-sectional
studies, cohort studies, comparative studies, validation
studies and evaluation studies, reporting CRA using
standardized models in patients of any age related to
caries data recorded by Decayed, Missing, Filled Tooth/
Surface (DMFT/S) or the International Caries Detection
and Assessment System (ICDAS) indices were included.
Only papers in English published from the 1st of January
2000 to the 31st of December 2017 were collected. This
time frame was chosen since no standardized CRA tools
were studied before the year 2000 as emerged from a
first evaluation made by two authors (GC and MGC).

Information sources and search strategy
Three different electronic databases were searched:
PubMed, Scopus® and Embase®. Two search strategies

were used; the first included a combination of MeSH
terms and key words: caries risk assessment, caries risk
assessment models, caries risk assessment tools, caries
risk epidemiology, caries risk profile, Cariogram, CAM-
BRA, PreViser, NUS-CRA, ADA caries risk assessment,
CAT caries risk assessment, AAPD caries risk assess-
ment and dental caries susceptibility. The second strat-
egy included the search string "((dentistry) OR (dental
caries) OR (caries)) AND ((caries risk assessment) OR
(Cariogram) OR (CAMBRA) OR (AAPD) OR (CAT) OR
(ADA) OR (nuscra) OR (NUS-CRA) OR (PreViser))
AND ((cross-sectional studies) OR (cohort analysis risk)
OR (cohort studies) OR (clinical trial) OR (clinical study)
OR (controlled clinical trial) OR (observational study))".

Study selection
Repeated papers were deleted after comparing the results
from the two different search strategies using the three
databases. Two authors (GB and MGC) independently examined all the abstracts of the papers (see Additional file 1
for the whole list). All the papers meeting the inclusion
criteria were obtained in the full-text format. The two authors independently assessed the papers to establish
whether each paper should or should not be included in
the systematic review (see Additional file 2 for the list of
the papers excluded at this stage).

Data collection
Data collection was carried out using an ad hoc designed
data extraction form without masking journal title or authors. Data were extracted by two authors (MGC, GC)
independently. For each paper the following data were
searched and recorded when available: a) the year of
publication and duration of the study; b) details of the
participants including sample size at baseline, age and
country of origin; c) caries data including actual caries
status, caries experience and caries increment measured
through DMFT/S or dmft/s or ICDAS; d) Caries risk
assessment including standardized model used and
categorization of the risk levels; e) sensibility and specificity of the CRA model.

Row data were requested to authors of longitudinal
studies to perform data synthesis and analysis.

Assessment of risk of bias and risk of bias across studies
The risk of bias assessment was conducted by two
authors (GC and MGC). The methodological quality of
the included studies was scored according to the
customized quality assessment tool developed by the
National Heart, Lung, and Blood Institute and Research
Triangle Institute International for Observational Cohort
and Cross-Sectional Studies since, as reported in the
result section no RCTs were obtain after studies' selection [17] (see Additional file 3 for quality assessment of

included studies). Disagreements between authors were resolved by discussion. Where this was not possible, other authors were consulted (PL).

Synthesis of the results
To facilitate a comparison of the results from different studies, the caries values were organized in two-by-two tables. Based on these tables, sensitivity and specificity were calculated, along with the corresponding 95% confidence intervals.

Results
This review provides a concise description of the findings of the included papers, structured around the association between the standardized CRA models, performed on children and/or adults, and the actual or the predicted caries status.

The search identified 3326 papers; after removing duplicates, 1934 papers were selected and, after reviewing titles, abstracts and texts, 32 papers were finally included: 16 on children, 12 on adults and 4 on both, 3 of which considered children and adults as a single sample and one as two different samples (Fig. 1). In order to record caries status (experience/prevalence/incidence), 9 papers used DMFT index or sub-components, 13 papers used DMFS index or sub-components and only 1 used the ICDAS. Four papers focused on primary teeth, 24 on permanent teeth and 4 on both dentitions. The majority of papers ($n = 31$) estimated the caries risk using the Cariogram as a single model or in comparison with

other models. No RCTs were included in the systematic review. All the considered longitudinal papers were comparative studies or validation studies or retrospective cohort studies or, finally, evaluation studies. All the included papers along with the quality assessment grade are reported in Table 2. Nineteen papers were classified as being of good quality, 9 papers of fair quality and only 4 of low quality.

Association between caries risk level and actual caries status in children
Two papers [18, 19] evaluated the association between caries prevalence (DMFS) and Cariogram 9 factors (hereinafter named Full Cariogram) in orthodontic patients. The low caries group at baseline displayed a statistically significant difference regarding caries increment and Cariogram level. Neither DMFT nor the number of caries lesions differed significantly in the Cariogram's risk categories (7 factors) in a sample of Chilean subjects [20]. Children with a cleft lip and/or palate and non-cleft controls classified in the Cariogram high-risk category had a higher caries experience [21]. A significant linear regression between mean dmft and caries risk categories assessed according to a form based on the Cariogram was found in children from low-income families ($p < 0.01$) [22]. A statistically significant association between caries experience and Cariogram categories was found ($p < 0.01$) in Indian children [23]. Caries experience and the presence of white spot lesions were statistically significantly associated with Cariogram categories in Greek pre-school

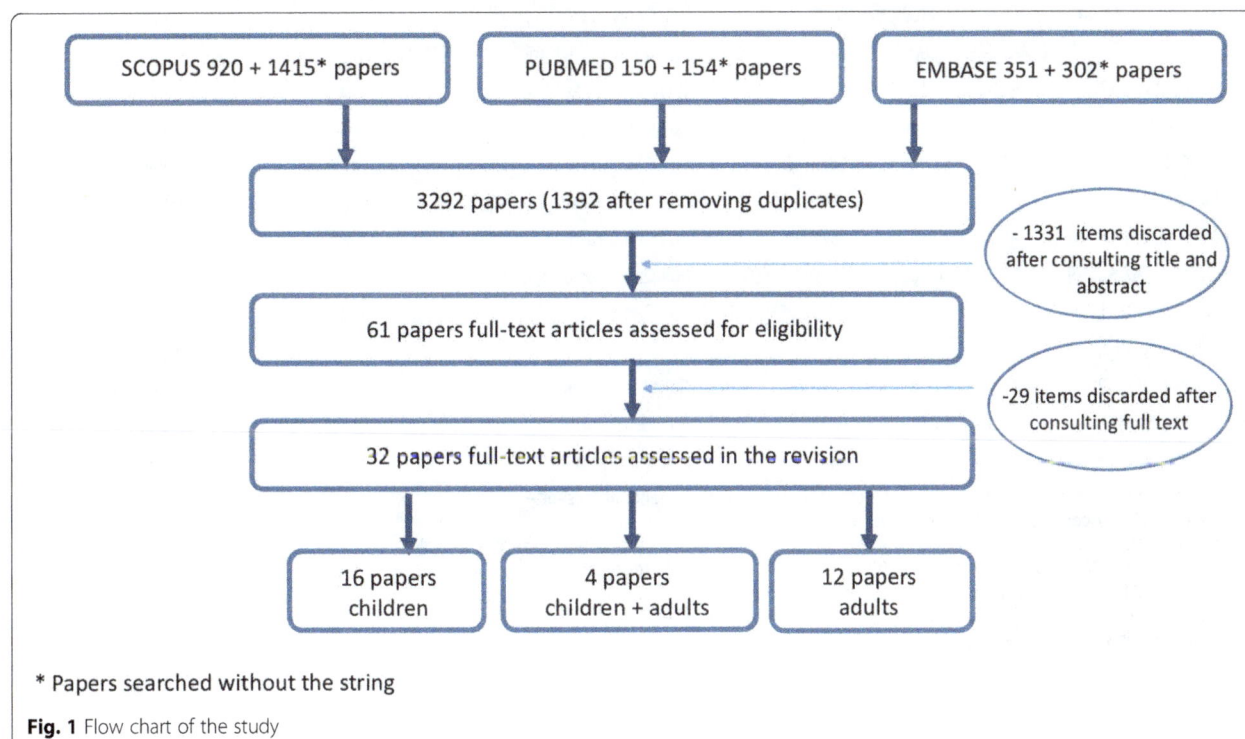
Fig. 1 Flow chart of the study

Table 2 Papers included. Association between standardized CRA and actual caries status and/or caries prediction

Authors (year)	Outcome	Subjects	Indices	Caries risk model	Statistical significance	Quality assessment
Children/Adolescents						
Gao[b], (2015) [8]	CI	544	dmft	Full Cariogram, CAT, CAMBRA, NUS-CRA	+	Good
Sundel, (2015) [21]	ACS	133	dmfs/DMFS	Full Cariogram	+	Good
Cabral, (2014) [22]	ACS	150	dmft/DMFT	Form based on Cariogram 7 factors	++	Poor
Kemparaj, (2014) [37]	CI	200	DMFT/S	Full Cariogram	+	Poor
Gao[b], (2013) [36]	CI	544	dmft	Full Cariogram, CAT, CAMBRA, NUS-CRA	+	Good
Zukanovich, (2013) [41]	CI	109	DMFS/DMFT	Full Cariogram, PreViser, CAT	+	Fair
Campus, (2012) [35]	CI	957	DFS	Cariogram 7 factors	+	Good
Hebbal, (2012) [23]	ACS	100	DMFT	Full Cariogram	++	Poor
Kavvadia, (2012) [24]	ACS	814	dmft	Full Cariogram	+	Fair
Gao, (2010) [16]	CI	1576	dmft	Full Cariogram	e	Good
Petersson[c],(2010b) [39]	CI	392	DMFS	Full Cariogram, Cariogram 6 factors	+	Good
Petersson, (2010a) [40]	CI	392	DMFS	Full Cariogram	+	Good
Campus, (2009) [25]	ACS	957	dmfs/DMFS	Cariogram 7 factors	++	Good
Holgerson, (2009) [15]	CI	125	dmfs/DMFS	Full Cariogram	+	Fair
Twetman, (2005) [33]	CI	64	DFS	Full Cariogram	++	Good
Petersson[a,b], (2004) [34]	CI	446	DFS	Full Cariogram	++	Good
Petersson[b], (2002) [32]	CI	446	DMFT/S	Full Cariogram	+	Good
Adults						
Petersson, (2015) [44]	CI	1295	DFT/DFTS	Full Cariogram	++	Good
Carta, (2015) [31]	ACS	480	ICDAS	Full Cariogram	++	Good
Chaffee, (2015) [45]	CI	4468	DFS	CAMBRA	+	Good
Chang (2014) [30]	CI	110	DMFT/S	Cariogram 7 factors	+	Good
Chang and Kim, (2014) [42]	ACS	102	DMFT	Full Cariogram	+	Good
Lee, (2013) [29]	ACS	80	DMFT	Full Cariogram, Cariogram 7/8 factors	+	Fair
Petersson, (2013) [7]	ACS	1295	DFT/S	Cariogram 8 factors	++	Good
Celik, (2012) [43]	CI	100	DMFT/S	Full Cariogram	+	Fair
Peker, (2012) [27]	ACS	90	DMFT/S	Full Cariogram	+	Fair
Sonbul, (2008) [28]	ACS	175	DMFS	Full Cariogram	+	Good
Ruiz Miravet, (2007) [26]	ACS	48	DMFT/S	Full Cariogram	++	Poor
Petersson[a,d], (2004) [34]	CI	208	DFS	Full Cariogram	++	Fair
Petersson[d], (2003) [1]	CI	208	DMFS /DFS/DFRS	Full Cariogram	++	Good
Both Children/Adults						
Giacaman, (2013) [20]	ACS	180	DMFT	Cariogram 7 factors	–	Poor
Almosa, (2012) [18]	ACS	89	DMFS	Full Cariogram	++	Fair
Al Mulla, (2009) [19]	ACS	100	DFS	Full Cariogram	++	Fair

ACS actual caries status, *CI* Caries Increment. Subjects: number of subjects at baseline
Statistical significance: - = $p > 0.05$ + = $p < 0.05$; ++ = $p \leq 0.01$
[a]Petersson, (2004) reported in both children and adults and describes data in two different samples
[b]Gao, (2013) and (2015), and Petersson, (2002) and (2004) respectively reported data for the same sample of children
[c]Petersson, (2010a) and (2010b) reported data for the same sample of children
[d]Petersson, (2003) and (2004) reported data for the same sample of elderly people
[e]Data not obtainable from the paper

children ($p < 0.01$) [24]. A significant linear trend between the five Cariogram categories and dmfs/DMFS scores was observed ($p < 0.01$) in Italian children [25].

Association between caries risk level and actual caries status in adults

Several papers focused on young adults and all of them reported an association between Cariogram categories and caries prevalence/experience/severity [7, 26, 27]. In Saudi Arabia [28], the mean caries prevalence in the high-risk group differed significantly from that recorded in the low-risk group ($p < 0.05$). A caries profile obtained from the Cariogram, including 7 and 8 factors, was compared to the Full Cariogram and correlated to caries experience: all models measured statistically significant associated risk levels to the caries experience [29]. The chance of avoiding caries was statistically significantly associated ($p < 0.01$) to the caries experience in a group of Korean adults [30]. Caries at ICDAS levels 5–6 and the presence of more than five missing teeth were statistically significant associated to the Cariogram scores (OR = 2.36, 95%CI = 1.83–3.03 and OR = 1.43, 95%CI = 1.13–1.82 respectively) in Italian adults [31].

Association between caries risk level and caries increment in children and adults

A total of 17 longitudinal papers investigated the validity of standardized CRA models to predict new caries lesions (Table 3). Twelve papers regarding children were included [15, 16, 32–41], nine of which used the Cariogram model and three compared different CRA models, including the Cariogram [36, 38, 41]. Six papers regarding adults were included, five of which used the Cariogram [1, 34, 42–44] and one the CAMBRA model [45].

In a two-year prospective study [32] subjects in the highest risk group developed a mean of about 10 times more caries lesions (DMFS) than the lowest risk group. The same authors compared [34] data from the previous study with those recorded in a group of adults/elderly people, showing a higher mean of caries increment per year for high-risk groups. The caries increment in children affected by Type 1 diabetes mellitus (ΔDMFS) was about eight times higher in the Cariogram highest risk category [33]. After five years from baseline, children classified at high risk (Full Cariogram) developed about four times more caries lesions [15] (study not included in Table 3). Five times more caries lesions were found in schoolchildren assessed by the Full Cariogram as running the highest risk compared with those with the lowest risk [40]. On the same sample, two different Cariogram models with and without saliva factors were tested. Both models revealed a statistically significant relationship with caries development ($p < 0.05$) at the two-year follow-up [39]. A prospective study (not included in Table 3) was conducted on preschool children with different risk assessment models, including the Full Cariogram [16]. One year after baseline the model showed a sensitivity/specificity lower values than the biopsychosocial models proposed by the authors. In Italian schoolchildren, the caries risk was assessed (7-factor Cariogram) and 2 years later the children classified as high risk developed caries lesions about as twice as much as those developed by children classified as low risk [35]. Full Cariogram, Previser and the Caries-risk Assessment Tool (CAT) were compared in children [41]. At the follow-up examination (3 years), only the Cariogram model successfully predicted new caries lesions. Full Cariogram, NUS-CRA, CAT and CAMBRA were assessed on preschool children [36]. After 1 year, using CAT and CAMBRA, the majority of children were considered to be at high risk, while, using the Full Cariogram and the National University of Singapore Caries Risk Assessment (NUS-CRA), almost 2/3 of the children were defined as very low or low risk. The CRA was evaluated in a sample of 12-year-old children using the Full Cariogram and dividing them into five groups of risk [37]. Two years later, children classified as very high risk at baseline developed about thirty times more caries lesions compared to children classified as very low risk. The same sample of three-year-old children from a previous study [36] was re-evaluated 18 months from baseline ($n = 462$) using the same risk assessment model; a gradient in caries increment from lower to higher risk groups was found using all programs [38].

Full Cariogram was evaluated in elderly people and, after 5 years, subjects with the highest risk profile had about three times more caries lesions compared to the lowest risk group [1]. Full Cariogram was assessed in two samples of young adults [43, 44]; after 2 years, subjects classified at very high risk at baseline developed caries lesions about as twice as much as those classified at very low risk; at the 3 year follow-up of the second sample [44], subjects with the highest risk profile had about seven times more caries lesions compared to those in the lowest risk group. The CAMBRA model was used to split a sample of young adults into four risk groups [45]; caries increment was more than three times higher in subjects classified as high risk than those classified at low risk.

Few of the included papers report data allowing the authors to calculate sensibility and specificity of the CRA models [15, 16, 32, 33, 35, 36, 44]. In Table 4 the available data for the Cariogram model are displayed. Sensibility values ranged from low (41.0) [32] to fairly low (52.0) [35], while specificity values were quite high, ranging from 71.0 [33] to 88.0 [15]. Moreover, wide Confidences Intervals are reported for both parameters, indicating that the reliability of the model differs in the different caries risk levels.

Table 3 Association between caries increment and caries risk model categories in longitudinal papers

Authors (year)	Age	Study time (years)	Subjects	Caries increments	Range Mean (Standard Deviation)				
				Cariogram	**0–20**	**21–40**	**41–60**	**61–80**	**81–100**
Gao (2013) [36]	C	1	485	dmft	2.67 (2.96)	2.02 (1.71)	1.56 (1.63)	0.77 (1.21)	0.34 (0.88)
Kemparaj (2014) [37]	C	2	200	DMFT	0.54 (1.2)	0.43 (1.32)	0.39 (1.04)	0.34 (0.80)	0.06 (0.09)
				DMFS	0.79 (1.73)	0.73 (1.55)	0.48 (1.72)	0.39 (1.20)	0.09 (1.12)
Celik (2012) [43]	A	2	100	DMFT	1.23 (0.86)	0.65 (0.81)	0.39 (1.02)	0.08 (0.28)	0 (0)
				DMFS	1.23 (0.86)	0.9 (0.97)	0.48 (1.6)	0.08 (0.28)	0 (0)
Petersson (2002) [32]	C	2	392	DMFT	1.67 (1.44)	1.46 (2.20)	1.07 (1.36)	0.42 (0.90)	0.23 (0.61)
				DMFS	2.58 (1.83)	2.62 (4.11)	1.47 (1.81)	0.53 (1.24)	0.27 (0.70)
Petersson (2015) [44]	A	3	982	DFT	1.00 (1.40)	0.84 (0.95)	0.82 (1.18)	0.53 (1.07)	0.24 (0.58)
Petersson (2010a) [40]	C	2	392	DMFS	3.00 ([a])	2.70 ([a])	1.50 ([a])	0.50 ([a])	0.20 ([a])
				DFS	1.99 (3.00)	1.7 (1.76)	1.59 (2.55)	0.85 (1.91)	0.29 (0.89)
Petersson (2004)[b] [34]	C	2	392	DFS	1.30 ([a])	1.30 ([a])	0.70 ([a])	0.30 ([a])	0.10 ([a])
	A	5	148	DFS	1.90 ([a])	1.00 ([a])	1.20 ([a])	0.40 ([a])	0 ([a])
Campus (2012) [35]	C	2	861	DS	1.20 ([a])	1.20 ([a])	0.10 ([a])	0.20 ([a])	0.10 ([a])
				Cariogram	**0–20**	**21–40**	**41–60**	**61–100**	
Chang and Kim (2014) [42]	C	1.3	64	DMFT	2.97 (5.2)	1.28 (1.5)	1.36 (2.2)	0.44 (0.7)	
				DMFS	5.81 (11.97)	1.28 (1.5)	3.27 (6.8)	0.44 (0.7)	
Petersson (2003) [1]	A	5		DMFS	16.21 (15.97)	7.36 (9.34)	7.96 (9.52)	5.23 (6.97)	
				Cariogram	**0–25**	**26–50**	**51–75**	**76–100**	
Twetman (2005) [33]	C	3	64	DFS	8 (10.8)	3.4 (2.6)	2.6 (3.7)	0 (0)	
				Cariogram	**0–20**		**21–80**	**81–100**	
Zukanovic (2013) [41]	C	3	70	DMFT	1.80 (1.79)		2.40 (2.36)	1.77 (1.88)	
				DMFS	5.00 (7.07)		4.71 (4.34)	2.54 (2.44)	
				Cariogram	**0–40**			**41–100**	
Holgerson (2009) [15]	C	5	125	dmfs/DMFS	2.40 (3.2)			0.10 (0.4)	
				Cambra	**High**		**Moderate**	**Low**	
Gao (2013) [36]	C	1	485	dmft	1.24 (1.58)		0.27 (0.68)	0.20 (0.76)	
Chaffee (2015) [45]	A	1.5	4468	DFT	1.74 ([a])		1.16 ([a])	1.01 ([a])	
				CAT	**High**		**Moderate**	**Low**	
Gao (2013) [36]	C	1	485	dmft	0.79 (1.31)		0.08 (0.28)	0 (0)	
Zukanovic (2013) [41]	C	3	70	DMFT	2.19 (2.33)		2.60 (1.82)	2.38 (1.92)	
				DMFS	4.54 (4.41)		3.80 (5.81)	3.13 (2.53)	
				NUS-CRA	**Very High**	**High**	**Moderate**	**Low**	**Very Low**
Gao (2013) [36]	C	1	485	dmft	2.18 (1.87)	2.10 (1.63)	1.26 (1.38)	0.85 (1.11)	0.17 (0.69)
				PreViser	**High**		**Moderate**	**Low**	
Zukanovic (2013) [41]	C	3	70	DMFT	2.35 (2.27)		1.92 (2.18)	2.18 (2.32)	
				DMFS	5.04 (4.75)		3.08 (2.87)	2.82 (3.19)	

A Adults, *C* Children

([a]) indicates that Standard Deviation data were not described in the paper. The decimal places reported are those reported in each paper
Petersson, (2004)[b] reports the increment for year of observation. Holgerson, (2009) and Petersson, (2010b) were excluded from the table since as no mean data for caries were present. Gao (2015) was excluded from the table as the data are the same as those reported for Gao, (2013)

In brief, the results of the present review show: all the included papers on children showed a statistically significant association between the risk levels and the actual caries status and/or the future increment. More than half of these papers, including the Cariogram model, were classified as being of good quality. The same positive association between the risk levels and the actual caries status and/or the future increment was reported in the included papers on adults. More than half of the papers were classified as being of good quality and all

Table 4 Sensitivity and specificity of the Cariogram model in children and adults

Authors (year)	Number of factors	Sample n	Age at baseline (years)	Sensibility % ($_{95\%}$Confidence Interval)	Specificity % ($_{95\%}$Confidence Interval)
Children					
Gao (2013) [36]	Full	485	3	66.4[a]	78.5[a]
Campus (2012) [35]	7	861	7–9	52.0 (18.6–94.6)	79.5 (99.2–54.7)
Gao (2010) [16]	Full	1782	3–6	70.5[a]	65.8[a]
Holgerson[b] (2009) [15]	Full	66[b]	2	46.0 (31.0–62.0)	88.0 (71.0–104.0)
Twetman (2005) [33]	Full	64	8–16	75.0[a]	71.0[a]
Petersson (2002) [32]	Full	392	10–11	41.0 (9.0–73.0)	79.8 (99.6–60.0)
Adults					
Petersson (2015) [44]	Full	1295	19	47.0 (11.9–89.2)	72.5 (33.5–94.8)

[a]Range not available
[b]Control group only

except one used the Cariogram. Three of four papers comprising children and adults found a positive association between the risk levels and the actual caries status and/or the future increment.

Discussion

Determining the validity of different caries risk assessment models to fit the actual caries status, analyzing cross-sectional papers, and to predict new caries lesions in the near future, analyzing longitudinal papers, was the aim of this systematic review. The CRA models that were examined were the reasoning-based (CAT, CAMBRA and ADA model) and algorithm-driven (Cariogram, NUS-CRA and PreViser).

The findings described enable to draw some conclusions.

All papers involving children [15, 16, 21–25, 32–41] assessed a statistically significant association between the risk level measured by the CRA model and the actual caries status or the caries increment in a follow-up examination. Eleven papers [16, 21, 25, 32–36, 38–40] of seventeen were classified as being of good quality, and all of them used the Cariogram as sole model or in conjunction with other models. Sensibility and specificity of the Cariogram model were evaluated in six papers [15, 16, 32, 33, 35, 36] and data showed that the model is not accurate in predicting caries lesion development. Furthermore, the validity of the Cariogram to evaluate the caries risk might be flawed: four papers [32, 34, 39, 40] involved the same population.

Papers carried out on adult populations [1, 7, 26–31, 34, 42–45] showed a positive association between the CRA model and caries data. Eight papers [1, 7, 28, 30, 31, 42, 44, 45] of thirteen were classified as being of good quality and all except one [45] used the Cariogram model. Sensibility and specificity of the Cariogram model were reported in one paper [44]; data confirm the low accuracy of the model. Within the three papers [18–20] involving both children and adults regarded as a single sample, two found a positive association between risk level and caries status and one [20] failed to find such an association. This last paper was evaluated as being of poor quality.

Different Cariogram models using from nine to seven factors were used. The excluded factors were salivary parameters, namely mutans streptococci, lactobacilli, salivary secretion rate and buffer capacity. Reduced Cariogram versions were statistically significant associated to caries data, in both cross-sectional and longitudinal papers [7, 21, 29, 30, 35], except for one paper [20].

Only three papers, two of good quality (reporting data on the same sample) [36, 38] and one fair, compared different risk models [41]: the Full Cariogram, CAT, CAMBRA and NUS-CRA were compared in two and the Full Cariogram, PreViser and CAT in the third one. The results showed that different CRA models assessed the risk differently, but, due to the small amount of available data, it is not possible to draw clear conclusions about the most effective method for predicting caries lesions.

The main limitation of this review is that the included papers do not form a homogeneous group and original databases are not available making it impossible to perform a meta-analysis. Different study populations (adults or children), different versions of the same standardized CRA model (Cariogram from seven to nine parameters), different indices used to measure carious lesions (dmfs/t, DMFS/T, DFS/T, DS, ICDAS) make the comparison of papers questionable and hamper the synthesis of results. This limitation cannot be overcome until papers with a standardized study design, outcome measurements and reporting of data will be carried out.

At present, only the Cariogram was used in papers of good quality to assess its efficacy in predicting caries development, while, for the other standardized CRA models, the lack of papers does not make it possible to draw conclusions on their effectiveness.

Conclusions

The evidence relating to the quality of existing CRA models in assessing and predicting caries lesions is limited; even if Cariogram was used in few studies of good quality carried out in children and adults, no sufficient evidence is available to affirm that the method is effective in caries assessment and prediction. The Full Cariogram and reduced versions, eight or seven factors, appear to produce similar results. Although other CRA models, such as CAT, CAMBRA, NUS-CRA and PreViser, might be effective in clinical settings, the scientific evidence to date is limited.

Abbreviations

AAPD: American academy of pediatric dentistry; ADA: American dental association; CAMBRA: Caries management by risk assessment; CAT: Caries risk-assessment tool; CRA: Caries risk assessment; DMFT/S: Decayed missed filled tooth/surface; ICDAS: International caries detection and assessment system; NUS-CRA: National university of singapore- caries risk assessment; PRISMA: Preferred reporting items for systematic reviews and meta-analyses; RCT: Randomized clinical trial

Acknowledgements

The authors want to thank the authors of the included longitudinal papers who provided data for the analysis.

Authors' contributions

MGC: selected the papers, performed the papers validity assessment and drafting the manuscript; GB: performed the search and selected the papers; FC: realized tables and figure and contributed to write the manuscript; PL: performed the final revision of the paper; LS: designed the paper; GC: was consulted in case of discussion between the examiners of the validity assessment and contributed to write the paper. All authors read and approved the final version of the manuscript.

Competing interests

The authors declare that they have no competing interests. There are no financial completing interests as we have not received any grants. The authors alone are responsible for the content and writing of the paper.

Author details

[1]Department of Biomedical, Surgical and Dental Sciences, University of Milan, Via Beldiletto 1, 20142 Milan, Italy. [2]WHO Collaboration Centre for Epidemiology and Community Dentistry, Via Beldiletto 1, 20142 Milan, Italy. [3]Department of Surgery, Microsurgery and Medicine Sciences, School of Dentistry University of Sassari, Viale San Pietro, 43 Sassari, Italy. [4]Department of Cariology, Institute of Odontology, The Sahlgrenska Academy, University of Gothenburg, Medicinaregatan 12 A-G, P.O. Box 450, 405 30 Gothenburg, Sweden.

References

1. Petersson GH, Fure S, Bratthall D. Evaluation of a computer-based caries risk assessment program in an elderly group of individuals. Acta Odontol Scand. 2003;61:164–71.
2. Trottini M, Bossu M, Corridore D, Ierardo G, Luzzi V, Saccucci M, Polimeni A. Assessing risk factors for dental caries: a statistical modeling approach. Caries Res. 2015;49:226–35.
3. Tellez M, Gomez J, Pretty I, Ellwood R, Ismail AI. Evidence on existing caries risk assessment systems: are they predictive of future caries? Community Dent Oral Epidemiol. 2013;41:67–78.
4. Senneby A, Mejare I, Sahlin NE, Svensäter G, Rohlin M. Diagnostic accuracy of different caries risk assessment methods. A systematic review. J Dent. 2015;43:1385–93.
5. Zhang Q, van Palenstein Helderman WH. Caries experience variables as indicators in caries risk assessment in 6-7-year-old Chinese children. J Dent. 2006;34:676–81.
6. Du Q, Yu M, Li Y, Du H, Gao W, Mei H, et al. Permanent caries experience is associated with primary caries experience: a 7-year longitudinal study in China. Community Dent Oral Epidemiol. 2016;45:43–8.
7. Petersson GH, Ericson E, Isberg PE, et al. Caries risk assessment in young adults: a 3-year validation of clinical guidelines used in public dental service. Acta Odontol Scand. 2013;71:1645–50.
8. Arrica M, Carta G, Cocco F, et al. Does a social/behavioural gradient in dental health exist among adults? A cross-sectional study. J Int Med Res. 2017;45:451–61.
9. American Dental Association. Caries diagnosis and risk assessment. A review of preventive strategies and management. J Am Dent Assoc. 1995;126:1s–24s.
10. Mejare I, Axelsson S, Dahlen G, Espelid I, Norlund A, Tranæus S, et al. Caries risk assessment. A systematic review. Acta Odontol Scand. 2014;72:81–91.
11. Aleksejūnienė J, Holst D, Brukienė V. Dental caries risk studies revisited: causal approaches needed for future inquiries. Int J Environ Res Public Health. 2009;6:2992–3009.
12. Doméjean S, Banerjee A, Featherstone JDB. Caries risk/susceptibility assessment: its value in minimum intervention oral healthcare. Br Dent J. 2017;223:191–7.
13. Senneby A, Mejàre I, Sahlin NE, Svensäter G, Rohlin M. Diagnostic accuracy of different caries risk assessment methods. A systematic review. J Dent. 2015;43:1385–93.
14. Bratthall D, Petersson GH. Cariogram–a multifactorial risk assessment model for a multifactorial disease. Community Dent Oral Epidemiol. 2005;33:256–64.
15. Holgerson PL, Twetman S, Stecksen-Blicks C. Validation of an age-modified caries risk assessment program (Cariogram) in preschool children. Acta Odontol Scand. 2009;67:106–12.
16. Gao XL, Hsu CY, Xu Y, Hwarng HB, Loh T, Koh D. Building caries risk assessment models for children. J Dent Res. 2010;89:637–43.
17. Quality Assessment Tool for Observational Cohort and Cross-Sectional Studies Available from: https://www.nhlbi.nih.gov/health-pro/guidelines/in-develop/cardiovascular-risk-reduction/tools/cohort
18. Almosa NA, Al-Mulla AH, Birkhed D. Caries risk profile using the Cariogram in governmental and private orthodontic patients at de-bonding. Angle Orthod. 2012;82:267–74.
19. Al Mulla AH, Kharsa SA, Kjellberg H, Birkhed D. Caries risk profiles in orthodontic patients at follow-up using Cariogram. Angle Orthod. 2009;79:323–30.
20. Giacaman RA, Miranda Reyes P, Bravo Leon V. Caries risk assessment in Chilean adolescents and adults and its association with caries experience. Braz Oral Res. 2013;27:7–13.
21. Sundell AL, Ullbro C, Marcusson A, Twetman S. Comparing caries risk profiles between 5- and 10- year-old children with cleft lip and/or palate and non-cleft controls. BMC Oral Health. 2015;15:85.
22. Cabral RN, Hilgert LA, Faber J, et al. Caries risk assessment in schoolchildren–a form based on Cariogram software. J Appl Oral Sci. 2014;22:397–402.
23. Hebbal M, Ankola A, Metgud S. Caries risk profile of 12 year old school children in an Indian city using Cariogram. Med Oral Patol Oral Cir Bucal. 2012;17:e1054–61.
24. Kavvadia K, Agouropoulos A, Gizani S, Papagiannouli L, Twetman S. Caries risk profiles in 2- to 6-year-old Greek children using the Cariogram. Eur J Dent. 2012;6:415–21.
25. Campus G, Cagetti MG, Sacco G, Benedetti G, Strohmenger L, Lingström P. Caries risk profiles in Sardinian schoolchildren using Cariogram. Acta Odontol Scand. 2009;67:146–52.

26. Ruiz Miravet A, Montiel Company JM, Almerich Silla JM. Evaluation of caries risk in a young adult population. Med Oral Patol Oral Cir Bucal. 2007;12:E412-8.

27. Peker I, Mangal T, Erten H, Gulcin A, Emre A, Gulcin A. Evaluation of caries risk in a young adult population using a computer-based risk assessment model (Cariogram). J Dent Sci. 2012;7:99-104.

28. Sonbul H, Al-Otaibi M, Birkhed D. Risk profile of adults with several dental restorations using the Cariogram model. Acta Odontol Scand. 2008;66:351-7.

29. Lee JH, Son HH, Kim HY, Chang J. Caries risk profiles of Korean dental patients using simplified Cariogram models. Acta Odontol Scand. 2013;71:899-905.

30. Chang J, Lee JH, Son HH, Kim HY. Caries risk profile of Korean dental patients with severe intellectual disabilities. Spec Care Dentist. 2014;34:201-7.

31. Carta G, Cagetti MG, Cocco F, Sale S, Lingström P, Campus G. Caries-risk profiles in Italian adults using computer caries assessment system and ICDAS. Braz Oral Res. 2015;29:S1806-83242015000100306.

32. Petersson GH, Twetman S, Bratthall D. Evaluation of a computer program for caries risk assessment in schoolchildren. Caries Res. 2002;36:327-40.

33. Twetman S, Petersson GH, Bratthall D. Caries risk assessment as a predictor of metabolic control in young type 1 diabetics. Diabet Med. 2005;22:312-5.

34. Petersson GH, Fure S, Twetman S, Bratthall D. Comparing caries risk factors and risk profiles between children and elderly. Swed Dent J. 2004;28:119-28.

35. Campus G, Cagetti MG, Sale S, Carta G, Lingström P. Cariogram validity in schoolchildren: a two-year follow-up study. Caries Res. 2012;46:16-22.

36. Gao X, Di Wu I, Lo EC, Chu CH, Hsu CY, Wong MC. Validity of caries risk assessment programmes in preschool children. J Dent. 2013;41:787-95.

37. Kemparaj U, Chavan S, Shetty NL. Caries risk assessment among school children in davangere city using cariogram. Int J Prev Med. 2014;5:664-71.

38. Gao XL, Lo ECM, Chu CH, Hsu SC. Caries risk assessment programmes for Hong Kong children. Hong Kong Med J. 2015;21:S42-S6.

39. Petersson GH, Isberg PE, Twetman S. Caries risk assessment in school children using a reduced Cariogram model without saliva tests. BMC Oral Health. 2010;10:5.

40. Petersson GH, Isberg PE, Twetman S. Caries risk profiles in schoolchildren over 2 years assessed by Cariogram. Int J Paediatr Dent. 2010;20:341-6.

41. Zukanovic A. Caries risk assessment models in caries prediction. Acta Med Acad. 2013;42:198-208.

42. Chang J, Kim HY. Does caries risk assessment predict the incidence of caries for special needs patients requiring general anesthesia? Acta Odontol Scand. 2014;72:721-8.

43. Celik EU, Gokay N, Ates M. Efficiency of caries risk assessment in young adults using Cariogram. Eur J Dent. 2012;6:270-9.

44. Petersson GH, Twetman S. Caries risk assessment in young adults: a 3 year validation of the Cariogram model. BMC oral health. 2015;15:17.

45. Chaffee BW, Cheng J, Featherstone JD. Baseline caries risk assessment as a predictor of caries incidence. J Dent. 2015;43:518-24.

10

Children's dental fear and anxiety: exploring family related factors

Lingli Wu[1] and Xiaoli Gao[2*]

Abstract

Background: Dental fear and anxiety (DFA) is a major issue affecting children's oral health and clinical management. This study investigates the association between children's DFA and family related factors, including parents' DFA, parenting styles, family structure (nuclear or single-parent family), and presence of siblings.

Methods: A total of 405 children (9–13 years old) and their parents were recruited from 3 elementary schools in Hong Kong. Child's demographic and family-related information was collected through a questionnaire. Parents' and child's DFA were measured by using the Corah Dental Anxiety Scale (CDAS) and Children Fear Survey Schedule-Dental Subscale (CFSS–DS), respectively. Parenting styles were gauged by using the Parent Authority Questionnaire (PAQ).

Results: DFA was reported by 33.1% of children. The mean (SD) CFSS-DS score was 29.1 (11.0). Children with siblings tended to report DFA (37.0% vs. 24.1%; $p = 0.034$) and had a higher CFSS-DS score (29.9 vs. 27.4; $p = 0.025$) as compared with their counterpart. Children from single-parent families had lower CFSS-DS score as compared with children from nuclear families ($\beta = -9.177$; $p = 0.029$). Subgroup analysis showed a higher CFSS-DS score among boys with siblings ($\beta = 7.130$; $p = 0.010$) as compared with their counterpart; girls' from single-parent families had a lower CFSS-DS score ($\beta = -13.933$; $p = 0.015$) as compared with girls from nuclear families. Children's DFA was not associated with parents' DFA or parenting styles ($p > 0.05$).

Conclusions: Family structure (nuclear or single-parent family) and presence of siblings are significant determinants for children's DFA. Parental DFA and parenting style do not affect children's DFA significantly.

Keywords: Dental fear, Dental anxiety, Children, Parents, Parenting styles, Family factors

Background

Dental fear and dental anxiety (DFA) refer to the strong negative feelings associated with dental treatment, whether or not the criteria for a diagnosis of dental phobia are met [1]. The reported prevalence of DFA among children and adolescents in different countries ranged from 5 to 33% [1–4]. Children with DFA often try all means to avoid or delay dental treatment, resulting in deterioration of their oral health [5]. They also demonstrate poor cooperation during dental visits, which compromises the treatment outcomes, creates occupational stress on dental staff, and causes discord between dental professionals and their parents [1]. DFA

acquisition in childhood may track into adulthood and is a significant predictor for dental avoidance in adulthood [6, 7]. Preventing and intercepting DFA during childhood is considered as a critical approach for improving people's oral health and dental experience [5].

It was speculated that parents' DFA might exerts an influence on their children's DFA through modeling and information [8]. Many adults with DFA may verbalize their fearful feelings in front of their children, creating a negative impression on dental treatment [5]. Most children at early school age begin to emulate their parents who are looked upon as models [9]. They are very likely to internalize their parents' values, attitudes and worldviews, which would gradually become a part of their own belief system [9]. There is moderate evidence to support the relationship between parental and child DFA [10]. An American study reported that over 40% of

* Correspondence: gaoxl@hku.hk
[2]Dental Public Health, Faculty of Dentistry, The University of Hong Kong, 3rd Floor, Prince Philip Dental Hospital, 34 Hospital Road, Sai Ying Pun, Hong Kong
Full list of author information is available at the end of the article

parents/guardians gave their children negative connotation about their previous dental visit [11]. This study also showed a shared anxiety between parents/guardians and their children, thus suggesting that parents played a key role in children's anxiety and fear development. In another study, parental dental anxiety was demonstrated as a significant indicator for children's dental anxiety ($\beta = 0.244$; $p = 0.016$) [12]. Despite the potential influence of parents, consensus is lacking regarding whether mother or father plays a more significant role in children's DFA. A previous study concluded that fathers deliver major information, such as danger, to children and play a mediating role for the transfer of dental fear from parents to children [13]. However, another study showed no significant difference between the influence of mothers and fathers on their children's DFA [14].

Parenting styles provided an environmental framework for children's psychosocial growth and were assumed to shape children's behaviors [15]. Baumrind identified three main styles of parenting, namely authoritative, authoritarian, and permissive [16]. This classification of parenting styles has served as a useful tool for investigating the influence of parenting on various issues concerning child development [16]. The relationship between parenting styles and children's dental fear has attracted some scholarly attention. A study measured parents' child-rearing attitudes and found that the subscale self-complaints (example item "My child's happiness needs a lot of sacrifice on my part") were associated with children's dental fear [17]. However, another study found no association between parenting styles and dental anxiety of children [18]. With limited evidence gleaned from very few studies, the association between parenting styles and children's DFA remains ambiguous.

In addition, a family dynamics model revealed that birth order could influence one's personality and behavior [19]. It has been reported that children's birth order partially determines their ability to cope with stresses in medical situations [20]. In the dental setting, only born children and first-born children were found to have a higher clinical situational DFA and were less cooperative than others [21, 22]. A study involving children of various age showed that more children reported to have DFA if their siblings reported DFA [23]. However, no association was found between children's DFA and the number of children in their families in another study [24]. The current evidence concerning how birth order and presence of siblings are associated with children's DFA remains scarce and inconsistent findings have been reported.

In view of the currently insufficient and contradictory evidence, this study aimed to investigate the association between children's DFA and a variety of family related factors, namely parents' DFA, parenting styles, family structure (single-parent or nuclear family), and presence of siblings.

Methods

Sample size calculation

The sample size was calculated by using G*Power version 3.1.9.2. Targeting a statistical power of 0.9 and a significant level of 0.05 and estimating 13.5% children have DFA [25], 373 subjects are needed to detect an effect size of 0.5.

Participant recruitment

The protocol of this study was reviewed by the Institutional Review Board (IRB) of the University of Hong Kong/Hospital Authority Hong Kong West Cluster. An ethical approval was obtained (#UW16–130).

A list of government-funded elementary schools was retrieved from the official website of the Education Bureau, Hong Kong Special Administrative Region (http://www.edb.gov.hk). Among a total of 454 schools, 5 were randomly selected and approached. Three out of the 5 elementary schools participated. Child-mother-father triads were recruited. The inclusion criteria were: (i) the school was a government-funded, co-educational school (i.e. mixed-sex school); (ii) the child was enrolled in Primary 4–6 of a participating school; (iii) the child was 9–13 years old; and (iv) the child and his/her both parents were literate and were able to complete questionnaires themselves. Children with severe systemic diseases or physical or psychological disabilities were excluded. All eligible children in the participating schools were approached. Children with informed written consent from both parents were recruited.

Questionnaires

Each participating family was asked to complete a set of four questionnaires. The questionnaires were distributed via class teachers and were completed by the participants at home on a self-administered basis. Clear instructions were given to avoid confusion. All questionnaires were completed anonymously. Each participating family was identified with a code and their names were not disclosed. The questionnaires were pretested among 6 families with diverse background to ensure relevance and clarity. Completing the questionnaires took approximately 20 min.

The first questionnaire, completed by parents, collected information on the child's demographic background (age, gender, and birth place), family socioeconomic status (family income, parents' education levels, parents' occupation, and housing condition), family structure (single-parent or nuclear family), presence of sibling, and the birth order of the child.

The second questionnaire was the Parental Authority Questionnaire (PAQ); a psychometric scale that assesses the authoritativeness, authoritarianism and permissiveness practiced by fathers and mothers, respectively, in rearing their children. This study used a short version comprising 20 items, which was adapted from the Buri's 30-item PAQ and showed adequate validity and internal consistency in children [26]. Test-retest reliability (the intraclass correlation) of Buri's PAQ were 0.77–0.92 and internal consistency (Cronbach alpha) were 0.74–0.87 [27]. The validity was adequate; authoritarianism was inversely related to permissiveness (mother: $r = -0.38$; father: $r = -0.50$; all $p < 0.0005$) and authoritativeness (mother: $r = -0.48$; father: $r = -0.52$; all p < 0.0005) and permissiveness was not significantly related to authoritativeness (mother: $r = 0.07$; father: $r = 0.12$; all $p > 0.10$) [27]. The Chinese version of PAQ was adopted [28]. There were 7 items for authoritativeness, 7 for authoritarianism, and 6 for permissiveness. Responses to each item are made on a 5-point Likert scale, ranging from "strongly disagree" to "strongly agree". The total score for each parenting style was calculated by summing scores of items in the corresponding parenting style. Among the three parenting styles (authoritative, authoritarian and permissive), the one with the highest mean score was regarded as the dominant parenting style for that parent. The PAQ was completed by the child him/herself, as instructed.

The third questionnaire was Corah Dental Anxiety Scale (CDAS) for measuring parents' DFA. CDAS has been widely used in research studies and its reliability, validity and usefulness have been documented [29]. The test-retest reliability (correlation coefficient) was 0.82 and the internal consistency (Kuder-Richardson Formula) was 0.86. The validity was moderate as shown by the correlations between the dentists' ratings and the patients' test scores. The scale was later translated into Chinese [30]. CDAS contains 4 items, where respondents choose a score closest to their respective dental situations. The score ranged from 1 (not anxious) to 5 (extremely anxious). The total score for 4 items ranges from 4 to 20, with a higher score indicating a higher DFA level. The anxiety level was classified as "low" (scores below 9), "moderate" (scores from 9 to 12), "high" (scores from 13 to 14), and "severe" (scores from 15 to 20) [29].

The fourth questionnaire was the Children Fear Survey Schedule Dental Subscale (CFSS-DS), which was used to assess child's DFA. CFSS-DS consists of 15 items on various anxiety stimuli [31]. To each item, the response ranges 1–5, from "not afraid at all" to "very much afraid". The total score ranges from 15 to 75. Children with a total CFSS-DS score below 32 are considered non-fearful; 32–39 is defined as moderate fearful; > 39 is defined as fearful [31]. CFSS-DS is deemed one of the most commonly used psychological scales for children. A Chinese version of CFSS-DS [32] was used in this study and was completed by the child him/herself. The test-retest reliability (intraclass correlation) of CFSS-DS was 0.71 and the internal consistency (Cronbach's alpha) was 0.85 [33]. The validity was good; higher mean CFSS-DS scores were found in children who were defined as uncooperative by using the Frankl Scale (standardized mean difference = 1.15; $p < 0.01$) [33]. All scales used can be found in Additional file 1.

Statistical analysis

The data analysis was performed by using Statistical Package for Social Sciences (SPSS) version 23.0. Participants' socio-demographic profile and family related factors were described. Parametric and non-parametric tests were used for comparing means/medians, whereas Chi-square tests were used for comparing proportions. Multiple linear regression models were constructed to test the associations after controlling for possible confounders. The collinearity among independent variables has been tested. In order to avoid possible collinearity, "mother's education" and "father's education" were converted to "parental education", defined as education level of mother or father, whichever is lower. The same conversion applied to "parental occupation". After such conversions, collinearity was ruled out because all the values of tolerance were well above 0.2. The stratified analysis by gender was also carried out to test the associations in boys and girls, respectively.

Results
Socio-demographic profile, family related factors and parenting styles
Among 881 eligible families approached, 405 participated and returned the questionnaires. The response rate was 46.0%. Most (71.0%) children were 10–11 year-old, with some 9 year-olds and 12–13 year-olds (Table 1). There were 188 (46.7%) boys and 215 (53.3%) girls. Most (90.3%) of them were born in Hong Kong. Around two-thirds (62.7%) of mothers were in the age group of 35–44 and two-thirds (60.7%) of fathers were 45 or above. Two-thirds (69.5%) of families had a moderate monthly income (HKD 10,000–39,999). Housing condition was classified into basic (tenement building, public permanent housing), moderate (home ownership scheme, village house, and dormitory) and good (owned or rent private housing estates). Around 61.5% lived in basic housing condition. The majority of mothers (74.3%) and fathers (72.8%) reported secondary school as their highest education level. Occupation is classified

Table 1 Socio-demographic profiles of participants

		n	%
Child's demographic			
Gender	Male	188	46.7
	Female	215	53.3
Age (years)	9	69	17.9
	10–11	274	71.0
	12–13	43	11.1
Place of birth	Hong Kong	355	90.3
	Other places	38	9.7
Parents' demographic			
Mother's age (years)	34 or below	45	12.1
	35–44	234	62.7
	45 or above	94	25.2
Father's age (years)	34 or below	7	2.0
	35–44	131	37.3
	45 or above	213	60.7
Socio-economic status of the family			
Family monthly income[a]	Low (<HKD10000)	71	20.4
	Moderate (HKD10000–39999)	242	69.5
	High (≥HKD40000)	35	10.1
Housing condition[b]	Basic	236	61.5
	Moderate	46	12.0
	Good	102	26.6
Mother's Education	Elementary school or below	33	8.7
	Secondary school	281	74.3
	Tertiary education or above	64	16.9
Father's Education	Elementary school or below	39	11.0
	Secondary school	257	72.8
	Tertiary education	57	16.1
Mother's Occupation[c]	Managerial or professional	25	6.4
	Clerical or skilled workers	51	13.0
	Service or labours	64	16.4
	Housewives	251	64.2
Father's Occupation[c]	Managerial or professional	56	20.2
	Clerical or skilled workers	97	35.0
	Service or labours	113	40.8
	Unemployed	11	4.0
Total		405	100.0

[a]Source: Wang LD-L, Lam WWT, Fielding R. 2016. Hong Kong Chinese parental attitudes towards vaccination and associated socio-demographic disparities. Vaccine. 34:1426–1429
[b]Housing condition was classified into basic (tenement building, public permanent housing), moderate (home ownership scheme, village house, and dormitory) and good (owned or rent private housing estates)
[c]Occupation is classified into managerial or professional (managers and administrators, professionals, self-employed), clerical or skilled workers (associate professionals, clerical support workers), service or labours (sales, unskilled laborers, service industry) and housewives/unemployed

into managerial or professional (managers and administrators, professionals, self-employed), clerical or skilled workers (associate professionals, clerical support workers), service or labours (sales, unskilled laborers, service industry) and housewives/unemployed. Two-thirds (64.2%) of mothers were housewives. Two-thirds (40.8%) of fathers were in the industry of "service or labours".

The majority (91.5%) of children were from nuclear families. Most (70.3%) children had siblings and more than half (55.9%) were the first child in the family. Among the three parenting styles, both parents scored the highest in authoritativeness. The means (SD) were 3.6 (0.8) and 3.6 (0.9) for mothers and for fathers respectively. This was followed by "authoritarian", for which the means (SD) were 3.1 (0.8) and 3.0 (0.9) for mothers and fathers respectively. The scores were the lowest in permissiveness, with a mean (SD) of 2.6 (0.8) and 2.8 (0.9) for mothers and fathers respectively. "Authoritative" was identified as the dominant parenting style for 68.6 and 72.1% mothers and fathers respectively; while 25.0% mothers and 18.0% fathers practiced authoritarian parenting. Only 6.4% mothers and 9.9% fathers were permissive.

Dental fear and anxiety (DFA) of child and parents

Table 2 shows children's responses to possible fearful events related to dental practice. Items that over 20% children felt "very much afraid" or "pretty much afraid" were "the dentist drilling" (32.1%), "the sight of dentist drilling" (24.3%), "having a stranger touch you" (23.6%), "hearing drilling sound" (22.5%) and "injection" (20.6%). As for their DFA level, 66.9% of the children were considered non-fearful, 15.3% were moderate and 17.8% were fearful. The mean (SD) total CFSS-DS score was 29.1 (11.0).

The DFA level of 43.4, 42.1, 11.6 and 2.8% mothers was considered low, moderate, high and severe respectively. As for fathers' DFA level, 54.7, 37.0, 6.6 and 1.7% were considered low, moderate, high and severe respectively. The means (SD) total CDAS score of mothers and fathers were 9.2 (3.0) and 8.2 (2.9) respectively.

Family related factors and children's DFA

No significant difference was found in children's DFA among all socio-economic subgroups (all $p > 0.05$). Table 3 shows the results of bivariate analysis between each family related factor and children's DFA. Parental DFA and parenting styles of both parents were not associated with children's DFA (all $p > 0.05$). Children having siblings tended to report DFA, as compared with single child (37.0% vs. 24.1%; $p = 0.034$). They also had a higher CFSS-DS score (29.9 vs. 27.4; $p = 0.025$). No significant

Table 2 Children's dental fear and anxiety (DFA)

Events/possible triggers	Not afraid at all	Very little fear	Moderate sfear	Pretty much afraid	Very much afraid
			n (%)		
Dentists	187 (47.3)	147 (37.2)	27 (6.8)	12 (3.0)	22 (5.6)
Doctors	276 (69.9)	83 (21.0)	16 (4.1)	9 (2.3)	11 (2.8)
Injections	122 (31.0)	139 (35.3)	52 (13.2)	26 (6.6)	55 (14.0)
Somebody examines your mouth	265 (67.3)	93 (23.6)	24 (6.1)	6 (1.5)	6 (1.5)
Having to open your mouth	334 (84.8)	44 (11.2)	7 (1.8)	3 (0.8)	6 (1.5)
Having a stranger touch you	100 (25.3)	120 (30.4)	82 (20.8)	37 (9.4)	56 (14.2)
Having somebody look at you	180 (45.8)	107 (27.2)	61 (15.5)	22 (5.6)	23 (5.9)
Dentist drilling	97 (24.6)	92 (23.3)	79 (20.0)	42 (10.6)	85 (21.5)
Sight of dentist drilling	168 (43.0)	76 (19.4)	52 (13.3)	36 (9.2)	59 (15.1)
Hearing drilling sound	155 (39.6)	92 (23.5)	56 (14.3)	30 (7.7)	58 (14.8)
Putting instruments in mouth	172 (43.8)	102 (26.0)	46 (11.7)	25 (6.4)	48 (12.2)
Choking	163 (42.0)	116 (29.9)	58 (14.9)	22 (5.7)	29 (7.5)
Having to go to the hospital	185 (47.4)	103 (26.4)	53 (13.6)	18 (4.6)	31 (7.9)
People in white uniform	302 (77.0)	56 (14.3)	15 (3.8)	8 (2.0)	11 (2.8)
Having the dentist clean your teeth	271 (69.0)	77 (19.6)	19 (4.8)	11 (2.8)	15 (3.8)
Mean (SD) of total CFSS-DS score			29.1 (11.0)		
Range of total CFSS-DS score			15.0–66.0		
Possible range of the scale			15.0–75.0		

Level of DFA	Non-fearful CFSS-DS score < 32	Moderate fear CFSS-DS score 32–39	Fearful CFSS-DS score > 39
		n (%)	
	245 (66.9)	56 (15.3)	65 (17.8)

difference was found in DFA scores of those who were first child in the family and others.

When multivariate analysis (linear regression) was conducted (Table 4), children from single-parent families were found with lower CFSS-DS score as compared with children from nuclear families ($\beta = -9.177$; $p = 0.029$). When stratified analysis was carried out for boys and girls separately (Model 2 and Model 3), it was found that (i) boys who had siblings had significantly higher DFA in contrast to those without siblings ($\beta = 7.130$; $p = 0.010$); (ii) boys whose family had a basic housing condition reported significantly lower DFA as compared with those under a good housing condition ($\beta = -7.752$; $p = 0.006$); and (iii) girls from single-parent families had lower DFA score as compared with girls from nuclear families ($\beta = -13.933$; $p = 0.015$).

Discussion

This study explored the possible associations between children's DFA and a variety of family related factors. The results showed that DFA was quite common an issue reported by around one third (33.1%) of children. In comparison with children from nuclear families,

children from single-parent families had lower DFA score. Subgroup analysis showed that boys' DFA was associated with "having siblings", whereas girls' DFA was lower when they were from "single-parent families". Children's DFA was however not associated with parents' DFA or parental styles.

Invasive procedures and dental pain were often reported as the most important causes of dental anxiety [5, 14]. Similarly, teenagers participating in this study tended to relate their DFA to injection and drilling; the latter also extended to stimuli (sound and sight) associated with drilling. It is worth noting that "having a stranger touch you" also appeared as a major fearful situation for the respondents. Our finding is somewhat in line with that of a previous study, in which "having a stranger touch you" was identified as the highest-ranked cause for dental fear, followed by "injection" and "choking" [34]. Although being touched by a stranger in the clinical scenario may not be unexpected and stressful to adult patients, it may impose considerable stress on adolescents. This highlights the importance of building rapport and trust with adolescent patient before starting any dental examination and treatment.

Table 3 Family related factors and Children's DFA

	No fear (CFSS-DS <32)	Moderate fear (CFSS-DS 32-39) n (%)	Severe fear (CFSS-DS >39)	Total CFSS-DS score Mean (SD)
Parental dental fear				
CDAS scale of mother				
Low anxiety	109 (69.4)	27 (17.2)	21 (13.4)	27.90 (10.02)
Moderate anxiety	90 (63.8)	20 (14.2)	31 (22.0)	29.72 (11.98)
High/sever anxiety	35 (66.0)	8 (15.1)	10 (18.9)	30.49 (10.62)
		$P = 0.411$		$P = 0.277$
CDAS scale of father				
Low anxiety	128 (70.3)	21 (11.5)	33 (18.1)	28.42 (11.75)
Moderate anxiety	78 (62.4)	22 (17.6)	25 (20.0)	29.80 (10.63)
High/sever anxiety	13 (56.5)	7 (30.4)	3 (13.0)	31.39 (11.10)
		$P = 0.141$		$P = 0.111$
Parenting style				
Mother dominant style				
Authoritative	167 (68.2)	33 (13.5)	45 (18.4)	28.91 (10.75)
Authoritarian	58 (63.7)	18 (19.8)	15 (16.5)	29.54 (11.64)
Permissive	16 (69.6)	2 (8.7)	5 (21.7)	28.87 (13.23)
		$P = 0.593$		$P = 0.853$
Father dominant style				
Authoritative	164 (66.9)	39 (15.9)	42 (17.1)	28.56 (10.63)
Authoritarian	42 (64.6)	10 (15.4)	13 (20.0)	30.52 (11.74)
Permissive	24 (70.6)	4 (11.8)	6 (17.6)	29.54 (13.22)
		$P = 0.952$		$P = 0.531$
Family characteristics				
Family structure				
Nuclear family	212 (66.3)	51 (15.9)	57 (17.8)	29.1 (11.1)
Single-parent family	23 (76.7)	3 (10.0)	4 (13.3)	26.3 (9.6)
		$p = 0.500$		$p = 0.167$
Having siblings				
Yes	158 (62.9)	45 (17.9)	48 (19.1)	29.9 (11.1)
No	85 (75.9)	10 (8.9)	17 (15.2)	27.4 (10.8)
		$p = 0.034*$		$p = 0.025*$
First child				
Yes	141 (70.5)	22 (11.0)	37 (18.5)	28.8 (11.4)
No	98 (62.8)	31 (19.9)	27 (17.3)	29.4 (10.4)
		$p = 0.065$		$p = 0.280$

p values for categorical outcomes were obtained from the Chi-square test. p values for continuous outcomes were obtained from the non-parametric test (Mann-Whitney U test or Kruskal-Wallis test)
*Significant difference

It was often speculated that parental DFA and parenting styles are associated with children's DFA. Such association was supported by a studies conducted in the US [12] and was however absent in our study sample. It is worth noting that our study focused on a slightly older age group as compared with the American study. There is a notion that older children's perception of dental treatment is more influenced by their actual dental experience such as painful procedure and professional's behaviors [17]. Fear toward unknown appears to be predominant during early childhood, but fears are usually linked to

Table 4 Determinants of DFA in children (CFSS-DS score)

		Model 1 (all children) β (95% CI)**	Model 2 (boys) β (95% CI)**	Model 3 (girls) β (95% CI)**
Age (years)	Continuous	−0.165 (−1.229, 0.899)	0.822 (− 1.339, 2.982)	− 0.838 (− 2.146, 0.470)
Gender	Male [#]			
	Female	2.554 (−0.088, 5.197)	—	—
Place of birth	Hong Kong[#]			
	Other places	−4.036 (− 8.848,0.776)	0.839 (− 6.055, 7.733)	− 6.143 (− 13.355, 1.068)
Family monthly income	Continuous	−0.098 (−1.342, 1.146)	− 1.057 (− 2.835, 0.721)	0.964 (− 0.925, 2.854)
Family housing condition	Good[#]			
	Moderate	−3.373 (− 8.068, 1.322)	−7.011 (− 13.943, − 0.079)	−2.977(− 9.927, 3.972)
	Basic	−3.247 (− 6.857,0.363)	− 7.752 (− 13.204, − 2.301)*	− 2.061 (− 7.240, 3.117)
Parental Education[##]	Continuous	−2.214 (− 5.415, 0.986)	−4.540 (− 9.825, 0.745)	−1.907 (− 6.314, 2.500)
Parental Occupation[##]	Unemployed/housewives[#]			
	Service /labours	3.223 (−0.014, 6.460)	5.646 (1.220, 10.071)*	1.309 (− 3.608, 6.225)
	Clerical/skilled workers	−0.434 (− 4.916, 4.048)	−5.057 (− 12.018, 1.904)	−0.509 (− 6.841, 5.822)
	Managerial/ professional	2.748 (− 6.035, 11.530)	15.713 (− 0.516, 31.942)	− 4.041 (− 15.161, 7.079)
Age of first dental visit	1–6 years-old [#]			
	7–11 years-old	−0.153 (− 3.857, 3.551)	−3.001 (− 8.119, 2.117)	3.416 (− 2.348, 9.179)
First visit as checkup	Checkup [#]			
	Treatment	−0.749 (− 3.844, 2.347)	1.520 (−3.098, 6.138)	− 1.885 (− 6.179, 2.409)
Having sibling	No [#]			
	Yes	3.386 (−0.210, 6.982)	7.130 (1.757, 12.503)*	1.147 (− 4.228, 6.523)
First child	No [#]			
	Yes	1.038 (−2.317, 4.394)	3.159 (−2.090, 8.408)	− 0.010 (− 4.761, 4.740)
Family structure	Nuclear family[#]			
	Single-parent family	−9.177(− 17.418,-0.936)*	− 4.564 (− 17.936, 8.808)	−13.933(− 25.136,-2.731)*
Mother's dominant parenting style	Authoritative [#]			
	Authoritarian	0.062 (−3.283, 3.407)	0.222 (−4.494, 4.938)	− 0.504 (− 5.392, 4.385)
	Permissive	2.277 (−4.071, 8.624)	0.651 (− 10.264, 11.566)	2.921 (−5.681, 11.523)
Father's dominant parenting style	Authoritative [#]			
	Authoritarian	0.099 (−3.662, 3.859)	0.720 (−4.730, 6.170)	0.383 (−5.239, 6.006)
	Permissive	1.689 (−2.723, 6.101)	4.298 (−1.834, 10.430)	−1.052 (− 7.703, 5.599)
Mother's dental fear	Continuous	0.209 (−0.251, 0.669)	0.388 (−0.267, 1.042)	0.044 (− 0.627, 0.716)
Father's dental fear	Continuous	0.298 (−0.178, 0.774)	0.310 (−0.344, 0.965)	0.310 (− 0.407, 1.027)
Constant		28.845(13.512, 44.177)	22.804(−5.129, 50.737)	37.964 (17.833,58.095)
		$R^2 = 0.095$	$R^2 = 0.224$	$R^2 = 0.117$

The results were obtained through multiple linear regressions using total CFSS–DS score of all children, CFSS–DS score of boys, and CFSS–DS score of girls as a dependent variable respectively. Independent variables are as above
*Significant difference between/among subgroups
**CI: confidence interval
[#]Reference group
[##]Parental education was defined as mother's or father's education, whichever is lower. The same conversion applied to "parental occupation"

body injures including various situations encounter in dental setting by 9 years of age [35]. A review also indicated that the relationship between parental and child' dental fear was obvious in children under 8 years old [10]. It is possible that parental DFA is not a direct factor to influence child's DFA when the child reached adolescence.

The finding that children in single-parent families reported less DFA is in congruence with a previous study [18] but contradict some others [36, 37]. In single-parent families, children may become more independent and are more likely to grow maturity and resilience [38]. Given these characteristics, they may cope better with the challenges and stressful situations, such as dental visit. Also, children in single-parent families may receive more attention from other caregivers, such as grandparents. This might also play a role in their growth and development. For instance, grandfathers were identified as an important figure who can affect the emotional transmission of dental fear among family members [13].

Given the gender difference in psychological development and socialization, stratified analysis was performed for boys and girls respectively. It was found that among boys, the impact of having sibling(s) was evident; those with sibling(s) reported significantly higher DFA. There is a notion that only-born children tend to internalize parents' expectations, turn predominantly mature, have higher self-esteem, and grow adult behavior due to their enhanced time interacting with adults [39]. On the other hand, there was an alternative theory describing personality of single-born children as more self-centered, demanding, shy, dependent and moody [40]. While the former lends support to our findings, the latter points to the possibility of higher DFA in single children, which was a finding of some other studies [21, 22]. There were also research studies suggesting no difference in the personalities of single child and their peers with siblings when judged by parents, teachers, and themselves [41]. Apart from personality traits, siblings' past dental experience and their positive or negative modeling might play an important role in shaping children's perception of dental care. The analysis for girls showed that living in a single family indicated a lower level of DFA, as compared with those in nuclear families. It is believed that girls are more adult-oriented [42]; therefore they may be more affected by parental factors and less by their siblings.

The findings of this study could be better interpreted by taking into consideration the methodological strengthens and limitations. Data were collected from a relatively large sample with diverse backgrounds. Well-established and validated psychometric scales were used to measure parenting styles and the DFA of children and their parents. For determining the parenting styles, different scales are available and can be completed by parents or children. Since parents may tend to give socially desirable answers and their perceptions may not truly reflect the reality, children's response is preferable. Although some items may seem abstract, reliable answers could be obtained from adolescents through proper wording of the questions. This study is cross-sectional in nature. Therefore, no temporal relationship can be established and our findings could

only suggest associations but not causation. The sample of this study was drawn from children in Hong Kong. Therefore, findings of this study cannot be directly extrapolated to other populations, although some useful implications can be drawn especially for populations of similar cultures and social context. Although the regression models suggested the impact of familial factors on children's DFA, the R^2 were low and the models only explained 9.5, 22.4, and 11.7% of the variance in DFA of all subjects, boys, and girls, respectively. This supports the notion that DFA is a complex phenomenon, in which many other factors, such as child's personality traits [43], past dental experiences [44], other life incidents/events [45], were involved.

To sum up, several implications can be derived from the findings of this study. The commonly neglected factors (e.g. "having a stranger touch you") that trigger DFA in children implies that dental personnel could consider spending some time wherever possible to establish trust with paediatric patients before proceeding to dental procedures. Previous research revolved around parents' DFA and consequently negative modeling on children. Our findings however suggest that the impact of family on the development of children's DFA is not as straightforward as previously speculated. In contrast to the assumption held by many people, our results showed that children's DFA is not associated with parents' DFA and parenting style. Instead, family structure (nuclear/single-parent family) and presence of siblings plays a significant role in children's DFA. To prevent and intercept DFA among children, it may be important to redirect the attention from parental influence to possible negative influence of siblings. Although children from nuclear family might benefit from such healthy family environment in many aspects of their personal growth, they are more likely to have DFA. Parents and clinicians are advised to be more sensitive to the signs of DFA in these children and make necessary efforts to prepare them for dental visits.

Conclusions

Family structure (nuclear or single-parent family) and presence of siblings are significant determinants for children's DFA. Parental DFA and parenting style do not affect children's DFA significantly.

Abbreviations
CDAS: Corah Dental Anxiety Scale; CFSS–DS: Fear Survey Schedule-Dental Subscale; DFA: Dental fear and anxiety; PAQ: Parent Authority Questionnaire; SPSS: Statistical Package for Social Sciences

Acknowledgements
The following people have contributed significantly to the subject recruitment, preparation of questionnaires, data collection, and data handling: CHU Sin Po, KWOK Hoi Ching Venus, LAI Wing Tak, LEE Hor Ching, MOK Kar Po Carolle, NGAN Ming Chun, WONG Wing Lam, YIP Chun Kit and YU Chak Fai.

Funding
This study was financially supported by the Faculty of Dentistry, The University of Hong Kong. The funding body played no role in the design of the study and collection, analysis, and interpretation of the data and in writing the manuscript.

Authors' contributions
LW contributed to the data analysis and manuscript preparation. XG contributed to the design of the work and supervised the data collection, data analysis, manuscript preparation and critical revisions. Both authors have read and approved the final version of the manuscript submitted for publication.

Competing interests
The authors declare that they have no competing interests.

Author details
[1]Department of Dentistry, Key Laboratory of Oral Diseases of Gansu Province, Northwest University for Nationalities, Lanzhou, China. [2]Dental Public Health, Faculty of Dentistry, The University of Hong Kong, 3rd Floor, Prince Philip Dental Hospital, 34 Hospital Road, Sai Ying Pun, Hong Kong.

References
1. Klingberg G, Broberg AG. Dental fear/anxiety and dental behaviour management problems in children and adolescents: a review of prevalence and concomitant psychological factors. Int J Paediatr Dent. 2007;17:391–406.
2. Chhabra N, Chhabra A, Walia G. Prevalence of dental anxiety and fear among five to ten year old children: a behaviour based cross sectional study. Minerva Stomatol. 2012;61:83–9.
3. Baier K, Milgrom P, Russell S, Mancl L, Yoshida T. Children's fear and behavior in private pediatric dentistry practices. Pediatr Dent. 2004;26: 316–21.
4. Gatchel RJ. The prevalence of dental fear and avoidance: expanded adult and recent adolescent surveys. J Am Dent Assoc (1939). 1989;118:591–3.
5. Gao X, Hamzah SH, Yiu CK, McGrath C, King NM. Dental fear and anxiety in children and adolescents: qualitative study using YouTube. J Med Internet Res. 2013;15:e29.
6. Crocombe LA, Broadbent JM, Thomson WM, Brennan DS, Slade GD, Poulton R. Dental visiting trajectory patterns and their antecedents. J Public Health Dent. 2011;71:23–31.
7. Milgrom P, Weinstein P. Dental fears in general practice: new guidelines for assessment and treatment. Int Dent J. 1993;43:288–93.
8. Rachman S. The conditioning theory of fear-acquisition: a critical examination. Behav Res Ther. 1977;15:375–87.
9. Newman BM. Development through life: a psychosocial approach (6th ed.). Pacific Grove, Calif.: Brooks/Cole Pub. Co. 1995.
10. Themessl-Huber M, Freeman R, Humphris G, MacGillivray S, Trezi N. Empirical evidence of the relationship between parental and child dental fear: a structured review and meta-analysis. Int J Paediatr Dent. 2010;20:83–101.
11. Boynes SG, Abdulwahab M, Kershner E, Mickens F, Riley A. Analysis of parental factors and parent-child communication with pediatric patients referred for nitrous oxide administration in a rural community health center setting. Oral Biol Dent. 2014;2:10.
12. Majstorovic M, Morse DE, Do D, Lim L, Herman NG, Moursi AM. Indicators of dental anxiety in children just prior to treatment. J Clin Pediatr Dent. 2014; 39:12–7.
13. Lara A, Crego A, Romero-Maroto M. Emotional contagion of dental fear to children: the fathers' mediating role in parental transfer of fear. Int J Paediatr Dent. 2012;22:324–30.
14. Olak J, Saag M, Honkala S, Nommela R, Runnel R, Honkala E, Karjalainen S. Children's dental fear in relation to dental health and parental dental fear. Stomatologija. 2013;15:26–31.
15. Burlaka V. Externalizing behaviors of Ukrainian children: the role of parenting. Child Abuse Negl. 2016;54:23–32.
16. Baumrind D. Current patterns of parental authority. Dev Psychol. 1971;4:1–103.
17. Ten Berge M, Veerkamp JS, Hoogstraten J, Prins PJM. Childhood dental fear in relation to parental child-rearing attitudes. Psy Report. 2003;92:43–50.
18. Krikken JB, Vanwijk AJ, Tencate JM, Veerkamp JS. Child dental anxiety, parental rearing style and dental history reported by parents. Eur J Paediatr Dent. 2013;14:258–62.
19. Sulloway FJ. Birth-order, sibling competition, and human behavior. In: Holcomb HR, editor. Conceptual challenges in evolutionary psychology: innovative research strategies. 3rd ed. Dordrecht, the Netherlands: Kluwer Academic; 2001.
20. Gould SJ. Dolly's fashion and louis's passion. (implications of the current fascination with the genetic sciences and its use in popular culture to explain moral and behavioral phenomena: cloned sheep and behavior of first-born judges who condemned louis xiv). Nat Hist. 1997;106:18.
21. Aminabadi NA, Sohrabi A, Erfanparast LK, Oskouei SG, Ajami BA. Can birth order affect temperament, anxiety and behavior in 5 to 7-year-old children in the dental setting? J Contemp Dent Pract. 2011;12:225–31.
22. Ghaderi F, Fijan S, Hamedani S. How do children behave regarding their birth order in dental setting? J dent (Shiraz,Iran). 2015;16:329–34.
23. Rantavuori K, Tolvanen M, Hausen H, Lahti S, Seppä L. Factors associated with different measures of dental fear among children at different ages. J Dent Child (Chic). 2009;76:13–9.
24. Peretz B, Nazarian Y, Bimstein E. Dental anxiety in a students' paediatric dental clinic: children, parents and students. Int J Paediatr Dent. 2004;14: 192–8.
25. Chellappah NK, Vignehsa H, Milgrom P, Lo GL. Prevalence of dental anxiety and fear in children in Singapore. Community Dent Oral Epidemiol. 1990;18:269–71.
26. Alkharusi H, Aldhafri S, Kazem A, Alzubiadi A, Al-Bahrani M. Development and validation of a short version of the parental authority questionnaire. Social Behavior And Personality. 2011;39:1193–208.
27. Buri JR. Parental authority questionnaire. J Pers Assess. 1991;57:110–9.
28. Zhou YJ, Liang BY, Cai Y. Chinese revision of Buri's parental authority questionnaire. Chin J Clin Psych. 2010;18:8–10.
29. Corah NL. Development of a dental anxiety scale. J Dent Res. 1969;48:596.
30. Guo B, Liu J, Yang F, Xie SJ, Que KH, Zhang Q. The prevalence of dental anxiety in the aged people. International journal of stomatology. 2007;34: 162–4.
31. Cuthbert MI. Melamed BG. A screening device: children at risk for dental fears and management problems. ASDC J Dent Child. 1982;49:432–6.
32. Lu JX, Yu DS, Luo W, Xiao XF, Zhao W. Development of Chinese version of children's fear survey schedule-dental subscale, Zhonghua kouqiang yixue zazhi = Chinese journal of stomatology 2011; 46: 218–221.
33. Ma L, Wang M, Jing Q, Zhao J, Wan K, Xu Q. Reliability and validity of the chinese version of the children's fear survey schedule-dental subscale. Int J Paediatr Dent. 2015;25:110–6.
34. Raadal M, Milgrom P, Weinstein P, Mancl L, Cauce AM. The prevalence of dental anxiety in children from low-income families and its relationship to personality traits. J Dent Res. 1995;74:1439–43.
35. Chapman HR, Kirby-Turner NC. Dental fear in children–a proposed model. Br Dent J. 1999;187:408–12.
36. Gustafsson A. Dental behaviour management problems among children and adolescents–a matter of understanding? Studies on dental fear,

personal characteristics and psychosocial concomitants Swed Dent J Suppl 2010:2 p preceding 1–46.

37. Suprabha BS, Rao A, Choudhary S, Shenoy R. Child dental fear and behavior: the role of environmental factors in a hospital cohort. J Indian Soc Pedod Prev Dent. 2011;29:95–101.

38. Spagnola M, Fiese BH. Family routines and rituals. Infants & Young Children. 2007;20:284–99.

39. Shen J, Yuan BJ. Moral values of only and sibling children in mainland China. The J Psychol. 1999;133:115–24.

40. Bögels SM, Brechman-Toussaint ML. Family issues in child anxiety: attachment, family functioning, parental rearing and beliefs. Clin Psychol Rev. 2006;26:834–56.

41. Falbo T, Poston DL Jr. The academic, personality, and physical outcomes of only children in China. Child Dev. 1993;64:18–35.

42. Crombie G. Gender differences: implications for social skills assessment and training. J Clin Child Psychol. 1988;17:116–20.

43. Halonen H, Salo T, Hakko H, Rasanen P. Association of dental anxiety to personality traits in a general population sample of finnish university students. Acta Odontol Scand. 2012;70:96–100.

44. Lee CY, Chang YY, Huang ST. The clinically related predictors of dental fear in taiwanese children. Int J Paediatr Dent. 2008;18:415–22.

45. Hagqvist O, Tolvanen M, Rantavuori K, Karlsson L, Karlsson H, Lahti S. Dental fear and previous childhood traumatic experiences, life events, and parental bonding. Eur J Oral Sci. 2015;123:96–101.

11

Glass hybrid restorations as an alternative for restoring hypomineralized molars in the ART model

Juliana de Aguiar Grossi[1], Renata Nunes Cabral[1], Ana Paula Dias Ribeiro[1,2] and Soraya Coelho Leal[1]* (iD)

Abstract

Background: This study aimed to evaluate the survival rate of glass hybrid restorations placed under the atraumatic restorative treatment (ART) technique in first permanent molars affected by molar incisor hypomineralization (MIH).

Methods: Sixty teeth with severe MIH associated to carious dentin lesions without pulp involvement were included. Treatments were performed by one trained dentist using the ART approach and restored with a glass hybrid restorative system (Equia Forte, GC®) on school premises. Treatments were evaluated after 6 and 12 months by an independent examiner using the modified ART criterion. Data analysis involved descriptive statistics and actuarial success analysis.

Results: The sample comprised 24 (54.54%) girls and 20 (45.45%) boys with a mean age of 10.55 (±1.25) years. In regard to the number of surfaces involved in the restorations, 29 (48.3%) comprised one surface and 31 (51.7%) two or more surfaces. Considering cavity extent, 25 (41%) presented dentin cavitation without cusp weakness, 23 (37.7%) with large dentin cavitation with cusp weakness and 13 (21.3%) with large dentin cavitation with the breakdown of one or more cusps. Only 4 teeth required local anesthesia. A success rate of 98.3% after 6 and 12 months was observed, as only one restoration failed. The only failure occurred in a restoration involving three or more sur-faces presenting the breakdown of all cusps.

Conclusion: Restorations using a glass hybrid restorative system and performed in the field with the ART technique proved, after 12 months of evaluation, to be an effective approach to preserving first permanent molars affected by MIH.

Keywords: Molar incisor hypomineralization, Atraumatic restorative treatment, Glass ionomer, Cavity size, Survival rate

Background

Molar incisor hypomineralization (MIH) is a relatively common condition, with its prevalence varying from 20% to 40% depending on the population studied [1, 2]. Due to its high prevalence, MIH should receive more attention, specially in developing more appropriate dental healthcare strategies to manage the problem [3]. However, it is believed that the real prevalence of MIH might not be known, as there are many methodological differences among studies carried out by different research groups [4].

MIH is defined as a developmental defect of the enamel of systemic origin that is observed in at least one of the first permanent molars, sometimes also affecting the permanent incisors [5]. Genetic variations, preterm and a number of childhood illness (such as acute otitis media, chicken pox and respiratory diseases during first years of life) are likely to be related to MIH [6]. Clinically, the lesions are characterized by demarcated opacities varying from white to a yellow/brown color surrounded by sound enamel [7]. The affected enamel is of normal thickness but of low quality in comparison with the sound enamel because of the presence of porosities that become progressively more severe as the color of the opacities changes; the darker the opacity, the lower the mineral content [6]. Often, because of masticatory forces, posteruptive breakdown of the affected enamel

* Correspondence: sorayaodt@yahoo.com
[1]Faculdade de Ciências da Saúde, Universidade de Brasília, Campus Universitário Darcy Ribeiro, Asa Norte, Brasília, DF 70910-900, Brazil
Full list of author information is available at the end of the article

is observed [5, 8], which may increase sensitivity in the region due to the exposure of the dentin below the fractured enamel.

Moreover, a significant association between MIH and dental caries was found [9, 10]. Also, MIH is considered a risk factor for dental caries in populations with a low prevalence of caries [11], meaning that children who are of low caries risk have a higher chance to present the disease if affected by MIH. Chemically, the defective enamel has a high amount of carbon and a low concentration of calcium and phosphorus when compared with sound enamel [5]. Jalevik et al. (2001) [12] observed that the presence of large porosities in the microstructure of the hypomineralized enamel affects the adhesive performance of composite resin, leading to the premature loss of restorations on MIH-affected teeth. Thus, these teeth end up requiring repeated interventions, making treatment more complex and challenging [7, 13, 14].

The management of MIH is challenging as the clinical appearance and individual need for treatment varies widely [15]. Many treatment options are described for the clinical management of MIH-affected teeth that present posteruptive breakdown, such as the use of steel crowns [16], composite resin, and glass ionomer cement (GIC) [2] and also exodontia followed by orthodontia. However, consensus regarding the best restorative option for this condition is lacking in the literature [7, 8, 13, 14]. Moreover, taking into account that in low socio-economic communities, the access to dental care is limited, it is worth testing alternative treatment models for severe MIH affected teeth in which the dental equipment is not needed.

Therefore, the objective of this paper was to evaluate the survival rate of restorations performed using a new glass hybrid restorative system placed according to the atraumatic restorative treatment (ART) technique in first permanent molars affected by MIH. The choice of the ART protocol relied on the fact that it can be applied in a conventional dental setting and in field conditions [17, 18].

Methods
Study population
The sample was composed of children aged 7 to 13 years, who were selected from a previous epidemiological survey of 1963 children from Paranoá, an underserved community located about 30 km from Brasilia, the capital of Brazil. Of these, 185 children had MIH. A survey of their treatment needs was undertaken, and those in need of restorative treatment on MIH-affected teeth were included in this clinical trial (Fig. 1). Cases in which endodontic treatment and/or dental extraction were indicated were excluded and referred to the Regional Hospital of Paranoá to receive treatment.

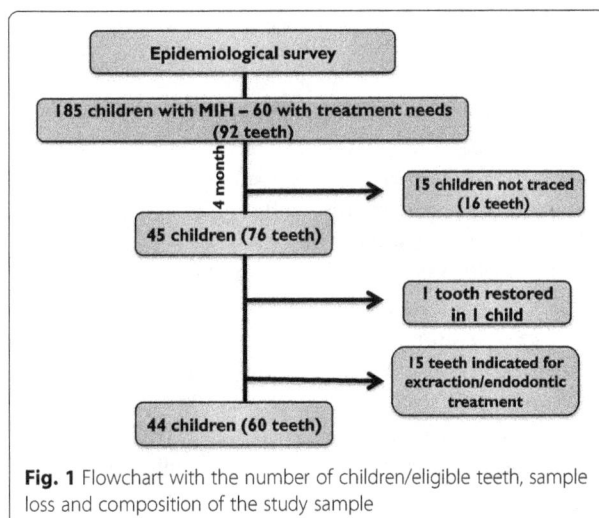

Fig. 1 Flowchart with the number of children/eligible teeth, sample loss and composition of the study sample

Parents or guardians of the selected children were interviewed by telephone regarding the socioeconomic status of the family and their knowledge of the oral health status of their children (Additional file 1).

Before the examinations were carried out, the study objectives were explained to the parents, who then signed an informed consent form. This study was approved by the Research Ethics Committee of the University of Brasilia, Brazil (CAAE-31973413.0.0000.0030) and registered as a clinical trial in the Brazilian Registry of Clinical Trials (REBEC-RBR-8drccq) with the support of the local Secretary of Education.

Selection of cases
To determine the treatment needs of the children with MIH-affected teeth, a trained and calibrated examiner performed the clinical examinations on the school premises using portable beds, a probe, a mirror, and artificial lighting. The Nyvad criterion [19] that differentiates active from inactive carious lesions at both cavitated and non-cavitated levels, and the EAPD criterion [20] were used respectively to record dental caries and MIH. The EAPD criterion registers enamel opacities, post-eruptive breakdown, atypical restorations and tooth loss due to MIH. But in this study, it was modified as enamel breakdown with and without dentin exposure was recorded separately. Prior to the study, the examiner had been extensively calibrated on using both criteria under the supervision of an expert. Discussions and practical exercises were carried out followed by the examination of 32 children who did not participate in the main study, until an acceptable intra-examiner reliability was obtained. Kappa values of 0.95 for dental caries and 0.85 for MIH were obtained. Those teeth which presented only opacities (mild MIH) and/or opacities with posteruptive breakdown limited to the enamel (moderate MIH) were

judged as not in need of invasive treatment. Teeth with posteruptive breakdown already involving dentin or those with atypical unsatisfactory restoration (severe MIH) in which there was a breakdown at the restorations margins, but that the restoration was working properly were classified as needing restoration and formed the sample of this study. MIH teeth in which pulpal exposure, fistulas, and abscesses were observed and those with major coronal destruction were indicated for endodontic treatment or exodontia. Radiographs were not used in addition to the clinical examination as all treatments were performed under field conditions. It is important to stress that the cases that were dubious, in which the examiners judged that a reliable diagnosis could not be performed without a radiograph, were excluded.

Clinical procedures

All the restorative treatment was carried out on school premises by a single dentist and an assistant, with the child lying on a portable bed. Before beginning treatment, both the operator and the assistant were trained to perform restorations using the glass hybrid restorative system and the ART protocol [21]. The training took place at the University Hospital of Brasília, where the operator performed several restorations under the super-vision of an expert.

The carious tissue was removed with sharp excavators (Kit ART, Duflex® - Rio de Janeiro, Brazil). In some cases, when the carious tissue was involving all the hypomineralized enamel, the total affected structure was removed. Therefore, there were situations in which the restoration was placed along an MIH affected border while in others, in sound enamel. The carious removal process followed the principles of Minimum Intervention Dentistry, where the tissue was removed selectively, depending on the cavity depth [22]. In addition, unsupported enamel was removed with a hatchet specifically developed for the ART approach. If the child complained of pain, local anesthesia was administered. Once the cavity was considered ready to receive the restoration, it was classified according to the number of surfaces involved: one surface and two or more surfaces. Cavities were also classified according to the Mount & Hume classification [23] as follows: dentin cavitation without cusp weakening; extensive dentin cavitation with cusp weakening; or very extensive cavitation with destruction of one or more cusps.

The cavity was then conditioned using the Cavity Conditioner® (GC, Leuven, Belgium) for 10 s. After washing the cavity with a cotton wool pellet soaked in water, the cavity was isolated with a cotton roll, and dried with dried cotton pellets. While the operator kept the environment dry, the assistant activated the glass hybrid

restorative system (Equia Forte®, GC Europe, Leuven, Belgium) in the mixer indicated by the manufacturer for 10 s. Immediately thereafter, the capsule containing the ready-to-use material was loaded into the appropriate applicator and inserted into the cavity. The material was pressed down for 40 s with a finger coated in petroleum jelly. The excess material was then removed, and the occlusion was checked using fine carbon paper. Dry cotton pellets were used to clean the surface, and the procedure was completed by applying a resinous and light-cured surface sealant (Equia Coat®, GC, Leuven, Belgium) for 20 s.

Evaluation

One examiner (dentist) evaluated the restorations on school premises after six and 12 months using the modified ART criterion (Table 1), in which only codes 0 and 1 are considered success [24].

Previous to start assessing the restorations, the examiner was trained in using the criterion at paediatric clinic at University of Brasilia, where the examiner evaluated a series of ART restorations up to a kappa higher than 0. 90 was obtained. Battery-illuminated dental mirrors (Kudos®, Hong Kong, China), CPITN probes, and compressed air aided in the evaluation.

Statistical analysis

The data were analyzed using Stata Software Version 14. 1. Descriptive statistics were used to present the results. The success rate of the MIH restorations was evaluated using the actuarial methods technique.

Results

Treatment needs

All the first permanent molars and incisors of the 185 children diagnosed with MIH during the epidemiological survey were evaluated regarding treatment needs for a total of 2200 teeth (740 M and 1480 incisors). MIH

Table 1 Codes used to assess the ART restorations and their description

Code	Criteria
0	Present, stisfactory
1	Present, slight deficiency at cavity margin less than 0.5 mm
2	Present, slight deficiency at cavity margin more than 0.5 mm
3	Present, fracture in the restoration
4	Present, fracture in the tooth
5	Present, overextension of approximal margin of 0.5 mm or more
6	Not present, most or all restoration is missing
7	Not present, other restorative treatment performed
8	Not present, tooth is not present
9	Unable to diagnose

characteristics were detected in 447 M and 158 incisors (27.5%), of which 82.65% were classified as not needing invasive treatment. Of those needing treatment (105 M and 1 incisor), 5.66% of the teeth ($n = 6$) were indicated for extraction, 7.54% ($n = 8$) were referred for endodontic treatment, and 86.80% ($n = 92$) for restoration. All teeth in need of treatment had associated carious lesions.

Characterization of lesions
Sixty teeth were restored: 31 upper molars (51.67%), 28 lower molars (46.67%) and a lower central incisor (1.67%).

Regarding MIH, all teeth were classified as severe: 57 teeth (95%) presented posteruptive breakdown with exposure of the dentin and three with (5%) unsatisfactory atypical restorations.

Considering the number of surfaces involved, 29 (48.3%) restorations involved only one surface. and 31 (51.7%) involved two or more surfaces. As for the extent of the cavity, 25 (41%) presented lesions in the dentin without compromise of the cusp, 23 (37.7%) had dentin lesions with cusp weakening, and 13 (21.3%) had dentin lesions with destruction of one or more cusps.

Pain
Both the presence of pain and the need for local anesthesia before the beginning of treatment were recorded. Nine children reported feeling pain (15%), but only two (4 teeth) required local anesthesia. No significant associations were found between the number of surfaces involved and pain, or between the number of surfaces involved and the use of anesthesia ($p > 0.05$, Chi2).

Success rate
Within 6 months of evaluation, one failure was recorded (Fig. 2g-i) and was classified as 6 using the modified ART criterion [24], which characterizes fracture of the restoration and/or tooth in need of repair. The remaining restorations were classified as codes 1 (54 restorations, 90%) (Fig. 2a-f) and 2 (five restorations, 8.33%), which indicates good condition or marginal wear of less than 0.5 mm with no need for repair, respectively.

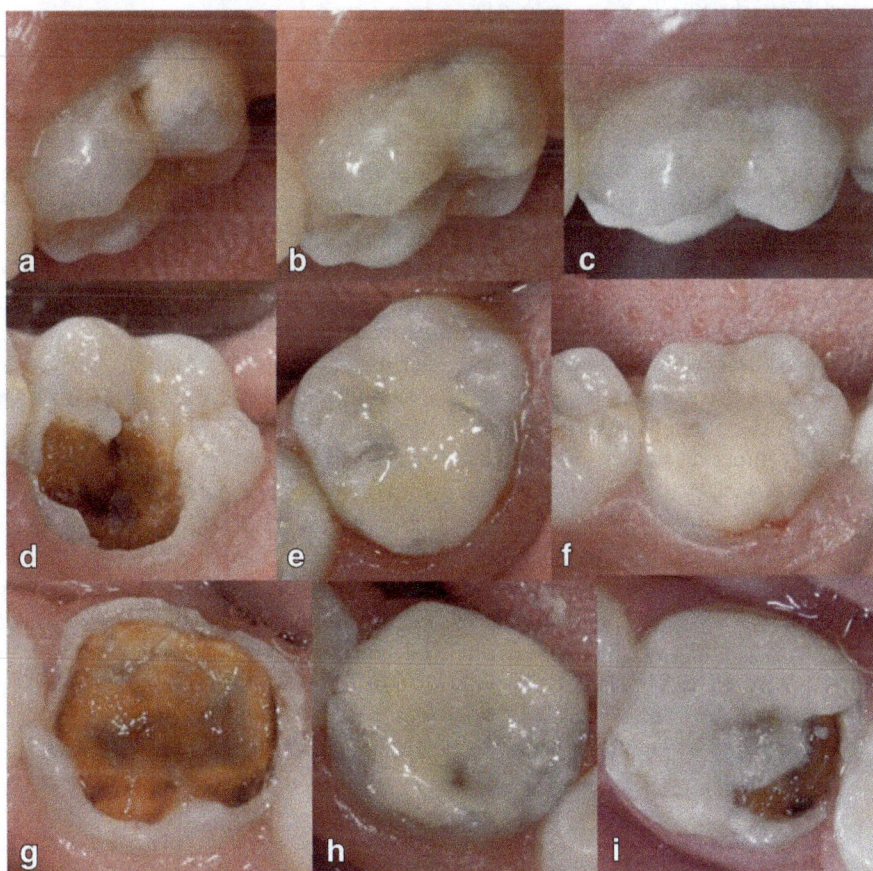

Fig. 2 12-month follow-up and restorative failure. **a**, **d**, **g** - initial aspect of MIH affected molars associated with carious lesions at baseline; **b**, **e**, **h** - clinical aspect of restorations immediately after being performed using the ART technique involving 1 surface (**b**), 2 surfaces (**e**) and all surfaces (**h**); **c**, **f**, **i** - clinical aspect of restorations after 12 months (**c** and **d**) and the only failure observed (**i**) which occurred after 6 months follow-up

During the 6- to 12-month follow-up period, no other failure was recorded. However, four children (five restorations) were censored during this time as they were not available for evaluation. It was observed that 42 (74.78%) restorations remained classified as code 1, and 12 (22.22%) restorations as code 2. The success rate was 98.3%, as noted below in Table 2.

Parent/Guardian social questionnaire

The questionnaire (Additional file 1) response rate was 63.64%. The data indicated that the sample was composed of children considered to be socially vulnerable based on their family income and the level of schooling of their guardian. The income of the families did not exceed two Brazilian minimum wages (71.42%), and the guardian's level of education, in more than half of the cases (53.57%), did not exceed eight years of study.

With regard to the oral health of the children, fewer than half of the interviewees reported being aware that their child had caries. Of those who said they knew, 53.57% said they had sought treatment, as opposed to 46.42% who had not. Of those who sought treatment, 17.85% sought private care, and 35.61% sought public service care. Of those who sought public care, only 44% were evaluated.

Discussion

This study aimed to evaluate the success rate of restorations in MIH-affected teeth using a new restorative material and the ART protocol. The results showed a high success rate after 12 months, proving that such a strategy is a viable option for managing the problem, even without conventional dental equipment.

The present study was conducted in Paranoá, a region that has one of the lowest human development indexes in the Federal District [25]. In this context, the vast majority of families depend on the public healthcare system for dental treatment. This information is supported by the number of teeth in need of treatment and by the parents' reports regarding the difficulties of obtaining treatment in the public service. This is not an unexpected result, since another study carried out in same region also revealed the limited access of this population to healthcare services, whether public or private [26].

Considering the vulnerability of this population, the use of the ART protocol in a school environment was, surely, the most suitable choice. ART is an approach that has

been used in other countries, broadening the population's access to healthcare services [18] and increasing the number of restorative procedures. In a study carried out in South Africa, the introduction of ART into the public service increased the number of teeth restored in both deciduous and permanent dentitions [27]. However, there is a lack of information about the performance of ART restorations in permanent teeth. Therefore, the restorations placed in this study must be carefully controlled, not only because of the nature of the procedure, but also due to the MIH affected tooth fragility. In this context, repair and even replacing the restorations might be needed in the future. In addition, the reduced need for local anesthesia in the ART approach is an advantage, especially when unaccompanied children are being treated. ART has proved to be especially important in the behavior management of children when the dentist is not pediatric specialist [17], as was the case in the present investigation. Of the 44 children treated, only two (four teeth) required local anesthesia during the procedure. The low need for local anesthesia related to ART is probably due to the exclusive use of hand instruments to access and clean the cavity, but this is a hypothesis that calls for further investigation.

The success of restorations after 12 months of follow-up was 98%, considered a high success rate. This result was better than that found by Fragelli et al. (2014) [2], in which a 78% success rate was achieved in restorations performed on teeth affected by MIH. The difference with respect to survival rates between the present investigation and the study performed by Fragelli et al., (2014) [2] may be due to the restorative technique and the type of restorative material used. In the present investigation, the restorations were placed using the ART technique, in which absolute isolation is not used, and a new encapsulated hybrid restorative system. Fragelli et al. (2014) [2] used a high viscosity glass ionomer cement that was hand mixed.

Regarding the type of material, this is the first clinical study to Equia Forte® (GC, Leuven, Belgium) for severely affected MIH teeth, making it impossible to compare these results with similar studies. However, Gurgan et al. (2015) [28] evaluated the clinical performance of Equia Fil® (GC, Leuven, Belgium) with a surface protector (Equia Coat®, GC, Leuven, Belgium), precursor of the Equia Forte®, for managing carious lesions in premolars and permanent molars for four years in comparison with

Table 2 Success of ART restorations in the 6- and 12-month periods

Interval (months)	Restorations evaluated in this period	Censored restorations	Restorations at risk during the period	Failures during the interval	Success rate during the interval	Cumulative success rate until the end of the observation period
6	60	0	60	1	0.983	0.983
12	54	5	54	0	1	0.983

the microhybrid composite resin. The authors showed that the clinical performance of Equia Fil® was similar to that of composite resin for both class I and class II restorations [28]. One of the differentials of this hybrid restorative system is the surface protection of the restorations, which is accomplished by applying a light-cure resin sealant that seems to improve the final smoothness of the restoration and reduce surface wear. The material used in the present study seems to have had a positive influence on the survival outcomes.

Composite resin was recently tested as a restorative material for MIH teeth in a clinical trial. After 12 months of control, the survival rate of the restorations performed with the self-etching adhesive system was 73% and 59% with the total-etching adhesive system [29]. Comparing the success rate obtained in the present study (98%) in the same period, better behavior of the hybrid system tested here was noted. These results can be partly explained by inherent differences in the sample, but also by the poor adhesion already observed between composite resin and enamel edges affected by MIH [13, 15]. The formation of tags after acid etching—an extremely important step in resin adhesion— is deficient and negatively affects the retention of the restoration [13, 29, 30]. Hence, the removal of all opacity [31, 32] has been recommended to allow the adhesion of the resin to sound enamel. However, this is an extremely invasive strategy, especially for those cases in which the entire crown of the tooth is affected and where the child is quite young. In the present study, opacities were only removed when there was carious tissue present or were located in unsupported enamel. Another management option would be steel crowns, which are widely used and recommended in the United States and Europe [16, 31]. However, these were not considered in this study, since they are not available on the Brazilian market.

As only one failure was detected during the observational period, more robust statistical analysis such as Kaplan Meier regression and Cox regression could not be applied. Initially, this aspect can be seen as a limitation, but it does stress the excellent results obtained in the present investigation. An observational analysis of the factors that influenced the success of the treatment showed that the only failure occurred in a cavity in which all surfaces were involved and which was already presenting the destruction of all cusps (Fig. 2g,). Because of this, we infer that any other type of restorative material placed with the direct technique would have had a greater chance of failure. Although direct restoration may be contraindicated in such a case, it was done because the child's mother could not afford private treatment and did not have time to take her child to the local hospital for free treatment. In general, although the results have been very promising, other studies using the

glass hybrid restorative system should confirm these data before recommending the system as the material of choice for direct restorations in teeth affected by MIH in young children, even in areas of masticatory effort.

This study presents has limitations. They include reduction in the initial sample, sample selection, and absence of a control group. Initially, the study identified 185 children with MIH, of whom 60 (92 teeth) had restorative needs. However, the implementation of the present investigation was only achieved 4 months after the epidemiological survey had been completed, and after the children had returned from their summer vacation, reducing the sample number to 45 children. Of these children, who initially presented 76 teeth with MIH and restoration needs, only 60 teeth could be treated (Fig. 1). This happened since 15 teeth were assessed at the moment of the intervention as in need of endodontics/exodontia, demonstrating the rapid destruction of teeth affected by MIH because of enamel porosity in association with carious lesions. Such results are supported by the literature and demonstrate the need for the early diagnosis of MIH. When restorative needs are already present, treatment must be performed as soon as possible [7, 30, 32, 33]. When not treated immediately, more complex therapies and greater costs are entailed, making the problem even more difficult to solve. Moreover, the power of the study can be questioned because of the number of restorations performed. However, the present investigation was able to include a greater number of affected teeth (60) in comparison with studies with a similar aim: 48 and 41 teeth respectively [2, 29]. This shows the difficulties of working with very specific conditions such as MIH.

Another limitation is the lack of a control group. This is justified by the fact that no consensus protocol exists regarding the treatment of MIH teeth [2, 7, 8, 16, 30, 31], which would indicate the best material/technique to be used as a comparison. Two systematic reviews that aimed to assess the modalities of treatments available to manage affected MIH teeth concluded that that there is a lack of information provided by long-term clinical trials with respect to the management of the condition, not allowing strong recommendations to be made with respect to the best protocol [14, 15].

Conclusion

The majority of MIH teeth did not need invasive treatment, and those that did need treatment required mostly direct restorations. Restoration using a glass hybrid restorative system and performed in the field with the ART technique proved to be an effective approach to preserving first permanent molars affected by MIH.

Abbreviations

ART: Atraumatic restorative treatment; DF: Federal District; EAPD: European Academy of Paediatric Dentistry; GIC: Glass ionomer cement; MIH: Molar incisor hypomineralization; SUS: Brazilian Public Health System

Acknowledgements

We would like to express our special thanks to: GC, which donated the restorative material for this research. Maria José Figueiredo Sé and Ana Luiza de Souza Hilgert, who started the initial epidemiological survey providing data for this study. Patrícia Bastos de Vasconcellos de Medeiros, who performed the on-site evaluation of the restorations after 6 and 12 months.

Authors' contributions

JAG performed the on-site restorations and identified the need for treatment. RNC carried out the survey of needs and of MIH. She accompanied the operator when restorations were being performed. APDR conducted the statistical analysis and interpreted the data of this study. SCL conceived, coordinated, and designed the study. All authors were involved in writing the paper and approved the final manuscript.

Competing interests

The authors declare that they have no competing interests.

Author details

[1]Faculdade de Ciências da Saúde, Universidade de Brasília, Campus Universitário Darcy Ribeiro, Asa Norte, Brasília, DF 70910-900, Brazil. [2]Department of Restorative Dental Sciences, College of Dentistry, University of Florida, 1395 Center Dr, Gainesville, FL 32610-0415, USA.

References

1. Soviero V, Haubek D, Trindade C, Da Matta T, Poulsen S. Prevalence and distribution of demarcated opacities and their sequelae in permanent 1st molars and incisors in 7 to 13 year-old Brazilian children. Acta Odontol Scand. 2009;67:170–5.
2. Fragelli CMB, Souza JF, Jeremias F, Cordeiro RCL, Santos-Pinto L. Molar incisor hypomineralization (MIH): conservative treatment management to restore affected teeth. Braz Oral Res. 2015;29:1–7.
3. Zhao D, Dong B, Yu D, Ren Q, Sun Y. The prevalence of molar incisor hypomineralization: evidence from 70 studies. Int J Paediatr Dent. 2017; https://doi.org/10.1111/ipd.12323.
4. Hernandez M, Boj JR, Espasa E. Do we really know the prevalence of MIH? J Clin Pediatr Dent. 2016;40:259–63.
5. Weerheijm KL, Jalevik B, Alaluusua S. Molar incisor hypomineralization. Caries Res. 2001;35:390–1.
6. Chawla N, Messer LB, Silva M. Clinical studies on molar incisor Hypomineralisation part 1: distribution and putative associations. Eur Arch Paediatr Dent. 2008;9:180–90.
7. Takahashi K, Correia ASC, Cunha RF. Molar incisor hypomineralization. J Clin Pediat Dent. 2009;33:193–8.
8. Lygidakis NA, Wong F, Vierrou AM, Alaluusua S, Espelid I. Best clinical practice guidance for clinicians dealing with children presenting with molar incisors hypomineralisation (MIH). An EADP policy document. Eur Arch Paediatr Dent. 2010;11:75–81.
9. Grossi JA, Cabral RN, Leal SC. Caries experience in children with and without molar-incisor Hypomineralisation: a case-control study. Caries Res. 2017;51:419–24.
10. Americano GC, Jacobsen PE, Soviero VM. Haubek D.- a systematic review on the association between molar incisor hypomineralization and dental caries. Int J Paediatr Dent. 2017;27:11–21.
11. Garcia-Margarit M, Catalá-Pizarro M, Montiel-Company JM, Almerich-Silla JM. Epidemiologic study of molar-incisor hypomineralization in 8-year-old Spanish children. Int J Paediatr Dent. 2014;24:14–22.
12. Jälevik B, Norén JG. Enamel hypomineralization of permanent first molars: a morphological study and survey of possible aetiological factors. Int J Paediatr Dent. 2000;10:278–89.
13. Jälevik B, Klingberg GA. Dental treatment, dental fear and behaviour management problems in children with severe enamel hypomineralisation of their permanent first molars. Int J Paediatr Dent. 2002;12:24–32.
14. Lygidakis NA. Treatment modalities in children with teeth affected by molar-incisor enamel hypomineralisation (MIH): a systematic review. Eur Arch Paediatr Dent. 2010;11:65–74.
15. Elhennawy K, Schwendicke F. Managing molar-incisor hypomineralization: a systematic review. J Dent. 2016;55:16–24.
16. Koch MJ, García-Godoy F. The clinical performance of laboratory fabricated crowns placed on first permanent molars with developmental defects. JADA. 2000;131:1285–90.
17. Frencken JE, Leal SC, Navarro MFL. 25 years atraumatic restorative treatment (ART) approach: a comprehensive overview. Clin Oral Invest. 2012;16:1337–46.
18. Luengas-Quintero E, Frencken JE, Muñúzuri-Hernández JA, Mulder J. The atraumatic restorative treatment (ART) strategy in Mexico: two-years follow up of ART sealants and restorations. BMC Oral Health. 2013;13:42.
19. Nyvad B, Machiulskiene V, Baelum V. Reliability of a new caries diagnostic system differentiating between active and inactive caries lesions. Caries Res. 1999;33:252–60.
20. Weerheijm KL, Duggal M, Mejare I, Papagiannoulis L, Koch G, Martens LC, Hallonsten AL. Judgement criteria for molar incisor hypomineralization (MIH) in epidemiologic studies: a summary of European meeting on MIH held in Athens, 2003. Eur J Paed Dent. 2003;3:110–3.
21. Frencken JE, Holmgren CJ. Atraumatic restorative treatment for dental caries. STI Book B.V: Nijmegen; 1999.
22. Schwendicke F, Frencken JE, Bjørndal L, Maltz M, Manton DJ, Ricketts D, Van Landuyt K, Banerjee A, Campus G, Doméjean S, Fontana M, Leal S, Lo E, Machiulskiene V, Schulte A, Splieth C, Zandona AF, Innes NP. Managing carious lesions: consensus recommendations on carious tissue removal. Adv Dent Res. 2016;28:58–67.
23. Lasfargues JJ, Kaleka R, Louis JJ. A new system of minimally invasive preparations: The Si/Sta concept. In: Roulet JF & Degrange M Adhesion: The Silent Revolution in Dentistry. Chicago: Quintessence; 2000. p. 107–151.
24. Farag AM, Van der Sanden WJ, Abdelwahab H, Frencken JE. Survival of ART restorations assessed using selected FDI and modified ART restoration criteria. Clin Oral Investig. 2011;15:409–15.
25. Atlas de Desenvolvimento Humano no Brasil. 2013. http://www.atlasbrasil.org.br/2013/pt/perfil_udh/22939. Accessed 20 Sept 2016.
26. De Amorim RG, Figueiredo MJ, Leal SC, Mulder J, Frencken JE. Caries experience in a child population in a deprived area of Brazil, using ICDAS II. Clin Oral Investig. 2012;16:513–20.
27. Mickenautsch S, Frencken JE. Utilization of the ART approach in a group of public oral health operators in South Africa: a 5-year longitudinal study. BMC Oral Health. 2009;21:9–10.
28. Gurgan S, Kutuk ZB, Ergin E, Oztas SS, Cakir FY. Four-year randomized clinical trial to evaluate the clinical performance of a glass ionomer restorative system. Oper Dent. 2015;40:134–43.
29. De Souza JF, Fragelli CB, Jeremias F, Paschoal MAB, Santos-Pinto L, Cordeiro RCL. Eighteen-month clinical performance of composite resin restorations with two different adhesive systems for molars affected by molar incisor hypomineralization. Clin Oral Invest. 2016; https://doi.org/10.1007/s00784-016-1968-z.
30. Garg N, Jain AK, Saha S, Singh J. Essentiality of early diagnosis of molar incisor Hypomineralization in children and review of its clinical presentation, etiology and management. Int J Clin Pediatr Dent. 2012;5:190–6.
31. William V, Messer LB, Burrow MF. Molar incisor Hypomineralisation: review and recommendations for clinical management. Pediatr Dent. 2006;28:224–32.
32. Fayle SA. Molar-incisor hypomineralisation: restorative management. Eur J Paediatr Dent. 2003;4:121–6.
33. Preusser SE, Ferring WC, Wetzel WE. Prevalence and severity of molar incisor hypomineralization in a region of Germany - a brief communi-cation. J Public Health Dent. 2007;67:148–50.

Panoramic radiographs and quantitative ultrasound of the radius and phalanx III to assess bone mineral status in postmenopausal women

Katarzyna Grocholewicz[1], Joanna Janiszewska-Olszowska[1*] ⓘ, Magda Aniko-Włodarczyk[2], Olga Preuss[2], Grzegorz Trybek[2], Ewa Sobolewska[3] and Mariusz Lipski[4]

Abstract

Background: Various mandibular indices have been developed to detect osteoporosis on panoramic radiographs. Quantitative ultrasound (QUS) is a low-cost, radiation-free method to assess bone status. The aim of this study was to compare mandibular morphometric analysis and QUS at the radius and proximal phalanx III finger.

Methods: The study involved 97 postmenopausal women, aged 48.5–71.5y (mean: 55.4). Mandibular morphometric analysis comprised: distance between upper and lower mandibular borders just behind the mental foramen (H), distance: mental foramen - inferior mandibular cortex (IM) and mandibular cortical width at the mental region (MCW). Then, ratios were calculated: MCW/IM = PMI (panoramic mandibular index), H/IM = MR (mandibular ratio). Mandibular cortical index (MCI) was used to classify the morphology of the mandibular cortex.
Bone mineral status assessed using QUS at the radius and proximal phalanx III finger was compared to population mean apical bone mass (T-score).
Linear regression analysis was used for correlations between continuous variables, Pearson's correlation coefficient r - for variables of normal distribution. Student's t-test was used to compare variables of normal distribution and for the latter - Mann-Whitney U-test. The level of significance was $p < 0.05$.

Results: Mandibular height was 13.42–34.42 mm. The mean mandibular cortical width was 3.31 mm. Mean values of PMI and MR were 0.33 and 2.57, respectively. Higher mean value of Ad-SoS was found in the radius than in the III finger. Phalanx T-score values were lower than those of the radius. T-score of the radius was < -1.0 in 22 patients, indicating osteopenia. Basing on phalanx T-score, osteopenia was found in 39 patients. Category C1 of Mandibular Cortical Index was found in 48 women, C2 - in 37 women and C3 - in 12 women. Higher scores of Mandibular Cortical Index were recorded in older women. MCI significantly correlated with the skeletal status ($p = 0.01$) as well as with H, MCW and MR. Phalanx T-score was not correlated to PMI, MR or MCW.

Conclusions: 1. Mandibular Cortical Index can be used as a screening tool for detecting osteoporosis.
2. Quantitative ultrasound at the phalanx III constitutes a reliable way of assessing bone status.

Keywords: Osteoporosis, Quantitative ultrasound, Panoramic radiograph, Radiomorphometric indices

* Correspondence: jjo@pum.edu.pl
[1]Department of Interdisciplinary Dentistry, Pomeranian Medical University in Szczecin, Al. Powstancow Wlkp. 72, 70-111 Szczecin, Poland
Full list of author information is available at the end of the article

Background

In 1993, osteoporosis was defined as a "disease characterized by low bone mass and microarchitectural deterioration of bone tissue, leading to enhanced bone fragility and a consequent increase in fracture risk". More recently, the National Institutes of Health (NIH) Consensus Development Panel on Osteoporosis defines osteoporosis as a skeletal disorder characterized by compromised bone strength predisposing a person to an increased risk of fracture. The gold standard in assessing bone mineral density (BMD) is dual-energy X-ray absorptiometry (DXA) [1]. The most recent and non-radiation exposure method of assessing bone mineral status is quantitative ultrasound (QUS). Quantitative ultrasound is a non-invasive and inexpensive method for estimating bone mineral status through measurements performed at skeletal sites with predominance of cortical bone, such as calcaneus (the most validated method) and most recently - proximal phalanges [2–5]. However, no studies reporting on correlations between findings on panoramic radiographs and QUS of the phalanx or radius have been found.

The oral implications of osteoporosis include loss of teeth, loss in alveolar bone height, erosion of inferior mandibular cortex, reduced mandibular inferior cortical width. The earliest suggestion of an association between osteoporosis and oral bone loss was made in 1960 [6–8].

Dental panoramic radiograph is one of the most popular radiographs, performed as a diagnostics image before dental treatment. An important advantage of panoramic radiographs is very low cost in comparison to the expensive DXA technique. Identifying women with low bone mineral density by using panoramic radiographs is a particular topic that has drawn the attention of researchers over the last decade [9]. Osteopenia can be identified by thinning of the cortex at the lower border of the mandible. A number of mandibular cortical indices, including the mandibular cortical index (MCI), panoramic mandibular index (PMI), mental index (MI), antegonial index (AI) and gonial index (GI) have been developed to assess and quantify the quality of mandibular bone mass and to observe signs of resorption on panoramic radiographs for identification of osteopenia [10–13].

The earlier the diagnosis of osteopenia or osteoporosis is made the better is for prophylaxis of bone fractures. The dentists may play an important role in early detection of increased bone fracture risk. Dental radiographs, especially panoramic images, have been used to predict low bone mineral density in patients. It is likely that the clinician may estimate the future risk of fractures and osteoporosis by dental panoramic radiographs [14–20].

The aim of this study was to evaluate the diagnostic efficacy of panoramic radiography using morphometric analysis in early detection of osteopenia and osteoporosis in post-menopausal women and to correlate it with the bone mineral status assessed by QUS at the radius and proximal phalanx III finger.

Methods
Study sample

The study involved 97 postmenopausal women, aged 48.5 to 71.5 years (mean age 55.4 years), who were patients of the Department of Integrated Dentistry of Pomeranian Medical University in Szczecin, Poland and had panoramic radiographs made using a Digital Panoramic System (Soredex Cranex 3D, Soredex, Finnland) and a computer (Windows - XP operating system, Service Pack – 3, 64 bit, flat screen LCD display). The panoramic radiographs were made in order to plan the dental treatment. Head position was standardized as much as possible.

The exclusion criteria were: previous diagnosis of osteoporosis, interview history of hysterectomy or oophorectomy, history of medication affecting bone metabolism such as glucocorticoids, anticonvulsants, excessive thyroxin doses, diseases altering bone metabolism such as hyperparathyroidism, multiple myeloma and estrogen replacement therapy.

Radiographic measurements

All the panoramic radiographs were analyzed on the screen of a monitor (2.3-Megapixel Medical Clinical Display, 1920 × 1200 native resolution, DICOM conformance) with subdued lighting condition. One researcher evaluated each image according to patient positioning, head alignment, film density as well as contrast and radiographs with distortion were excluded. All the radiographs were re-analyzed by the same observer after 2 weeks interval. On each radiograph, the following radiomorphometric measurements were made (Fig. 1):

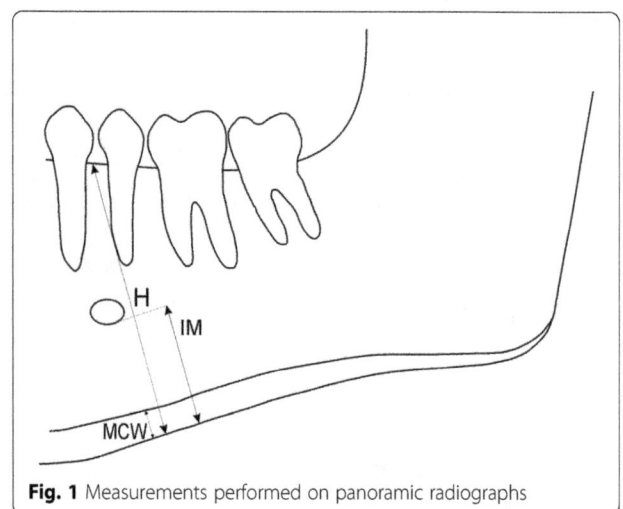

Fig. 1 Measurements performed on panoramic radiographs

1. Mandibular height (H): the distance between the lower and upper border of mandible, measured just behind the mental foramen
2. IM: distance between the mental foramen and the inferior mandibular cortex
3. Mandibular cortical width at the mental region (MCW): mandibular cortical thickness measured on the line perpendicular to the bottom of the mandible at the middle of the mental foramen.

Based on these measurements panoramic mandibular index (PMI) and mandibular ratio (MR) were calculated. Panoramic mandibular index PMI, was calculated according to Benson et al. [18] as the ratio of MCW/IM,. MR, an indicator of alveolar crest resorption degree developed by Wical and Swoope [19], was calculated as the ratio H/IM.

Moreover, a morphological classification of the mandibular cortical bone has been proceeded on panoramic radiographs. Mandibular cortical index (MCI) according to Klemetti et al. [20] was used to assess morphological changes in the inferior cortex of the mandible. Mandibular cortical shapes were analysed by observing the mandible distally from the mental foramina bilaterally and by categorizing them into one of the following three groups as previously described by Klemetti et al. [20]: "C1 – the endosteal margin of the cortex is even and sharp on both sides (Fig. 2); C2 - the endosteal margin shows semilunar defects (lacunar resorption) or endosteal cortical residues on one or both sides, mild to moderate cortex erosion (Fig. 3); C3 – the cortical layer forms heavy endosteal cortical residues and clearly porous, severely eroded cortex" (Fig. 4).

Ultrasound bone measurements
In all women, bone mineral density was assessed using an ultrasound bone sonometer Omnisens 7000S (Sunlight Medical Inc.). Measurements were made in the third distal part of radius and distal metaphysis of the proximal phalanx III finger of the non-dominant hand. The sonometer measures the Amplitude-dependent Speed of Sound - Ad-SoS, expressed in m/s. The result of QUS was related to the mean values in population and showed as a number of standard deviations from mean apical bone mass of young adults of the same sex (T-score). In the assessment of the skeletal system the most useful is to compare the results of the study with a mean apical bone mass of the population (T-score). According to World Health Organization, the following criteria were applied to assess osteoporosis: T-score $\pm$ 1.0 was considered normal; $-2.5 \leq$ T-score < -1.0 was a sign of osteopenia; T-score < -2.5 indicated osteoporosis.

Statistical analysis
The results were analyzed using the statistical package STATISTICA 6.0. Linear regression analysis was used to check for correlations between continuous variables. Pearson's correlation coefficient r was calculated between variables of normal distribution. Student's t-test was used to analyse statistical significance of differences between variables of normal distribution and for the latter - Mann-Whitney U-test was used. The level of significance has been established at $p < 0.05$.

Results
The results of measurements and radiomorphometric indices of the mandible are summarized in Table 1. Raw data is provided as an additional Excel file. Mandibular height ranged between 13.42 and 34.42 mm. The mean mandibular cortical width was 3.31 mm. Mean values of PMI and MR were 0.33 and 2.57, respectively.

The parameters describing the skeletal status are summarized in Table 2. Higher mean value of Ad-SoS was observed in the distal part of radius than in the proximal phalanx III finger.

T-score values were lower for the phalanx than for the radius.

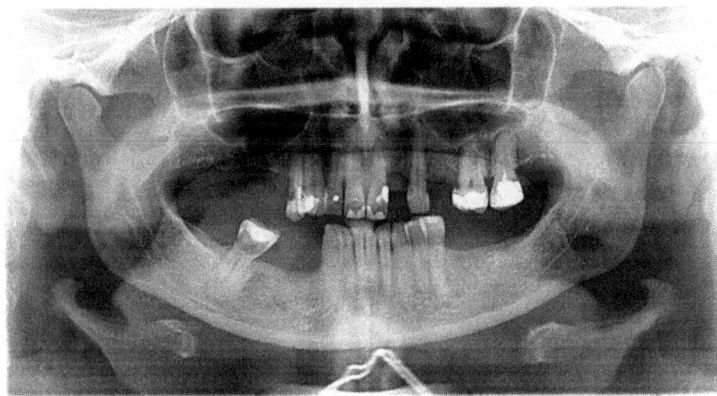

Fig. 2 Panoramic radiograph with C1 category of MCI

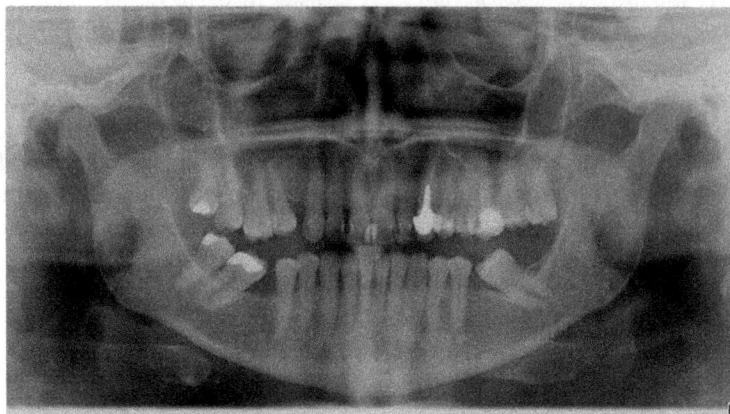

Fig. 3 Panoramic radiograph with C2 category of MCI

Ultrasonographic measurements showed that the T-score of the radius was < – 1.0 in 22 patients, indicating greater than a physiological loss of bone mass, meaning osteopenia. However, basing on the phalanx T-score, osteopenia was found in 39 patients. These results are presented in Table 3.

Category C1 of Mandibular Cortical Index was found in 48 women, category C2 in 37 women and category C3 in 12 women. Higher categories of Mandibular Cortical Index were recorded in older women (Table 4).

Table 5. shows the distribution of patients in each MCI group, according to the phalanx and radius T-score. Phalanx T-score revealed more women with low bone mass and, therefore, it was used for the determination of changes in bone.

The analysis of results obtained revealed 39 patients with osteopenia according to the phalanx T-score. The highest porosity inferior cortex (C3) was observed in 12 patients and in 10 of them phalanx T-score was < – 1. The mild eroded cortex (C2) was observed in 37 women and 13 of them showed osteopenia. Correlations between MCI and bones parameters indicated that in patients with a reduction of

bone mass, the mandibular cortex shape was characterized by a higher porosity.

Mandibular Cortical Index significantly correlated with the skeletal status and mandibular height, mandibular cortical width as well as mandibular ratio. These relationships are presented in Table 6.

The Ad-SoS and T-score in phalanx, mandibular height, Mandibular Ratio and Mandibular Cortical Width were significantly lower in patients with higher category of MCI.

In women with C3 category of mandibular cortical index, phalanx Ad-SoS, phalanx T-score and the mandibular cortical width were significantly lower than in women with C2 and C1 category.

The present study showed correlations between mandibular cortical shape (MCI) and the status of bones as well as MR and MCW. Phalanx T-score was not correlated with other indexes relating radiomorphometric measurements PMI, MR and MCW (Table 7).

Discussion

Panoramic radiography is frequently performed before dental treatment, especially in older patients, to assess

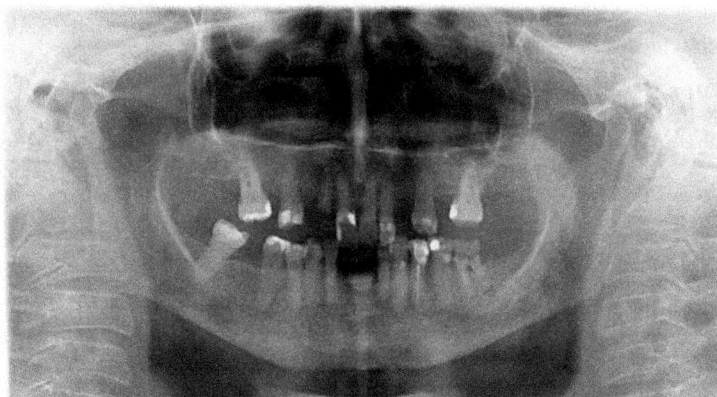

Fig. 4 Panoramic radiograph with C3 category of MCI

Table 1 Distribution of radiomorphometric measurements and mandibular indices

Parameter	n	Mean	Median	Minimum	Maximum	SD
H (mm)	97	25.22	25.58	13.42	34.42	3.20
IM (mm)	97	9.96	9.85	6.42	15.23	1.61
MCW (mm)	97	3.31	3.38	1.69	5.38	0.67
PMI	97	0.33	0.33	0.05	0.52	0.07
MR	97	2.57	2.54	1.51	3.78	0.40

Table 3 Distribution of the study group according to T-score values

Parameter	T-score ≥ -1 n	T-score < -1 n	Total n
Phalanx	58	39	97
Radius	75	22	97

not only dental status but also the status of bones. Many studies suggested that incidental findings detected on these radiographs might be helpful to identify patients with low bone mineral density [13–17, 21]. This is the first study to compare measurements from panoramic radiographs and the radiation-free method of QUS of the phalanx and radius.

No correlations between MCW and phalanx as well as between Ad-SoS and phalanx T-score were found in the present study. Moreover, both PMI and MR proved to be ineffective in the screening of osteopenia/osteoporosis in women. These results are consistent with those by other authors, who emphasized poor utility of PMI and MR, but usefulness of MCI and MCW as screening tools for osteoporosis. Bhatnagar et al. [22] found a weak correlation between PMI and BMD. The same study showed that the degree of mandibular cortical shape erosion significantly correlated with BMD and concluded that the combined mandibular cortical findings (mandibular cortical shape erosion and mandibular cortical width) on panoramic radiographs were effective indicators of osseous changes in postmenopausal osteoporosis.

A similar evaluation was performed by Benson et al. [23], who used PMI to compensate for the vertical magnification that differs among various panoramic machines, but found a very weak correlation between the index and BMD in spite of the fact that PMI is inclusive of other variable i.e., half mandibular width. Therefore Benson et al. [23] used MCW, instead of PMI as an effective indicator. Klemetti et al. [23] also found that linear correlation of the panoramic mandibular index with all bone mineral density values was weak. Patients with reduced bone mass showed lower height of mandible and thereupon also MR.

Stagraczynski et al. [24] showed that PMI and MR are not adequate radiological markers of vertebral bone loss in postmenopausal women. However, measurements of the distance between the inferior margin of the mental foramen and the inferior mandibular cortex did correlate with the degree of lumbar BMD deficiency.

Lee et al. [25] concluded that simple visual estimation of the mandibular inferior cortex width on panoramic radiographs might be useful for identifying postmenopausal women with low BMD. In similar studies Ohtsuki et al., [26] as well as Horner and Devlin [27] also found that mandibular cortical width significantly correlated with BMD,.

The lower specificity of cortical width in identifying low BMD, comparing to cortical shape was confirmed in the study by Khojastehpour et al. [28]. They demonstrated significant associations between BMD and MCW and MCI and concluded that postmenopausal women with thin or eroded mandibular inferior cortex may have an increased risk of low BMD or osteoporosis. Bollen et al. [29] observed that subjects with a self-reported history of osteoporotic fractures tend to have increased resorption and thinning of the mandibular lower cortex. In a study by Gulsahi et al. [30], it was stated that patients with C3 type of MCI should be considered as high-risk individuals for osteoporosis irrespective of age and gender. The usefulness of a visual estimation of the mandibular cortical bone integrity from panoramic radiographs for identifying postmenopausal women at high risk for osteoporosis has been confirmed by Geary et al. [31] as well as Alapati et al. [32].

Some authors emphasize that more lengthy training and experience in using the MCI would be needed for it to be effective as a diagnostic tool in general dental practice [33, 34].

In most studies, the diagnosis of osteoporosis is based on bone mineral density measured by dual-energy X-ray absorptiometry (DXA), but this technique is not a

Table 2 The skeletal status in examined women

Parameter	N	Mean	Median	Minimum	Maximum	SD
Phalanx Ad-SoS (m/s)	97	3941	3976	3337	4384	194
Phalanx T-score	97	−0.65	−0.4	−3.60	2.30	1.26
Radius Ad-SoS (m/s)	97	4152	4160	3853	4601	130
Radius T-score	97	−0.18	−0.2	−3.2	4.4	1.33

Table 4 MCI categories according to the age

MCI	n	Age (years)				SD
		Mean	Median	Minimum	Maximum	
C1	48	54.8	54	48.5	67	4.3
C2	37	55.3	54	50	69	4.7
C3	12	58.5	55.5	50	71.5	7.9
Total	97	55.4	54	48.5	71.5	5.0

Table 5 Distribution of subjects in individual Mandibular Cortical Index groups according to the phalanx and radius T-score

MCI	Phalanx T-score ≥ – 1 n	Radius T-score ≥ – 1 n	Phalanx T-score < – 1 n	Radius T-score < – 1 n
C1	32	41	16	7
C2	24	28	13	9
C3	2	6	10	6

Table 7 Pearson's correlation coefficients

Characteristics	Pearson's correlation coefficient r	p value
MCI versus phalanx Ad-SoS	−0.22	< 0.05
MCI versus phalanx T-score	−0.27	< 0.05
MCI versus MR	0.25	< 0.05
MCI versus MCW	−0.26	< 0.05

practical and economical one [22–25, 27, 28]. Quantitative ultrasound at the hand phalanges has been less popular [2–5], so far, but the present study indicates, it constitutes a reliable method of assessing bone status.

Recently, studies have been published describing the use of radiomorphometric indicators with CBCT and computerized estimation of the risk of osteoporosis [35–37]. This could be a promising direction in the development of dental diagnostics for identifying women with low bone mineral density. However, CBCT to evaluate the bone density of jaws, despite the lower radiation dose and cost, is not useful when absolute values are taken into consideration; a conversion ratio needs to be applied [38].

Table 6 Mean values of observed parameters according to Mandibular Cortical Index

Parameter	C1 n = 48		C2 n = 37		C3 n = 12	
	Mean	SD	Mean	SD	Mean	SD
Phalanx Ad-SoS (m/s)	3965	187	3955	201	3799	151
			p=0.01			
	p=0.002					
Phalanx T-score	-0.44	1.11	-0.6	1.4	-1.68	1.03
			p=0.01			
	p=0,001					
H (mm)	25.41	3.06	25.65	3.39	23.16	2.51
			p=0.01			
	p=0.005					
MR	2.58	0.42	2.60	0.37	2.46	0.45
			p=0.047			
MCW	3.44	0.67	3.31	0.62	2.84	0.68
			p=0.044			
	p=0.02					

Conclusions

The present study showed a correlation between mandibular cortical shape and bone status. MCI can be effectively assessed on panoramic radiographs, hence could be used as a screening tool for determining osteoporosis. This index, very simple for evaluation, may possibly be used as a potential screening tool in identifying individuals with osteoporosis. As routinely requested in dental offices, dental panoramic radiography has an important role in referring patients for osteoporosis investigation.

The simple method of quantitative ultrasound at the hand phalanges constitutes a reliable way of assessing bone status.

Abbreviations

Ad-SoS: Amplitude-dependent Speed of Sound; AI: Antegonial index; BMD: Bone mineral density; DXA: Dual-energy X-ray absorptiometry; GI: Gonial index; H: Mandibular height just behind the mental foramen; IM: Distance between the mental foramen and the inferior mandibular cortex; MCI: Mandibular cortical index; MCW: Mandibular cortical width at the mental region; MI: Mental index; MR: Mandibular ratio (H/IM); NIH: National Institutes of Health; PMI: Panoramic mandibular index; PMI: Panoramic mandibular index (MCW/IM); QUS: Quantitative ultrasound

Authors' contributions

KG: study design, data analysis and interpretation, writing manuscript, JJO: participation in literature review and selection, participation in writing manuscript, MAW: participation in literature review, GT: participation in literature review and in final corrections, critical revising for intelectual content, OP: participation in final manuscript corrections, ES: participation in final manuscript corrections, critical revising for intelectual content, ML: critical revising for intelectual content. All authors read and approved the final manuscript.

Authors' information

KG is a practising specialist in prosthetic dentistry, head of Department of Interdisciplinary Dentistry, JJO is a practising orthodontist associate professor Department of Interdisciplinary Dentistry, MAW, OP and GT are dental surgeons, ES is a specialist in prosthetic dentistry, Head of Department of Dental Prosthetics and ML is a specialist in restorative dentistry and endodontics, Head of Department of Preclinical Conservative Dentistry and Preclinical Endodontics.

Competing interests

The authors declared that they have no competing interests.

Author details

[1]Department of Interdisciplinary Dentistry, Pomeranian Medical University in Szczecin, Al. Powstancow Wlkp. 72, 70-111 Szczecin, Poland. [2]Department of Oral Surgery, Pomeranian Medical University in Szczecin, Szczecin, Poland. [3]Department of Dental Prosthetics, Pomeranian Medical University in Szczecin, Szczecin, Poland. [4]Department of Preclinical Conservative Dentistry and Preclinical Endodontics, Pomeranian Medical University in Szczecin, Szczecin, Poland.

References

1. Szulc P, Bouxsein ML. Vertebral Fracture Initiative. Part I: Overview of osteoporosis: Epidemiology and clinical management. https://www.iofbonehealth.org/sites/default/files/PDFs/Vertebral%20Fracture%20Initiative/IOF_VFI-Part_I-Manuscript.pdf.
2. Motta AC, de Macedo LD, Santos GG, Guerreiro CT, Ferrari T, de Oliveira TF, et al. Quantitative ultrasound at the hand phalanges in patients with bisphosphonate-related osteonecrosis of the jaws. Braz Oral Res. 2015;29:1–9.
3. Høiberg MP, Rubin KH, Hermann AP, Brixen K, Abrahamsen B. Diagnostic devices for osteoporosis in the general population: a systematic review. Bone. 2016;92:58–69.
4. Drozdzowska B, Pluskiewicz W, Tarnawska B. Panoramic-based mandibular indices in relation to mandibular bone mineral density and skeletal status assessed by dual energy X-ray absorptiometry and quantitative ultrasound. Dentomaxillofac Radiol. 2002;31:361–7.
5. Pluskiewicz W, Halaba Z, Chelmecka L, Drozdzowska B, Sonta-Jakimczyk D, Karasek D. Skeletal status in survivors of acute lymphoblastic leukemia assessed by quantitative ultrasound at the hand phalanges: a longitudinal study. Ultrasound Med Biol. 2004;30:893–8.
6. Hildebolt CF. Osteoporosis and oral bone loss. Dentomaxillofac Radiol. 1997;26:3–15.
7. Dervis E. Oral implications of osteoporosis. Oral Surg. Oral med. Oral Pathol Oral Radiol Endod. 2005;100:349–56.
8. Grocholewicz K, Bohatyrewicz A. Oral health and bone mineral density in postmenopausal women. Arch Oral Biol. 2012;57:245–51.
9. Yasar F, Sener S, Yesilova E, Akgünlü F. Mandibular cortical index evaluation in masked and unmasked panoramic radiographs. Dentomaxillofac Radiol. 2009;38:86–91.
10. Devlin H, Horner K. Mandibular radiomorphometric indices in the diagnosis of reduced skeletal bone mineral density. Osteoporos Int. 2002;13:373–8.
11. Govindraju P, Chandra P. Radiomorphometric indices of the mandible - an indicator of osteoporosis. J Clin Diagn Res. 2014;8:195–8.
12. Klemetti E, Kolmakov S, Kröger H. Pantomography in assessment of the osteoporosis risk group. Scand J Dent Res. 1994;102(1):68–72.
13. Taguchi A, Suei Y, Ohtsuka M, Otani K, Tanimoto K, Ohtaki M. Usefulness of panoramic radiography in the diagnosis of postmenopausal osteoporosis in women. Width and morphology of inferior cortex of the mandible. Dentomaxillofac Radiol. 1996;25:263–7.
14. Tözüm TF, Taguchi A. Role of dental panoramic radiographs in assessment of future dental conditions in patients with osteoporosis and periodontitis. N Y State Dent J. 2004;70:32–5.
15. Taguchi A, Tsuda M, Ohtsuka M, Kodama I, Sanada M, Nakamoto T, et al. Use of dental panoramic radiographs in identifying younger postmenopausal women with osteoporosis. Osteoporos Int. 2006;17:387–94.
16. Nakamoto T, Taguchi A, Ohtsuka M, Suei Y, Fujita M, Tanimoto K, et al. Dental panoramic radiograph as a tool to detect postmenopausal women with low bone mineral density: untrained general dental practitioners' diagnostic performance. Osteoporos Int. 2003;14:659–64.
17. Taguchi A, Suei Y, Sanada M, Ohtsuka M, Nakamoto T, Sumida H, et al. Validation of dental panoramic radiography measures for identifying postmenopausal women with spinal osteoporosis. Am J Roentgenol. 2004;183:1755–60.
18. Benson BW, Prihoda TJ, Glass BJ. Variations in adult cortical bone mass as measured by a panoramic mandibular index. Oral Surg Oral Med Oral Pathol. 1991;71:349–56.
19. Wical KE, Swoope CC. Studies of residual ridge resorption. I. Use of panoramic radiographs for evaluation and classification of mandibular resorption. J Prosthet Dent. 1974;32:7–12.
20. Klemetti E, Kolmakow S. Morphology of the mandibular cortex on panoramic radiographs as an indicator of bone quality. Dentomaxillofac Radiol. 1997;26:22–5.
21. Gaur B, Chaudhary A, Wanjari PV, Sunil M, Basavaraj P. Evaluation of panoramic radiographs as a screening tool of osteoporosis in post menopausal women: a cross sectional study. J Clin Diagn Res. 2013;7:2051–5.
22. Bhatnagar S, Krishnamurthy V, Pagare SS. Diagnostic efficacy of panoramic radiography in detection of osteoporosis in post-menopausal women with low bone mineral density. J Clin Imaging Sci. 2013;3:23.
23. Klemetti E, Kolmakov S, Heiskanen P, Vainio P, Lassila V. Panoramic mandibular index and bone mineral densities in postmenopausal women. Oral Surg Oral Med Oral Pathol. 1993;75:774–9.

24. Stagraczynski M, Kulczyk T, Podfigurna A, Meczekalski B. Estimation of mandibular bone status and lumbar bone mineral density in postmenopausal women. Pol Merkur Lekarski. 2016;4:79–83.

25. Lee K, Taguchi A, Ishii K, Suei Y, Fujita M, Nakamoto T, et al. Visual assessment of the mandibular cortex on panoramic radiographs to identify postmenopausal women with low bone mineral densities. Oral Surg Oral Med Oral Pathol Oral Radiol Endod. 2005;100:226–31.

26. Ohtsuki H, Kawakami M, Kawakami T, Takahashi K, Kirita T, Komasa Y. Risk of osteoporosis in elderly individuals attending a dental clinic. Int Dent J. 2017;67:117–22.

27. Horner K, Devlin H. The relationship between mandibular bone mineral density and panoramic radiographic measurements. J Dent. 1998;26:337–43.

28. Khojastehpour L, Afsa M, Dabbaghmanesh MH. Evaluation of correlation between width and morphology of mandibular inferior cortex in digital panoramic radiography and postmenopausal osteoporosis. Iran Red Crescent Med J. 2011;13:181–6.

29. Bollen AM, Taguchi A, Hujoel PP, Hollender LG. Case-control study on self-reported osteoporotic fractures and mandibular cortical bone. Oral Surg Oral Med Oral Pathol Oral Radiol Endod. 2000;90:518–24.

30. Gulsahi A. Osteoporosis and jawbones in women. J Int Soc Prev Community Dent. 2015;5:263–7.

31. Geary S, Selvi F, Chuang SK, August M. Identifying dental panoramic radiograph features for the screening of low bone mass in postmenopausal women. Int J Oral Maxillofac Surg. 2015;44:395–9.

32. Alapati S, Reddy RS, Tatapudi R, Kotha R, Bodu NK, Chennoju S. Identifying risk groups for osteoporosis by digital panoramic radiography. Contemp Clin Dent. 2015;6:S253–7.

33. Jowitt N, MacFarlane T, Devlin H, Klemetti E, Horner K. The reproducibility of the mandibular cortical index. Dentomaxillofac Radiol. 1999;28:141–4.

34. Calciolari E, Donos N, Park JC, Petrie A, Mardas N. Panoramic measures for oral bone mass in detecting osteoporosis: a systematic review and meta-analysis. J Dent Res. 2015;94:17S–27S.

35. Muramatsu C, Horiba K, Hayashi T, Fukui T, Hara T, Katsumata A, et al. Quantitative assessment of mandibular cortical erosion on dental panoramic radiographs for screening osteoporosis. Int J Comput Assist Radiol Surg. 2016;11:2021–32.

36. Alonso MB, Vasconcelos TV, Lopes LJ, Watanabe PC, Freitas DQ. Validation of cone-beam computed tomography as a predictor of osteoporosis using the Klemetti classification. Braz Oral Res. 2016;30

37. Barngkgei I, Halboub E, Almashraqi AA, Khattab R, Al HI. IDIOS: an innovative index for evaluating dental imaging-based osteoporosis screening indices. Imaging Sci Dent. 2016;46:185–202.

38. Cassetta M, Stefanelli LV, Pacifici A, Pacifici L, Barbato E. How accurate is CBCT in measuring bone density? A comparative CBCT-CT in vitro study. Clin Implant Dent Relat Res. 2014;16:471–8.

Perceived oral health and its association with symptoms of psychological distress, oral status and socio-demographic characteristics among elderly in Norway

Kari Elisabeth Dahl[1]* ⓘ, Giovanna Calogiuri[1] and Birgitta Jönsson[2,3]

Abstract

Background: There is poor knowledge about the extent to which psychological distress influences oral health in older people in Norway. The aim of this study was two-fold: i) to describe the oral health of Norwegian elderly and their levels of psychological distress; and ii) to examine the relationship of psychological distress with self-rated oral health, while controlling for oral status and socio-demographic characteristics, in Norwegian elderly.

Methods: Data were retrieved from a national cross-sectional survey conducted by Statistics Norway in 2012 and included information about self-rated oral health, psychological distress (measured using the Hopkins Symptom Checklist 25; HSCL-25), gender, age, civil status, smoking, self-reported number of teeth present and dental attendance for 949 non-institutionalised adults aged 65 years or older. Logistic regression was used to establish whether psychological distress predicts self-rated oral health, controlling for socio-demographic characteristics and oral status.

Results: Around 27% of the elderly reported having poor oral health, and 8 % had a HSCL-25 mean score ≥ 1.75, which indicates higher levels of psychological distress. Among the symptoms listed in the HSCL-25, the most frequently reported problems were lack of energy (1.7 ± 0.8) and difficulties falling and staying asleep (1.6 ± 0.7). The likelihood of reporting poor oral health was independently associated with having a mean HSCL-25 score ≥ 1.75 (OR = 1.89; 95% CI = 1.14–3.15), even when smoking (OR = 1.83; 95% CI = 1.17, 2.87) and having fewer than 20 teeth (OR = 3.49; 95% CI = 2.56, 4.76) were taken into account.

Conclusion: Most of the Norwegian elderly in our sample perceived themselves to have good oral health and reported relatively low levels of psychological distress. Higher levels of psychological distress can influence the oral health of the elderly independently of other factors such as smoking and having reduced number of teeth. Dental care professionals should consider screening their elderly patients for psychological distress and individualise the information about dental care for this specific population.

Keywords: Ageing, Mental health, Depression, Older adults, Epidemiology

* Correspondence: kari.dahl@inn.no
[1]Department of Public Health, Faculty of Social and Health Sciences, Inland Norway University of Applied Sciences, Hamarveien 112, 2418 Elverum, Norway
Full list of author information is available at the end of the article

Background

As in other European countries, in Norway an increasing decline in fertility rates and increased life expectancy are resulting in an increase of the proportion of older people which represent a potential burden to society and a challenge to public health institutions [1](WHO). Compared with other European countries, only Poland, Iceland and Ireland have fewer elderly people than Norway [2]. However the population age is increasing at varying rates. For example, the proportion of the Norwegian population aged 65 years and older in 2015 was 16.3%, an increase from 8.4% in 2006. In order to ensure people's quality of life and to minimise increased public costs, it is important to understand how to promote good health among the increasing number of older citizens.

One challenge in becoming elderly is maintaining good oral health, especially for fragile or cognitively impaired older persons, which is one of the reasons why elderly people have received increasing attention from researchers and health policy makers [3]. To maintain good oral health is, an important component of a healthy ageing [4]. A number of dental conditions are associated with older age, such as dry mouth (xerostomia), root caries, and periodontal disease [5–7]. Periodontitis, which may result in tooth loss, is still a common disease and its prevalence is reported by European and US studies to range from 31% to 76% [8–10]. Furthermore, its prevalence and severity increase with age [6, 7]. During recent decades, a reduction in the prevalence of edentulousness and the prevalence and incidence of tooth loss has occurred in many countries [11, 12]. Despite these observed declining trends in edentulousness, the mean number of lost teeth increases with increasing age and a substantial proportion of the current older generations experience tooth loss [11, 13]. Furthermore, studies have confirmed the expected positive associations between tooth loss and reduced perceived oral health [13, 14].

While most of the elderly have good mental health and psychological well-being, many are at increased risk of developing mental disorders [15]. Symptoms of psychological distress are common and serious, causing significant disruption in daily living. Mental disorders account for circa 7.4% of the global burden of disease and will probably steadily increase in the future [16]. Psychological distress is often under-recognised and under-treated in primary care [17]. Psychological distress is so widespread that it can be considered one of the most common health problems in Norway [18]. It is estimated that about 30% of the Norwegian population experience high levels of psychological distress at some time during their lifetime [18]. Psychological distress is highly prevalent in the elderly and often has negative consequences on their everyday life, such as leading to a reduced quality of life [19]. Increased psychological distress might also have a negative impact on the elderly's health-related behaviours, including their dietary patterns as well as their dental hygiene behaviours, which can in turn lead to poor oral health [20]. Symptoms of psychological distress have been found to be associated with tooth loss and use of dental care services in the U.S. [21] and in a Finnish populations [22, 23]. However, in Norway, knowledge about how non-institutionalised older adults perceive their oral health and how often they have check-ups still remains scanty [24]. Furthermore, little is known about the extent to which psychological distress affects the oral health of Norwegian elderly [21, 24].

The aim of this study was two-fold: i) to describe Norwegian elderly's self-rated oral health and levels of psychological distress; and ii) to examine the relationship between psychological distress and self-rated oral health while controlling for oral status, smoking, dental attendance and sociodemographic characteristics.

Methods

Study population

The data for this study were retrieved from a national Norwegian cross-sectional study conducted by Statistics Norway (SSB) in 2012: "The Living Conditions study – Health, health care and social contact" [25]. A representative random sample of 10,000 Norwegians aged 16 years and older was drawn, stratified by gender, age group and region of residence, from SSB's demographic/population database BEREG, a database that is updated from The Central Population Register. Of the total drawn from the database, 229 persons had died or were living abroad, consequently, these were not invited to participate, giving a gross sample of 9771 (100% of the invited participants) persons of whom 4111 declined to participate (42%) giving a net samples of 5660 people (58%). For this study, only respondents aged 65 years and above were used for the analyses ($n = 949$).

The samples were balanced in respect of gender, age and region of residence where everyone in the household was considered as one unit [25].

Data collection process

Persons in the study were invited to participate by a letter from the SSB, which provided information in Norwegian regarding the purpose of the study, the procedures and actions taken to ensure confidentiality and stating that they would be contacted by telephone for an interview. Data collection involved a combination of a phone interview and a follow-up self-administered questionnaire. Before the interview started, all respondents consented to participate. The follow-up questionnaire was sent to the participants two to three weeks after the phone interview and could be completed either on paper or on a web site.

Instruments

Self-reported oral health, which was the dependent variable in the study, was assessed with one question in the follow-up questionnaire: "How do you perceive your dental health to be?" Five response options were provided: "Very poor", "poor", "neither poor nor good", "good", or "Very good".

Psychological distress, which was the primary predictor in this study, was assessed using the Hopkins Symptoms Checklist – 25 (HSCL-25). HSCL-25 is a shortened version of an original 90 items questionnaire (HSCL-90) and is one of the most commonly used questionnaires to measure the prevalence of mild psychological distress in the population [26–29]. A Norwegian version of this instrument has been validated and used

for research and clinical purposes since the late 1980s [30]. The scale consists in one question followed by 25 statements that describe symptoms of two major components of psychological distress, Anxiety and Depression: "Specify how much each problem has plagued you or caused trouble during the past 14 days? Each statement was rated by the participants on a four point Likert scale", with each symptom being rated on a 4-point scale (1= "Not at all", 2 = "A little", 3= "Quite a bit", and 4 = "Extremely"). The first ten items in the HSCL-25 questionnaire concern anxiety symptoms and the following 15 items concern depression symptoms. A total mean score ≥ 1.75 indicates psychological distress at a case level [31]. The overall internal consistency for the HSCL-25 was high (alpha = 0.95). All individual items of the HSCL-25 are presented in Table 1.

Other control variables in this study include oral status, smoking, dental attendance, and sociodemographic

Table 1 Proportions of responses to each item on the Hopkins Symptom Checklist-25 ($n = 949$)

Item	Not at all	A little	Quite a bit	Extremely	Mean (SD)
1. Headache	73.9	22.1	2.6	0.5	1.3 (0.6)
2. Tremor	86.0	9.7	1.8	0.6	1.2 (0.4)
3. Lassitude or dizziness	66.2	27.9	4.1	0.5	1.4 (0.7)
4. Nervousness, restlessness	66.5	29.0	3.2	0.7	1.4 (0.6)
5. Suddenly scared for no reason	88.3	9.3	1.8	0.2	1.1 (0.4)
6. Increasingly fearful or anxious	85.7	11.1	2.2	0.1	1.2 (0.6)
7. Palpitations, heart beat running away	77.9	18.2	1.8	0.2	1.3 (06)
9. Bouts of anxiety or panic	91.7	6.5	0.8	0.2	1.1 (0.4)
10. So restless that it is difficult to sit still	84.7	12.9	1.3	0.5	1.2 (0.5)
11. Lack of energy, everything goes slower than usual	40.8	20.2	9.5	2.0	1.7 (0.8)
12. Blaming yourself for things	63.5	30.2	4.6	0.7	1.4 (0.7)
13. Tearfulness	76.0	20.0	2.8	0.7	1.3 (0.5)
14. Thoughts about taking your life	96.3	2.4	0.7	0	1.0 (0.2)
15. Poor appetite	90.1	7.9	1.3	0.3	1.1 (0.5)
16. Difficulty falling asleep, staying asleep	55.6	33.6	7,6	2.5	1.6 (0.7)
17. Sense of hopelessness about the future	74.4	22.1	2.4	0.6	1.3 (0.5)
18. Depressed, melancholy	78.4	18.4	1.8	0.4	1.2 (0.6)
19. Feeling of loneliness	74.3	21.1	3.5	0.5	1.3 (0.6)
20. Loss of sexual desire and interest	53.5	29.7	9.7	3.8	1.6 (0.8)
21. Feeling of being cheated in a trap or trapped	93.8	5.0	0.5	0.4	1.0 (0.3)
22. Very worried or upset	70.3	25.6	3.4	0.4	1.3 (0.6)
23. No interest in anything	87.2	10.5	1.4	0.4	1.1 (0.5)
24. Feeling everything is an effort	75.2	20.2	3.1	0.9	1.3 (0.6)
25. Feeling useless	79.3	17.1	2.6	0.9	1.2 (0.5)
Anxiety mean score					1.2 (0.3)
Depression mean score					1.3 (0.3)
HSCL-25 total mean score					1.3 (0.3)

When numbers in columns do not equal 100%, there is internal drop-out in the questionnaire characteristics. Oral status was assessed with one variable: Number of teeth present. "Roughly, how many of your own teeth do you have left?" which was answered by choosing one of four response options: 1) "20 teeth or more", 2) "10–19 teeth", 3) "1–9 teeth", and 4) "none". Two variables assessed habits that could have an impact on dental status and oral health: Smoking habits and dental attendance. Smoking was assessed with the question: "Do you smoke?" to which the respondents answered "yes" or "no". Dental attendance was assessed with the question: "When did you last visit a dentist?", which were answered by choosing one of five response choices: 1) "6 month ago or less", 2) "7-12 months ago", 3) "1–2 years ago" 4) "more than two years but less than five years ago", 5) "more than 5 years ago".

Gender, Age group (65–74 years and 75+ years), and Civil Status (i.e. living with partner or Single) were used as selected sociodemographic characteristics.

Statistical analysis

Descriptive statistics was used to address the first objective of our study. Self-rated oral health was dichotomised: 1) Good oral health (comprising the response alternatives "Very good" and "Good"), and 2) Poor oral health (comprising the response alternatives "Neither good nor poor", "Poor" and "Very poor"). The individual items of the HSCL-25 and the Anxiety and Depression components are presented as means (M) and standard deviations (SD), while the total score of the HSCL-25 is presented as prevalence of individuals with mean score above or below the 1.75 cut-off, i.e. individuals with lower or higher levels of psychological distress [31].

In order to address the second objective of our study, logistic regressions were performed. Before performing the Logistic regression analysis, the responses to self-assessed number of teeth present were collapsed into two categories (20 teeth and more vs. 0–19 teeth) and dental attendance into two categories (within 6–12 months vs. more than 12 months). Those variables that were significant in the univariate analysis were included in a multivariable logistic regression analysis in order to examine the extent to which Psychological distress predicted Self-reported oral health while controlling for the respondents' sociodemographic characteristics, oral health status, smoking habits and dental attendance. The associations are presented as odds ratios (ORs) and 95% confidence intervals (95% CI). The Hosmer-Lemeshow goodness-of-fit test was used to examine whether the final model adequately fitted the data. The significance was set at $p > 0.05$. All data analyses were performed using the Statistical Package for the Social Sciences (SPSS, Version 24.0, IBM Armonk, NY).

Results

The participants' ages ranged between 65 to 96 years, with the median age being 69 years (quartile deviation 68–73 years). The sample consisted of 54.4% (514) women and 45.6% (431) men. A total of 71.3% ($n = 674$) rated their oral health as good or very good and 28.7% (271) rated their oral health as very poor, poor, or neither good nor poor. There were no differences between men and women on how they rated their oral health (χ^2 0.093, df 1, $p = 0.760$) or between age groups (χ^2 0.130, df1, $p = 0.718$).

The individual HSCL-25 items are presented in Table 1. Missing values for each question varied from 0.2% to 3.3%, with the highest internal loss for the item concerning 'Loss of sexual desire and interest' (3.3%). For 23 of the 25 items, the missing values were under 1.0%.

In the overall sample, the total mean score of the HSCL-25 was 1.3 ± 0.32. The overall score for the Anxiety component was 1.2 ± 0.3, the mean score for the Depression component was 1.3 ± 0.3. Eight per cent of the participants had a total HSCL-25 mean score above the 1.75 cut-off, indicating higher levels of psychological distress, while the prevalence of those having a mean score above the 1.75 cut-off for Anxiety was 6.3% and Depression was 10.4%. Among the various symptoms listed in the HSCL-25, "Lack of energy" (1.7 ± 0.8), "Difficulties falling and staying asleep" (1.6 ± 0.7), and "Loss of sexual desire and interest" (1.6 ± 0.8) were rated with the highest mean scores. Women had significantly higher HSCL-25 mean scores than men (1.32 ± 0.33 and 1.26 ± 0.30, respectively; ANOVA: F = 7.46, $p = 0.006$), and the elderly in the oldest age group had significantly higher HSCL-25 mean scores than the youngest age group mean (1.36 ± 0.34 and 1.27 ± 0.30, respectively; ANOVA: F = 5.99, $p = 0.003$).

In Table 2, predictors of self-reported oral health are presented. Totals of 65.4% and 89.2% were living with partner and were non-smokers, respectively. Moreover, totals of 65.9% and 83.2% had 20 teeth or more and attended a dentist annually, respectively.

In the univariable analysis, the likelihood of perceiving poor oral health was increased for individuals who had symptoms of psychological distress, lived alone, smoked, had fewer than 20 teeth, and for persons' who had not attended the dentist within the past year.

When the model was adjusted for all variables in a multivariable model, the participants who had higher levels of psychological distress were 1.89 times more likely to report poor oral health, even when other factors were controlled. Smokers were 1.83 times more likely to perceive poor oral health than non-smokers and those with fewer than 20 teeth were 3.49-times more likely to perceive poor oral health than those with more teeth. In the final model, living alone and not having attended the

Table 2 Predictors of self-rated poor oral health among elderly Norwegian adults

Variables	Categories	Crude measures		Univariable			Multivariable[a]		
		N	Poor self-rated oral health %	OR	95% CI	P	OR	95% CI	P
HSCL-25 diagnose	Mean score > 1.75	75	45.3	2.21	1.37–3.57	0.001	1.89	1.14–3.15	0.014
	Mean score ≤ 1.75 (reference)	870	27.2	1.00			1.00		
Civil status	Single	327	33.9	1.47	1.09–1.97	0.009	1.16	0.85–1.59	0.345
	Living with partner (reference)	618	25.9	1.00			1.00		
Smoker	Yes	102	46.1	2.36	1.55–3.59	< 0.001	1.83	1.17–2.87	0.008
	No (reference)	843	26.6	1.00			1.00		
Number of teeth	0–19	322	47.2	3.79	2.82–5.09	< 0.001	3.49	2.56–4.76	< 0.001
	≥ 20 (reference)	623	19.1	1.00			1.00		
Dental attendance	> 12 month	153	35.3	1.48	1.02–2.13	0.037	0.93	0.62–1.40	0.746
	6–12 month (reference)	786	27.0	1.00			1.00		

OR = Odds ratio; 95% CI = 95% confidence Interval. [a]Model adjusted for the interaction between HSCL-25 diagnose, civil status, smoking, number of teeth, and dental visits

Discussion

dentist within the past year were not significantly associated with poor oral health. The goodness-of-fit of measurement used in the model was an acceptable fit on the Omnibus test of model coefficient (χ^2 92.98, $p > 0.001$) and Hosmer and Lemeshow test (χ^2 2.61, $p = 0.760$). The factors used as predictor in the model explained 13.5% of the variance of perceived poor oral health (Nagelkerke's R^2 0.135).

Discussion

The first objective of our study was to describe oral health and psychological distress among Norwegian elderly. The majority of the elderly in our sample were non-smokers, had 20 teeth or more, and had attended a dental check-up within the past 12 months. Nearly one-third of the elderly reported having poor oral health, and 8% had higher levels of psychological distress. Among the symptoms listed in the HSCL-25, the most frequently reported problems were lack of energy and difficulties falling and remaining asleep. There were no differences between men and women, or between age groups, in the extent to which they rated their oral health, though women and those in the oldest age group showed higher levels of psychological distress than men and those in the youngest age group, respectively. The second objective of our study was to examine the relation of psychological distress with perceived oral health, controlling for sociodemographic characteristics, smoking, oral status, and dental attendance. The likelihood of reporting poor oral health was independently associated with higher levels of psychological distress while controlling for the other independent variables. Smoking and, especially, having fewer than 20 teeth were also highly significant predictors of poor oral health.

Nearly 66% of the elderly in our sample had 20 teeth or more, confirming the high proportion of elderly

people in Norway who retained their natural teeth, as shown in earlier studies [14, 32–34], which is considered essential to maintain adequate chewing function and normal oral health-related quality of life [35, 36].

In line with our findings, a study carried out in nine European countries showed that the occurrence of symptoms of depression in older people living at home varied between 8.0 and 23.6%, with a higher prevalence in women than in men [37]. Although we found the prevalence of Norwegian elderly with higher levels of psychological distress was somewhat low, symptoms such as lack of energy and difficulties falling and remaining asleep were commonly reported. Such symptoms might give an indication of mood and psychological distress and should therefore be regarded in light of their possible impact on the elderly's oral health. Furthermore, the prevalence of psychological distress is likely to increase in future, alongside the increase in the ageing population, and this represents a challenge in Norway and other countries [38, 39].

Our findings relative to the association of psychological distress with oral health are consistent with the literature. Previous studies have in fact found an increased risk for impaired oral health among adults with anxiety and depressive symptoms [21, 22]. For example, in a Finnish study [23], elderly with symptoms of anxiety or depression were almost twice as likely to experience poor oral health. Women with high rates of depressive symptoms had more negative attitude toward preserving their natural teeth, used sugary products more frequently and did not attend for dental check-ups regularly, compared with non-depressed women. Further, depressive symptoms were associated with edentulousness among non-smoking men and symptoms of anxiety were significantly associated with lower tooth brushing frequency [21, 23]. Similarly, in a study on a U.S.

population, Okoro et al. found that adults with psycho-logical disorders such as depression and anxiety were less likely to attend oral health services and to have tooth loss or had one or more teeth removed than those without such disorder, after controlling for multiple con-founders [21].

Higher levels of psychological distress are often associ-ated with loss of energy and might result, for example, in less effective dental hygiene and difficulty following-up routines such as general dental care attendance. Dry mouth is a common complaint in older people, persons suffering from dryness of the mouth are likely to experi-ence several oral problems, including high levels of caries, in addition to difficulties in chewing, eating and commu-nicating [36]. The appetite often declines alongside inter-est in cooking meals. This can lead to more pronounced loss of energy due to lack of nutrition [20] and such per-sons show less interest in socialising with other people.

In our study, we also found that the highest adjusted odds ratios were observed for having fewer than 20 teeth, which is also in line with the literature [33, 40, 41]. Musacchio et al. [42] found that tooth loss impacts on general health and is a risk factor for malnutrition, disability, loss of self-sufficiency, and deterioration in quality of life, and having fewer teeth was associated with social lifestyle factors in a population of elderly Ital-ians. Despite an increasing number of people retaining their natural teeth throughout life, the prevalence of oral diseases increases among the institutionalised elderly, their objective need for dental treatment is therefore even greater than before [38, 43].

Ekback et al. [39] showed that elderly persons missing many teeth were less likely to be satisfied with their oral condition than those missing only a few or no teeth. In-dividuals who perceived they had poor general health, smoked daily, had tooth loss, experienced toothache, had difficulties with chewing, and reported bad breath were less likely than their counterparts to be satisfied with their oral health status.

Implications of our findings

Our findings underline the necessity for dental profes-sionals to be aware of elderly people's levels of psycho-logical distress, as this can have a negative impact on oral health and oral-health related quality of life. Conse-quently, dental care professionals should consider screening their elderly patients for psychological distress. Moreover, the importance of oral care for older people with psychological distress needs to be emphasised by dental professionals, to reduce the possibility of poorer oral health and deterioration of quality of life in this population.

As tooth loss has a negative impact on how people perceive their oral health is essential in order to

maintain adequate chewing function and higher stan-dards of oral health related quality of life [36]. Regular oral health care check-ups are important for helping eld-erly people maintain their natural teeth through periods when they are in poor health [44, 45]. Therefore, it is important that systematic dental care services for older adults are accessible and affordable [45, 46].

Strength and weaknesses of the present study

The HSCL 25 has been used to assess psychological dis-tress in a number of age and cultural contexts [31, 47, 48]. The way in which the HSCL-25 questionnaires is administrate differs slightly. For example, statements can be delivered face-to-face by a trained interviewer or, like in the present study, the instrument can be self-administered. This may account for some differences in the overall HSCL scores, though evidences suggest that the method of delivery should not have a major im-pact on the total scores. Nonetheless, in view of this methodological difference, the main emphasis in this analysis has been on the patterns of association rather than absolute differences in the questionnaire scores. Our study is subject to several limitations. First, all data are self-reported. The HSCL-25 was however found to perform well in assessing the symptom severity of anx-iety and depression distress among non-elderly in gen-eral, and it could therefore be considered as a suitable and valid measure for elderly people. A critical issue in the clinical application of HSCL-25 is to identify cut-off points on the scale that can be used to support decisions about whether further clinical examination is necessary. In our study, the 1.75 cut-off was applied, which has previously shown high validity in a Swedish population [31] and which can be expected to be fairly similar to Norwegian populations in terms of language and cultural context. Another limitation is that the participants' oral status (number of remaining teeth) was self-reported and thus might not correspond to the actual remaining number of natural teeth. However, previous studies have shown a close agreement between self-reported and clin-ically measured dentition status. [49, 50]. The use of only clinical measures to assess oral health of individuals has been criticized because they fail to consider func-tional and psychosocial aspects of health and do not ad-equately reflect the functioning, concerns and perceived needs of individuals [51, 52]. It is hereby of interest also to include patients` assessment of their wellbeing in the term oral health. In addition, there is a growing interest in dentistry also to assess the influence of oral health on daily life, often labelled oral health-related quality of life (OHRQoL) [52, 53].

Furthermore, tooth loss is considered as an effective marker of the population oral situation. [54]. One of the major limitation of this study relates to possible self-selection bias. The participants in this study were probably healthy elderly living at home, able to manage themselves in everyday life, while the ill or less independent elderly who were unable or did not wish to participate might have affected the responses and the results. In a study by Vehkalahti et al., poor oral health have been shown to be a major factor in this kind of population study of the elderly [55]. Thus, taking into account that missing values and drop -out have poorer health, the present findings that differences in dental attendance were mainly related to presence or absence of natural teeth may only relate to healthy women.

Conclusions

Most of the Norwegian elderly in our sample rated their oral health to be good and relatively few showed higher levels of psychological distress. Higher levels of psychological distress can negatively influence the elderly's oral health, though other factors such as smoking and tooth loss are even stronger predictors of poor oral health. Dental care professionals should consider screening their elderly patients for psychological distress and customize the information about dental care and dental hygiene for this specific population.

Abbreviations
HSCL-25: Hopkins Symptom Checklist-25

Acknowledgements
The numerous participants for their efforts in completing the questionnaires. We would also like to thank Statistic Norway (SSB) who conduced the data collection and for letting use the data. This study was supported by Inland University of Applied Sciences in Norway and TkNN in Tromsø, Norway.

Funding
The study was funded by Department of Public Health, Inland Norway University of Applied Sciences (Elverum, Norway). The Public Dental Health Service. Competence Centre of Northern Norway (Tromsø, Norway); and the Department of Periodontology, Institute of Odontology, The Sahlgrenska Academy, University of Gothenburg (Gothenburg, Sweden).

Authors' contributions
KED did the data processing, contributed to data analysis, interpretation of findings, and to manuscript writing. GC contributed to interpretation of the findings and manuscript writing. BJ did the data processing, carried out data analysis, contributed to interpretation of findings, and manuscript writing. All authors have read and approved the final manuscript.

Competing interests
The authors declare that they have no competing interests.

Author details
[1]Department of Public Health, Faculty of Social and Health Sciences, Inland Norway University of Applied Sciences, Hamarveien 112, 2418 Elverum, Norway. [2]The Public Dental Health Service. Competence Centre of Northern Norway (TkNN), Tromsø, Norway. [3]Institute of Odontology, Department of Periodontology, The Sahlgrenska Academy, University of Gothenburg, Gothenburg, Sweden.

References
1. World report on ageing and health [http://apps.who.int/iris/bitstream/10665/186463/1/9789240694811_eng.pdf?ua=1].
2. Statisticks Norway: Befolkning/nøkkeltall. In. http://www.ssb.no/befolkning/nokkeltall/befolkning last updated 17. November 2016: Statistisk sentralbyrå-SSB, Oslo; 2015.
3. Guarnizo-Herreño CC, Watt RG, Pikhart H, Sheiham A, Tsakos G. Socioeconomic inequalities in oral health in different European welfare state regimes. J Epidemiol Community Health. 2013; jech-2013-202714
4. Langballe E, Evensen M. Eldre i Norge: Forekomst av psykiske plager og lidelser (Older Adults in Norway: Prevalence of Mental Problems and Disorders). Oslo: Folkehelseinstituttet; 2011.
5. Petersen PE, Bourgeois D, Ogawa H, Estupinan-Day S, Ndiaye C. The global burden of oral diseases and risks to oral health. Bull World Health Organ. 2005;83(9):661–9.
6. Eke PI, Wei L, Borgnakke WS, Thornton-Evans G, Zhang X, Lu H, McGuire LC, Genco RJ. Periodontitis prevalence in adults≥ 65 years of age, in the USA. Periodontology 2000. 2016;72(1):76–95.
7. López R, Smith PC, Göstemeyer G, Schwendicke F. Ageing, dental caries and periodontal diseases. J Clin Periodontol. 2017;44(S18):S145–52.
8. Hugoson A, Sjödin B, Norderyd O. Trends over 30 years, 1973–2003, in the prevalence and severity of periodontal disease. J Clin Periodontol. 2008; 35(5):405–14.
9. Holtfreter B, Kocher T, Hoffmann T, Desvarieux M, Micheelis W. Prevalence of periodontal disease and treatment demands based on a German dental survey (DMS IV). J Clin Periodontol. 2010;37(3):211–9.
10. Eke PI, Dye BA, Wei L, Slade GD, Thornton-Evans GO, Borgnakke WS, Taylor GW, Page RC, Beck JD, Genco RJ. Update on prevalence of periodontitis in adults in the United States: NHANES 2009 to 2012. J Periodontol. 2015;86(5): 611–22.
11. Müller F, Naharro M, Carlsson GE. What are the prevalence and incidence of tooth loss in the adult and elderly population in Europe? Clin Oral Implants Res. 2007;18(s3):2–14.
12. Norderyd O, Koch G, Papias A, Kohler AA, Helkimo AN, Brahm C-O, Lindmark U, Lindfors N, Mattsson A, Rolander B. Oral health of individuals aged 3-80 years in Jonkoping, Sweden during 40 years (1973-2013). Swed Dent J. 2015;39(2):69–86.
13. Ramsay S, Whincup P, Watt R, Tsakos G, Papacosta A, Lennon L, Wannamethee S. Burden of poor oral health in older age: findings from a population-based study of older British men. BMJ Open. 2015;5(12):e009476.
14. Gülcan F, Nasir E, Ekbäck G, Ordell S, Åstrøm AN. Change in oral impacts on daily performances (OIDP) with increasing age: testing the evaluative properties of the OIDP frequency inventory using prospective data from Norway and Sweden. BMC oral health. 2014;14(1):59.
15. Mental health and older adults: Fact sheet [http://www.who.int/mediacentre/factsheets/fs381/en/].
16. Murray CJ, Vos T, Lozano R, Naghavi M, Flaxman AD, Michaud C, Ezzati M, Shibuya K, Salomon JA, Abdalla S. Disability-adjusted life years (DALYs) for 291 diseases and injuries in 21 regions, 1990–2010: a systematic analysis for the global burden of disease study 2010. Lancet. 2013;380(9859):2197–223.
17. Ólafsdóttir M, Marcusson J, Skoog I. Mental disorders among elderly people in primary care: the Linköping study. Acta Psychiatr Scand. 2001;104(1):12–8.
18. Mykletun A, Knudsen AK, Mathiesen KS. Psykiske lidelser i Norge: Et folkehelseperspektiv. In: Oslo: Nasjonalt folkehelseinstitutt; 2009.
19. Charney D, Reynolds IIIC, Lewis L, Lebowitz B, Sunderland T, Alexopoulos G. Consensus development panel of the depression and bipolar support alliance.(2003). Depression and bipolar support alliance consensus statement on the unmet needs in diagnosis and treatment of mood disorders in late life. Arch Gen Psychiatry. 2003;60(7):664–72.

20. Pekka P, Pirjo P, Ulla U. Influencing public nutrition for non-communicable disease prevention: from community intervention to national programme-experiences from Finland. Public Health Nutr. 2002;5(1A):245–52.

21. Okoro CA, Strine TW, Eke PI, Dhingra SS, Balluz LS. The association between depression and anxiety and use of oral health services and tooth loss. Community Dent Oral Epidemiol. 2012;40(2):134–44.

22. Anttila S, Knuuttila M, Ylöstalo P, Joukamaa M: Symptoms of depression and anxiety in relation to dental health behavior and self-perceived dental treatment need. Eur J Oral Sci 2006, 114(2):109–114.

23. Anttila S, Knuuttila MLE, Sakki TK. Relationship of depressive symptoms to edentulousness, dental health, and dental health behavior. Acta Odontol Scand. 2001;59(6):406–12.

24. Birkeland A, Natvig GK. Coping with ageing and failing health: a qualitative study among elderly living alone. Int J Nurs Pract. 2009;15(4):257–64.

25. Amdam S, Vrålstad S. Levekårsundersøkelsen 2012. Helse, omsorg og sosial kontakt (Living Conditions 2012. Health, Care and Social Network). In: Statistics Norway; 2012.

26. Derogatis LR, Lipman RS, Rickels K, Uhlenhuth EH, Covi L. The Hopkins symptom checklist (HSCL): a self-report symptom inventory. Behav Sci. 1974; 19(1):1–15.

27. Lipman RS, Covi L, Shapiro AK. The Hopkins symptom checklist (HSCL): factors derived from the HSCL-90. J Affect Disord. 1979;1(1):9–24.

28. Schauenburg H, Strack M. Measuring psychotherapeutic change with the symptom checklist SCL 90 R. Psychother Psychosom. 1999;68(4):199–206.

29. Parloff MB, Kelman HC, Frank JD. Comfort, effectiveness, and self-awareness as criteria of improvement in psychotherapy. Am J Psychiatr. 1954;111(5): 343–52.

30. Tambs K, Røysamb E. Selection of questions to short-form versions of original psychometric instruments in MoBa. Norsk epidemiologi. 2014;24(1–2)

31. Nettelbladt P, Hansson L, Stefansson C-G, Borgquist L, Nordström G. Test characteristics of the Hopkins symptom check List-25 (HSCL-25) in Sweden, using the present state examination (PSE-9) as a caseness criterion. Soc Psychiatry Psychiatr Epidemiol. 1993;28(3):130–3.

32. Åstrøm A, Haugejorden O, Skaret E, Trovik T, Klock K. Oral impacts on daily performance in Norwegian adults: validity, reliability and prevalence estimates. Eur J Oral Sci. 2005;113(4):289–96.

33. Åstrøm A, Haugejorden O, Skaret E, Trovik T, Klock K. Oral impacts on daily performance in Norwegian adults: the influence of age, number of missing teeth, and socio-demographic factors. Eur J Oral Sci. 2006;114(2):115–21.

34. Trovik T, Berge T. Do tooth gaps matter? Evaluation of self-assessments: a pilot study. J Oral Rehabil. 2007;34(11):814–20.

35. Kikutani T, Yoshida M, Enoki H, Yamashita Y, Akifusa S, Shimazaki Y, Hirano H, Tamura F. Relationship between nutrition status and dental occlusion in community-dwelling frail elderly people. Geriatr Gerontol Int. 2013;13(1):50–4.

36. Willumsen T, Fjaera B, Eide H. Oral health-related quality of life in patients receiving home-care nursing: associations with aspects of dental status and xerostomia. Gerodontology. 2010;27(4):251–7.

37. Copeland J, Beekman A, Braam AW, Dewey ME, Delespaul P, Fuhrer R, Hooijer C, Lawlor BA, Kivela S-L, Lobo A. Depression among older people in Europe: the EURODEP studies. World Psychiatry. 2004;3(1):45–9.

38. Samson H, Strand GV, Haugejorden O. Change in oral health status among the institutionalized Norwegian elderly over a period of 16 years. Acta Odontol Scand. 2008;66(6):368–73.

39. Ekbäck G, Åstrøm AN, Klock K, Ordell S, Unell L. Variation in subjective oral health indicators of 65-year-olds in Norway and Sweden. Acta Odontol Scand. 2009;67(4):222–32.

40. Shimazaki Y, Soh I, Saito T, Yamashita Y, Koga T, Miyazaki H, Takehara T. Influence of dentition status on physical disability, mental impairment, and mortality in institutionalized elderly people. J Dent Res. 2001;80(1):340–5.

41. Steele JG, Sanders AE, Slade GD, Allen PF, Lahti S, Nuttall N, Spencer AJ. How do age and tooth loss affect oral health impacts and quality of life? A study comparing two national samples. Community Dent Oral Epidemiol. 2004;32(2):107–14.

42. Musacchio E, Perissinotto E, Binotto P, Sartori L, Silva-Netto F, Zambon S, Manzato E, Chiara Corti M, Baggio G, Crepaldi G. Tooth loss in the elderly and its association with nutritional status, socio-economic and lifestyle factors. Acta Odontol Scand. 2007;65(2):78–86.

43. Henriksen BM, Ambjørnsen E, Axéll T. Dental caries among the elderly in Norway. Acta Odontol Scand. 2004;62(2):75–81.

44. Samson H, Berven L, Strand GV. Long-term effect of an oral healthcare programme on oral hygiene in a nursing home. Eur J Oral Sci. 2009;117(5): 575–9.

45. World Health Organization. International consortium in psychiatric epidemiology. Cross-national comparisons of the prevalences and correlates of mental disorders. Bull World Health Organ. 2000;78:413–26.

46. Petersen PE, Yamamoto T. Improving the oral health of older people: the approach of the WHO global oral health Programme. Community Dent Oral Epidemiol. 2005;33(2):81–92.

47. Strand BH, Dalgard OS, Tamb K, Rogneerud M. Measuring the mental health status of the Norwegian population: a comparison of the instruments SCL-25, SCL 10, SCL 5 and MHI-5 (SF 36). Nord J Psychiatry. 2003;57(2):113–8.

48. Sandanger I, Moum T, Ingebrigtsen G, Dalgard O, Sørensen T, Bruusgaard D. Concordance between symptom screening and diagnostic procedure: the Hopkins symptom Checklist-25 and the composite international diagnostic interview I. Soc Psychiatry Psychiatr Epidemiol. 1998;33(7):345–54.

49. Pitiphat W, Garcia RI, Douglass CW, Joshipura KJ. Validation of self-reported oral health measures. J Public Health Dent. 2002;62(2):122–8.

50. Helø LA. Comparison of dental health data obtained from questionnaires, interviews and clinical examination. Eur J Oral Sci. 1972;80(6):495–9.

51. Tsakos G, Marcenes W, Sheiham A. The relationship between clinical dental status and oral impacts in an elderly population. Oral health & preventive dentistry. 2004;2(3).

52. Locker D. Clinical correlates of changes in self-perceived oral health in older adults. Community Dent Oral Epidemiol. 1997;25(3):199–203.

53. Dahl KE, Wang NJ, Holst D, Ohrn K. Oral health-related quality of life among adults 68-77 years old in Nord-Trondelag, Norway. Int J Dent Hyg. 2011;9(1): 87–92.

54. Kassebaum N, Bernabé E, Dahiya M, Bhandari B, Murray C, Marcenes W. Global burden of severe tooth loss: a systematic review and meta-analysis. J Dent Res. 2014;93(7_suppl):20S–8S.

55. Vehkalahti M, Siukosaari P, Ainamo A, Tilvis R. Factors related to the non-attendance in a clinical oral health study on the home-dwelling old elderly. Gerodontology. 1996;13(1):17–24.

Rapid urease test (RUT) for evaluation of urease activity in oral bacteria in vitro and in supragingival dental plaque ex vivo

Gunnar Dahlén[*], Haidar Hassan, Susanne Blomqvist and Anette Carlén

Abstract

Background: Urease is an enzyme produced by plaque bacteria hydrolysing urea from saliva and gingival exudate into ammonia in order to regulate the pH in the dental biofilm. The aim of this study was to assess the urease activity among oral bacterial species by using the rapid urease test (RUT) in a micro-plate format and to examine whether this test could be used for measuring the urease activity in site-specific supragingival dental plaque samples ex vivo.

Methods: The RUT test is based on 2% urea in peptone broth solution and with phenol red at pH 6.0. Oral bacterial species were tested for their urease activity using 100 μl of RUT test solution in the well of a micro-plate to which a 1 μl amount of cells collected after growth on blood agar plates or in broth, were added. The color change was determined after 15, 30 min, and 1 and 2 h. The reaction was graded in a 4-graded scale (none, weak, medium, strong). Ex vivo evaluation of dental plaque urease activity was tested in supragingival 1 μl plaque samples collected from 4 interproximal sites of front teeth and molars in 18 adult volunteers. The color reaction was read after 1 h in room temperature and scored as in the in vitro test.

Results: The strongest activity was registered for *Staphylococcus epidermidis*, *Helicobacter pylori*, *Campylobacter ureolyticus* and some strains of *Haemophilus parainfluenzae*, while known ureolytic species such as *Streptococcus salivarius* and *Actinomyces naeslundii* showed a weaker, variable and strain-dependent activity. Temperature had minor influence on the RUT reaction. The interproximal supragingival dental plaque between the lower central incisors (site 31/41) showed significantly higher scores compared to between the upper central incisors (site 11/21), between the upper left first molar and second premolar (site 26/25) and between the lower right second premolar and molar (site 45/46).

Conclusion: The rapid urease test (RUT) in a micro-plate format can be used as a simple and rapid method to test urease activity in bacterial strains in vitro and as a chair-side method for testing urease activity in site-specific supragingival plaque samples ex vivo.

Keywords: Rapid urease test, Supragingival dental plaque, Urease activity, Oral microbiota

* Correspondence: dahlen@odontologi.gu.se
Department of Oral Microbiology and Immunology, Institute of Odontology,
Sahlgrenska Academy, University of Gothenburg, Box 450, SE 40530
Gothenburg, Sweden

Background

Urease is an enzyme that hydrolyses urea (carbamide) into ammonia and carbon dioxide and is produced by several bacterial species. Detection of urease activity has become an important tool for the diagnosis of *Helicobacter pylori* infections in association with chronic gastritis, which increases the risk of developing peptic ulcer [1, 2]. Several oral bacterial species have been shown to produce urease e.g. *Streptococcus salivarius, Actinomyces naeslundii, Haemophilus parainfluenzae* [3, 4] although the understanding on the variation in the activity between species and strains is limited. Furthermore, the extent of urease production in vivo by the dental plaque bacteria is still unclear.

Urea is delivered in the gingival crevicular fluid (GCF) and in all salivary gland secretions at concentrations ranging from 3 to 10 mM in healthy individuals [5, 6]. Several studies have shown that urea in such concentrations can increase the baseline pH of the dental biofilm (plaque) and may significantly counteract the effects of glycolytic acidification in the plaque [7, 8]. Ammonia could also be produced by the hydrolysis of a number of amino acids. The net pH change in plaque is not only a result of ureolysis but other factors are also involved [8]. Urease activity in the plaque in situ has been measured indirectly by quantifying the amount of ammonia formed using Nessler's reagent [9–11]. Nessler's reagent is slow and estimates the ammonia concentration as well as the urease activity indirectly, however it is not suitable as a chair side method.

The rapid urease test (RUT) is a simple method used for the diagnosis of *H. pylori* infections [12] and which also has been used for measuring the urease activity in dental plaque samples ex vivo. In such studies focusing on the presence of *H. pylori* in the dental plaque, it was argued that *H. pylori* were the only dental plaque bacteria able to rapidly produce detectable amounts of urease [13]. The knowledge of the extent and rate of urease production in oral bacteria is limited. The first aim of this study was to use RUT to screen and grade the urease activity in oral bacterial species/strains in vitro. For that purpose, the RUT method was modified into a micro-plate format for the semi-quantification of bacterial urease activity by visual scoring. The second aim was to test if this RUT method could be used as a simple and rapid chair-side test to screen for site differences of urease activity in ex vivo plaque.

Methods

Bacteria

As seen in Table 1, the bacterial strains used for in vitro evaluation of RUT included both laboratory reference strains (Culture Collection, University of Gothenburg, CCUG, Sweden; American Type Culture Collection,

ATCC) and own clinical isolates (Oral Microbiology, Gothenburg, Sweden, OMGS). *Campylobacter ureolyticus, H. pylori, Staphylococcus epidermidis* strains were used as positive controls and *Enterococcus faecalis, Escherichia coli, Pseudomonas aeruginosa* and *Staphylococcus aureus* strains as negative controls according to their known present or absent ureolytic activity [14]. In addition, oral bacterial species e.g. *A. naeslundii, H. parainfluenzae* and *S. salivarius* with documented ureolytic capacity were included [3, 4]. Furthermore, we also included a number of strains commonly associated with supragingival and subgingival dental plaque (see Table 1). Fresh clinical isolates of *A. naeslundii, H. parainfluenzae* and *S. salivarius* from saliva samples in the oral microbiological diagnostic laboratory of the department, identified using common laboratory methods [14], were used for evaluation of bacterial strain variability (Table 2).

Urease test

The NCTC micro method (National Collection of Type Cultures, NCTC, Public Health England, UK) of RUT used for detection of *H. pylori* in stomach samples [15, 16] was modified into a micro-plate format and used for the estimation of urease positive bacteria. Urease-broth (Bakt lab, Sahlgrenska hospital, Gothenburg, Sweden) was used in volumes of 100 µl in 96-hole micro-titer plates (Nunc, Copenhagen, Denmark). The nutrient broth contained 2% urea, pH 6.8, and phenol red as an indicator. The broth has an orange color, which turns yellow at a lower pH and pink to red then purple at alkaline pH.

In vitro evaluation of urease activity in bacterial strains

The bacterial strains shown in Table 1 (including the urease positive and negative control strains) were grown on Brucella-blood agar plates aerobically for 2 days or, in the case of anaerobic species, anaerobically for 5–7 days at 36° C. Colonies from the plates were harvested by scraping a loopful (1 µl Inoculation loop, Sarstedt, Nümbrecht, Germany) of colony cells, which were suspended into the urea-broth and incubated at 36 °C. The color change was read after 15 min, and 30 min, and 1 and 2 h. The visual color change was graded as no reaction (0) for no color change (or noted as 'changed to yellow as a result of acid production'), + denoted a weak reaction with a shift to pink color, ++ denoted a moderate reaction with a shift towards red and +++ a strong reaction with a clear purple color.

S. epidermidis (OMGS 3949), *C. ureolyticus* (CCUG 7319), *S. salivarius* (OMGS 3945) and *A. naeslundii* (OMGS 2466) were used as positive controls, and *E. coli* (OMGS 3935) as a negative control, in experimental series performed in order to further evaluate the method's dependency on time and temperature. To test the time dependency, the plates were left on the bench

Table 1 Bacterial species tested for urease activity with the RUT test, read after 1 h incubation at 36 °C

Bacterial species	Origin or strain designation[a]	Urease activity[b]
Actinomyces naeslundii	OMGS 2466	+
Actinomyces naeslundii	OMGS 1923	0
Actinomyces oris	OMGS 2683	+
Campylobacter gracilis	CCUG 27720	+
Campylobacter rectus	OMGS 1236	+
Campylobacter ureolyticus	CCUG 7319	+++
Enterococcus faecalis	ATCC19433	0
Escherichia coli	OMGS 3935	0
Fusobacterium nucleatum	OMGS 2685	0
Haemophilus parainfluenzae	CCUG 12836 T	0
Haemophilus. parainfluenzae	OMGS 199/11	++
Haemophilus parainfluenzae	OMGS 202/11	+++
Haemophilus parainfluenzae	OMGS 203/11	+++
Helicobacter pylori	ATCC 43504	+++
Lactobacillus casei/paracasei	OMGS 3184	0
Lactobacillus. salivarius	CCUG 55845	0
Lactobacillus fermentum	OMGS 3182	+
Porphyromonas gingivalis	OMGS 2860	0
Prevotella intermedia	OMGS 2514	0
Pseudomonas aeruginosa	OMGS 3943	0
Rothia dentocariosa	OMGS 1956	0
Streptococcus mitis	CCUG 31611	+
Streptococcus mutans	OMGS 2482	0
Streptococcus salivarius I	OMGS 3944	0
Streptococcus salivarius II	OMGS 3945	+
Streptococcus sanguinis	OMGS 2478	0
Staphylococcus aureus	OMGS 3947	+
Staphylococcus epidermidis	OMGS 3949	+++
Tannerella forsythia	ATCC43037	0

[a]ATCC and CCUG means reference strains, OMGS means clinical isolates from the department collection
[b]The visual color change was graded as no reaction (0) for no color change, + denoted a weak reaction with a shift to pink color, ++ denoted a moderate reaction with a shift towards red and +++ a strong reaction with a clear purple color

Table 2 Reactions from the clinical oral isolates in the RUT method read after 1 h. Cells were obtained from agar plates by scraping (1 μl)

Bacteria	No reaction No of strains (%)	Weak No of strains (%)	Moderate No of strains (%)	Strong No of strains (%)
Streptococcus salivarius (N = 8)	4 (50%)	2 (25%)	2 (25%)	0 (0%)
Actinomyces naeslundii (N = 8)	7 (87.5%)	1 (12.5%)	0 (0%)	0 (0%)
Haemophilus. parainfluenzae (N = 5)	1 (20%)	0 (0%)	0 (0%)	4 (80%)

and were read every hour for another 4 h and finally after 24 h. The temperature dependency was tested at similar time points after incubation of the plates at the temperature's 20, 25 and 36 °C. All experiments were performed in triplicate.

The same bacterial strains were used to test RUT for the dependence of glucose and lowered pH during the bacterial growth before inoculation in the urea test broth. The strains were incubated in a peptone broth containing 0.1, 0.5 or 1.0% glucose for 1–2 days. The final pH was measured and the bacterial cells were harvested by centrifugation and a loopful (1 µl) amount was then used to test the urease activity with the RUT method. The reaction was followed and read after 1 h.

The strain variability in urease activity was tested by using fresh clinical isolates of *S. salivarius* (8 strains), *A. naeslundii* (8 strains) and *H. parainfluenzae* (5 strains) and using both cells obtained from agar plates (1 µl) and from a pellet (1 µl) after broth culture.

Ex vivo evaluation of urease activity in dental plaque

Eighteen volunteers (11 females and 7 males, mean age ± SD of 37.3 ± 15.4, range 25–69) among students and laboratory personnel at the Institute of Odontology, University of Gothenburg, participated in the test. They had a DMFT±SD (Decayed Missed Filled Teeth ±Standard deviation) of 9.7 ± 5.54. No further specific inclusion criteria were considered necessary for evaluating the RUT method on dental plaque ex vivo. The subjects were instructed not to brush their teeth 2 days prior to the test and not to eat or drink anything except water 2 h prior to the test. They all participated voluntarily and gave an informed consent.

Individual supragingival plaque samples were collected by scraping with a curette from interproximal sites between the lower incisors (site 31/41), between the upper incisors (site 11/21), between the upper left first molar and second premolar (site 26/25), and between lower right second premolar and molar (site 45/46) on 18 adult individuals. A loopful (1 µl) amount of plaque from each respective site was added to 100 µl of urea broth in a 96-hole plate and left in room temperature. The color reaction was read after 1 h and was graded similar to the bacterial in vitro tests.

Statistical analysis

Non-parametric Mann-Whitney test were used to analyse the difference of urease activity of the interproximal supragingival plaque between the sites. The statistical analysis were performed using Microsoft® Excel® for Mac (Version 14.4.8, 2011) and KaleidaGraph® (version 4.1.2, Synergy Software. 2011). It was considered statistically significant if the *p*-value was < 0.05.

Results
Urease evaluation in vitro

Distinct reactions were obtained after 1 h at 36 °C using bacteria grown on agar plates (Table 1). Strong, purple and rapid reactions (+++) were seen for *C. ureolyticus*, *H. parainfluenzae* (two strains), *H. pylori* and *S. epidermidis*, which had already turned purple after 15 min. One strain of *H. parainfluenza* showed a slower, moderate reaction (++) whereas another showed no reaction after 1 h. Weak and pink color reactions (+) only were registered for some strains of *Actinomyces* spp., *Campylobacter* spp., *Lactobacillus* spp., alpha-streptococci and *S. aureus*. No reaction (0) was obtained from the anaerobic periodontal disease associated species; e.g. *Porphyromonas gingivalis*, *Tannerella forsythia*, *Fusobacterium nucleatum* and *Prevotella. intermedia* or opportunistic strains tested; e.g. *P. aeruginosa*, *E. faecalis* and *E. coli*.

The time dependency tests showed that both slow and rapid urease-producing bacteria could clearly be distinguished after 1 h incubation in the RUT-medium. Strong positive strains (*H. pylori*, *C. ureolyticus*, *S.epidermidis* and *H. parainfluenzae*) showed a color change to purple within 15 min. The color change was otherwise gradual and slow for urease positive oral strains with minor, insignificant changes from 1 h to 2 h. Bacterial strains that did not change colors within 2 h were registered as negative. From these findings it was decided to read the reactions after a fixed time (1 h) for the strains (Table 1) and plaque samples (Fig. 1). Moreover, the effect of temperature (20, 25, or 36 °C) was only marginal on the color reaction (data not shown) and, thus, the final color reaction was read after 1 h at room temperature in all further in vitro and ex vivo experiments.

The urease activity in cells cultured in broth with a glucose concentration < 1% was generally weaker than in cells after plate culture. The influence of pH during growth was found to be negligible in the interval between 6.0 and 7.5 but a yellow color developed for some streptococcal strains with a pH < 5.0 in the broth before harvesting.

Tests using several strains of the same species showed strong urease activity after 1 h (+++) in 4 strains (80%) of *H. parainfluenzae* and a moderate (++) and a weak reaction (+) in 2 strains (25%) respectively of *S. salivarius*. No reaction (0) was seen for 7 of the 8 strains of *A. naeslundii* tested, while one strain showed a weak positive reaction. The result was the same regardless if the cells were grown on agar or in broth (Table 2) and illustrates the phenotypic variability between the strains of the same species.

Ex vivo urease plaque test

Interproximal supragingival plaque samples collected from the interproximal site of the lower central incisors

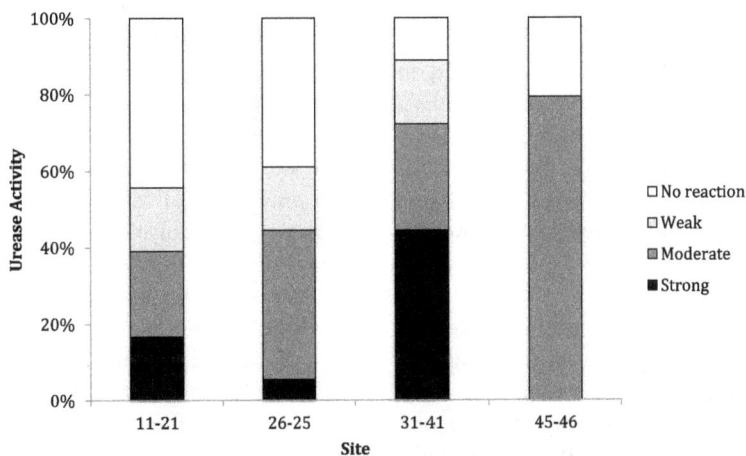

Fig. 1 Urease activity (% of samples) in plaque samples from between upper (interproximal site 11/12) and lower (interproximal site 31/41) central incisor and from the mesial aspect of upper left (interproximal site 26/25) and lower right (interproximal site 45/46) first molar of 18 adult volunteers

(31/41) showed significantly higher urease activity than samples from the interproximal sites of upper central incisors (11/12) ($p < 0.05$), upper left first molar and premolar (26–25) ($p < 0.05$) and lower right first molar and premolar (45–46) ($p < 0.001$). The differences between the three latter sites were not significant. The frequency of the RUT scores for each of the 4 sites is shown in Fig. 1.

Discussion

Urea agar or broth test has been used routinely in bacteriological laboratories to test bacterial strains for urease activity. The broth test is described in most manuals in clinical microbiology [14]. It is a simple, reliable, and rapid test that is used in vivo/ex vivo for diagnostic purpose to detect urease positive *H. pylori* in peptic ulcers [15]. For the detection of *H. pylori* infections, both in-house and commercial variants of RUT have been developed [15–17]. The present study found that a NCTC modified micro-titer plate method of the rapid urease test (RUT) could be used to screen and semi-quantify the urease activity among bacterial strains in vitro and as a chair-side method for assessing the site specific ureolytic activity in dental plaque samples ex vivo.

A strong reaction was noticed already after 15 min for bacteria with the most expressed urease activity such as *H. pylori, C. ureolyticus* and *S. epidermidis,* which are not normally considered as resident in the dental plaque. Some oral streptococci e.g. *S. salivarius* and *S. mitis* showed weak urease activity. Others like *A. naeslundii,* more commonly found in the dental plaque also showed a weak activity. Both streptococci and *Actinomyces* strains needed 1–2 h to show some reaction. Longer incubation time may affect the outcome of the test due to bacterial growth and acid production from sugars or ammonia production by amino acid degradation

(arginolysis). One hr. was therefore chosen as a reliable incubation time that could be used also for chair-side tests. Furthermore, tests performed at 20, 25 and 36 °C showed that temperature had a limited effect on the urease reaction and there was no difference between the results obtained from plate and broth cultured bacterial cells. Also, except for strong acidogenic species giving slightly yellow color in the in vitro test if the cell material used for inoculation had a low pH (≤ 5), similar results were obtained from cells grown with or without glucose before the RUT test. These findings suggest that the production of urease by bacteria is a stable and conserved characteristic for many bacterial species, which is generally not affected by environmental factors such as temperature and the presence of glucose or the broth. They further suggest that for ex vivo estimation of the plaque urease activity, RUT should be used on patients who have abstained from sugar-containing food or drinks for at least 2 h. Also, the amount of bacterial cells and plaque material for ex vivo test using RUT, may affect the outcome. There is, however, no ideal and standardized way to collect dental plaque. We evaluated the use of a loopful (1 μl) and found the amount to give minor, non-significant variations only when repeated in triplicates.

Many oral bacteria are described in the literature as being ureolytic. Much focus has been paid on *S. salivarius* and *A. naeslundii* [8], which have been claimed to play an important role in the dental plaque ecology by reducing the plaque acidity and thereby having anti-cariogenic effects [7, 18–20]. Other streptococci have not been shown to have this capacity. Most of the referred studies are performed in models in vitro and the phenotypic expression of the involved genes encoding for the enzyme activity may vary due to the environment

[21–23]. This may be one reason why the ureolytic capacity was not a common feature for the phenotype of the strains of *S. salivarius* and *A. naeslundii* tested in the present study. The low activity of the *A. naeslundii* strains may be explained by several taxonomic revisions of this species (previously named Genospecies I and II) [24, 25]. Genospecies II (previously called *A. viscosus*) is now called *A. oris* and the strain tested here showed a positive reaction, while those classified as *A. naeslundii* had a weaker capacity.

For *H. parainfluenzae*, which are not implicated in caries disease but more associated with gingivitis [26, 27], 4 out of 5 strains showed a strong and rapid urease activity (Table 2). No urease activity seen for one strain may be due to different biotypes. In a recent publication, strains of the genus *Haemophilus* and especially *H. parainfluenzae* were significantly more prevalent in the dental plaque of children with a high urease activity and it was concluded that they were major contributors of the urease enzyme for the alkali production in the plaque [28]. Thus, previous and present findings suggest that *H. parainfluenzae* may be of greater importance to the alkalization of the dental plaque through ureolysis than streptococci and *Actinomyces* spp.

It is worth notice that *F. nucleatum*, *P. gingivalis*, *P. intermedia* and *T. forsythia*, all associated to periodontal disease were negative for ureolytic activity. This is of no surprise due to the fact that the periodontal pocket normally is slightly alkaline [29], and there is less need for the acid intolerant bacteria to neutralize acids compared to the acidogenic supragingival environment.

It is important to note that also some other bacterial species such as *Campylobacter* spp. (*C. ureolyticus* in particular) and *H. pylori* showed a rapid ureolytic activity, giving a positive purple reaction within 15 min. They are normally considered to belong to the gastrointestinal and not to the oral microbiota. However, *C. ureolyticus* as well as *H. pylori* are intermittently found in the dental plaque from the subgingival area and in periodontal diseases when DNA probes or PCR methodology are used for the analyses [30, 31]. The strong and rapid reaction of these two bacteria indicate a putative significant contribution to the net urease activity in the plaque, even when present in lower numbers compared to other but predominant plaque bacteria, with a considerably lower urease activity. According to a recently published review the RUT method has also been used for the detection of *H. pylori* in dental plaque [13]. In view of our finding of many urease positive species that can be present in the dental plaque, this must be considered doubtful.

One advantage with the RUT method applied for plaque samples is the possibility to use it site-specifically. The screening of four different sites in a group of adult individuals showed a strong activity in the mandibular anterior region of > 70% of the individuals. This activity was significantly higher than in plaque samples from the other sites of the dentition tested. It is well known that the teeth in the mandibular anterior region are characterized by a low caries experience and high prevalence of calculus, related to low and high pH, respectively. Ureolysis may therefore have a biological impact on both periodontitis and caries. This study did, however, not consider the clinical status of the included individuals. It did, however, show that the method could be used as a chair side method for site-specific urease activity measurements, which could be of interest for the evaluation the individual susceptibility to dental diseases.

Conclusions

This study evaluated the usefulness of a simple test (Rapid urease test, RUT) for the assessment and semi-quantification of the ureolytic activity in various bacterial species in vitro as well as in dental plaque samples ex vivo. Bacteria with strong, moderate, weak or no activity were distinguished. Strains of *Haemphilus parainfluenzae*, but not of other common plaque bacteria tested, showed strong and rapid urease activity. Dental plaque from mandibular anterior teeth frequently showed a significantly higher urease activity ex vivo than plaque from other sites. It can be concluded that the RUT method can be used as a simple and rapid method in order to assess urease activity in bacteria in vitro and in plaque samples ex vivo.

Abbreviations
ATCC: American Type Culture Collection; CCUG: Culture Collection University of Gothenburg; DMFT: Decayed Missed Filled Teeth; GCF: Gingival crevicular fluid; NCTC: National Collection of Type Culture; OMGS: Oral Microbiology Gothenburg Sweden; RUT: Rapid urease test

Funding
This study was supported by a TUA-Grant from the Public Dental Health Service, VG region, Sweden (TUAGBG-67191).

Author's contributions
GD – contributed to design, planning and writing of the manuscript. HH- contributed to the clinical sampling, data calculations and revised the manuscript. SB – planned and contributed to most of the laboratory work and revised the manuscript. AC – contributed to the conception, planning and design of the study and critically revised the manuscript. All authors have read and approved the manuscript.

Competing interests
The authors declare that they have no competing interests.

References

1. Wildner-Christensen M, Lassen AT, Lindebjerg J, Schaffalitsky De Muckadell OB. Diagnosis of *Helicobacter pylori* in bleeding peptic ulcer patients, evaluation of urea-based tests. Digestion. 2002;66:9–13.
2. Tang JH, Liu NJ, Cheng T. Et al endoscopic diagnosis of Helicobacter infection by rapid urease test in bleeding peptic ulcers: a prospective case-control study. J Clin Gastroenterol. 2009;43:131–9.
3. Salako NO, Kleinberg I. Incidence of selected ureolytic bacteria in human dental plaque from sites with differing salivary access. Arch Oral Biol. 1989; 34:787–91.
4. Chen YY, Weaver CA, Burne RA. Dual functions of *Streptococcus salivarius* urease. J Bacteriol. 2000;182:4667–9.
5. Golub LM, Borden SM, Kleinberg I. Urea content of gingival crevicular fluid and its relation to periodontal diseases in humans. J Periodontal Res. 1971;6: 243–51.
6. Al-Nowaiser A, Roberts GJ, Trompeter RS, Wilson M, Lucas VS. Oral health in children with chronic renal failure. Pediatr Nephrol. 2003;18:39–45.
7. Kleinberg I. Effect of urea concentration on human plaque in situ. Arch Oral Biol. 1967;12:1475–84.
8. Bowen WH. The Stephan curve revisited. Odontology. 2013;101:2–8.
9. Shu M, Morou-Bermudez E, Suarez-Perez E, Rivera-Miranda C, Browngardt CM, Chen Y-YM, Magnusson I, Burne RA. The relationship between dental caries status and dental plaque urease activity. Oral Microbiol Immunol. 2007;22:61–6.
10. Nascimento MM, Gordan VV, Garvan CW, Browngardt CM, Burne RA. Correlation of oral bacterial arginine and urea catabolism with caries experience. Oral Microbiol Immunol. 2009;24:89–95.
11. Toro E, Nascimento MM, Suarez-Perez E, Burne RA, Elias-Boneta A, Morou-Bermudez E. The effect of sucrose on plaque and saliva urease levels in vivo. Arch Oral Biol. 2010;55:249–54.
12. Goh KL, Parasakthi N, Peh SC, Puthucheary SD, Wong NW. The rapid urease test in the diagnosis of *Helicobacter pylori* infection. Singap Med J. 1994;35:161–2.
13. Anand PS, Kamath KP, Anil S. Role of dental plaque, saliva and periodontal disease in *Helicobacter pylori* infection. World J Gastroenterol. 2014;20:5639–53.
14. Barrow GI, Feltham RKA. Cowan and Steel's manual for the identification of medical bacteria. 3rd ed. Cambridge: Cambridge University Press; 2004.
15. Said RM, Cheah P-L, Chin S-C, Goh K-L. Evaluation of a new biopsy urease test: Prontodry, for the diagnosis of *Helicobacter pylori* infection. Eur J Gastroenterol Hepatol. 2004;16:195–9.
16. Boromeo M, Lambert JR, Pinkard KJ. Evaluation of the "CLO-test" to detect *Campylobacter pyloridis* infection. J Clin Patol. 1987;40:701–2.
17. Levin DA, Watermayer G, Mohamed N, Epstein DP, Hiatshwayo SJ, Metz DC. Evaluation of a locally produced rapid urease test for the diagnosis of *Helicobacter pylori* infection. S Afr Med J. 2007;97:1281–4.
18. Hassan H, Lingström P, Carlen A. Plaque pH in caries-free and caries-active young individuals before and after frequent rinses with sucrose and urea solution. Caries Res. 2015;49:18–25.
19. Biswas SD. Effect of urea on pH, ammonia, amino acids and lactic acid in the human salivary sediment system incubated with varying levels of glucose. Arch Oral Biol. 1982;27:683–91.
20. Sissons CH, Hancock EM. Urease activity in *Streptococcus salivarius* at low pH. Arch Oral Biol. 1993;38:507–16.
21. Yaling L, Tao H, Jingyi Z, Xuedong Z. Characterization of the *Actinomyces naeslundii* ureolysis and its role in bacterial aciduricity and capacity to modulate pH homeostasis. Microbiol Res. 2006;161:304–10.
22. Morou-Bermudez E, Burne RA. Analysis of urease expression in *Actinomyces naeslundii* WVU45. Infect Immun. 2000;68:6670–6.
23. Liu Y, Hu T, Jiang J, Zhou X. Regulation of urease gene of *Actinomyces naeslundii* in biofilms in response to environmental factors. FEMS Microbiol Lett. 2008;278:157–63.
24. Johnson JL, Moore LVH, Kaneko B, Moore WEC. *Actinomyces georgiae* sp. Nov. *Actinomyces gerencseriae* sp. Nov., designation of two genospecies of *Actinomyces naeslundii*, and inclusion of *A. naeslundii* serotypes II and III and *Actinomyces viscosus* serotype II in *A. naeslundii* genospecies 2. Int J Syst Bacteriol. 1990;40:273–86.
25. Henssage U, Do T, Radford DR, Gilbert SC, Clark D, Beighton D. Emended description of *Actinomyces naeslundii* and descriptions of *Actinomyces oris* sp. Nov. and *Actinomyces johnsonii* sp. Nov., previously identified as *Actinomyces naeslundii* genospecies 1,2 and WVA 963. Int J Syst Evolution Microbiol. 2009;59:509–16.
26. Liljemark WF, Bloomquist CG, Uhl LA, Schaffer EM, Wolff LF, Pihlstrom BL, Bandt CL. Distribution of oral Haemophilus species in dental plaque from a large adult population. Infect Immun. 1984;46:778–86.
27. Socransky SS, Haffajee AD. Periodontal microbial ecology. Periodontol. 2000; 2005(38):135–87.
28. Morou-Bermudez E, Rodriguez S, Bello AS, Dominguez-Bello MG. Urease and dental plaque microbial profiles in children. PLoSONE. 2015;10(9):e0139315. https://doi.org/10.1371/journal.pone0139315.
29. Marsh PD, Martin MV. Oral Microbiology. 5th ed. Edinburgh: Churchill Livingstone; 2009.
30. Appelgren L, Dahlen A, Eriksson C, Suksuart N, Dahlen G. Dental plaque pH and ureolytic activity in children and adults of a caries population. Acta Odont Scand. 2014;72:194–201.
31. Bouziane A, Ahid S, Abougal R, Ennibi O. Effect of periodontal therapy on prevention of gastric *Helicobacter pylori* recurrence: a systematic review and meta-analysis. J Clin Periodontol. 2012;39:1166–73.

Relations among obesity, family socioeconomic status, oral health behaviors, and dental caries in adolescents: the 2010–2012 Korea National Health and nutrition examination survey

Jin Ah Kim[1†], Hayon Michelle Choi[2†], Yunhee Seo[3] and Dae Ryong Kang[4*] (ID)

Abstract

Background: The purpose of this study was to examine the relationships among obesity, family socioeconomic status, oral health behaviors, and dental caries and to identify possible differences in factors related with dental caries according to gender among a representative sample of Korean adolescents.

Methods: Data were obtained from the Korean National Health and Nutrition Examination Survey, which was conducted between 2010 and 2012. This nationally representative cross-sectional survey included approximately 10,000 individuals, including adolescents, each year as a survey sample, and collected information on socioeconomic status, health-related behaviors, quality of life, healthcare utilization, anthropometric measures, biochemical and clinical profiles for non-communicable diseases, and dietary intake via three component surveys (health interview, health examination, and nutrition survey). The health interview and health examination were conducted by trained staff members. A total of 1646 adolescents of ages 13 to 18 years old were included in this study; there were 879 males and 767 females. Data were analyzed by t-test, X^2-test, and univariate and multivariate logistic regression analyses using SAS 9.4 and 'R' statistical software for Windows to account for the complex sampling design.

Results: In males, significant associations between family income and dental caries on permanent teeth were noted after adjusting for confounding variables; the odds ratios and 95% confidence intervals thereof were 0.43(0.24–0.76), 0.41(0.24–0.70), and 0.28(0.16–0.49) for low-middle, middle-high, and high family income, respectively. Smoking experience showed a significant association with dental caries on permanent teeth in females. Oral health behaviors, such as tooth brushing frequency, were associated with dental caries in only male adolescents. There was no association between obesity and dental caries on permanent teeth in either male or female adolescents.

Conclusion: The present study demonstrated that factors associated with dental caries in adolescents differ according to gender. Therefore, gender-specific interventions may be warranted to improve dental health among adolescents.

Keywords: Dental caries, Adolescent, Oral health, Cross-sectional study

* Correspondence: dr.kang@yonsei.ac.kr
[†]Jin Ah Kim and Hayon Michelle Choi contributed equally to this work.
[4]Center of Biomedical Data Science / Institute of Genomic Cohort, Wonju College of Medicine, Yonsei University, 20 Ilsan-ro, Wonju, Gangwon-do 26426, Korea
Full list of author information is available at the end of the article

Background

Rapid development of modern society and improvement in income status are affecting human health, particularly obesity rates, which have doubled over the past 30 years [1]. Obesity rates in adolescents have been increasing steadily since the 1980s [1]. A serious concern, adolescent obesity has been shown to be closely related to risk factors for chronic diseases, such as hyperlipidemia, hypertension, diabetes, and fatty liver, in adulthood [2, 3]. Furthermore, previous studies have shown that obesity is significantly correlated with dental caries on permanent teeth in adults and adolescents [4, 5]. According to the national statistics of Korea, the incidence rate of dental caries in Korean adolescents is 38%, with a decayed, missing, and filled teeth index (DMFT) score of 1.91, which is higher than the average score of 1.6 among Organization for Economic Cooperation and Development countries. Additionally, statistics indicate that one third of all dental patients in Korea are adolescents [6]. Considering the high rate of obesity and prevalence of dental caries in adolescents, we suspect that there may be a relationship between obesity and dental caries. In addition to obesity, family socioeconomic status may be a risk factor for dental caries in adolescents. Among the factors affecting dental caries in adults, socioeconomic status could be the major risk factor. Previous studies on adults have reported that individuals from lower socioeconomic status tend to exhibit a higher number of risk factors for dental caries than those of higher socioeconomic status [7]. Based on these prior studies, it can be inferred that family economic status can affect dental caries in adolescence.

Building healthy dental care habits in adolescence is important, since dental health at this time is related to dental health throughout one's entire life. A previous study showed that women have better oral hygiene habits than men [8]. Therefore, identifying possible differences in oral health behaviors in relation to dental caries on permanent teeth according to gender can help with developing oral health policies through which to prevent dental caries on permanent dental caries.

Although it is important to confirm the relationships among obesity, family socioeconomic status, oral health behaviors, and dental caries in adolescents, studies on dental caries in adolescents in relation to these factors are limited in Korea. Herein, the hypothesis of this study was that obesity, family socioeconomic status, and oral health behaviors would be related to dental caries on permanent teeth in adolescents. Therefore, the present study was performed to identify associations among obesity, socioeconomic status, oral health behaviors, and dental caries and to find out possible differences in factors related with dental caries according to gender among adolescents in a large sample from the Korean population using data from the Korea National Health and Nutrition Examination Survey (KNHANES).

Methods
Data collection and measurement
The Korea National Health and Nutrition Examination Survey (KNHANES) is a national surveillance system that has been assessing the health and nutritional status of Koreans since 1998. Based on the National Health Promotion Act, the surveys have been conducted by the Korea Centers for Disease Control and Prevention (KCDCP). This nationally representative cross-sectional survey includes approximately 10,000 individuals each year as a survey sample, and collects information on socioeconomic status, health-related behaviors, quality of life, healthcare utilization, anthropometric measures, biochemical and clinical profiles for non-communicable diseases, and dietary intakes with three component surveys: health interview, health examination and nutrition survey. The health interview and health examination are conducted by trained staff members, including physicians, dentists, medical technicians, and health interviewers, at a mobile examination center, and dieticians who visit the homes of the study participants for follow up. This study includes data from the KNHANES between 2010 and 2012. In total, 1829 individuals aged 13–18 years were targeted for the survey, and 1646 participants with complete data were evaluated in the present study.

Demographic and socioeconomic variables
In the present study, demographic and socioeconomic status were assessed according to age, gender, alcohol experience, smoking experience, monthly household income, and residential area. Monthly household income levels were divided into quartiles in consideration of the number of family members. Based on the results, the first group was defined as the lowest income group and the fourth group as the highest income group: specifically, quartiles comprised 10 thousand ~ 1 million won, 1.01–2 million won, 2.01–2.8 million won, and 2.81–5 million won or more. Sixteen living areas were categorized as rural and urban.

Oral health behaviors
Experience of a dental checkup within a year and whether adolescents brushed their teeth regularly after every meal (breakfast, lunch, and dinner) were assessed.

Anthropometric measurements
Body weight and height were measured to the nearest 0.1 kg and 0.1 cm, respectively, whilst participants were wearing light indoor clothing without shoes. Body mass index (BMI) was calculated using the following

formula: BMI = body weight (kg)/height^2 (m^2). In general, the BMI (kg/m^2) cut-off points for overweight and obese are set at 25 and 30, respectively, in adults. However, in children and adolescents, "overweight" is defined as a BMI (kg/m^2) $\geq$ the sex–age-specific 95th BMI percentile and "at risk for overweight" as 85th $\leq$ BMI <95th percentile [9, 10]. Based on these references, we defined "obesity" as a BMI (kg/m^2) $\geq$ the sex–age-specific 95th BMI percentile.

Data analysis

Data were analyzed by t-test, X^2-test, and univariate and multivariate logistic regression analysis using the SAS statistical software package for Windows (version 9.4) to account for the complex sampling design. Two-sided p-values < 0.05 were considered to indicate a statistically significant difference, and weight estimates were also considered.

Results

Table 1 shows the general characteristics, family socio-economic status, and oral health behaviors of the study population divided according to gender. The age of the male participants who exhibited permanent tooth decay was 15.81 ± 0.11 years old, while that of male participants who did not was 15.47 ± 0.08 years old (p-value = 0.011). The incident rates of permanent tooth decay were higher in both males and females of low income status than those of high income status (p-value< .001). Drinking experience was significantly more common in male adolescents with permanent decay that in those without permanent decay; this was not observed in females (Male: p-value = 0.010; Female: p-value = 0.206). Smoking experience, however, was more common in both male and female adolescents with permanent decay than those without (Male: p-value = 0.004; Female: p-value < .001).

Table 1 Characteristics of the study population

| Variables | Incidence of permanent tooth decay | | | | | |
| | Male | | | Female | | |
	No	Yes	p-value§	No	Yes	p-value§
Age (years) †	15.47 ± 0.08	15.81 ± 0.11	0.011	15.50 ± 0.08	15.59 ± 0.14	0.603‡
Income (quartiles)						
Q1 (lowest)	56 (9.16)	49 (19.44)	<.001	64 (11.19)	40 (21.86	<.001
Q2	140 (22.91)	67 (26.58)		142 (24.83)	58 (31.69)	
Q3	179 (29.29)	74 (29.36)		176 (30.77)	50 (27.32)	
Q4 (highest)	236 (38.62)	62 (24.60)		190 (33.22)	35 (19.13)	
Obesity						
Normal	528 (84.75)	212 (82.81)	0.500	523 (89.86)	160 (86.49)	0.118
Obesity	95 (15.25)	44 (17.19)		59 (10.14)	25 (13.51)	
Living area						
Rural	336 (53.93)	135 (52.73)	0.536	323 (55.50)	105 (56.76)	0.745
Urban	287 (46.07)	121 (47.27)		259 (44.50)	80 (43.24)	
Drinking experience						
No	403 (65.32)	141 (55.29)	0.010	388 (67.36)	113 (61.41)	0.206
Yes	214 (34.68)	114 (44.71)		188 (32.64)	71 (38.59)	
Smoking experience						
No	489 (79.25)	170 (66.93)	0.004	524 (90.97)	153 (83.15)	<.001
Yes	128 (20.75)	84 (33.07)		52 (9.03)	31 (16.85)	
Dental checkup within a year						
No	400 (64.62)	187 (73.33)	0.001	321 (55.44)	119 (64.32)	0.103
Yes	219 (35.38)	68 (26.67)		258 (44.56)	66 (35.68)	
Tooth brushing after every meal						
No	430 (70.382)	194 (76.98)	0.029	281 (48.78)	94(51.09)	0.315
Yes	181 (29.62)	58 (23.02)		295 (51.22)	90 (48.91)	

†Data are presented as mean ± standard error or number (percentages), estimated mean and its standard error using sampling weight for complex sample
‡Using t-test of coefficient of estimates complex sample general linear model
§P-values < 0.05 indicate a statistically significant difference

Oral health behaviors showed significant associations with permanent decay in males, but not in females (*p*-value = 0.001). More specifically, male adolescents who had undergone a dental checkup within a year or brushed after every meal comprised a lower number of survey participants with permanent dental decay (dental checkup: 73.33% [No], 26.67% [Yes]; tooth brushing after every meal: 76.98% [No], 23.02% [Yes]).

Figures 1 and 2 present the odds ratios and 95% confidence intervals (CIs) from univariate logistic regression analyses of obesity, socioeconomic status, and oral health behaviors in relation to incidence of dental cries on permanent teeth for male and female adolescents separately. Both drinking and smoking experience were significantly associated with dental caries in male adolescents. However, only smoking experience was associated with dental caries in female adolescents.

Table 2 presents the odds ratios and 95% CIs from multiple logistic regression analyses of obesity, socioeconomic status, and oral health behaviors in relation to incidence of dental cries on permanent teeth for male and female adolescents separately. An association was detected between household income and permanent dental decay in male adolescents after all adjusting for variables. The odds ratios and 95% CIs thereof were 0.43 (0.24–0.76), 0.41 (0.24–0.70), and 0.28 (0.16–0.49) for the low-middle, middle-high, and high income groups, respectively. The association between smoking experience and dental cries on permanent teeth remained after adjustment for all variables in female adolescents (2.50

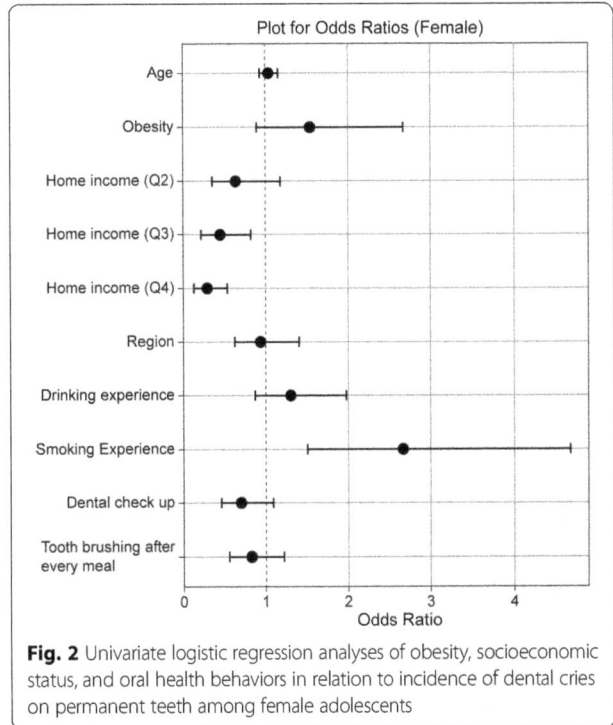

Fig. 2 Univariate logistic regression analyses of obesity, socioeconomic status, and oral health behaviors in relation to incidence of dental cries on permanent teeth among female adolescents

[1.36–4.58]). Although not significant, a similar trend was observed for male adolescents. Oral health behaviors, such as tooth brushing after every meal, showed associations with dental caries in only male adolescents. The odds ratio and CI for male survey participants who brushed after every meal was 0.63 (0.41–0.96). While our results suggested an association between oral health behaviors and dental cries on permanent teeth in Korean adolescents, we noted no association between obesity and dental cries on permanent teeth in either the male or female adolescent groups.

Discussion

This study was conducted to examine the associations among obesity, family socioeconomic status, oral health behaviors, and dental caries and to disclose possible differences in factors related with dental caries according to gender among Korean adolescents. Herein, we found that several socioeconomic characteristics and oral health behaviors were associated with dental caries and that these results differed significantly depending on gender among Korean adolescents. Nevertheless, we noted no association between obesity and dental caries. Therefore, our hypothesis that there would be a relationship between obesity and dental caries was not supported.

Previous studies have asserted that frequent consumption of mono and disaccharide sugars is the predominant cause of both obesity and dental caries [11, 12]. Soft drink consumption has also been shown to be a risk factor for obesity and dental caries among children and adolescents

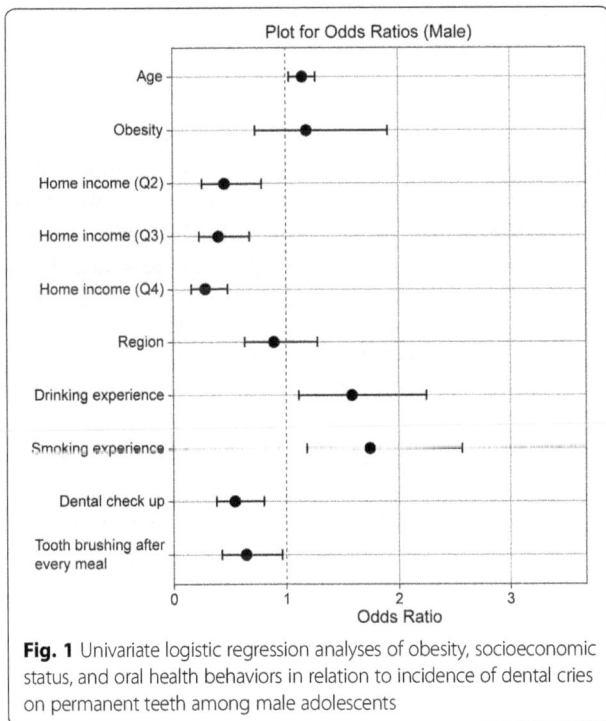

Fig. 1 Univariate logistic regression analyses of obesity, socioeconomic status, and oral health behaviors in relation to incidence of dental cries on permanent teeth among male adolescents

Table 2 Multivariate logistic regression analyses of obesity, socioeconomic status, and oral health behaviors on incidence of dental cries on permanent teeth

Variables	Dental caries incidence in male		Dental caries incidence in female	
	OR (95% CI)	p-value[†]	OR (95% CI)	p-value[†]
Age (years)	1.09 (0.95–1.24)	0.215	0.97 (0.84–1.12)	0.641
Obesity				
Non-obesity	1.00		1.00	
Obesity	1.37 (0.83–2.28)	0.221	1.52 (0.82–2.80)	0.179
Income (quartiles)				
Q1 (lowest)	1.00		1.00	
Q2	0.43 (0.24–0.76)	0.003	0.68 (0.37–1.27)	0.229
Q3	0.41 (0.24–0.70)	0.001	0.47 (0.25–0.90)	0.022
Q4 (highest)	0.28 (0.16–0.49)	<.001	0.31 (0.15–0.62)	0.001
Living area				
Rural	1.00		1.00	
Urban	0.77 (0.53–1.13)	0.183	1.12 (0.72–1.73)	0.624
Drinking experience				
No	1.00		1.00	
Yes	1.14 (0.71–1.83)	0.577	0.97 (0.57–1.62)	0.892
Smoking experience				
No	1.00		1.00	
Yes	1.54 (0.97–2.44)	0.065	2.50 (1.36–4.58)	0.003
Dental checkup within a year				
No	1.00		1.00	
Yes	0.67 (0.44–1.01)	0.055	0.67 (0.43–1.04)	0.075
Tooth brushing after every meal				
No	1.00		1.00	
Yes	0.63 (0.41–0.96)	0.033	0.98 (0.65–1.47)	0.921

†P-values < 0.05 indicate a statistically significant difference

[13]. For these reasons, the Comprehensive Improvement Plans for School Food Service (2007~2011) and policies targeting the prohibition of beverage sales in school were enacted to prevent obesity caused by foods in Korea. Through these national efforts, adolescent obesity caused by sugar consumption and an unbalanced diet has been relatively controlled [14]. However, obesity caused by other factors, such as decreased physical activity and increased sedentary time, has been increasing [15]. As our study revealed that adolescent obesity is not related to dental caries, which are affected by sugary diets, and in light of the results of the studies above, taken altogether, this suggests that adolescent obesity in Korea is presently related more with a lack of exercise than diet.

Previous studies have explained that low socioeconomic status can be an impediment to oral health, because of the high cost of dental services, the low availability of dental insurance, poorer living conditions, less knowledge about the negative consequences of health-compromising behaviors, and greater psychological stress among adults [16–

19]. Also, much of the literature has reported that socioeconomic status and smoking are correlated. Similarly, smoking experience among adolescents has been found to increase with lower parental socioeconomic status [19], further threatening the oral health of adolescents because of lots of hazardous substances in cigarettes. It is suggested that parents with good socioeconomic status are more likely to be interested in health education, including smoking cessation and abstinence. Like previous studies, the results of the present study support that higher household socioeconomic status could be a protective factor against dental caries in adolescents and that smoking experience is related to dental caries. Also, interestingly, we discovered that smoking experience was more strongly associated with dental caries in female adolescents than in male adolescents. According to Statistics Korea [20], the prevalence of smoking has decreased from 12.8% in 2009 to 7.8% in 2015 among adolescents. However, these rates are much higher than those in Australia (5.6%), Finland (5.0%), and Canada (1.9%), as well as other

Asian countries, such as China (6.9%), Singapore (6.0%), and Japan (1.7%) [21]. Furthermore, smoking rates have increased significantly among female adolescents in Korea (3.2%) [21], a rate much higher than those in Canada (1.7%), China (2.2%), and Japan (1.1%) [20].Therefore, we suggest that it may be necessary to develop measures targeting dental health among adolescents of low socioeconomic status, so that they can live healthy lives even when they become adults. Moreover, oral health policies targeting female adolescents should stress the dental problems associated with smoking.

Oral health behaviors, such as an annual dental checkups and daily tooth brushing after every meal, are very important to reducing teeth plaque and calculus. Adolescent brushing habits, such as tooth brushing, interdental tooth brushing, and use of floss, are important, because they can affect oral health in adulthood. A previous study that examined the number of tooth brushings after every meal for 761 adolescents reported that 77.7% of the adolescent participants brushed their teeth after every meal [22]. In the present study, 27.7% of the male adolescents brushed their teeth after every meal, while 50.7% of the female adolescents brushed their teeth after every meal. Similarly, the percentage of female adolescents who underwent dental checkups within a year was higher than that in male adolescents. These results suggest better oral health behaviors among female adolescents of Korea than their male counterparts. According to a previous study that described the percentage of adolescents who brushed their teeth after lunch and factors related therewith, 40.6% of adolescents did not use floss, and 43.7% did not even know how to floss at all [23]. Ostberg [24] and Watt [25] asserted that oral health education in schools can expect only a short-term effect, because it does not consider individual characteristics. Therefore, attempts to strengthen oral hygiene education should be tailored to the individual's knowledge and oral health condition.

As the data for this study were derived from the KNHANES, the largest representative survey in Korea, the present results are considered to accurately reflect the oral health statuses of and factors related to dental caries among Korean adolescents, particularly owing to the large sample size. However, as this was a cross-sectional study, a cause-and-effect relationship between variables cannot be inferred. Therefore, we suggest the need for a school-based cohort study to clarify the factors affecting dental caries among adolescents.

Conclusions

This study revealed associations between family socioeconomic status or oral health behavior and dental cries on permanent teeth in Korean male adolescents. In female adolescents, we noted associations between family socioeconomic status or smoking experience and dental caries. Unexpectedly, obesity was not found to be related to dental caries. In light of our results, we suggest that oral health interventions tailored to the individual gender may help in improving dental health among adolescents.

Abbreviations
BMI: Body mass index; CI: Confidence interval; DMFT: Decayed, missing, and filled teeth index; KCDCP: Korea Centers for Disease Control and Prevention; KNHANES: Korea National Health and Nutrition Examination Survey

Authors' contributions
JAK and HMC, co-first authors, were major contributors in the conception of the study, the analysis and interpretation of the data, and in writing the manuscript. Yunhee Seo YS contributed to the interpretation of the data and critically reviewed the manuscript. DRK conceived of the study and was a major contributor to the analyses and interpretation of the data and in writing the manuscript. All authors read and approved the final manuscript.

Competing interests
The authors declare that they have no competing interests.

Author details
¹College of Nursing Science, Kyung Hee University, Seoul, Korea. ²Graduate School of Public Health, Seoul National University, Seoul, Korea. ³Graduate School of Public Health, Ajou University, Suwon, Korea. ⁴Center of Biomedical Data Science / Institute of Genomic Cohort, Wonju College of Medicine, Yonsei University, 20 Ilsan-ro, Wonju, Gangwon-do 26426, Korea.

References
1. World Health Organization. Obesity and overweight.2015. Available at: http://www.who.int/mediacentre/factsheets/fs311/en/. Accessed 5 Apr 2017.
2. Sinha R, Fisch G, Teague B, Tamborlane WV, Banyas B, Allen K, et al. Prevalence of impaired glucose tolerance among children and adolescents with marked obesity. N Engl J Med. 2002;346:802–10.
3. Rizzo AC, Goldberg TB, Silva CC, Kurokawa CS, Nunes HR, Corrente JE. Metabolic syndrome risk factors in overweight, obese, and extremely obese Brazilian adolescents. Nutr J. 2013;12(1):1–7.
4. Hayden C, Bowler JO, Chambers S, Freeman R, Humphris G, Richards D, et al. Obesity and dental caries in children: a systematic review and meta-analysis. Community Dent Oral Epidemiol. 2013;41(4):289–308.
5. Bailleul-Forestier I, Lopes K, Souames M, Azoguy-Levy S, Frelut ML, Boy-Lefevre ML. Caries experience in a severely obese adolescent population. Int J Paediatr Dent. 2007;17:358–63.
6. National Health Insurance Corporation, health insurance review & assessment service. National health insurance statistical yearbook. 2014. Available at: http://www.nhis.or.kr/bbs7/boards/B0159/16094. Accessed 5 Apr 2017.

7. Singh A, Rouxel P, Watt RG, Tsakos G. Social inequalities in clustering of oral health related behaviors in a national sample of British adults. Prev Med. 2013;57(2):102–6.

8. Mamai-Homata E, Koletsi-Kounari H, Margaritis V. Gender differences in oral health status and behavior of Greek dental students: a meta-analysis of 1981, 2000, and 2010 data. J Int Soc Prev Community Dent. 2016;6(1):60.

9. Barlow SE, Dietz WH. Obesity evaluation and treatment: expert committee recommendations. The Maternal and Child Health Bureau, Health Resources and Services Administration and the Department of Health and Human Services. Pediatrics. 1998;102:E29.

10. Wang Y, Beydoun MA, Liang L, Caballero B, Kumanyika SK. Will all Americans become overweight or obese? Estimating the progression and cost of the US obesity epidemic. Obesity. 2008;16(10):2323–30.

11. World Health Organization. Joint WHO/FAO expert Consultation.Nutrition and the prevention of chronic diseases Tech Rep Ser 916 Diet.

12. Harrington S. The role of sugar-sweetened beverage consumption in adolescent obesity: a review of the literature. J Sch Nurs. 2008;24(1):3–12.

13. Sohn W, Burt BA, Sowers MR. Carbonated soft drinks and dental caries in the primary dentition. J Dent Res. 2006;85(3):262–6.

14. Ministry of Education. Ministry of Education, Comprehensive Improvement Plans for School food service (2007~2011) and policy of prohibition of beverage sales. 2011.Available at: http://www.moe.go.kr/boardCnts/view. do?boardID=294&lev=0&statusYN=W&s=moe&m=0503&opType= N&boardSeq=34263. Accessed 5 Apr 2017.

15. Janssenm I, Katzmarzykl-E PT, Boyce WF, Vereecken C, IVlulvihillE C, Robertsfi, C, Currie C. Comparison of overweight and obesity prevalence in school-aged youth from 34 countries and their relationships with physical activity and dietary patterns. Obes Rev 2005;6(2):123–132.

16. Park JB, Han K, Park YG, Ko Y. Association between socioeconomic status and oral health behaviors: the 2008-2010 Korea national health and nutrition examination survey. Exp Ther Med. 2016;12(4):2657–64.

17. Peres MA, Peres KG, de Barros AJD, Victora CG. The relation between family socioeconomic trajectories from childhood to adolescence and dental caries and associated oral behaviours. J Epidemiol Community Health. 2007;61(2):141–5.

18. Chen E. Why socioeconomic status affects the health of children: a psychosocial perspective. Curr Dir Psychol Sci. 2004;13:112–5.

19. Hanson MD, Chen E. Socioeconomic status and health behaviors in adolescence: a review of the literature. J Behav Med. 2007;30(3):263–85.

20. Ministry of Education, Ministry of Health and Welfare, Korea Centers for Disease Control and Prevention. The tenth Korea youth risk behavior web-based survey. Available at: http://www.index.go.kr/potal/main/ EachDtlPageDetail.do?idx_cd=2829. Accessed 5 Apr 2017.

21. World Health Organization. Tob Control country profiles.Available at: http://www. who.int/tobacco/surveillance/policy/country_profile/en. Accessed 5 Apr 2017.

22. do Carmo Matias Freire M, Sheiham A, Hardy R. Adolescents' sense of coherence, oral health status, and oral health-related behaviours. Community Dent Oral Epidemiol. 2001;29(3):204–12.

23. Korea Centers for Disease Control and Prevention. Major results of Korea National Health and nutrition examination survey. 2007. Available at: https:// knhanes.cdc.go.kr/knhanes/eng/index.do. Accessed 5 Apr 2017. https:// knhanes.cdc.go.kr/knhanes/sub04/sub04_03.do?classType=7

24. Östberg AL. Adolescents' views of oral health education. A qualitative study. Acta Odontol Scand. 2005;63(5):300–7.

25. Watt R, Fuller S, Harnett R, Treasure E, Stillman-Lowe C. Oral health promotion evaluation–time for development. Community Dent Oral Epidemiol. 2001;29(3):161–6.

16

Lead exposure may affect gingival health in children

Borany Tort[1], Youn-Hee Choi[1][*] (iD), Eun-Kyong Kim[2], Yun-Sook Jung[1], Mina Ha[3], Keun-Bae Song[1] and Young-Eun Lee[4]

Abstract

Background: Several studies have reported the harmful effects of lead poisoning. However, the relationship between lead exposure and oral health of children has not been well defined. The aim of this study was to investigate the relationship between blood lead level (BLL) and oral health status of children.

Methods: A total of 351 children (aged 7–15 years) were recruited from the pilot data of the Korean Environmental Health Survey in Children and Adolescents, which was designed to examine environmental exposure and children's health status in South Korea. Blood samples were taken to determine BLLs and oral examinations were performed to assess oral health parameters, including community periodontal index (CPI), gingival index (GI), and plaque index (PI). Information regarding socioeconomic status, oral hygiene behavior, and dietary habits was collected from parents and guardians.

Results: The participants were divided equally into four quartiles, with quartile I comprised of children with the lowest BLLs. There were significant differences for PI ($p < 0.05$) among the quartile groups. Using logistic regression models, we found a significant relationship between BLL and oral health parameters. The crude odds ratios for CPI, GI, and PI in the third quartile were 5.24 (95% CI: 1.48-18.56), 4.35 (95% CI: 1.36-13.9), and 4.17 (95% CI: 1.50-11.54), respectively, while the age and gender-adjusted odds ratios were 7.66 (95% CI: 1.84-31.91), 6.80 (95% CI: 1.80-25.68), and 3.41 (95% CI: 1.12-10.40), respectively. After adjustments for age, gender, parent education level, and frequency of tooth brushing, the adjusted odds ratios were 7.21 (95% CI: 1.72-30.19), 6.13 (95% CI: 1.62-23.19), and 3.37 (95% CI: 1.10-10.34), respectively.

Conclusions: A high BLL might be associated with oral health problems in children, including plaque deposition and gingival diseases.

Keywords: Gingivitis, Pathology, Oral hygiene

Background

Lead is a heavy metal widely employed in automobiles, gasoline, lubricants, and decolorizing agents, including other applications such as agriculture as an insecticide [1]. In the medical field, lead is used to produce antifungal agents and provide radiation protection [2]. However, reports of symptoms of lead poisoning are common and have been known since at least the second century B.C, with such poisoning in lead industrial workers and children first reported in the nineteenth century [3].

The detrimental effects of lead poisoning are related to the amount of lead accumulated in the body and blood lead level (BLL) is considered to be associated with physical health, mental health, the immune system, and functional growth [4]. Also, lead exposure has been reported to have an impact on human intelligence and social behavior, with life-long adverse effects [5, 6].

In addition to these general health risks, lead exposure can have harmful effects on oral health. Such exposure can affect enamel formation leading to caries production, delayed dental enamel formation, worsened dental fluorosis, and periodontal bone loss, as well as increased tooth loss in men [7–14]. A study by Saraiva et al. found that BLL was significantly associated with periodontal health in adult participants [15]. Another study conducted with Thai children living in a shipyard industrial area showed that there was a significantly positive correlation between high BLL and periodontal problems, including the presence of deep pockets, particularly teeth 16 and 46 [16].

* Correspondence: cyh1001@knu.ac.kr
[1]Department of Preventive Dentistry, School of Dentistry, Kyungpook National University, 2177 Dalgubeol-daero, Jung-gu, Daegu 700-412, Republic of Korea
Full list of author information is available at the end of the article

Children tend to absorb more lead into their bodies than adults because of a higher rate of metabolism as well as a physical tendency to inhale lead from polluted air. Moreover, child gastrointestinal organs seem to absorb lead more easily [17]. Although some studies have speculated regarding a possible relationship between BLL and dental caries in children [18, 19], few have assessed the association between BLL and periodontal status in child subjects. The aim of present study was to investigate the relationship between BLL and oral health status in Korean children.

Methods

Study population

A total of 351 children ranging from 7 to 15 years old living in two cities in South Korea (Incheon city and Cheonan city) were recruited from the participants of the pilot study of the Korean Environmental Health Survey in Children and Adolescents [20]. That study aimed to show the environmental exposure and health of Korean children who were sampled with a national representativeness by use of a questionnaire survey, clinical tests, and physical examinations in 2011 and 2012. Of 351 subjects, 137 agreed to participate, were undertook oral health examination, and included in this study. The present study was approved by the institutional review board of a university hospital (IRB No. DKUH 2012-10-003-001). Parents or guardians of the subjects provided written informed consent for their participation, and completed questionnaires regarding their socioeconomic status and the oral hygiene behaviors of their children.

Measurement of blood lead levels

Whole blood (3–5 ml) was drawn from the subjects and sealed in a heparin containing tube. Lead levels were determined using atomic absorption spectrophotometry (800 Zeeman correction; Spectral AA, Varian, NSW, Australia) at a commercial laboratory. The coefficient of variation of the blood lead measurements was 4.9%.

Oral health examinations

Oral health examinations were conducted by 1 dentist and 2 dental hygienists trained according to the World Health Organization (WHO) guidelines on oral health surveys [21]. The dentist performed oral examinations using a dental mirror and periodontal probe under artificial light with the subject in a portable dental chair in order to detect decayed, missing, and filled surfaces of permanent teeth (DMFT), and also determined community periodontal index (CPI), gingival index (GI), and plaque index (PI) values [21–24]. The CPI, GI, and PI values of teeth 11, 16, 26, 31, 36, and 46 were assessed in the present study. CPI was scored as follows: 0 (healthy), 1 (bleeding following probing), 2 (presence of

dental calculus). Because the presence of dental calculus is not an indicator of periodontal health in children, 11 participants whose CPI scores of six representative teeth were only 0 and 2 were excluded in the analysis for CPI. Also participants whose one of CPI scores of six representative teeth was 1 regardless of the rest were classified as having CPI score of 1. Given that children scarcely have periodontitis and are likely to have pseudo-periodontal pockets due to tooth eruption, CPI scores of 3 and 4 were not used.

Socioeconomic status and oral hygiene behavior

Information regarding potential covariates was obtained from questionnaires completed by parents and guardians. We surveyed socioeconomic variables including family income, parent education level, father and mother's occupations, oral hygiene behaviors such as frequency of tooth cleaning and frequency of intake of sugar-containing sweets, dental treatment demands, and history of decayed teeth.

Statistical analysis

The subjects were divided into 4 equal quartiles based on measured BLL, with quartile I comprised of children with the lowest BLLs. Analysis of variance (ANOVA) and a Chi-square test were used to compare the covariates and oral health parameters among the quartiles. One crude and two adjusted logistic regression models were used to explore the relationship between BLL and oral health parameters. Two adjusted odds ratios (OR) were calculated.

The first model adjusted for age and gender, and the other added parent education level, and frequency of tooth brushing additionally as confounders. SPSS (ver. 20.0, IBM, NY, USA) was utilized for the analyses, with statistical significance considered at $p < 0.05$.

Results

Table 1 shows the average measured BLLs according to demographic characteristics, socioeconomic status, oral hygiene behavior, dietary habits, and clinical oral parameters. The mean age of the subjects was 10.9 ± 2.1 years and 69 were girls (50.4%). Overall mean BLL was 1.25 ± 0.43 µg/dl, ranging from 0.36 to 2.90 µg/dl. There were no statistically significant differences observed among those factors.

Table 2 shows the distribution of demographic characteristics, socioeconomic status, oral health behavior, and dietary habits of the subjects after dividing into the BLL quartiles. Based on measured BLL, the study population was divided into equal quartile groups (I, II, III, and IV), with quartile I composed of subjects with the lowest BLLs. There were no statistically significant differences observed among the quartile groups.

Table 1 Mean blood lead level according to socioeconomic status and oral hygiene behavior in school-age children

	N	Pb (μg/dl) Mean ± SD
Total participants	137	1.25 ± 0.43
Grade		
Elementary	100	1.35 ± 0.43
Middle	37	0.99 ± 0.32
Gender		
Male	68	1.33 ± 0.43
Female	69	1.19 ± 0.43
Family income (×10,000 won/month)[a]		
< 200	17	1.18 ± 0.38
200-399	47	1.20 ± 0.36
400-599	46	1.31 ± 0.46
> 600	23	1.25 ± 0.52
Level of parent's education[a]		
≤ High school	61	1.29 ± 0.39
College/university	70	1.22 ± 0.48
Graduate school	5	1.22 ± 0.17
Father's occupation		
Professional	17	1.18 ± 0.38
White collar/service	47	1.20 ± 0.36
Blue collar	46	1.31 ± 0.46
Unemployed	23	1.25 ± 0.52
Mother's occupation		
Professional	24	1.31 ± 0.50
White collar/service	39	1.23 ± 0.42
Blue collar	11	1.21 ± 0.34
Unemployed	63	1.23 ± 0.40
Frequency of tooth cleaning		
≤ once a day	3	1.20 ± 0.12
2-3 times/day	101	1.29 ± 0.44
> 4 times/day	33	1.17 ± 0.40
Intake of sugar-containing sweets		
< Once a day	23	1.26 ± 0.40
Once a day	71	1.25 ± 0.44
2-3 times/day	43	1.27 ± 0.45
Dental treatment demand (1 year)		
Yes	80	1.27 ± 0.45
No	56	1.23 ± 0.41
History of decayed teeth		
Yes	63	1.31 ± 0.40
No	74	1.21 ± 0.46
CPI index		
0	34	1.19 ± 0.39
≥ 1	92	1.29 ± 0.44

Table 1 Mean blood lead level according to socioeconomic status and oral hygiene behavior in school-age children *(Continued)*

	N	Pb (μg/dl) Mean ± SD
Gingival index		
≤ 1	39	1.20 ± 0.41
2-3	98	1.28 ± 0.44
Plaque index		
≤ 2	56	1.15 ± 0.46
3	81	1.33 ± 0.40

Abbreviations: *Pb* lead
[a]Some answers were missing

Distribution of oral health parameters according to the BLL quartiles is shown in Table 3. Participants with a higher BLL were more likely to have a high PI value ($p < 0.015$). There were no other statistically significant differences.

Results of logistic regression analysis for the association between BLL and oral health parameters are shown in Table 4. A significant association was found in the third quartile between BLL and all oral health parameters. Subjects quartile III had a crude OR of 5.24 (95% CI: 1.48-18.56), 4.35 (95% CI: 1.36-13.9), and 4.17 (95% CI: 1.50-11.54) for CPI, GI, and PI, respectively, while those in the fourth quartile had a crude OR of 3. 14 [95% CI: 1.14-8.41] for PI.

We constructed an age and gender adjusted model, which showed that subjects in the third quartile had an OR of 7.66 (95% CI: 1.84-31.91), 6.80 (95% CI: 1.80-25. 68), and 3.41 (95% CI: 1.12-10.40) for CPI, GI, and PI, respectively, while those in the second quartile had an OR of 3.29 [95% CI: 1.06-10.19] for GI.

Finally, following adjustments for age, gender, parent education level, and frequency of tooth brushing, subjects in the third quartile had an OR of 7.21 (95% CI: 1. 72-30.19), 6.13 (95% CI: 1.62-23.19), and 3.37 (95% CI: 1.10-10.34) for CPI, GI, and PI respectively, while those in the second quartile had an OR of 3.44 [95% CI: 1.00-11.90] and 3.58 [95% CI: 1.12-11.40] for CPI and GI, respectively.

Discussion

The aim of the present study was to investigate the relationship between BLL and oral health in children. We recruited subjects from participants in the CHEER study, a national representative study performed in Korea that focused on the influence of living environment on the well-being of children. We found that higher BLLs were positively correlated with worse oral health measurements, including CPI, GI, and PI. Furthermore, in logistic regression analysis, that effect was maintained after adjusting for age, gender, parent education level, and frequency of tooth brushing.

Table 2 Distribution of demographic characteristics, socioeconomic status, oral health behavior, and dietary habits of children according to blood lead level quartiles

	Total (n = 137)	Quartile I (n = 35)	Quartile II (n = 34)	Quartile III (n = 34)	Quartile IV (n = 34)
	No. (%)	No. (%)	No. (%)	No. (%)	No. (%)
Age (years, mean ± SD)	10.9 ± 2.1	12.4 ± 1.7	11.1 ± 2.1	10.2 ± 1.9	9.8 ± 1.8
Gender					
Male	68 (49.6)	12 (34.3)	17 (50.0)	19 (55.9)	20 (58.8)
Female	69 (50.4)	23 (65.7)	17 (50.0)	15 (44.1)	14 (41.2)
Family income (10,000 won/month)[a]					
< 200	17 (12.8)	4 (11.4)	8 (24.2)	1 (2.9)	4 (12.9)
200-399	47 (35.3)	14 (40.0)	11 (33.3)	14 (41.2)	8 (25.8)
400-599	46 (34.6)	9 (25.7)	12 (36.4)	11 (32.4)	14 (45.2)
> 600	23 (17.3)	8 (22.9)	2 (6.1)	8 (23.5)	5 (16.1)
Parent's education[a]					
≤ High school	61 (44.9)	11 (31.4)	19 (55.9)	11 (33.3)	20 (58.8)
College/university	70 (51.5)	24 ()	13 (38.2)	19 (57.6)	14 (41.2)
Graduate school	5 (3.7)	–	2 (5.9)	3 (9.1)	–
Father's occupation					
Profession	50 (36.5)	10 (28.6)	12 (35.3)	13 (38.2)	15 (44.1)
White collar/Service	45 (32.8)	15 (42.9)	8 (23.5)	10 (29.4)	12 (35.3)
Blue collar	34 (24.8)	8 (22.9)	11 (32.4)	10 (29.4)	5 (14.7)
Unemployed	8 (5.8)	2 (5.7)	3 (8.8)	1 (2.9)	2 (5.9)
Mother's occupation					
Profession	24 (17.5)	6 (17.1)	3 (8.8)	10 (29.4)	5 (14.7)
White collar/Service	39 (28.5)	10 (28.6)	8 (23.5)	9 (26.5)	12 (35.3)
Blue collar	11 (8.0)	1 (2.9)	6 (17.6)	2 (5.9)	2 (5.9)
Unemployed	63 (46.0)	18 (51.4)	17 (50.0)	13 (38.2)	15 (44.1)
Frequency of tooth cleaning					
≤ Once a day	3 (2.2)	–	1 (0.7)	2 (5.9)	–
2-3 times/day	101 (73.7)	25 (71.4)	24 (17.5)	27 (79.4)	25 (73.5)
> 4 times/day	33 (24.1)	10 (28.6)	9 (26.5)	5 (14.7)	9 (26.5)
Sugar-containing sweets intake					
< Once a day	23 (16.8)	5 (14.3)	5 (14.7)	7 (20.6)	6 (17.6)
Once a day	71 (51.8)	18 (51.4)	22 (64.7)	16 (47.1)	15 (44.1)
2-3 times/day	43 (31.4)	12 (34.3)	7 (20.6)	11 (32.4)	13 (38.2)
Dental treatment demand (1 year)					
Yes	80 (58.8)	20 (57.1)	21 (61.8)	17 (50.0)	22 (66.7)
No	56 (41.2)	15 (42.9)	13 (38.2)	17 (50.0)	11 (33.3)

[a]Some answers were missing

The mean BLL of the children enrolled in this study was 1.25 ± 0.43 μg/dl and ranged from 0.36 to 2.90 μg/dl, which was lower than noted in previous studies conducted in China (5.56 μg/dL) and the United States (2.30 μg/dL) [19, 25]. However, even with this relatively low concentration of lead, we found evidence of its adverse effects on the oral health of our subjects.

Our results are consistent with those of previous studies of adults. According to a study conducted by El-Said et al. that focused on the risk of gingivitis in lead-exposed workers, gingivitis is related to lead sulfide, a product of the reaction between lead and hydrogen sulfide during food fermentation, which can produce gum irritation [26]. According to their study, the risk of gingivitis in exposed workers

Table 3 Distribution of oral health parameters according to blood lead level quartiles

	Total (n = 137) No. (%)	Quartile I (n = 35) No. (%)	Quartile II (n = 34) No. (%)	Quartile III (n = 34) No. (%)	Quartile IV (n = 34) No. (%)	P-value
Presence of dental caries						
DMFT (mean ± SD)	1.5 ± 1.9	1.4 ± 1.5	1.7 ± 2.3	1.1 ± 1.5	1.7 ± 2.1	0.477[a]
History of dental caries (DMFT ≥1)						
Yes	63 (46.0)	11 (31.4)	17 (50.0)	18 (52.9)	17 (50.0)	0.252[*]
No	74 (54.0)	24 (68.6)	17 (50.0)	16 (47.1)	17 (50.0)	
Community periodontal index						
mean ± SD	1.1 ± 0.8	0.9 ± 0.8	1.2 ± 0.7	1.2 ± 0.7	1.1 ± 0.8	0.358[a]
0	34 (27.8)	13 (41.9)	7 (23.3)	4 (12.1)	10 (31.3)	0.083
≥ 1	92 (73.0)	18 (58.1)	23 (76.7)	29 (87.9)	22 (68.8)	
Gingival index						
mean ± SD	2.1 ± 0.9	1.8 ± 0.9	2.1 ± 0.8	2.3 ± 0.7	2.0 ± 0.9	0.150[a]
≤ 1	37 (28.5)	15 (42.9)	8 (23.5)	5 (14.7)	11 (32.4)	*0.061*[*]
2-3	98 (71.5)	20(57.1)	26 (76.5)	29 (85.3)	23 (67.6)	
Plaque index						
mean ± SD	2.6 ± 0.5	2.4 ± 0.5	2.6 ± 0.5	2.7 ± 0.4	2.7 ± 0.5	*0.015*[a]
≤ 2	56 (40.9)	21 (60.0)	15 (44.1)	9 (26.5)	11(32.4)	*0.025*[*]
3	81 (59.1)	14 (40.0)	19 (55.9)	25 (73.5)	23 (67.6)	

Abbreviations: DMFT decayed/missing/filled surfaces of permanent teeth, CPI community periodontal index, GI gingival index, PI plaque index
*p-value obtained from χ²-test
[a]Data analyzed by ANOVA
Italics are statistically significant (p<0.05)

Table 4 Association between blood lead level (quartiles) and oral health parameters

		Model 1 OR	95%CI	Model 2 OR	95%CI	Model 3 OR	95%CI
CPI (outcome)							
Lead level	Quartile I	Ref.		Ref.		Ref.	
	Quartile II	2.37	0.79-7.18	3.14	0.93-10.55	*3.44*	*1.00-11.90*
	Quartile III	*5.24*	*1.48-18.56*	*7.66*	*1.84-31.91*	*7.21*	*1.72-30.19*
	Quartile IV	1.59	0.57-4.47	2.38	0.69-8.21	2.65	0.75-9.44
GI (outcome)							
Leadlevel	Quartile I	Ref.		Ref.		Ref.	
	Quartile II	2.44	0.86-6.88	*3.29*	*1.06-10.19*	*3.58*	*1.12-11.40*
	Quartile III	*4.35*	*1.36-1.90*	*6.80*	*1.80-25.68*	*6.13*	*1.62-23.19*
	Quartile IV	1.57	0.59-4.19	2.50	0.77-8.19	2.81	0.83-9.47
PI (outcome)							
Leadlevel	Quartile I	Ref.		Ref.		Ref.	
	Quartile II	1.90	0.73-4.95	1.66	0.61-4.52	1.60	0.58-.40
	Quartile III	*4.17*	*1.50-11.54*	*3.41*	*1.12-10.40*	*3.37*	*1.10-10.34*
	Quartile IV	*3.14*	*1.14-8.41*	2.47	0.80-7.60	2.37	0.76-7.38

Model 1: Unadjusted model
Model 2: Model adjusted for age and gender
Model 3: Model adjusted for age, gender, parent education level, and frequency of tooth brushing
Abbreviations: CI confidence interval, CPI community periodontal index, GI gingival index, PI plaque index, OR odds ratio, Ref reference quartile
Italics are statistically significant (p<0.05)

was 4.82 times higher than in non-exposed workers. Arora et al. also reported that cumulative lead exposure might increase the risk of tooth loss in adults [14].

Although the biological link between lead exposure and periodontal disease has not been clearly elucidated, an increase in reactive oxygen species (ROS) has been suggested to be a factor, as ROS are generated by lead exposure and known to cause oxidative stress [27]. Lee et al. reported an association between BLL and oxidative stress in adults [28]. ROS can also cause damage to proteins and DNA, as well as lipid peroxidation [29], and an increased level can lead to damage to gingival, periodontal ligament, and alveolar bone tissues [30]. Furthermore, lead in blood has been suggested to disturb the function of the salivary gland, which may contribute to plaque accumulation [31]. For example, heavy metals such as lead imitate calcium in some ways. Therefore lead may interfere with calcium metabolism which can alter normal cell function acutely and perturbation of calcium-metabolism may cause disorder of salivary gland function [32–34]. Available evidences showed that administration of lead resulted in 30-40% diminishment of salivary flow rates in rats [31]. However, there was no study to support this hypothesis in case of people. These factors might explain the results of our study.

The current study has some limitations. First, since the subjects of our study were recruited from only 2 cities in South Korea, the findings are not representative of the overall Korean population. In addition, since this is a cross-sectional study, the results must be cautiously interpreted because this is not causality but association study. As for another limitation, final sample size was not enough to have statistical power when including several confounders in logistic regression models resulting in non-significant association at the stratum of the fourth quartile. However, this result provides meaningful evidence that relatively higher blood lead in children was associated with poorer gingival health. Despite these limitations, to the best of our knowledge, this is the first epidemiologic study to present results regarding the effects of lead exposure on periodontal health in children in Korea.

Conclusions

In conclusion, our findings indicate a relationship between BLL and oral health problems in children, especially gingivitis. Because of the adverse effects on oral health, attention must be paid even in cases with a low BLL and strategies devised to lower lead levels in children.

Abbreviations

ANOVA: Analysis of variance; BLL: Blood lead level; CHEER: Children's Health and Environment Research; CPI: Community periodontal index; DMFT: Decayed, missing, and filled surfaces of permanent teeth; GI: Gingival index; OR: Odds ratios; PI: Plaque index; WHO: World Health Organization

Acknowledgments

The authors thank Heesun Yang whose institution is department of Public Health, Graduate School of Dankook University for statistical analysis of linearity test. The authors also wish to thank the subjects and their parents for their kind cooperation.

Funding

This research was supported by Grants-in-Aid for Children's Health and Environment Research from the Ministry of Environment of Korea. This research was supported by Basic Science Research Program through the National Research Foundation of Korea funded by the Ministry of Education (NRF-2016R1D1A3B03934825).

Authors' contributions

Authors YHC and MH contributed to the design of the study, data interpretation, and manuscript revisions. KBS and YEL gathered the data. YSJ and EKK did statistical analysis. BT drafted the manuscript. All authors read and approved the final manuscript.

Competing interests

The authors declare that they have no competing interests.

Author details

[1]Department of Preventive Dentistry, School of Dentistry, Kyungpook National University, 2177 Dalgubeol-daero, Jung-gu, Daegu 700-412, Republic of Korea. [2]Department of Dental Hygiene, College of Science and Technology, Kyungpook National University, 386 Gajangdong, Sangju 742-711, Republic of Korea. [3]Department of Preventive Medicine, Dankook University College of Medicine, 119, Dandae-ro, Dongnam-gu, Cheonan-si, Chungnam 330-714, Republic of Korea. [4]Department of Dental Hygiene, Daegu Health College, 15 Youngsong-Ro, Buk-Gu, Daegu 702-722, Republic of Korea.

References

1. Rom WN, Markowitz SB. Environmental and occupational medicine. 4th ed. Philadelphia: Wolters Kluwer/Lippincott Williams & Wilkins; 2007.
2. Milne GWA. Gardner's commercially important chemicals: synonyms, trade names, and properties. New Jersey: Wiley; 2005.
3. Meyer PA, Brown MJ, Falk H. Global approach to reducing lead exposure and poisoning. Mutat Res. 2008;659:166–75.
4. Craft-Rosenberg M, Pehler SR. Encyclopedia of family health. Los Angeles: SAGE Publications; 2011.
5. Koller K, Brown T, Spurgeon A, Levy L. Recent developments in low-level lead exposure and intellectual impairment in children. Environ Health Perspect. 2004;112:987–94.
6. Ekvall S, Ekvall VK. Pediatric nutrition in chronic diseases and developmental disorders: prevention, assessment, and treatment. USA: Oxford University Press; 2005.
7. Bowen WH. Exposure to metal ions and susceptibility to dental caries. J Dent Educ. 2001;65:1046–53.
8. Moss ME, Lanphear BP, Auinger P. Association of dental caries and blood lead levels. JAMA. 1999;281:2294–8.
9. Weiss B, Anderson D, Marrs T. Aging and vulnerability to environmental chemicals: age-related disorders and their origins in environmental exposures. Royal Soc Chem. 2012;
10. Whitney E, Rolfes SR. Understanding nutrition. Boston: Cengage Learning; 2007.
11. Gerlach RF, Cury JA, Krug FJ, Line SR. Effect of lead on dental enamel formation. Toxicol. 2002;175:27–34.
12. Leite GA, Sawan RM, Teofilo JM, Porto IM, Sousa FB, Gerlach RF. Exposure to lead exacerbates dental fluorosis. Arch Oral Biol. 2011;56:695–702.
13. Dye BA, Hirsch R, Brody DJ. The relationship between blood lead levels and periodontal bone loss in the United States, 1988-1994. Environ Health Perspect. 2002;110:997–1002.
14. Arora M, Weuve J, Weisskopf MG, Sparrow D, Nie H, Garcia RI, Hu H. Cumulative lead exposure and tooth loss in men: the normative aging study. Environ Health Perspect. 2009;117:1531–4.

15. Saraiva MC, Taichman RS, Braun T, Nriagu J, Eklund SA, Burt BA. Lead exposure and periodontitis in US adults. J Periodontal Res. 2007;42:45–52.

16. Youravong N, Teanpaisan R. The periodontal health of lead-exposed children living in a shipyard industrial area. Toxicol Ind Health. 2015;31:459–66.

17. American Academy of Pediatrics Committee on Environmental Health. Lead exposure in children: prevention, detection, and management. Pediatr. 2005;116(4):1036.

18. Campbell JR, Moss ME, Raubertas RF. The association between caries and childhood lead exposure. Environ Health Perspect. 2000;108:1099.

19. Gemmel A, Tavares M, Alperin S, Soncini J, Daniel D, Dunn J, et al. Blood lead level and dental caries in school-age children. Environ Health Perspect. 2002;110:A625.

20. Ha M, Kwon HJ, Leem JH, Kim HC, Lee KJ, Park I, Lim YW, Lee JH, Kim Y, Seo JH, Hong SJ, Choi YH, Yu J, Kim J, Yu SD, Lee BE. Korean environmental health survey in children and adolescents (KorEHS-C): survey design and pilot study results on selected exposure biomarkers. Int J Hyg Environ Health. 2014;217:260–70.

21. World Health Organization. Oral health surveys: basic methods. 4th ed. Geneva: World Health Organization; 1997.

22. Larmas M. Has dental caries prevalence some connection with caries index values in adults. Caries Res. 2010;44:81–4.

23. Löe H. The gingival index, the plaque index and the retention index systems. J Periodontol. 1967;38(Suppl):610–6.

24. Mueller HP. Periodontology: the essentials. Stuttgart: Thieme; 2011.

25. Li MM, Cao J, Xu J, Cai SZ, Shen XM, Yan CH. The national trend of blood lead levels among Chinese children aged 0-18 years old, 1990-2012. Environ Int. 2014;71:109–17.

26. El-Said KF, El-Ghamry AM, Mahdy NH, El-Bestaw NA. Chronic occupational exposure to lead and its impact on oral health. J Egypt Public Health Assoc. 2008;83:451–66.

27. Hsu PC, Liu MY, Hsu CC, Chen LY, Guo YL. Lead exposure causes generation of reactive oxygen species and functional impairment in rat sperm. Toxicol. 1997;122:133–43.

28. Lee DH, Lim JS, Song K, Boo JDR Jr. Graded associations of blood lead and urinary cadmium concentrations with oxidative-stress-related markers in the U.S. population: results from the third National Health and nutrition examination survey. Environ Health Perspect. 2006;114:350–4.

29. Yetkin-Ay Z, Cadir B, Uskun E, Bozkurt FY, Delibas N, Gultepe FM, et al. The periodontal status of indirectly lead-exposed apprentices working in autorepair workshops. Toxicol Ind Health. 2007;23:599–606.

30. Chakraborty S, Tewari S, Sharma RK, Narula SC, Ghalaut PS, Ghalaut V. Impact of iron deficiency anemia on chronic periodontitis and superoxide dismutase activity: a cross-sectional study. J Periodontal Implant Sci. 2014;44:57–64.

31. Watson GE, Davis BA, Raubertas RF, Pearson SK, Bowen WH. Influence of maternal lead ingestion on caries in rat pups. Nat Med. 1997;3:1024–5.

32. Pounds JG. Effect of lead intoxication on calcium homeostasis and calcium-medicated cell function. Neurotoxicology. 1984;5:295–332.

33. Simons TJB. Lead-calcium interactions in cellular lead toxicity. Neurotoxicology. 1993;14:77–86.

34. Craan A, Nadon G, P'an AYS. Lead flux through kidney and salivary glands of rats. Am J Phys. 1984;247:F773–83.

17

Agony resulting from cultural practices of canine bud extraction among children under five years in selected slums of Makindye

Fiona Atim[1,2]* ⓘ, Teddy Nagaddya[1], Florence Nakaggwa[1], Mary Gorrethy N-Mboowa[1], Peter Kirabira[1] and John Charles Okiria[1]

Abstract

Background: Canine Bud Extraction (CBE) is a process of removing or gouging children's healthy canine tooth buds embedded underneath the gum using traditional unsterilized tools. The practice of CBE commonly known as false teeth removal continues to be an adopted cultural intervention of choice, in the prevention of morbidity and mortality from common childhood illnesses. However, it is a practice against the rights of the children with serious consequences. While CBE is associated with the perceived myth of curative gains, the agony emanating from the cultural practice exposes children to ill-health conditions such as dehydration, malnutrition, blood-borne diseases like HIV/AIDs, septicemia, fever and death. This research sought to understand the factors underpinning the practice of CBE among urban slum dwellers.

Method: A cross-sectional study was conducted from five randomly selected slums in Makindye division; 298 household heads or guardians with children below 5 years, who had ever suffered from false teeth were interviewed. The variables measured included guardians' socio-demographic profiles, determinants of CBE, common childhood illnesses assumed to be treated with CBE and the reported side-effects associated with the practice.

Results: Of the 298 respondents with children who had ever suffered from "false teeth" interviewed, 56.7% had two or more children below 5 years and 31.9% were from the central region. The proportion of households practicing CBE was 90.3%; 69.8% of the caretakers mentioned that it was done by traditional healers and for 12.1% by trained health workers (dentists). Number of children (OR = 2.8, 95% CI: 1.1–7.2) and the belief that CBE is bad (OR = 0.1, 95% CI: < 0.001, $p < 0.001$) had a statistically significant association with CBE. Additionally, number of children ($\chi2 = 4.9$, $p = 0.027$) and 2 sets of beliefs (CBE treats diarrhea ($\chi2 = 12.8$, $p = 0.0017$) and CBE treats fever ($\chi2 = 15.1$, $p = 0.0005$) were independent predictors of CBE practice. A total of 55.7% respondents knew that there were side effects to CBE and 31% mentioned death as one of them.

Conclusion: The high proportion of households practicing CBE from this study ought to awaken the perception that the practice is ancient. CBE in this community as the study suggests was strongly driven by myths. The strong belief that CBE is bad provides an opportunity for concerted effort by primary health care providers, policy makers and the community to demystify the myths associated with false teeth and the gains of CBE.

Keywords: Canine bud extraction, Cultural practices, Children slums

* Correspondence: atimfio@gmail.com; fatim@ciu.ac.ug
[1]Clarke International University (CIU) formerly International Health Sciences University (IHSU), Plot 4686, St. Barnabas Road Kisugu-Namuwongo, P.O Box 7782, Kampala, Uganda
[2]St. Lawrence University, Kampala, Uganda

Background

Canine Bud Extraction is a process of removing or gouging children's healthy canine tooth buds embedded underneath the gum using traditional unsterilized tools. Many terms or names are used to mean Canine Bud Extraction which include; Infant Oral Mutilation (IOM), germectomy, Tooth Bud Extraction (TBE), and Deciduous Canine Tooth Bud Extraction (DCBE) [1]. Canines are also called eye teeth or cuspids used to ripe and tear tough foods and create bifurcation between the front teeth and back teeth [2] ill health conditions associated with CBE constitute greater than (75%) causes of under-five mortality in Sub-Saharan Africa with Uganda taking the lead. However, it is a practice against the rights of the children leading to serious health consequences [3] . The practice of CBE is known to have emanated from Northern Uganda [4] as the remedy for "false teeth". The concept of false teeth is believed to be brought about by traditional healers who in their attempts to find the causes of diarrheal diseases and fevers in children found that un-erupted canines together with tooth buds was an abnormal occurrence and were identifies as the causes of diarrhea, vomiting and fever in children, and that extracting them would relieve the children from those diseases [5]. Literature available indicates that CBE was rampant in the 1980's and 1990's [1, 6–8]. However, current literature shows that the practice is now common among African migrants to western countries [1, 5].

History of canine bud extraction

The practice of CBE is a superstitious belief whose origin is unknown. CBE is evident in most of the African and Sub-Saharan African countries with the first cases being recorded as early as 1932 among the Nilotic tribes [1] Some of the countries known to practice CBE include; Chad, Kenya, Somalia, Tanzania, Rwanda, Sudan, Congo, Uganda and the United Kingdom because of immigration [4–7, 9–11] other western countries where CBE was reported include; Sweden, Norway, France, New Zealand and Australia.

A survey conducted in 2013 among offspring of Ethiopian immigrants indicated that the prevalence of missing canines and poor dentition (poor teeth formation) is higher among emigrants from Ethiopia than those from Israel living in the same low socio-economic status [12].

Reports received in 2009 from DR. Congo former Zaire showed that CBE was common among people from Aru and Kivu areas and this practice was introduced from Uganda during Idi Amin's regime when Ugandan refugees entered Congo; the same experience was seen in Burundi and Rwanda [6]. A report in 2013 [12] indicates that the prevalence of CBE varied in African countries with Sudan having 22%, Tanzania 37.4%, and Uganda 17.2% among other African countries.

Studies conducted in Uganda show high prevalence of CBE. A study by Tirwomwe [13] in six districts of Uganda (Kabale, Mbale, Kampala, Arua, Gulu and Masindi) indicates an overall prevalence of 29.3%. However, findings of another study indicate that the prevalence of CBE was high in Northern Uganda with 55.1% in Gulu and 41.0% in Arua; in Masindi, the prevalence was at 36.1%, Kabale 21.8% and Mbale 22.5% [1, 5, 14]. Furthermore, a study carried out in Western Uganda [13] among children under 5 years, indicated that false teeth cause diarrhea, acute respiratory infection, fever and loss of appetite. Other key signs and symptoms of the same were believed to be treated with dental surgery which is done by traditional healers. It also suggested that conditions associated with false teeth which leads to CBE constitutes greater than (75%) causes of under-five mortality in the country and other Sub- Saharan African and East African countries; the practice is also associated with the fact that most health seeking behavior for the condition is directed to local traditional healers present in the local communities.

Study site context

The study was conducted in the slum areas of Makindye Division because most of the studies conducted on CBE have mainly been in hospitals, villages, Peri-urban settings and urban areas. The slum areas were also selected by the fact that they harbor the urban poor from different regions from Uganda and constitute different nationalities.

Methods

A cross sectional study design was used where 298 respondents consented before being interviewed; both qualitative and quantitative methods of data collection were used to obtain information regarding the above stated study. A researcher/interviewer administered questionnaire was used and translation to the local language made to accommodate those who were not able to communicate in English. The study was done in households with children under the age of 5 years who had ever suffered from "false teeth" living in the five randomly selected slums within (Namwongo Zone A, Kisugu central Zone, Kibuli Kisaga, Kikubamutwe, Wabigalo project Zone) known to be characterized by slums in Makindye Division, Kampala. These are characterized by urban neighborhoods of the lowest socio-economic level populated by migrants in to the city within informal settlements. The decision about CBE is not necessarily made by parents, but rather caretakers of children under the age of 5 years.

The researcher used stratified sampling technique using probability proportionate to population size to determine the number of households to be included in the study. Probability proportionate to sample size reduces on the chances of selecting more members from a larger group as opposed to a smaller group. This was used since the selected slums did not have equal number of households and household heads.

The study area was first stratified by village, eligible population in each slum by village determined, and the number of household. Proportionate number of household was determined, and simple random sampling used to select the households to be included in the study. For each household visited, a household head/caregiver found with a child below 5 years was included in the study and where there was no eligible participant, the next household found with the eligible participant was considered. The households had to have children below 5 years because the practice of CBE is common among children below the age of 5 years.

Prior to data collection, clearance to collect data was sought from the University Research Scientific Committee of International Health Sciences University and the respective heads of the selected villages. Informed consent was also sought from the study participants where participation was voluntary and the choice to withdraw from the study at any point in time observed. Data collected was cleaned on a daily basis to promote good quality data.

Participants' demographic characteristics (Table 1)

A total of 298 study participants were enrolled for the study with Namuwongo 102 (34.2%) contributing the highest number of respondents and Wabigalo 28(9.4%) the least. Most of the study participants were female 262 (87.9%), aged 26–31 years 115(38.6%), had primary level education 108(36.2%), were catholic 118(39.6%) and married 22(76.2%); 188(63.1%) were employed and 169(56.7%) had two or more children below 5 years old. The highest proportion of the respondents was from the central region 95 (31.9%).

Relationship between canine bud extraction and socioeconomic factors

From Table 1, the odds of CBE were lower among females compared to male respondents (OR:0.5, 95% CI:0.1–2.3), primary (OR:0.4, 95% CI:0.1–1.7), secondary (OR:0.3, 95% CI:0.1–1.6) and tertiary (OR:0.2, 95% CI:0.0–1.2) education levels compared to no education, all listed religions compared to catholic religion, and in central (OR:0.7, 95% CI:0.3–2.0) compared to western tribes. The odds of CBE were higher in all age groups compared to 14–19 years old (almost 3 times higher in age groups 32–38 years (OR:2.8, 95% CI:0.3–28.8) and 39 years or older (OR:2.7, 95% CI:0.2–30.8)), married and those separated, widowed or divorced compared to single respondents, 20% higher among those employed (OR:1.2, 95% CI:0.6–2.7) compared

to unemployed respondents, 2.3 times higher among respondents who had 2 or more children below 5 years compared to those who only had 1 child (OR:2.3, 95% CI:1.1–5.1) and 4 times higher among respondents of northern tribes compared to Western tribes (OR: 4.1 95% CI: 0.8–20.8); All foreign tribes had practiced CBE. Only number of children below 5 years was significantly associated with CBE (p-value = 0.036).

Proportion of households that practiced CBE

Up to 269 (90.3%) of the respondents with children who had ever suffered from "false teeth" reported subjecting their children to canine bud extraction (CBE); only 29 (9.7%) respondents reported not subjecting their children to canine bud extraction. Participants were further asked where they sought the canine bud extraction services and a majority (69.8%) mentioned that they had gone to traditional healers; 12.1% of the study participants had their children's canine buds extracted by a health worker. The children had their teeth extracted at 3 years (48%), 2 years (33.2%), 4 years (12.4%), 1 year (6%) and 5 years (0.3%).

With regards to instruments used during CBE, 82 (27.5%) reported that bicycle spokes were used, 71 (23.8%) said that surgical/razor blades were used, 54 (18.1%) mentioned nails, and 33 (11.1%) mentioned knives; 19.5% did not know what had been used during the CBE process, 56.9% of these had gone to traditional healers.

Those who reported not performing canine bud extraction were asked what they had done about the false teeth; 24 (82.8%) of them said that the children's teeth had been scrubbed while 5 (17.2%) had sought medical attention. Among the things used for scrubbing were herbal medicines (used by 21 respondents), honey and garlic (used by 3 respondents).

Knowledge

All research participants reported having ever heard about CBE. The sources of information mentioned by the study participants on the CBE practice included 22 (7.4%) from traditional healers, 10 (3.4%) from health workers, 24 (8.1% from spouses, 50 (16.8%) from friends 71 (23.8%) from neighbors and 121 (40.6%) from other relatives (see Table 2 for more details).

More than half of the research participants (55.7%) reported knowing the side effects of canine bud extraction whereas 44.3% said they did not know of any side effects of CBE; of those who reported side effects, 17 (10.4%) mentioned included death, 51 (31.3%) poor dentition (which meant funny shaped teeth and overcrowding of teeth in the mouth by the participants), 26 (16%) failure to develop canine teeth, 34 (20.9%) exposure to infections, 16 (9.8%) severe pain and 19 (11.7%) over bleeding. Respondents were asked to verify several statements

Table 1 Study Participants' characteristics

Characteristic	Frequency ($N = 298$)	Percentage	Unadjusted OR (95% CI)	P-value
Zone				
Namuwongo	102	34.2	1	
Kisugu central	88	29.5	0.4 (0.2–1.1)	0.089
KibuliKisaga	48	16.1	2.0 (0.4–9.6)	0.407
Kikubamutwe	32	10.7	1.3 (0.3–6.3)	0.765
Wabigalo	28	9.4	0.7 (0.2–2.9)	0.630
Sex				
Male	36	12.1	1	
Female	262	87.9	0.5 (0.1–2.3)	0.376
Age				
14–19	6	2.0	1	
20–25	59	19.8	1.3 (0.1–12.4)	0.834
26–31	115	38.6	1.7 (0.2–15.9)	0.635
32–38	75	25.2	2.8 (0.3–28.8)	0.387
39+	43	14.4	2.7 (0.2–30.8)	0.432
Education level				
None	52	17.5	1	
Primary	108	36.2	0.4 (0.1–1.7)	0.186
Secondary	106	35.6	0.3 (0.1–1.6)	0.178
Tertiary	32	10.7	0.2 (0.0–1.2)	0.078
Religion				
Catholic	118	39.6	1	
Protestant	90	30.2	0.5 (0.2–1.4)	0.183
Muslim	58	19.5	0.5 (0.2–1.4)	0.165
Other	32	10.7	0.3 (0.1–1.2)	0.084
Marital status				
Single	36	12.1	1	
Married	227	76.2	1.1 (0.3–3.2)	0.922
Sep/div/wid[1]	35	11.7	4.3 (0.5–40.1)	0.207
Employment				
Unemployed	110	36.9	1	
Employed	188	63.1	1.2 (0.6–2.7)	0.600
Tribe				
Western	57	19.1	1	
Northern	61	20.5	4.1 (0.8–20.8)	0.081
Central	95	31.9	0.7 (0.3–2.0)	0.553
Eastern	64	21.5	1.7 (0.5–5.5)	0.415
Other	21	7.1	–	–
No of children				
One	129	43.3	1	
Two or more	169	56.7	2.3 (1.1–5.1)	0.036[a]

[a]Statistically significant at $p = 0.05$, 1 *sep/div/wid* separated/widow/divorced

Table 2 Multivariate analysis of relationship between CBE and knowledge and perception factors using stepwise selection

Characteristic	Total $N = 298$	%	Unadjusted OR (95% CI)	P-value	Adjusted OR (CI)[b]	P-value
CBE Information source						
Friend	50	16.8	1			
Neighbor	71	23.8	1.3 (0.4–3.8)	0.654		
Health worker	10	3.4	1.5 (0.2–13.4)	0.735		
Traditional healer	22	7.4	1.6 (0.3–8.5)	0.565		
Spouse	24	8.1	1.1 (0.3–4.9)	0.860		
Relative	121	40.6	2.3 (0.9–6.7)	0.128		
Know side effects						
No	136	45.6	1			
Yes	162	54.4	0.4 (0.2–1.0)	0.062		
CBE leads to poor dentition						
Disagree	45	15.1	1			
Agree	170	57.1	0.6 (0.2–2.3)	0.497		
Don't know	83	27.8	0.6 (0.2–2.3)	0.443		
CBE treats fever						
Disagree	11	3.7	1			
Agree	275	92.3	17.1 (4.7–61.6)	< 0.001[a]		
Don't know	12	4.0	1.7 (0.3–8.8)	0.538		
CBE treats diarrhea						
Disagree	11	3.7	1		1	
Agree	281	94.3	7.5 (2.0–27.6)	0.003[a]	1.2 (0.1–19.6)	0.875
Don't know	6	2.0	0.1 (0.0–1.4)	0.086	0.02 (0.0–1.0)	0.051
CBE treats malaria						
Disagree	15	5.0	1	1	1	
Agree	186	62.4	4.8 (1.4–17.3)	0.015[a]	2.8 (0.2–44.5)	0.461
Don't know	97	32.6	2.6 (0.7–9.4)	0.152	2.7 (0.2–48.3)	0.497
CBE treats cough						
Disagree	49	16.4	1		1	
Agree	111	37.3	2.4 (0.7–8.7)	0.181	1.3 (0.3–6.5)	0.766
Don't know	138	46.3	0.7 (0.3–2.0)	0.523	0.5 (0.1–2.1)	0.347
CBE treats vomiting						
Disagree	14	4.7	1		1	
Agree	195	65.4	3.8 (0.9–15.4)	0.060	3.7 (0.5–27.1)	0.192
Don't know	89	29.9	1.6 (0.4–6.5)	0.515	2.6 (0.4–18.4)	0.325
Consider CBE bad						
No	181	60.7	1		1	
Yes	117	39.3	0.1 (0.1–0.4)	< 0.001[a]	0.1 (0.0–0.4)	< 0.001[a]
No of children						
One	129	43.3	1		1	
Two or more	169	56.7	2.3 (1.1–5.1)	0.036[a]	2.8 (1.1–7.2)	0.038[a]

[a]Statistically significant at $p = 0.05$, [b]Adjusted for diarrhea treats CBE, malaria treats CBE, vomiting treats CBE, consider CBE bad and number of children

regarding CBE; 94.3, 92.3, 65.4, 62.4 and 37.3% agreed with the statements "CBE treats diarrhea", "CBE treats fever", "CBE treats vomiting", "CBE treats malaria" and "CBE treats cough" respectively; 57.15% agreed with the statement "CBE leads to poor dentition" (see Table 2 for more details).

Concerning knowledge about the place where CBE is done, 69.8% mentioned traditional healers, 15.1% community elders, 12.1% health workers and 0.3% had the practice done by themselves (self).

Cultural beliefs

In all, 178 (59.7%) respondents reported that they had cultural beliefs related to false teeth while 120 (40.3%) said that they did not have such beliefs. Of those who reported the existence of cultural beliefs, 120 (66.3%) did not know the beliefs, 13 (7.3%) said that false teeth were caused by germs, 36 (20.2%) claimed that they are caused by "stepping on false teeth when pregnant", and 8 (5.1%) indicated that it was a family disease. Respondents were further asked whether the canine bud extraction practice was a taboo in their cultures; 267 (89.6%) said that it was not and only 31 (10.4%) said that it was. The reasons given for why CBE practice was a taboo were "it is a foreign cultural practice" mentioned by 10 respondents and "CBE kills" mentioned by 6 respondents and "it is associated with witchcraft" mentioned by 15 respondents.

Perception

Most of the respondents 173, (58.1%) perceived CBE to be a good practice, yet 22.1% thought that it was a bad practice, 15.1% thought that it should be banned while 4.7% believed that it was a very painful practice.

Multivariate analysis of relationship between CBE and knowledge and perception factors

From Table 2, the odds of the CBE practice were 60% lower among respondents who knew the side effects (OR:0.4, 95% CI:0.2–1.0) compared to those who did not know, 40% lower among those who believed that CBE causes poor dentition (OR:0.6, 95% CI:0.2–2.3) compared to those who disagreed with this, 90% lower among those who considered CBE a bad practice (OR:0.1, 95% CI:0.1–0.4) compared to those who did not, and 90 and 30% lower among respondents who did not know whether CBE caused diarrhea (OR:0.1 95% CI:0.0–1.4) and cough (OR:, 95% CI:0.3–2.0) respectively compared to those who disagree with the statement. Furthermore, the odds of CBE practice were higher among those who believed that CBE treats fever (OR:17.1, 95% CI:4.7–61.6), diarrhea (OR:7.5, 95% CI:2.0–27.6), malaria (OR:4.8, 95% CI:1.4–17.3), cough (OR:2.4, 95% CI:0.7–8.7) and vomiting (OR:3.8, 95% CI:0.9–15.4) compared to those who disagreed with these notions. After adjusting for the effect of diarrhea treats CBE, malaria treats CBE, vomiting treats CBE, consider CBE bad and number of children, the odds of CBE practice remained higher in these groups compared to those who disagreed. Only perception of CBE as a bad practice and a number of children remained associated with CBE.

Additionally, belief that CBE treats diarrhea (χ^2 = 12.8, p = 0.0017), number of children (χ^2 = 4.9, p = 0.027) and CBE treats fever (χ^2 = 15.1, p = 0.0005) remained independent predictors of CBE practice even after multivariate analysis.

Discussion

Majority of the study participants were female (87.9%), who were first time mothers and aged 26–31 years (38.6%) with a primary level education; the practice of CBE was high among the less educated which is different from the findings of [15] where the highly educated had practiced CBE the more. However, the former finding is in line with [16] where (36.2%), were Catholics, (39.6%) married, (76.2%); 63.1% were employed and 56.7% had two or more children below 5 years old. The highest proportion of the respondents were from the central region 95, (31.9%).

Proportion of households that practiced CBE

The proportion of households that practiced CBE was high at 269 (90.3%) which is higher than what is reflected in other sources [1]. The caregivers of the study participants were further asked where they sought the canine bud extraction services and a majority 69.8% mentioned that they had gone to traditional healers; 12.1% of the study participants had had their children's canine buds extracted by a health worker. The children had their teeth extracted at 3 years 48%, 2 years 33.2%, 4 years 12.4%, 1 year 6% and 5 years 0.3%. With regards to instruments used during CBE, 82 (27.5%) reported that bicycle spokes were used, 71 (23.8%) said that surgical/razor blades were used, 54 (18.1%) mentioned nails, and 33 (11.1%) mentioned knives; 19.5% did not know what had been used during the CBE process, 56.9% of these had gone to traditional healers.

Knowledge

The study revealed that 94.3% of the mothers know that CBE treats diarrhea [OR = 7.5 (2.0–27.6)]. These results are similar with that of a study that was conducted in Ethiopia where 68.7% of the study participants said that diarrhea was the major cause of canine tooth bud removal [17] and in a cross-sectional study in North West Ethiopia where 84.5% of mothers preferred canine tooth bud removal for the treatment of diarrhea [3]. This could be due to poor attitudes as reflected in another study in Kenya which revealed that the Maasai knew that diarrhea causing diseases were brought about by the canine tooth buds, despite having received sensitization interventions jointly run by the University of Nairobi, Kenya Medical Research Institute and the Kenya Medical Training College, among others [18]. This may be due to poor attitudes towards the practice of extraction of milk teeth.

The study revealed that 92.3% of the mothers know that CBE is the traditional treatment for fever [OR = 17.1 (4.7–61.6)]. Dr. Graham et al., [19] the study also revealed that there are strong cultural beliefs that the swelling in the area of the gums is associated with un-erupted cuspids which is the cause of persistent fever.

It should not be a surprise in the unindustrialized world to associate disease conditions that cause fever to be teething since febrile conditions are among the leading causes of morbidity and mortality, and hence subject their infants to oral mutilation techniques. In this regard, the basis for canine bud extraction would be presumed alleviation of fever among the young children [12] this was related to a study by Graham et al. [19] among household heads in western Uganda (Bushenyi district) where the cause of false teeth was mainly attributed to natural causes such as excessive or prolonged fever rather than to supernatural causes [12] .These findings suggest that canine bud extraction is still being practiced, which reflects ignorance of, and/or a negative reaction towards the nationally and globally recommended Western allopathic medicine for good oral health.

The study also revealed that 62.4% of the mothers know that CBE treats malaria [OR = 4.8 (1.4–17.3)]. Other findings suggest that education on simple hygiene will counteract some infectious conditions such as malaria, and that families with a good understanding of the causes of malaria could foresee that the relatively rough traditional practices might become less attractive [20]. Malaria being the leading cause of morbidity and mortality in Nakawa division, the children's risks to undergo these procedures are extensive and may stretch from septicemia and probable HIV transmission to potential death. There is, therefore, a need for precise strategies concerning management of suspected cases within Nakawa as a suburb of Kampala capital city.

Cultural beliefs and CBE
With the era of globalization people move from one part of the world to another, immigrants are interested in cultural socialization while teaching their children about their ethnic customs and traditions [4] considered as a way of identification. Even for those who are educated they still regard traditional beliefs when it comes to ill health. With no exception this study showed that immigrants and people who were coming from Northern Uganda neighboring South Sudan were 4 times more likely to practice CBE compared to Western tribes and all participants from foreign tribes had practiced CBE, this is in line with previous studies [2].

More than half of the respondents reported that they had cultural beliefs related to false teeth, they believed that false teeth were caused by germs, caused by "stepping on false teeth when pregnant", and that it was a

family disease. On the other hand, some respondents still believed that it was a taboo practicing CBE in their culture saying, *"it is a foreign cultural practice"...and "it is associated with witchcraft".*

However, no significant association was established between the socio-cultural factors like the cultural belief concerning the cause of "false teeth" and was rather seen to be caused by group influence since majority admitted being drawn to the practice by their neighbors. Tribe of the respondents and whether the practice was considered a taboo in the study respondents' cultures was not one of the factors associated to the practice. Furthermore, the study findings also indicate that majority of the respondents perceive CBE as a good practice hence the high proportion of households practicing CBE observed.

The custom of canine bud removal has detrimental consequences on children's general health and dental care [2] in that some children are reported never to have teeth grow in places where the canine bud was extracted. Parents of such children exposed to canine bud extraction are also emotionally traumatized especially if they did not consent to CBE, which was done on their children in the name of cultural norms by their relatives or in-laws.

Conclusion
A refined approach in communication on dental health is required by professional dentists and the Ministry of health in educating parents, guardians and caregivers, as they are key players in upholding cultural norms and traditions. There is need to sensitize health workers particularly those it the lower cadres who may be more likely to practice quackery about the consequences of conducting CBE. The child's rights should always be prioritized.

Abbreviations
CBE: Canine bud extraction; DCBE: Deciduous canine bud extraction; IHSU-REC: International Health Sciences University-Research Ethics Committee; IOM: Infant oral mutilation; TBE: Traditional bud extraction

Acknowledgements
We would like to acknowledge the International Health Sciences University Ethics Committee (IHSUREC) for the data collection approval letter, the study participants and data enumerators for the great job done.

Funding
Authors have no financial relationships related to this article.

Authors' contributions
FA conceptualized and designed the study, participated in the performance of the research, participated in data collection and data entry, drafted the initial manuscript and approved the final manuscript. TN wrote the initial manuscript and reviewed and approved the final manuscript. FN, MGM and Dr. PK designed the data collection instrument, participated in data analysis, and reviewed the final manuscript. Dr. JCO supervised and edited the final manuscript. All authors read and approved the final manuscript.

Competing interests

The authors declare that they have no competing interests.

References

1. Seligman CG, Seligman BZ. Pagan tribes of the Nilotic Sudan, vol. 132. London: George Routledge and Kegan Paul; 1965.
2. Levine, J.B. Prosthodontics. 2017 [cited 28th Mar 2018]; Available from: https://www.sharecare.com/doctor/dr-jonathan-levine.
3. Teshome A, Andualem G, Seifu S, Tsegie R. Knowledge, Attitude and Practice of Mothers towards Canine Tooth Bud Removal and Associated Factors among Mothers Visiting Dental Clinic of Gondar University Hospital, Ethiopia. J Community Med Health. 2016;6:396.
4. Iriso R, Accorsi S, Amone J, Fabiani M, Ferrarese N, Lukwiya M, Rosolen T, Declih S. 'Killer' canines: the morbidity and mortality of ebino in northern Uganda. Trop Med Int Health. 2000;5(10):706–10.
5. Girgis S, Gollings J, Longhurst R, Cheng L. Infant oral mutilation – a child protection issue? Br Dent J. 2016;220:357–60.
6. Matee MI, van Palenstein Helderman WH. Extraction of 'Nylon' teeth and associated abnormalities in Tanzanian Children. Afr Dent J. 1991;5:21–5.
7. Hassanali J, Amwayi P, Muriithi A. Removal of deciduous canine tooth buds in Kenyan rural Maasai. East Afr Med J. 1995;72(4):207–9.
8. Mutai J, Muniu E, Sawe J, Hassanali J, Kibet P, Wanzala P. Socio-cultural practices of deciduous canine tooth bud removal among Maasai children. Int Dent J. 2010;60(2):94–8.
9. Abusinna IM. Lugbara teeth germectomy of canines for the newborn babies. A magico-religious phenomena in some African tribes. Egypt Dent J. 1979;25(3):209–14.
10. MMA W. Traditional practices as a cause of infant morbidity and mortality in Juba area (Sudan). Ann Trop Pediatr. 1987;7:18–21.
11. Benzian H. World Dental Development Fund: Rwanda Project. Rwanda: Developing Dentistry; National survey on oral health; 2003.
12. Davidovich E, Kooby E, Shapira J, Ram D. The traditional practice of canine bud removal in the offspring of Ethiopian immigrants. BMC Oral Health. 2013;13(34):1472–6831.
13. Tirwomwe JF, Agwu E, Ssamula M. The Magnitude of tooth bud extraction in Uganda. Int J Med Med Sci. 2013;5(10):450–5.
14. Holand G, Mamber E. Extraction of canine tooth buds: prevalence and associated dental abnormalities in a group of Ethiopian Jewish Children. Int J Paediatr Dent. 1994;4(1):25–30.
15. Sebudde S. False teeth still a public health problem among children in Kanungu district - South Western Uganda Academic Journals, 2006. Educ Res Rev. 2006;1(5):156–61.
16. Kahabuka FK, Mugonzibwa EA, Mwalutambi S, Kikwilu EN. Diseases and conditions falsely linked with "Nylon teeth" myth: a cross section study of Tanzania adults. Tanzan J Health Res. 2015;1:1–10.
17. Barzangi J, Unell L, Soderfeldt B, Bond J, Musse I, Arnup K. Infant dental enucleation: a literature review on a traditional remedial practice in East Africa. Acta Odontol Scand. 2014;72(3):168–78.
18. Dagnew MB, Damena M. Traditional child health practices in communities in north-west Ethiopia. Trop Dr. 1990;20:40–1.
19. Graham EA, Domoto PK, Lynch H, Egbert MA. Dental injuries due to African traditional therapies for diarrhoea. West J Med. 2000;173:135–7.
20. Nuwaha F, Okware J, Hanningtone T, Mwebaze C. False teeth 'ebiino' and millet disease 'oburo' in Bushenyi district in Uganda. Afr Health Sci. 2007;7:25–32.

The dental perspective on osteogenesis imperfecta in a Danish adult population

Kirstine Juhl Thuesen[1], Hans Gjørup[2], Jannie Dahl Hald[3], Malene Schmidt[4], Torben Harsløf[3], Bente Langdahl[3] and Dorte Haubek[1*] ⓘ

Abstract

Background: To report on dental characteristics and treatment load in Danish adult patients with osteogenesis imperfecta (OI).

Methods: Oral examination of 73 patients with OI was performed and OI type I, III, and IV were represented by 75.3%, 8.2%, and 16.4%, respectively. Patients were diagnosed as having dentinogenesis imperfecta (DI) if they had clinical and radiological signs of DI. In the data analysis, mild OI (type I) was compared to moderate-severe OI (type III and IV).

Results: Discoloration of teeth was prevalent in patients with moderate-severe compared to mild OI (83.3% vs. 5.5%, $p < 0.001$). Cervical constriction and pulpal obliteration were frequent findings in patients with moderate-severe OI (61.1% and 88.9%, respectively), whereas pulp stones and taurodontism were diagnosed in patients with mild OI only (29.1% and 9.1%, respectively). DI was found in 24.7% of OI patients and considerably more frequent in patients with moderate-severe (94.4%) compared to mild OI (1.8%) ($p < 0.001$). The number of teeth with artificial crowns was significantly higher in patients with moderate-severe OI than in patients with mild OI (median 1.5, range 0–23 vs. median 0, range 0–14) ($p < 0.001$). The number of teeth with fillings in patients with mild OI was significantly higher than in patients with moderate-severe OI (mean 9.7, SD 5.1, median 9.0, range 1–21 vs. mean 5.0, SD 4.4, median 4.0, range 0–16) ($p < 0.001$).

Conclusions: One fourth of patients with OI had DI, and the vast majority of them had moderate-severe OI. Whereas discoloration of teeth, cervical constriction and pulp obliteration were frequent findings in patients with moderate-severe OI, pulp stones and taurodontism were found in patients with mild OI only. In patients with moderate-severe OI, the dental treatment load was dominated by prosthetic treatment, whereas restorative treatment with fillings was more prevalent in patients with mild OI.

Keywords: Collagen, Dentinogenesis imperfecta, Dental treatment load, Radiographic findings

Background

Osteogenesis imperfecta (OI) is a rare hereditary connective tissue disorder with different degrees of severity. The prevalence of OI in Denmark is estimated to 11 per 100.000 [1]. According to Sillence [2], type I is classified as a phenotype with low degree of deformity and near to normal stature, type II is the most severe form with perinatal death, type III is the most severe type with high degree of deformity and a very short stature, and type IV is the moderately affected phenotype with a severity between OI type I and III. The majority of OI cases are caused by autosomal dominant mutations in one of the two genes, COL1A1 and COL1A2 [3–5] that encode the α1(I) and the α2(I) chains of collagen type I, which is an important component in bone and dentine. Collagen mutations can lead to either quantitative or qualitative collagen abnormality, i.e., a reduced amount of structurally normal collagen respective the formation of an abnormally structured collagen [6].

In addition to OI, some patients have dentinogenesis imperfecta (DI) which is a hereditary dentine disorder characterized by greyish-blue to brown discoloration of

* Correspondence: dorte.haubek@dent.au.dk
[1]Section for Pediatric Dentistry, Department of Dentistry and Oral Health, Health, Aarhus University, Vennelyst Boulevard 9, 8000 Aarhus C, Denmark
Full list of author information is available at the end of the article

teeth and pulp obliteration [7]. DI is currently subdivided into three subtypes. DI type I is associated with OI and is caused by mutations in the genes, *COL1A1* and *COL1A2* encoding collagen type I. DI type II and III are caused by mutations in the gene encoding dentine sialophosphoprotein (*DSPP*) [7], and not found in OI patients. In DI, the enamel appears normal in structure, but is vulnerable due to the underlying abnormal dentine. Structurally, dentine is composed of hydroxyapatite, an organic phase composed primarily of type I collagen and water. Due to mutations in the genes encoding collagen type I, defects in the dentine occur [8]. In patients with DI type I, both dentitions are typically affected, but the primary dentition is usually more severely affected than the permanent dentition [9].

The aim of the present study was to report on dental characteristics and treatment load in adult Danish patients with OI.

Methods
Study population
The present study is based on a dental investigation of 73 patients with genetically-verified OI, recruited in a cross-sectional clinical study originally based on 85 Danish adult patients with OI [10]. With the overall aim to investigate medical aspects of OI in adult patients, the inclusion criteria were clinically confirmed diagnosis of OI and an age ≥ 18 years. Exclusion criteria were comorbidity of cancer, treatment with glucocorticoids equivalent to 5 mg prednisolone or more within the last 3 months, other metabolic bone diseases, renal diseases, or hepatic diseases. The final diagnosis of OI was based on consensus between three investigators (JDH, TH, and BL). The classification of OI in subtypes was based on criteria by Sillence and coworkers [2]. The recruitment of patients took place from 2010 to 2013 through databases at university hospitals and regional hospitals in Denmark and by advertisements in the Journal of the Danish OI Patient Society, DFOI.

Among the 85 patients with OI included in the clinical study, two were excluded due to lack of teeth, and ten did not participate for various reasons, leaving 73 participants for the dental assessment. Among the 73 participants, 63 (86.3%) had a skin biopsy taken during the medical study or previously. Skin biopsy was not obtained in 10 patients, either because they were unwilling to undergo the procedure, due to infection in the laboratory, or the procedure was not possible for logistic reasons [11].

Clinical and radiological dental examination
A dental examination was performed at Department of Dentistry and Oral Health, Aarhus University, including the recording of the teeth present in the oral cavity and the previous dental treatment carried out. Fillings in

teeth were recorded as well as artificial crowns, bridges, and the use of removable dentures. As a part of the investigation, clinical photos were obtained. A full-mouth periapical survey with digital intraoral radiographs, using GX 1000 dental X-ray© (Gendex, Des Plaines, IL, USA) as well as a digital panoramic radiograph, using the digital radiographic equipment Planmeca Promax© (Planmeca Oy, Helsinki, Finland), were obtained.

In the evaluation of the dental hard tissues, an assessment of the radiographs included: The number of teeth present, signs of obliterated pulp chamber, presence of pulp stone, short root, cervical constriction, and the dental treatment load. The recorded findings were obtained by a consensus among three co-authors (DH, HG, and KJT) after assessing clinical recordings, radiological signs, and evaluation of clinical photos.

The clinical signs of DI are increased translucency of enamel and greyish-blue to brown discoloration of teeth. In addition, abnormal radiographic signs like large pulp chambers in teeth under development and eruption, early and advanced or total pulp obliteration of fully developed teeth, short roots, cervical constriction, pulp stones, and taurodontism have been reported [12–15].

Statistics
In the data analysis, the mild OI (type I) was compared to moderate-severe OI (type III and IV). Descriptive statistics were used to summarize all data. Differences according to the severity of OI were evaluated by students t-test or Fischer's exact test as appropriate. Data analysis was performed using STATA 11.0 (StataCorp, College Station, Texas). In the present study, p-values < 0.050 were considered statistically significant.

Results
Seventy three patients (mean age: 45.4 years (SD 14.5)) with OI underwent a clinical and radiological dental examination, meaning 85.9% of the original clinical study population. According to OI severity, 55 (75.3%) patients had mild OI (type I) and 18 (24.7%) patients had moderate-severe OI (6 OI type III and 12 OI type IV). The group of 73 patients consisted of 53.4% women and 46.6% men ($p = 0.424$). According to OI severity, the mean age of patients with mild OI was 46.2 years (SD 2.1) and 42.9 years (SD 2.4) for the patients with moderate-severe OI ($p = 0.400$).

The quantitative collagen defect was associated with DI in only one out of 38 patients, all having mild OI, and the qualitative collagen defect was associated with DI in 17 out of 18 patients, all having moderate-severe OI ($p < 0.001$) (Table 1).

The distribution of patients with OI according to OI severity and dental characteristics is presented in Table 2. Discoloration of teeth, either as greyish or brownish color,

Table 1 OI severity and the presence of DI according to collagen I abnormality

OI severity	Presence of DI	Collagen types			
		Normal	Quantitative[a]	Qualitative[b]	Unknown
Mild	÷ DI	3	37	4	10
	+ DI	0	1	0	0
Moderate-severe	÷ DI	0	0	1	0
	+ DI	0	0	17	0

[a]Deviation in the amount of collagen I in skin biopsy
[b]Deviation in the structure of collagen I in skin biopsy

was found more often in patients with moderate-severe OI than in patients with mild OI (15 out of 18 (83.3%) vs. 3 out of 55 (5.5%)) ($p < 0.001$) (Table 2, Fig. 1, d and f), and also pulp obliteration (16 out of 18 (88.9%) vs. 4 out of 55 (7.3%) ($p < 0.001$)) and short roots (9 out of 18 (50%) vs. 4 out of 55 (7.3%) ($p < 0.001$)) appeared more often in patients with moderate-severe OI than in patients with mild OI (Fig. 2, a, b and e). Cervical constriction appeared in patients with moderate-severe OI only (11 out of 18 (61.1%) patients) ($p < 0.001$) (Table 2, Fig. 2, c). In contrast, pulp stones and taurodontism were found in patients with mild OI only (16 out of 55 (29.1%) ($p = 0.008$) and 5 out of 55 (9.1%) ($p = 0.322$), respectively) (Table 2, Fig. 2, d and f).

Patients with both discoloration and radiological signs of DI were diagnosed as having DI, being a total of 18 of 73 (24.7%) patients with OI. Among these 18 patients with DI, 1 (1.4%) had mild OI and 17 (94.4%) had moderate-severe OI ($p < 0.001$) (Table 2).

The number of teeth present in the oral cavity of patients with OI varied from 5 to 32 teeth (mean: 25.8, SD 5.0). The mean number of teeth present in patients with mild OI was 26.0 (SD 5.5; range 5–32), and not significantly different from the mean number of teeth present in patients with moderate-severe OI (mean: 25.3, SD 3.9; range 16–32) ($p = 0.657$). The mean number of teeth present in the group of patients with DI was not significantly different to the mean number in the group of patients without DI (mean: 25.4 (SD 3.9) and mean: 25.9 (SD 5.4), respectively) ($p = 0.686$).

The overall dental treatment load, including fillings and artificial crowns, is illustrated in Fig. 3. The number of teeth with fillings in patients with OI varied from 0 to 21 teeth and was in patients with mild OI (mean 9.7, SD 5.1, median 9.0, range 1–21) significantly higher than in patients with moderate-severe OI (mean 5.0, SD 4.4, median 4.0, range 0–16) ($p < 0.001$). The median number of filled teeth relative to the total number of teeth present was in the mild OI group 0.38 (range 0.04–0.80) and in moderate-severe OI 0.15 (range 0–0.64) ($p = 0.001$).

Thirty-two out of 73 (43.8%) patients with OI were treated with artificial crowns with the median number of crowns being 2.0 (range 1–23). Eleven out of 18 (61.1%) patients with moderate-severe OI had teeth treated with artificial crowns compared to 21 out of 55 (38.2%) patients with mild OI ($p = 0.107$). The median number of teeth with artificial crowns in patients with moderate-severe OI was 1.5 (range 0–23) and was 0 (range 0–14) in patients with mild OI ($p < 0.001$). The median number of teeth with artificial crowns relative to the total number of teeth present in mild OI group was 0 (range 0–0.6) and in the moderate-severe OI group 0.01 (range 0–0.9) ($p = 0.001$).

In total, eight patients had removable dentures (Table 3). In the mild OI group, two patients had a complete maxillary denture and one of these also had a partial mandibular denture. In addition, five patients with mild OI and one patient with moderate-severe OI had a removable partial denture.

Table 2 Dental characteristics in 73 patients with OI

OI severity	Mild		Moderate-Severe		
	OI type I	OI type III	OI type IV	OI type III and IV	
	($n = 55$)	($n = 6$)	($n = 12$)	($n = 18$)	P*
Diagnosed with DI (%)	1 (1.8)	5 (83.3)	12 (100)	17 (94.4)	< 0.001
Discoloration of teeth (%)[a]	3 (5.5)	5 (83.3)	10 (83.3)	15 (83.3)	< 0.001
Pulp obliteration (%)	4 (7.3)	4 (66.7)	12 (100)	16 (88.9)	< 0.001
Short root (%)	4 (7.3)	4 (66.7)	5 (41.7)	9 (50)	< 0.001
Pulp stone (%)[b]	16 (29.1)	0	0	0	0.008
Cervical constriction (%)	0	6 (100)	5 (41.7)	11 (61.1)	< 0.001
Taurodontism (%)[c]	5 (9.1)	0	0	0	0.322

The figures are number of patients with the specified type of dental characteristic, and the percentages in the respective OI severity groups are given in parentheses
*P-value according to Fischer's exact test. OI type I (mild) compared to OI type III and IV (moderate-severe)
[a]Missing data in one patient with mild and three patients with moderate-severe OI
[b]Missing data in one patient with mild and one patient with moderate-severe OI
[c]Missing data in one patients with mild OI

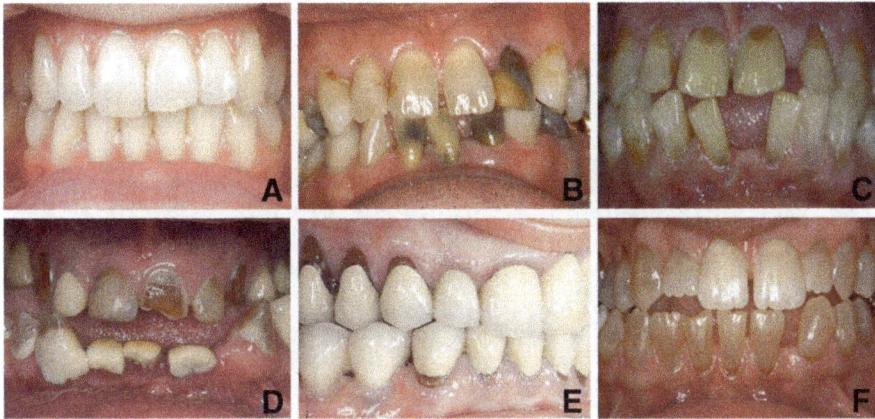

Fig. 1 The variation of the dental view of patients with OI. **a** OI type I without DI. **b** OI type I without DI, discoloration induced by endodontic therapy. **c** OI type III without DI. **d** OI type III with DI, including dental calculus accumulation. **e** OI type IV with DI, treated with artificial crowns. **f** OI type IV with DI

Discussion

The present cross-sectional study shows that DI is mainly found in the patients with qualitative collagen defects and moderate-severe OI and rarely seen in patients with quantitative defects and mild OI. Prosthetic treatment with artificial crowns and fixed partial dentures was carried out more often in the group of patients with moderate-severe OI compared to patients with mild OI. In the latter group of patients, conventional fillings and removable dentures were predominant.

A cross-sectional design was chosen in the present study. Although it has limitations, this type of study design is useful in studies on small populations, characterized by a rare disease, as it adds to the existing knowledge of the rare disease more than case reports do. The present study aimed at including a representative sample of adults with OI living in Denmark [10]. The majority of adult OI patients are routinely followed in Denmark on one of the three university hospitals in Aarhus, Odense or Hvidovre. Participants were recruited by advertisements in the Danish OI magazine, through regional hospitals, databases and Center for Rare Diseases, leading to the participation of both patients with mild and moderate-severe OI. A high participation rate of patients with mild OI was found (75.3%). In a previous Danish study by Lund and coworkers (1998), the participants were all referred patients to the Department of Clinical Genetics, Rigshospitalet, Copenhagen, Denmark, thus a

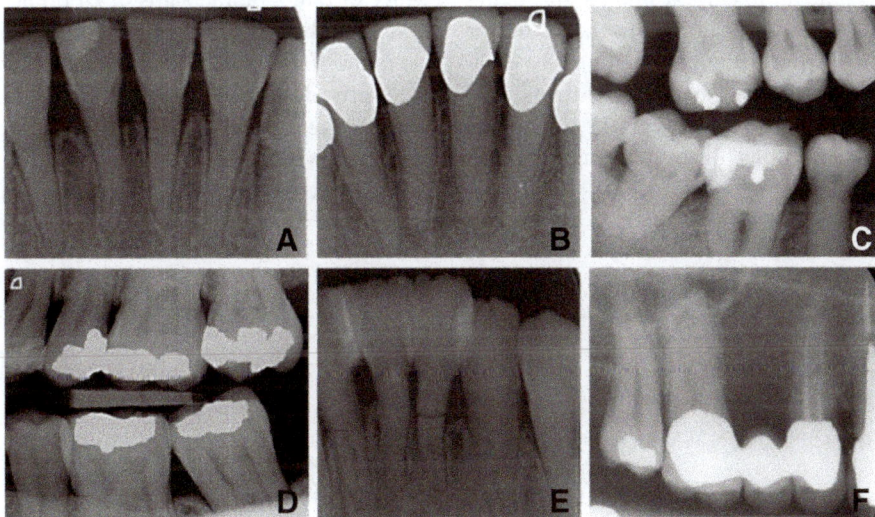

Fig. 2 The variation of radiographic signs of DI as seen on dental radiographs of patients with OI. **a** OI type IV with DI, incisor with short root and pulp obliteration. **b** OI type IV with DI, incisor with pulp obliteration and treated with artificial crowns. **c** OI type III with DI, molars and premolars with cervical constriction. **d** OI type I, pulp stones in 26, 27, 36 and 37. **e** OI type III with DI, incisor with pulp obliteration and root fractures. **f** OI type I, taurodontism

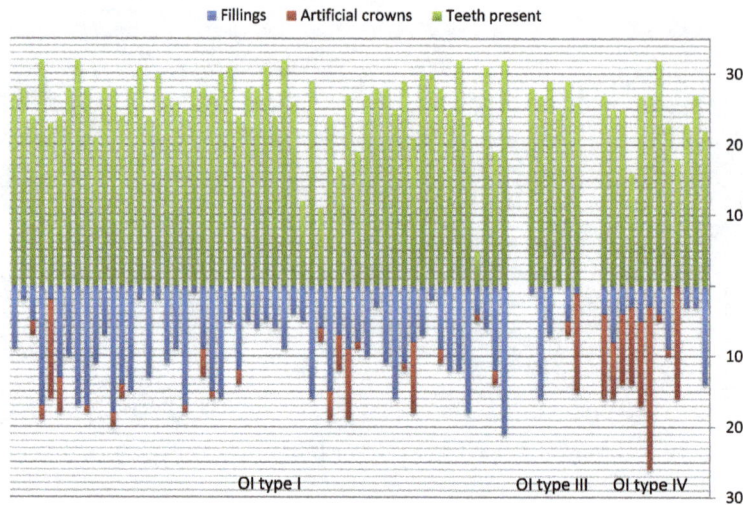

Fig. 3 Illustration of the dental treatment load in 73 patients with OI. For the individual patient, the number of teeth present and the number of teeth treated with fillings respective artificial crowns are illustrated

relative high frequency of patients with moderate-severe OI (43.2%) was included in that study [14]. The broad representation of all OI types, including a high number of patients with mild OI, is a strength of the present study. Though, concerning the representativity of the study population, some severely affected patients might having been unable to travel for the participation in the investigation, but on the other hand some mildly affected patients might having been too busy to participate in a time-consuming investigation. Thus, the study population is likely to reflect the relative distribution of OI types.

The dental characteristics of OI patients were assessed based on clinical examination, clinical photos and radiographs. Due to physical proportions, shortness of the neck and immobility, some patients with OI were challenging to examine. On the other hand, OI patients were very cooperative and willing to take part in the procedures needed to establish the diagnostic material collected in the present study.

The frequency of obliterated pulp, short roots, pulp stone, cervical constriction and taurodontism in various populations and patients groups varies when searching through the literature. No validated methods, based on specific definitions for diagnosing dental findings as obliterated pulp, pulp stones, and cervical constriction are available, except for taurodontism [16]. Thus, the overall radiographic diagnosis was based on visual assessment of the radiographs, and reached after consensus between the involved coworkers.

As both Saeves and coworkers [12] and Malmgren and coworkers [13] point out, normally colored teeth and absence of radiographic signs of DI do not necessarily indicate the absence of dentin abnormalities, which might be found if a histological examination was included. This is clearly described by Andersson and coworkers [15]. Hence, the diagnosis of DI may vary according to the parameters and tests on which the diagnosis is based. It is well-known that the number of tests, on which a

Table 3 The type of prosthetic treatment in 73 patients with OI

OI severity	Mild		Moderate-Severe		
	OI type I	OI type III	OI type IV	OI type III and IV	
	(n = 55)	(n = 6)	(n = 12)	(n = 18)	P*
Artificial crown (%)	21 (38.2)	2 (33.3)	9 (75)	11 (61.1)	0.107
Tooth-supported bridge (%)	6 (10.9)	0	3 (25)	3 (16.7)	0.680
Implant (%)	2 (3.6)	0	4 (33.3)	4 (22.2)	0.030
Implant-supported bridge (%)	1 (1.8)	0	2 (16.7)	2 (11.1)	0.435
Removable denture (%)	7 (12.7)	0	1 (8.3)	1 (5.6)	0.435

The figures are number of patients with the specified type of treatment, and the percentages in the respective OI severity groups are given in parentheses
*P-value according to Fischer's exact test. OI type I (mild) compared to OI type III and IV (moderate-severe)

diagnosis is based, is affecting the number of patients found. On the other hand, the assessment of dental agenesis on radiographs is, for example, a valid method. But in the present study population on adults, which included elderly individuals with a highly reduced number of teeth, our information on the reason(s) for the absence of teeth was sparse. Thus, dental agenesis was not assessed in the present study.

DI was diagnosed in 24.7% of the patients with OI. This corresponds roughly to the previous Danish study by Lund and coworkers [14] who reported the prevalence of DI to be 28% of the study group and a recent Swedish study by Andersson and coworkers [15], who reported the prevalence of DI to be 29% when based on a clinical and radiographic diagnostics. In a Norwegian study by Saeves and coworkers [12], the frequency of DI was 19%. The Norwegian study group consisted of 94 participants aged 25 years or older. In contrast, the appearance of DI was reported to be 42% in the Swedish study by Malmgren and coworkers [13] and raised to 48% in the above-mentioned Swedish study when histological assessment was included [15]. However, all patients in the Swedish studies were referred to a specialized diagnostic unit, thus may have included more patients with moderate-severe types of OI. The mild OI group in the two Swedish studies had a high DI prevalence (28% and 31%, respectively) compared to the present study (1.8%). Major differences in the composition of the various study populations mentioned above, and the recruitment of them, are likely to explain the differences between the results obtained. Furthermore, the patients of the Swedish studies were aged 0.3 to 20 years. In the present Danish study, the patients were adults, and consequently all had permanent dentition. Malmgren and coworkers point out that in the mixed dentition the permanent teeth were less affected than the primary teeth in terms of both discoloration and attrition [13]. Thus, the inclusion of children may explain the higher prevalence of DI in some previous studies [13–15] compared to the present and the Norwegian studies on adults only [12]. In this context, it is, however, an important point that the thickness of enamel of permanent teeth is twice that of primary teeth. Dentine dysplasia is visible through translucent enamel. Although not real, DI in the permanent dentition may 'seem milder' than in the primary dentition.

In the present study, pulp stones were found in patients with mild OI only (16 out of 55 (29.1%)) (Table 2). Contrary, pulp stones were most frequently found in patients with moderate-severe OI in the study by Lund and coworkers (moderate-severe OI: 10 out of 12 (83%); mild OI: 18 out of 30 (60%)) [14]. In the Swedish study by Malmgren and coworkers [13], pulp stones were rare (4.2%). But the presence of artificial crowns complicates the possibility of detecting pulp stones on radiographs.

As patients with moderate-severe OI often are characterized by DI and treatment with artificial crowns, this may explain the finding of no pulp stones in patients with moderate-severe OI in our study. Furthermore, the physiological obliteration of the pulp by age is 'accelerated' in patients with moderate-severe OI, and by age this phenomenon might gradually blur the possibility of diagnosing pulp stones. In addition, pulp stones are prevalent in the normal population (20.7%) [17], and this proportion is similar to the findings in patients with OI type I in the present study.

An evaluation of the dental treatment load according to OI severity showed an obvious tendency toward significantly more advanced treatment, such as fixed prosthetics, carried out in the group of moderate-severe OI patients compared to patients with mild OI, where conventional fillings and removable dentures were the predominant treatment types preformed. As the majority of patients with moderate-severe OI also had DI, it is likely that DI is the main reason for the more comprehensive use of fixed prosthetics. The health care system in Denmark gives patients with dental anomalies, like DI, the possibility to receive financial support when they are in need of dental treatment. This regulation might explain the more advanced and expensive treatments performed in patients with moderate-severe OI. In contrast, treatment with conventional fillings because of caries is only minimally supported by the health care system.

In the study by Saeves and coworkers [12], they found that the mean number of filled teeth was 13.5 in OI type I, and 11.0 in type III and IV. It is mentioned that some patients also had implants and artificial crowns carried out, but detailed information on the extent is not provided. In the present study, the mean number of filled teeth was 9.7 in OI type I, and 5.0 for type III and IV. The mean number of teeth with artificial crowns was 1.4 in OI type I, and 6.1 for type III and IV. In addition, implants were present in one third of patients with OI type III and IV in contrast to 5% in patients with type I. According to O'Connel and Marini, theoretically the binding of resin may be compromised, but clinically it appears successful [9]. Thus, composite fillings can be made also in patients with OI if enamel is present. The difference in treatment load may therefore be because of prevalent crown fractures and decay in teeth affected by DI, but might also be influenced by the previously mentioned possibility for governmental financial support when teeth are affected by DI. The relatively high number of fillings and low number of crowns in the mild OI group without DI can be explained by either less severe decay of the dentition or by patient's omission of the expensive prosthetic treatment options, which is without governmental financial support, when teeth are not affected by DI. These questions remain unanswered by the present cross-sectional study.

Conclusions

One fourth of patients with OI had DI, and the vast majority of them had moderate-severe OI. Whereas discoloration of teeth, cervical constriction and pulp obliteration were frequent findings in patients with moderate-severe OI, pulp stones, and taurodontism were found in patients with mild OI only. In patients with moderate-severe OI, the dental treatment load was dominated by prosthetic treatment including implant-based prostheses, whereas restorative treatment with fillings was more prevalent in patients with mild OI. Governmental financial support seems to facilitate the choice of prosthetic treatment in patients with DI.

Abbreviations

COL1a1: Gene encoding collagen type 1a1; *COL1a2*: Gene encoding collagen type 1a2; DI: Dentinogenesis imperfecta; *DSPP*: Gene encoding dentine sialophosphoprotein; Fig.: Fig.; OI: Osteogenesis imperfecta; p: *P*-value according to Fischer's exact test; SD: Standard deviation; vs.: Versus

Acknowledgements
We wish to thank chair-side assistant Ann Katholm at Department of Dentistry and Oral Health, Aarhus University for her help in patient management and efficient assistance during the study. The staff at Section of Oral Radiology, Department of Dentistry and Oral Health, Aarhus University is acknowledged for the collaboration during the radiographic examinations. We also thank dental hygienist, Rikke Frandsen at Department of Maxillofacial Surgery, Aarhus University Hospital for skillful clinical assistance.

Funding
This work was supported by Central Region of Denmark, Osteoporoseforeningen, Denmark, The Danish Association for Public Dentists (TNL/DOFT/ATO), Denmark and Care4BrittleBones Foundation. The role of the funding agencies was solely financial support, and the agencies were not involved in the design of the study or collection, analysis, and interpretation of data or in writing the manuscript.

Authors' contributions
JDH, TH, BL recruited the patients for a clinical-medical study on OI. DH and HG designed and established the aims of the present study. JDH, TH, BL, HG and DH wrote the research protocol. MS and HG clinically examined the study population. KJT, HG, DH contributed to the interpretation of the dental data. KJT has written the first draft of the manuscript. All authors have taken part in finalizing and have approved the submitted version of the manuscript.

Authors' information
Not applicable.

Competing interests
The authors declare that they have no competing interests.

Author details
[1]Section for Pediatric Dentistry, Department of Dentistry and Oral Health, Health, Aarhus University, Vennelyst Boulevard 9, 8000 Aarhus C, Denmark. [2]Center for Oral Health in Rare Diseases, Department of Maxillofacial Surgery, Aarhus University Hospital, Noerrebrogade 44, 8000 Aarhus C, Denmark. [3]Department of Endocrinology and Internal Medicine, Aarhus University Hospital, Tage-Hansens Gade 2, Aarhus, Denmark. [4]Aarhus Municipal Dental Service, Groendalsvej 2, 8000 Aarhus C, Denmark.

References
1. Andersen PE, Hauge M. Congenital generalised bone dysplasias: a clinical, radiological, and epidemiological survey. J Med Genet. 1989;27:37–44.
2. Sillence DO, Senn A, Danks DM. Genetic heterogeneity in osteogenesis imperfecta. J Med Genet. 1979;16:101–16.
3. Forlino A, Cabral WA, Barnes AM, Marini JC. New perspectives on osteogenesis imperfecta. Nat Rev Endocrinol. 2011;7:540–57.
4. Marini JC, Forlino A, Bächinger HP, Bishop NJ, Byers PH, Paepe AD, Fassier F, Fratzl-Zelman N, Kozleff KM, Krakow D, Montpetit K, Semler O. Osteogenesis imperfecta. Nat Rev Dis Primers. 2017;3:17052.
5. Van Dijk FS, Sillence DO. Osteogenesis imperfecta: clinical diagnosis, nomenclature and severity assessment. Am J Med Genet A. 2014;164A: 1470–81.
6. Lund AM, Müller J, Skovby F. Anthropometry of patients with osteogenesis imperfecta. Arch Dis Child. 1999;80:524–8.
7. Barron MJ, McDonnell ST, MacKie I, Dixon MJ. Hereditary dentine disorders: dentinogenesis imperfecta and dentine dysplasia. Orphanet J Rare Dis. 2008;3:31.
8. Malmgren B, Lindskog S. Assessment of dysplastic dentin in osteogenesis imperfecta and dentinogenesis imperfecta. Acta Odontol Scand. 2003;61: 72–80.
9. O'Connell AC, Marini JC. Evaluation of oral problems in an osteogenesis imperfecta population. Oral Surg Oral Med Oral Pathol. 1999;87:189–96.
10. Hald JD, Folkestad L, Harsløf T, Lund AM, Duno M, Jensen JB, Neghabat S, Brixen K, Langdahl B. Skeletal phenotypes in adult patients with osteogenesis imperfecta – correlation with *COL1A1/COL1A2* genotype and collagen structure. Osteoporos Int. 2016;27:3331–41.
11. Hald JD, Folkestad L, Swan CZ, Wanscher J, Schmidt M, Gjørup H, Haubek D, Leonard C-H, Larsen DA, Hjortdal JØ, Harsløf T, Duno M, Lund AM, Jensen J-EB, Brixen K, Langdahl B. Osteogenesis imperfecta and the teeth, eyes, and ears - a study of non-skeletal phenotypes in adults. Osteoporos Int. 2018. https://doi.org/10.1007/s00198-018-4663-x.
12. Saeves R, Wekre LL, Ambjørnsen E, Axelsson S, Nordgaarden H, Storhaug K. Oral findings in adults with osteogenesis imperfecta. Spec Care Dentist. 2009;29:102–8.
13. Malmgren B, Norgren S. Dental aberrations in children and adolescents with osteogenesis imperfecta. Acta Odontol Scand. 2002;60:65–71.
14. Lund AM, Jensen BL, Nielsen LA, Skovby F. Dental manifestations of osteogenesis imperfecta and abnormalities of collagen I metabolism. J Craniofac Genet Dev Biol. 1998;18:30–7.
15. Andersson K, Dahllöf G, Lindahl K, Kindmark A, Grigelioniene G, Åström E, Malmgren B. Mutations in *COL1A1* and *COL1A2* and dental aberrations in children and adolescents with osteogenesis imperfecta – a retrospective cohort study. PLoS One. 2017;12(5). https://doi.org/10.1371/journal.pone.0176466.
16. Ruprecht A, Batniji S, El-Neweihi E. The incidence of taurodontism in dental patients. Oral Surg Oral Med Oral Pathol. 1987;63:743–7.
17. Tamse A, Kaffe I, Littner MM, Shani R. Statistical evaluation of radiologic survey of pulp stones. J Endod. 1982;10:455–8.

Morphology of palatally displaced canines and adjacent teeth, a 3-D evaluation from cone-beam computed tomographic images

Rosalia Leonardi[1*], Simone Muraglie[1], Salvatore Crimi[2], Marco Pirroni[3], Giuseppe Musumeci[4] and Rosario Perrotta[5]

Abstract

Background: The goal of this study was to investigate in patients with unilateral palatally displaced canine (PDC) the morphology of maxillary teeth from cone-beam computed tomography (CBCT) scans both on the PDC side and non-PDC side using a "surface matching" technique.

Methods: CBCT images from 28 patients (mean age 16.04 ± 1.77 years) with unilateral PDC were selected. Each tooth in this study was segmented and then rendered into a 3D model using Mimics Research software and the root length was measured. Afterwards, 3D deviation analysis between the PDC and non-PDC side was carried out using Geomagic Control X software.

Results: Statistically significant differences ($p \leq 0.001$) were obtained when comparing the root lengths and volumes of lateral incisors from the PDC side, non-PDC side and control group. In accordance with the findings of 3D deviation analysis, statistically significant differences between the patients and control group were obtained for the lateral incisors and canines ($p \leq 0.0001$) and greater differences were found for the tooth crowns and root tips.

Conclusions: Lateral incisors adjacent to PDCs have shorter roots than contra-lateral lateral incisors. Furthermore, there were morphological differences between lateral incisors and canines in subjects with unilateral PDCs.

Keywords: Cone-beam computed tomography, Surface-to-surface matching, Digital dentistry, Palatally displaced canine, Teeth morphologhy

Background

Maxillary canine impaction occurs in the general population with a reported prevalence ranging from 0.27 to 2.4%, depending on the population [1–3]. This condition affects female patients 2 to 3 times more frequently than males [4].

Although numerous possible factors are under assessment, it is certain that buccally displaced canines (BDC) and palatally displaced canines (PDC) are characterized by different etiopathogeneses [4–6]. Whilst, BDC is thought to be one result of insufficient space in the maxilla for the eruption of the maxillary canine, the etiology of PDC is still unclear and varied reasons have been postulated [4, 6, 7].

Besides the several causes of PDCs, the most debated opinions of respected researchers are the genetic theory [6, 7] and the guidance theory [4, 8]. Nonetheless, both theories agree on the important role played by the adjacent lateral incisor, as normal canine eruption is guided by the lateral incisor root of sufficient length (guidance theory), whereas small or peg-shaped lateral incisors are associated genetically to PDC (genetic theory).

Several studies of dental casts have already described a higher risk of PDCs in patients with tooth crown size reduction [9–13]. Furthermore, recently, two more studies utilizing cone-beam computed tomography (CBCT) [14] and multi-slice spiral computed tomography (CT) [15], demonstrated that the lateral incisors adjacent to PDCs are smaller and the roots are shorter compared to those adjacent to normal canines. Another study [16] evaluating the crown-root angulation of the lateral incisor adjacent to PDCs on panoramic images, indicated that its

* Correspondence: rleonard@unict.it
[1]Department of Orthodontics, Policlinico Universitario "Vittorio Emanuele", University of Catania, Catania, Italy
Full list of author information is available at the end of the article

root was angled more mesially compared to the lateral incisor adjacent to the normally erupted canine. So, according to this latter finding, the roots of lateral incisors contiguous to PDCs seem to show a deviation in form. However, as the authors stated themselves [16], their study has some limitations, in that measurements from panoramic X-rays tend to overestimate the mesial angulation of lateral incisors compared to a three-dimensional image, such as CBCT, thereby revealing an inherent error in using a two dimensional image to depict three-dimensional structures.

Therefore, although there is no consensus about the exact etiology of palatally impacted canines, it appears that the adjacent lateral incisor highlights an important role, either because its eruption and size are controlled by the same genes that control the eruption of the canine (genetic theory) or because its position in the arch influences the canine's eruption path [16].

Recent advances in computer technologies and the rapid growth in the use of 3D imaging techniques provide more accurate evaluations and comparisons of anatomical structures. So, 3D 'surface-to-surface' matching of maxillary teeth from CBCT-derived models, could make morphological differences observable between homologous teeth from the two semi-arches as well as providing precise measurements of tooth sizes (volumes, widths and heights).

As no study, to our knowledge, has evaluated maxillary central and lateral incisors as well as first premolars adjacent to PDCs with the surface-volume matching technique, the aims of this study were to investigate in patients with unilateral PDC:

- the dimensions and morphologies of the central and lateral maxillary incisors, canines and first premolars from CBCT images both on the PDC side and non-PDC side;
- to do 'surface point-to-point' matching of teeth on the PDC side and non-PDC side (canines with a normal eruptive patterns);
- to compare these findings with a control sample of patients with no PDC.

The null hypothesis of this study was that there are no differences in either tooth morphologies or sizes on the PDC side and non-PDC side.

Methods

To determine the sample size, a power analysis was carried out (DSS Research, Washington, USA) which indicated that data from 18 participants would yield a confidence level of 95% and a Beta error level of 25%, making it sufficient to determine statistically significant differences.

So, the study group (SG) consisted of CBCT images from 28 consecutive patients (12 boys and 16 girls) who had been referred (between January 2016 and July 2017) to a private X-ray practice specialising in CBCT from large record pools. The scans were de-identified to protect patient confidentiality and ethic approval was obtained from the Ethic Committee of Policlinico Vittorio Emanuele, Catania, (reference number #4217). Also, a written informed consent was obtained from all patients included in this study. All procedures performed in this study involving human participants were in accordance with the ethical standards with the 1964 Helsinki declaration and its later amendments or comparable ethical standards.

The inclusion criteria were: good quality scan, sufficient field of view (FOV) for including the entirety of maxillary teeth, and the presence of a unilateral maxillary canine impaction.

The exclusion criteria were: movement artifacts, patients affected by cleft palate, dentofacial deformities, teeth anomalies (except for the PDC) or agenesis, caries, fillings, restorations, and conspicuous abrasions on the cusps and edges, buccal or midalveolar impacted canines, severe root resorption and teeth with dilacerated roots.

The mean age of the patients at the time of the CBCT scans was 16.04 ± 1.77 years.

These patients were age-and-gender matched with 25 subjects (11 boys and 14 girls, mean age??), affected by third molar impaction, who served as the control group (CG). The inclusion and exclusion criteria were the same as the SG plus the absence of PDC.

All CBCT images were taken with the NewTom 3G (QR SRL, Verona, Italy) device (110 kV, 6.19 mAs, 0.25 mm voxel size, and 8-mm aluminum filtration) with the patient in maximum intercuspation and Frankfort horizontal plane parallel to the floor following common CBCT imaging protocols [17].

All the data sets were exported and converted using the Digital Imaging and Communications in Medicine (DICOM).

To obtain 3D surface mesh models of the teeth and measure the root lengths of every single tooth (central incisor, later incisor, canine and first premolar of the maxillary arch), the DICOM-formatted images were volume rendered with Mimics (Mimics Research, version 19.0.0.347, Materialise NV, Liege, Belgium). Surface mesh models were further analyzed with reverse engineering software (Geomagic Control X, version 2017.0.0, 3D Systems, USA) to calculate the total volume of every single tooth model and to achieve a point-to-point surface analysis between the 3D models of the teeth on the PDC and non-PDC sides. The scanning, segmentation, and model fabrication protocols used in this study were previously validated and described [17–19].

Briefly, the work-flow to obtain root lengths, volumes and surface-to-surface matching is described below in seven steps:

Step 1- Generating the segmentation mask: to develop the segmentation mask (Fig. 1a), we used the 'automatic threshold' function of the Mimics Research software. The threshold was adjusted scan by scan to automatically detect the Hounsfield values and boundaries of all the teeth. During generation, the pulpal tissue of each tooth was included in the volumes to minimize the errors in discriminating dentin from pulpal tissue as an added source of variation (Fig. 1b). Then, The selected mask was then cropped into eight segments providing axial, sagittal and frontal views, by using the 'Crop Mask' function of the software, to obtain pure segmentation masks of every single tooth (Fig. 1c). Thereafter, the quality and precision of the single tooth mask was improved first by manually erasing, slice by slice, in the sagittal and axial views, the excess parts of the segmentation mask outside the tooth contour: for example the parts of the other teeth included in the mask during the cropping process. Later, the mask was smoothed and finely adjusted by using the interactive 'Contour Edit'

function, to improve quality and contour delineation. To avoid errors during the procedures, the PDC-side masks were colored blue while the non-PDC-side tooth masks were colored red.

Step 2- Segmentation: After generating the segmentation mask for each single tooth, to obtain the three-dimensional surface models of the teeth in this study, each mask was rendered into a three-dimensional model using the '3D calculation' function (Fig. 1d-e).

Step 3- Measurements: the root length was measured for each tooth, (i.e. the surface distance between the labial cement enamel junction and the root apex) (Figs. 2 and 5).

The measurements were made with the Mimics measurement tools, with a precision of 0.1 mm, directly on the rendered digital tooth models. The images were magnified by 300% to facilitate better visuals and to avoid errors during the point selections. The image was reoriented with the buccal surface of the tooth crown facing out of the computer screen, and the tooth standing vertically in the coronal and sagittal views. Then, using the surface measuring tool of the Mimics software, 4 points were identified on the buccal surface of the tooth

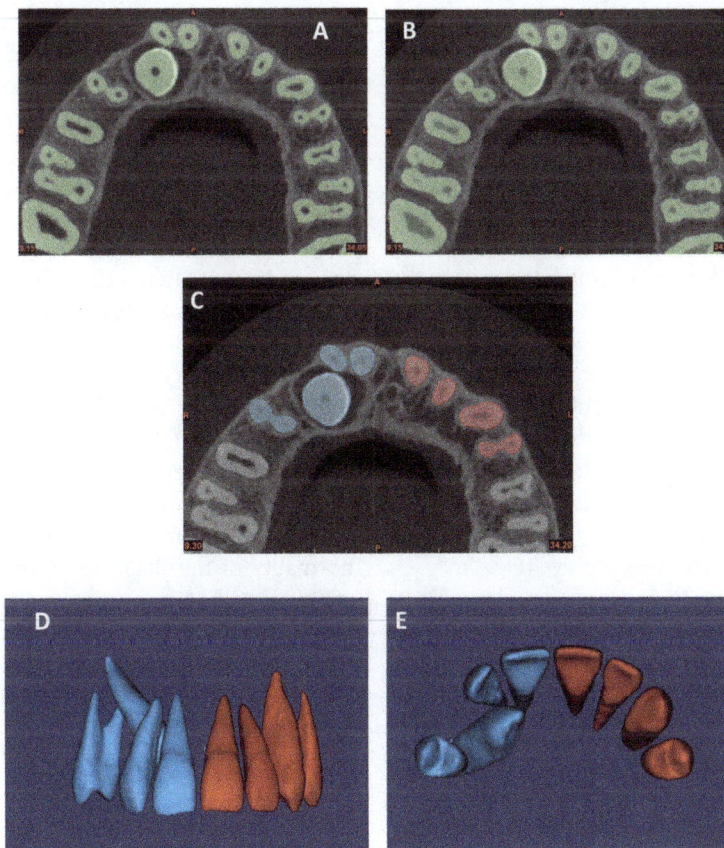

Fig. 1 Generation of the segmentation mask (**a**, **b**) using the 'automatic threshold' function of the software; pure segmentation masks (**c**); 3D surface models of the teeth (**d**, **e**)

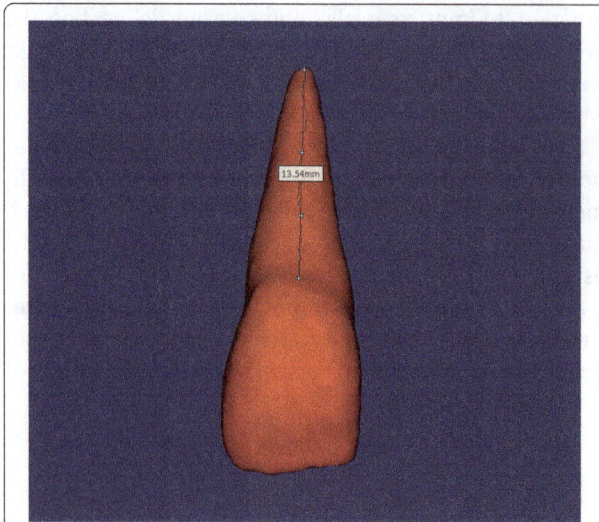

Fig. 2 The root lengths of each tooth were measured by selecting 4 points: the most apical point of the CEJ, two points respectively 4 mm and 8 mm apical to the CEJ level and a point at the apical foramen

root. These points were: the most apical point of the CEJ, two points respectively 4 mm and 8 mm apical to the CEJ level and a point at the apical foramen level. Each point was selected at the horizontal midpoint of the root surface. (Fig. 2).

Step 4- Mirroring: The 3D tooth models were exported to Geomagic Control X software as a stereo-lithographic format file (.stl) and the non-PDC side teeth were mirrored by converting their image orientation (Fig. 3a).

Step 5- First registration, point-based: a manual point-based superimposition selected the same 3 points on the surface of the specular tooth models to align the mirrored non-PDC side teeth models with the PDC-side teeth models. These points were the buccal and palatinal cusp tips and the deepest vestibular point at the cement enamel junction (CEJ) level, for the first premolar (Fig. 3b), the cusp tip and the mesial and distal points on the largest diameter of the crown for the canine (Fig. 3c); the deepest vestibular point at the CEJ level and the mesial and distal points on the largest diameter of the crown for the permanent incisive (Fig. 3d).

Step 6- Final registration: to enhance superimposition quality, a final registration was performed using the 'Best fit alignment' option in the Geomagic Control X software. The reference data-set was obtained, setting the precision of the registration to at least 0.2 mm (tolerance type: '3D Deviation') and the percentage of surface registration polygons to the maximum 100% (Fig. 3 e-f).

Step 7- 3D Deviation analysis: after superimposition, 3D surface deviation analysis was carried out with the Geomagic Control X software automatically calculating the means and maximum values of the distances

between the specular 3D crown models, measured between 100% of the surface mesh points, and representing them on a color analysis map. These values were visually displayed on a color map which showed the deviation in different colors (blue for maximum negative, red for maximum positive, green for the range tolerance). Distances greater than 0.3 mm are represented in red or blue while distances within the tolerance range (+ 0.3 to − 0.3 mm) are represented in green (Fig. 4 a-b). This map shows the surface distance (Euclidean distance) distributions between the entirety of the segmented tooth's surface points on the PDC side and its corresponding segmented tooth points on the non-PDC side.

The maximum deviation was set to 1.5 mm.

After the deviation analysis, the percentage (%) was calculated for all the deviation values within the tolerance range (− 0.3 to + 0.3 mm). These values indicated the matching percentage between the pairs of corresponding tooth models.

To minimize random and systematic errors, all the digital measurements on CBCT images were performed by a single examiner, with 25 years of orthodontic experience (R.L.). The examiner analyzed only 5 CBCT images each day to avoid fatigue. The CBCT images were examined in blind sequence.

To determine intra-observer error, 20 CBCT images were randomly selected and all the measurements repeated 6 weeks after the first examination by the same specialized operator with no knowledge of the first measurements.

Statistical analysis

All measurements were recorded on Microsoft Excel® spreadsheet (Microsoft, Redmond, WA, USA) and analyzed using SPSS® version 24 Statistics software (IBM Corporation, 1 New Orchard Road, Armonk, New York, USA).

Intra-examiner reliability was assessed using Dahlberg's formula [20] (method error = $\sqrt{\Sigma d_2/2n}$, where d is the difference between the two measurements of a pair, and n is the number of samples).

The Kolmogorov–Smirnov test was used to test the normality of the data. As all the data was normally distributed with homogeneous variance, parametric tests were used to evaluate the volumetric and linear data from the PDC side and non-PDC side. A paired t-Test was used to compare the root lengths and volumes of teeth from the PDC side and non-PDC side. Measurements of the PDC side, non-PDC side and control group were further analyzed by one-way Analysis of Variance (ANOVA) to evaluate if they were statistically significant to accept or reject the null hypothesis. The mesh percentages from the PDC sample and control sample were compared by t-test.

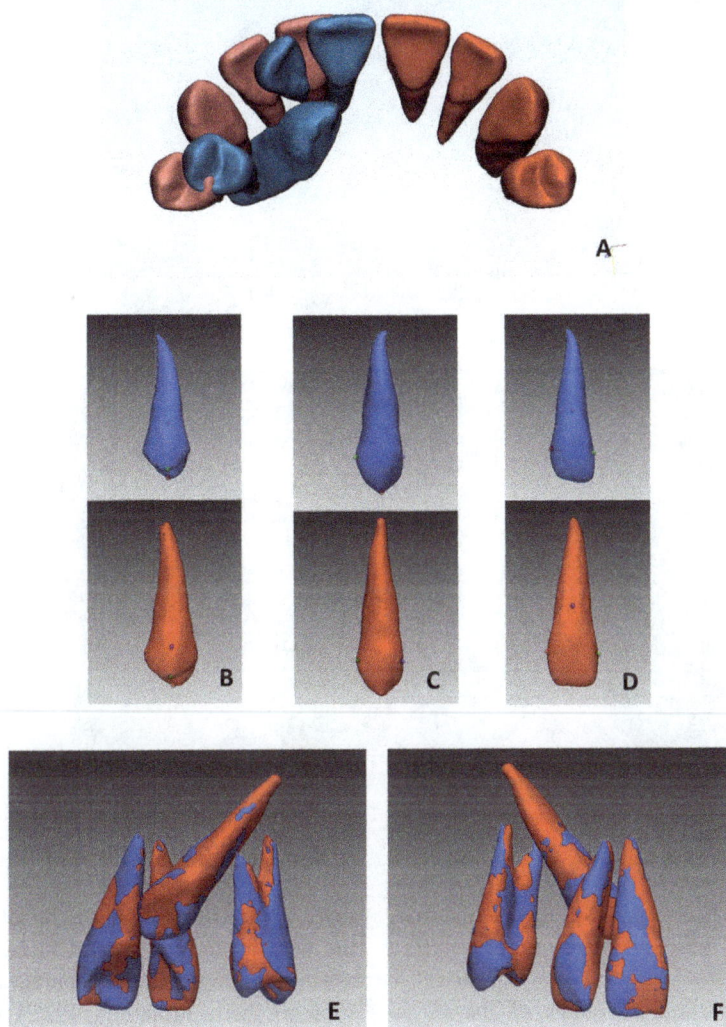

Fig. 3 3D tooth models (blue PDC side, red normal side) (**a**); selection of 3 points on the surface of the specular tooth models (**b**, **c**, **d**) (see text for points) for the first alignment; second alignment using the 'best fit' function of the software, palatal view (**e**) and vestibular view (**f**)

The significance level was set at $p \leq 0.05$. p values less than 0.05 were considered statistically significant.

Results

Of the 28 patients with unilaterally impacted canines, 13 were on the right side and 15 on the left. The intra-examiner reliability of the measurements showed a high correlation with Dahlberg's values not greater than 0.99 ($p < 0.000$) for both the volumetric and linear measurements.

The descriptive statistics for the root lengths (mm) and volumes (mm^3) of subjects with palatally displaced canines (PDC side and non-PDC side) and controls are shown in Table 1. Lateral incisors adjacent to PDCs showed a mean root length of 10.43 ±

0.72 mm, and this being shorter than that of the lateral incisor from the non-PDC side of the same patient (11.43 ± 0.78 mm), and from the control group (10.71 ± 0.86 mm). On average, lateral incisors adjacent to PDCs were shorter by 1 mm when compared to those on the non-PDC side of the same subject, and were 0.48 mm shorter compared to controls, these differences being statistically significant ($P \leq 0.001$), (Fig. 5). Even though there were some differences in tooth root lengths were obtained for the other teeth, they were only statistically significant for the first premolar ($P \leq 0.05$) which was shorter than those of controls.

As for volume, the most noticeable finding was that lateral incisors from the PDC side were smaller (308.26mm^3)

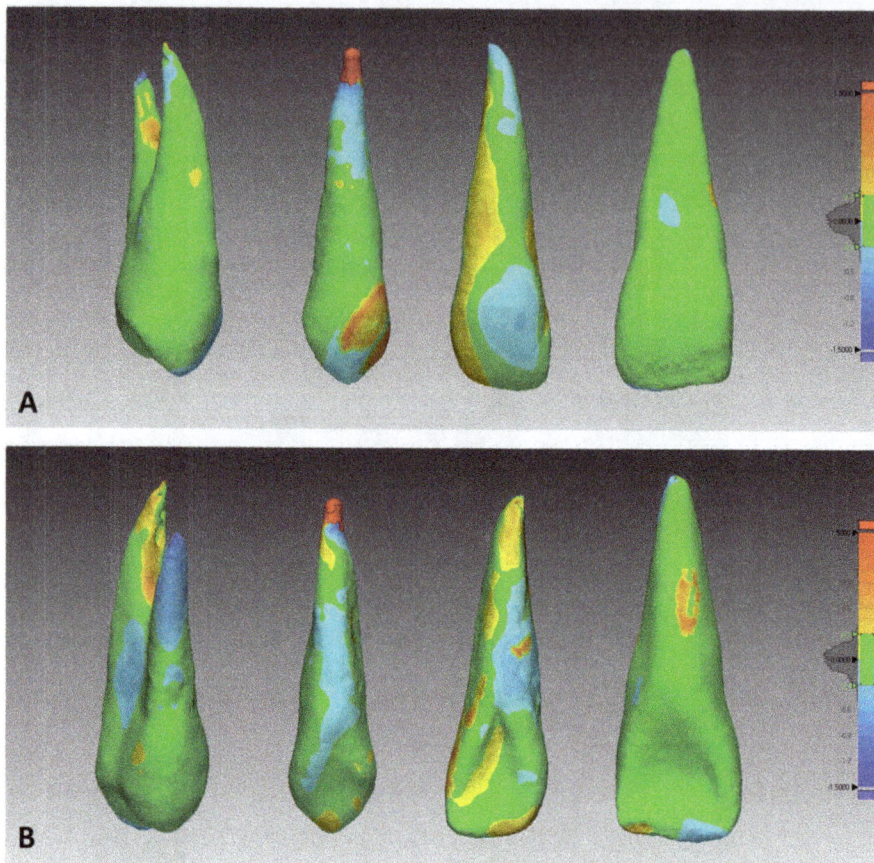

Fig. 4 Deviation analysis between the specular tooth models from the PDC side and non-PDC side. The colored map shows the deviations (negative blue, positive red) between the mesh models. **a**) vestibular view, **b**) palatal view

compared to the non-PDC side (361,43 mm^3) and these differences being statistically significant ($P \leq$ 0.0001) (Table 1).

The descriptive statistics and P values of the mesh matching percentages of subjects with unilateral PDCs versus controls are shown in Table 2. The percentage of mesh matching according to the 'surface-to-surface' analysis for the control group ranged from 84.75 for the first premolar to 85.37 for the central incisor, whilst for the

PDC group from 71.48 for the lateral incisor to 84.13 for the central incisor. Lateral incisors and canines showed the lowest matching percentages of the upper teeth in subjects with unilateral PDCs compared to controls. That is to say that the percentage differences in mesh point matches for lateral incisors and canines in the study group were lower than controls, demonstrating that there are some morphological mismatches of these teeth in subjects with palatally displaced canines.

Table 1 Mean Values and standard deviations (±). Comparison between PDC side, non-PDC side and control group for both radicular length (mm) and volume (mm^3)

		PDC		Non-PDC		P value	Control		P value
Root length	Central incisor	11.72	±0.67	11.71	±0.71	NS	11.63	±0.73	NS
	Lateral incisor	10.43	±0.72	11.43	±0.78	*	10.71	±0.86	†
	Canine	14.88	±1.37	14.84	±1.16	NS	14.63	±0.82	NS
	First premolar	11.07	±0.95	11.19	±0.95	NS	10.46	±0.64	*
Volume	Central incisor	402.23	±27.90	403.72	±24.34	NS	399.38	±21.03	NS
	Lateral incisor	308.26	±35.68	361.43	±31.41	*	351.26	±12.13	‡
	Canine	558.97	±49.30	553.68	±38.63	NS	544.47	±36.36	NS
	First premolar	383.26	±32.01	390.54	±29.92	NS	371.05	±27.56	NS

P value based on one-way ANOVA. *NS* non significant; *$P \leq 0.05$; † $P \leq 0.001$; ‡ $P \leq 0.0001$

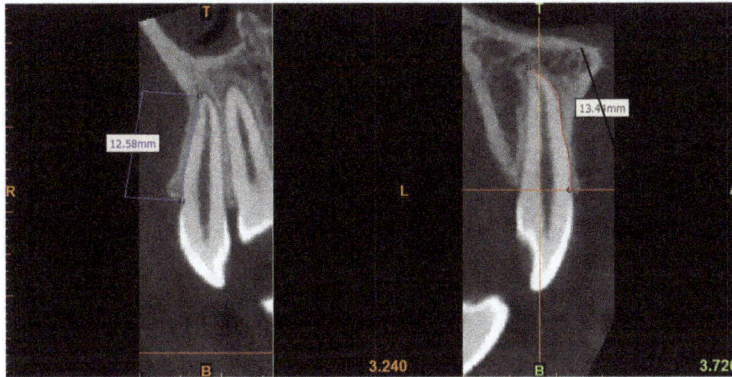

Fig. 5 CBCT scan of an upper lateral incisor on the palatally displaced canine side (Right) and of an upper lateral incisor on the non-palatally displaced canine side (Left). Measurements of the root lengths in millimeters at root surfaces from the labial cement enamel junction to the root apex

Statistically significant differences between the two groups were obtained for the lateral incisors and canines ($P \leq 0.0001$).

Therefore, 3D tooth symmetry using deviation analysis corroborated that tooth morphology (crown and root) on the PDC side and in controls not only differed for lateral incisors but also for palatally displaced canines. Interestingly, these differences were more evident at the root tips and in most of the crowns, according to the color-coded map, where red and blue areas highlighted the higher deviations.

Discussion

This investigation tested the assumption that upper tooth dimensions and morphologies for subjects with palatally displace canines differ from those of the teeth adjacent to normally erupted canines in the same subject and to those of controls. Our findings demonstrate, for the first time, that lateral incisor and displaced canine morphologies and dimensions on the PDC side differ from those on the non-PDC side and controls.

About 50 years ago, Miller [21] and Bass [22] independently observed that the prevalence of palatal displacement was greater when lateral incisors were congenitally missing. They concluded that the absence of

the lateral incisor denied the canine its guidance, permitting it to migrate palatally. These conclusions, were based on clinical impressions from viewing a number of patients in the clinic and not from a disciplined study of a large sample of affected patients vs an appropriate random control group.

Currently, the two most popular theories reported in the literature that have gained some degree of consensus worldwide, are the guidance theory [8, 22–25] and the genetic theory [4, 8, 9, 23, 26–29], which both share the belief that certain genetic features occur in association with the cause of palatal displacement of the maxillary canine. However, insofar there is no single and exclusive cause [30].

The results from this investigation seem to support shorter root lengths and reduced volumes of the upper lateral incisors involved in PDC as it can exert a powerful local influence.

Our results corroborate previous findings on lateral incisor root length [14, 15] being shorter on the PDC side. Additionally, for the first time a deviation in 3D tooth morphology of lateral incisors and canines of subjects with unilateral palatally displaced canines was demonstrated, as established by reverse engineering. Regarding lateral incisor root length, the results of our study demonstrated that its root was shorter on average by 1.00 mm compared to the contra-lateral side of the upper jaw, and by 0.48 mm compared to the lateral incisor root lengths of controls. Our findings substantiate previous studies [14, 15] which highlighted that lateral incisors had shorter mean length ranging from 0.78 mm [15] to 2.1 mm [14] and a smaller crown volume [15] on the PDC side.

By contrast, there were no statistically significant differences in root lengths or volumes for the maxillary central incisors, canines and first premolars (except for the length of the first premolar) between the three groups.

Table 2 Comparison between study group and control group for matching

		Mean and standard deviation (±)			
		Sample group		Control group	P value
Matching	Central incisor	84.13	±3.37	85.37	±2.52	NS
	Lateral incisor	72.48	±2.64	83.49	±2.02	*
	Canine	77.20	±2.27	83.21	±2.13	*
	First premolar	81.45	±3.14	82.75	±3.10	NS

P value based on independent t-test. NS non significant; *$P \leq 0.0001$

As far as volume is concerned, the lateral incisor on the palatally displaced canine side, showed a statistically significant smaller volume when compared to the lateral incisor on the non-displaced canine side and to lateral incisors from the control sample. However these findings are hardly comparable to the only previous study [15] because that investigation's data referred only to crowns and not to entire teeth.

The most noticeable and evident findings of our study concern the difference in surface-to-surface matching of upper teeth obtained from PDC patients and those of the control group. For the first time, a mesh analysis is presented, i.e. a 3D surface–to–surface matching from the affected and unaffected sides of PDC patients which was compared to data from the control sample. Interestingly, upper lateral incisors and canines from the PDC group displayed a lower percentage of matching when compared to homologous teeth of the control sample. Since the tolerance range was set at − 1.5 to + 1.5 mm, it is improbable that these mis-matchings were due to extreme curvature of the lateral incisor and canine roots. In fact this study was designed only to detect subtle differences which can hardly be appreciated by visual assessment, so CBTC scans with extreme variation in tooth morphologies were not included in the sample. Indeed, several previous studies have well documented a significant association between tooth morphology (lateral incisors and displaced canines) and palatally displaced canine [10, 14, 15, 23], however none of these studies has reported morphological differences, of small entities between homologous teeth from the PDC side and non-PDC side. The 3D surface-to-surface matching technique which was used in our research can reveal any differences, even small, in morphology and tooth size.

According to our results it may be suggested that individuals with shorter maxillary lateral incisor roots and morphological differences in the lateral incisors and canines (crowns and roots) are vulnerable to impaired eruption of the canine. Furthermore, before beginning orthodontic treatment, clinicians should be aware of both shorter lateral incisor root lengths and lateral incisor and canine dimorphism both in crowns and roots.

There are some limitations to this study in that the palatally impacted canine group from the radiology practice did not represent the general population. In fact, there is a tendency for clinicians to only refer patients with more severely impacted canines or other complicated cases for cone-beam volumetric tomography. Another weakness of the study, that puts this investigation at a risk of bias, is that researcher was obviously not blinded, when generating the segmentation masks for PDC and non-PDC-side.

Conclusions

The lateral incisors adjacent to palatally displaced canines have significantly shorter roots than contra-lateral lateral incisors adjacent to normally erupted canines. Furthermore, there are also differences in lateral incisor and canine morphologies in subjects with PDCs compared to controls.

Furthermore, this study provides new evidence that even the dimorphism of a small entity of permanent lateral incisor is involved in the canine palatal displacement process, besides the already described tooth anomalies.

Abbreviations
3D: Three-dimensional; ANOVA: One-way Analysis of Variance; BDC: Buccally displaced canine; CBCT: Cone beam computed tomography; CEJ: Cement-enamel junction; CG: Control group; FOV: Field of view; PDC: Palatally displaced canine; SG: Study group

Authors' contributions
RL: study concept and design, drafting manuscript, critical revision, final approval of the version to be published. SM: analysis and interpretation of data, application of digital technologies, final approval of the version to be published. SC: analysis and interpretation of data, final approval of the version to be published. GM: analysis and interpretation of data, final approval of the version to be published. MP: acquisition of data, final approval of the version to be published. RP: study concept and design, critical revision, final approval of the version to be published.

Competing interest
The authors declare that they have no competing interests.

Author details
[1]Department of Orthodontics, Policlinico Universitario "Vittorio Emanuele", University of Catania, Catania, Italy. [2]Department of Maxillofacial Surgery Policlinico G Martino, University of Messina, Messina, Italy. [3]Private practice, Bologna, Italy. [4]Department of Biomedical and Biotechnological Sciences, Human Anatomy and Histology Section, School of Medicine, University of Catania, Catania, Italy. [5]Department of Plastic Surgery, Director of the Master's Degree in Plastic Surgery, University of Catania, Catania, Italy.

References
1. Grover PS, Lorton L. The incidence of unerupted permanent teeth and related clinical cases. Oral Surg Oral Med Oral Pathol. 1985;59:420–5.
2. Kramer RM, Williams AC. The incidence of impacted teeth. A survey at Harlem hospital. Oral Surg Oral Med Oral Pathol. 1970;29:237–41.
3. Dachi SF, Howell FV. A survey of 3,874 routine full-mouth radiographs. I A study of retained roots and teeth. Oral Surg Oral Med Oral Pathol. 1961;14:916–24.
4. Becker A, Chaushu S. Etiology of maxillary canine impaction: a review. Am J Orthod Dentofac Orthop. 2015;148:557–67.
5. Mercuri E, Cassetta M, Cavallini C, Vicari D, Leonardi R, Barbato E. Dental anomalies and clinical features in patients with maxillary canine impaction. Angle Orthod. 2013;83:22–8.
6. Peck S, Peck L, Kataja M. Concomitant occurrence of canine malposition and tooth agenesis: evidence of orofacial genetic fields. Am J Orthod Dentofac Orthop. 2002;122:657–60.
7. Pirinen S, Arte S, Apajalahti S. Palatal displacement of canine is genetic and related to congenital absence of teeth. J Dent Res. 1996;75:1742–6.
8. Becker A. In defense of the guidance theory of palatal canine displacement. Angle Orthod. 1995;65:95–8.
9. Becker A, Sharabi S, Chaushu S. Maxillary tooth size variation in dentitions with palatal canine displacement. Eur J Orthod. 2002;24:313–8.

10. Chalakkal P, Thomas AM, Chopra S. Comparison between the dimensions of lateral incisor crowns adjacent to unerupted palatally displaced and nondisplaced canine. World J Orthod. 2010;11:245–9.

11. Paschos E, Huth KC, Fassler H, Rudzki-Janson I. Investigation of maxillary tooth sizes in patients with palatal canine displacement. J Orofac Orthop. 2005;66:288–98.

12. Yan B, Sun Z, Fields H, Wang L, Luo L. Etiologic factors for buccal and palatal maxillary canine impaction: a perspective based on cone-beam computed tomography analyses. Am J Orthod Dentofac Orthop. 2013; 143:527–34.

13. Anic-Milosevic S, Varga S, Mestrovic S, Lapter-Varga M, Slaj M. Dental and occlusal features in patients with palatally displaced maxillary canines. Eur J Orthod. 2009;31:367–73.

14. Liuk IW, Olive RJ, Griffin M, Monsour P. Maxillary lateral incisor morphology and palatally displaced canines: a case-controlled cone-beam volumetric tomography study. Am J Orthod Dentofac Orthop. 2013;143:522–6.

15. Kim Y, Hyun HK, Jang KT. Morphological relationship analysis of impacted maxillary canines and the adjacent teeth on 3-dimensional reconstructed CT images. Angle Orthod. 2017;87(4):590–7.

16. Kanavakis G, Curran KM, Wiseman KC, Barone NP, Finkelman MD, Srinivasan S, Lee MB, Trotman CA. Evaluation of crown-root angulation of lateral incisors adjacent to palatally impacted canines. Prog Orthod. 2015;16:4.

17. Forst D, Nijjar S, Flores-Mir C, Carey J, Secanell M, Lagravere M. Comparison of in vivo 3D cone-beam computed tomography tooth volume measurement protocols. Prog Orthod. 2014;15:69.

18. Shahbazian M, Jacobs R, Wyatt J, Willems G, Pattijn V, Dhoore E, VANL C, Vinckier F. Accuracy and surgical feasibility of a CBCT-based stereolithographic surgical guide aiding autotransplantation of teeth: in vitro validation. J Oral Rehabil. 2010;37:854–9.

19. Shaheen E, Khalil W, Ezeldeen M, Van de Casteele E, Sun Y, Politis C, Jacobs R. Accuracy of segmentation of tooth structures using 3 different CBCT machines. Oral Surg Oral Med Oral Pathol Oral Radiol. 2017;123:123–8.

20. Dahlberg G: Statistical methods for medical and biological students: G. Allen & Unwin ltd; 1940.

21. Miller WB, McLendon WJ, Hines FB 3rd. Two treatment approaches for missing or peg-shaped maxillary lateral incisors: a case study on identical twins. Am J Orthod Dentofac Orthop. 1987;92:249–56.

22. Bass TB. Observations on the misplaced upper canine tooth. Dent Pract Dent Rec. 1967;18:25–33.

23. Becker A, Smith P, Behar R. The incidence of anomalous maxillary lateral incisors in relation to palatally-displaced cuspids. Angle Orthod. 1981;51:24–9.

24. Becker A. The orthodontic treatment of impacted teeth, 2nd edt. London: Informa Healtcare UK Ltd; 2007.

25. Miller BH. The influence of congenitally missing teeth on the eruption of the upper canine. Dent Pract Dent Rec. 1963;13:497–504.

26. Peck S, Peck L, Kataja M. The palatally displaced canine as a dental anomaly of genetic origin. Angle Orthod. 1994;64:249–56.

27. Leonardi R, Barbato E, Vichi M, Caltabiano M. Skeletal anomalies and normal variants in patients with palatally displaced canines. Angle Orthod. 2009;79:727–32.

28. Leonardi R, Peck S, Caltabiano M, Barbato E. Palatally displaced canine anomaly in monozygotic twins. Angle Orthod. 2003;73:466–70.

29. Sajnani AK. Permanent maxillary canines - review of eruption pattern and local etiological factors leading to impaction. J Investig Clin Dent. 2015;6:1–7.

30. Kokich VG, Mathews DP. Surgical and orthodontic management of impacted teeth. Dent Clin N Am. 1993;37:181–204.

20

Can a brief psychological intervention improve oral health behaviour? A randomised controlled trial

U. Wide*⊙, J. Hagman, H. Werner and M. Hakeberg

Abstract

Background: Dental caries is a major public health issue affecting a large proportion of the general population. The disease is associated with behavioural factors and is thus preventable to a high degree. Individuals may need assistance to be able to change their oral health behaviour. There is a lack of such interventions for adults affected by severe caries. The aim of the study was to evaluate the effect of Acceptance and Commitment Therapy (ACT), a form of cognitive behavioural therapy, on oral health behaviour in young adults with poor oral health.

Methods: The study included a two group parallel randomised controlled trial at general dental clinics, with young adults, 18–25 years of age, ≥ two manifest proximal dental caries lesions ($n = 135$); 67 were treated with ACT and 68 with standard disease information only, respectively. Primary outcomes: oral health behaviours (tooth-brushing, flossing, use of toothpicks, and additional fluoride use). The CONSORT principles for RCTs were used, including intention-to-treat and per protocol analyses. The Chi-square, Mann-Whitney, and Wilcoxon Signed Rank tests were applied, including effect sizes.

Results: The study groups did not differ with regard to oral health behaviour variables at baseline. The intervention group improved all their oral health behaviours significantly over time (effect sizes, 0.26–0.32), while the control group showed improved behaviours on two measures (flossing and additional use of fluoride, effect sizes, 0.22–0.23).

Conclusions: By testing a psychological intervention on young adults (18–25 years of age) with a high prevalence of caries, we found an immediate positive effect with improved oral health behaviours.

Keywords: Acceptance and commitment therapy, Cognitive behaviour therapy, Psychological intervention, Caries, Young adults, Oral health behaviours, Randomised controlled trial

Background

Dental caries is a major public health issue, affecting around 60–90% of children, adolescents and adults worldwide [1]. Dental caries is associated with negative consequences and costs to sufferers and oral care providers [2, 3]. Moreover, dental caries is largely related to behavioural factors, such as oral hygiene, fluoride exposure and dietary habits. Thus, dental caries may be treated and prevented with behavioural interventions at the individual level.

Recent research in public health stresses the social determinants of oral health and inequalities in health, and the need for structural interventions to improve health and reduce health inequalities [4–6]. However, the dental care practice also needs effective methods to help individuals with poor oral health to change their behaviour.

One recent systematic review found evaluations and, to some degree, positive effects of behavioural interventions for adult individuals in the field of dentistry, mainly for older adults affected by periodontitis (besides

* Correspondence: ulla.wide@gu.se
Department of Behavioral and Community Dentistry, Institute of Odontology, The Sahlgrenska Academy, University of Gothenburg, P.O. Box 450, SE-40530 Gothenburg, Sweden

caries, the other major oral disease) [7]. Similar findings were reported by Newton and Asimakopoulou for behaviour interventions in improving oral hygiene related behaviour in patients with periodontitis [8]. However, a systematic review found no behavioural interventions for dietary change in adult patients with dental caries [9]. Thus, less is known about behavioural interventions for adults affected by caries. Young adults develop health behaviour habits for their adult lives, and possibly for their children, and are therefore an important group to target for behavioural interventions. Authors have emphasised the need to use stringent interventions based on accepted theory from the behavioural sciences (the field of health psychology) to affect oral health behaviour changes [10, 11].

Different theory-based interventions for behaviour change has been developed, and to some degree tested for oral health problems. The present study was designed to evaluate a brief psychological intervention, Acceptance and commitment therapy (ACT), delivered by a psychologist in general dentistry, as a means to help young adult patients with poor oral health to make behavioural changes to improve their oral health.

ACT is a recently developed psychological method [12], a form of Cognitive Behaviour Therapy (CBT), that has been used with positive results in the treatment of health problems, such as pain, tinnitus and addiction [13, 14]. ACT interventions have been developed in brief formats for primary care, a setting similar to general dentistry, but has, to our knowledge, not been tested in general dentistry. The rationale of ACT is to increase psychological flexibility, thus facilitating the individual to maintain functional behaviours, and to change dysfunctional behaviours, in order to live in accordance with chosen individual life values [15]. The intention of using ACT in the present study was to contribute to behaviour change by focusing on how health-related behaviour could be relevant to valued life directions, by addressing also the psychological flexibility of the individual.

Methods
The aim and design of the study
The aim of the study was to evaluate the effect of ACT on oral health behaviours in young adults with poor oral health. Hypothesis: A brief psychological intervention (ACT) improves oral health behaviours (such as tooth-brushing and flossing) more than standard information alone.

The present analysis is part of a larger clinical trial evaluating the effect of ACT on oral health behaviours, oral health (caries, gingivitis), sugar consumption, psychological distress, general health behaviour and the ability to handle stress. In the present analysis the primary outcomes were oral health behaviours (flossing, toothpick use, tooth-brushing, additional fluoride use).

The study was a two group parallel randomised controlled trial with an allocation ratio 1:1. The study was approved by the Regional Ethical Review Board in Gothenburg (Reg. no. 840–12).

Participants
The participants were recruited between 2013 and 2014 at two Public Dental Service clinics in Region Västra Götaland, Sweden. Inclusion criteria: 18–25 years of age, ≥ two manifest proximal dental caries lesions. Exclusion criteria: Psychiatric/neuropsychiatric diagnosis, such as depression, psychosis, autism spectrum disorder, mental retardation, substance abuse. Participants needed to have good understanding of Swedish which was assessed by the research coordinator. A power analysis was performed to determine the sample size. The calculation was made for gingivitis (mean ratio of bleeding surfaces) and the assumption of detecting a 20% reduction with an alpha of 0.05 and a power of 0.80. The number of participants needed was 53 individuals per group. Thus, including dropouts, the sample was determined to require at least 130 participants, 65 per group. Power calculations were repeated with other outcome variables (plaque, caries, oral health behaviours), but these did not change the minimum number of participants needed to detect a relevant difference between groups.

Potentially eligible individuals were screened (first screening) while at their ordinary routine dental examination, and were invited to participate in the trial. The research coordinator at the dental clinic contacted individuals interested in participating, and after a second screening/confirmation of the inclusion/exclusion criteria, the individual received written information about the trial. The study participants were asked for and provided written consent. The second screening resulted in 186 eligible patients. Of these, 51 declined to participate, the most common reasons being "not interested" and "lack of time" (see Fig. 1). The final sample consisted of 135 participants (acceptance rate 72.6%).

Procedure and allocation strategy
Individuals included in the study answered baseline questionnaire using a touch-screen computer. Clinical data were obtained from their most recent ordinary dental examination. All participants then received standardised oral health information, provided verbally by a registered dental nurse using a brochure on oral health behaviour and caries. The information, including the brochure, was at the time of the study used at all public dental service clinics in Region Västra Götaland, Sweden.

The participants were then randomised by an independent research coordinator, either to the Intervention

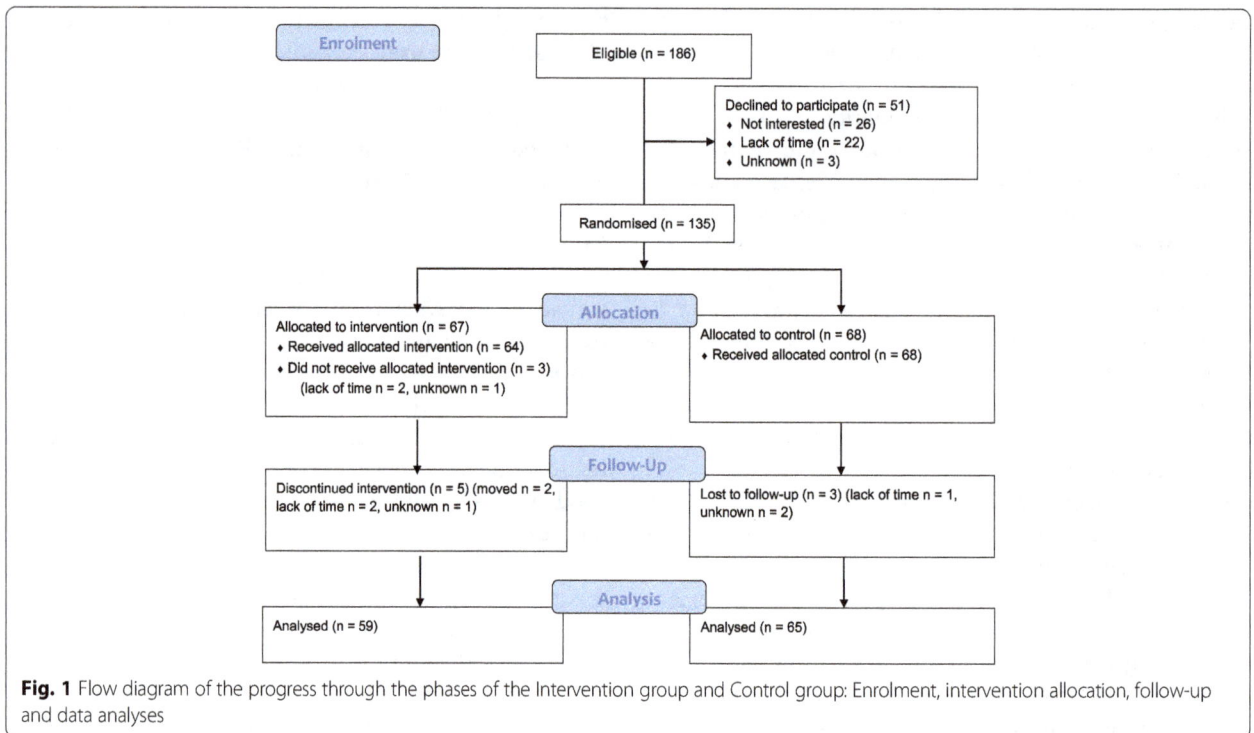

Fig. 1 Flow diagram of the progress through the phases of the Intervention group and Control group: Enrolment, intervention allocation, follow-up and data analyses

(ACT plus information) or Control (information alone) group, using a block randomisation procedure including stratification by gender and smoking (randomly permuted blocks within strata [16]). As an allocation strategy, the research coordinator used sealed opaque envelopes that had been prepared in advance by another research coordinator and placed in four boxes according to the stratification strategy. The allocation list was kept in a locked safety box, only available to the independent research coordinator.

Participants allocated to intervention were scheduled for two appointments with the psychologist 2 weeks apart (see below for description of the intervention). Participants answered follow-up questions at the clinic 3 weeks after baseline. (See Fig. 1, Flow chart according to CONSORT [17]).

At the two dental clinics, the study involved general practitioners (dentists and dental hygienists), a research coordinator, dental nurses and a clinical psychologist. All treatments and examinations were performed at the respective clinic.

Measures

Clinical measure of oral health: data on dental caries lesions (number and type) according to accepted standards (D1-D3, secondary caries), including assessment of caries on four surfaces, with proximal caries assessed on radiographs [18]. A summarised score of the number of surfaces with manifest caries (D3 and secondary caries) was calculated.

Sociodemographic characteristics were measured with questions about: age, gender, ethnicity (Swedish-born, including other Nordic country; foreign-born), mother's country of birth (Swedish-born, including other Nordic country; foreign-born), housing (rented flat; own flat/house; other), mother's education (primary; secondary; university).

Self-rated oral health was captured with the question 'How do you rate your oral health?', with four response alternatives (poor; fair; good; very good).

Oral health behaviour was assessed with questions about tooth-brushing, flossing, use of toothpicks, and use of additional fluoride (besides toothpaste), with six response alternatives: three times a day or more; twice a day; once a day; several times a week; once a week; more seldom/never. One question measured dental care attendance, where the five response alternatives were dichotomised into often (twice a year; once a year) vs. seldom (every other year; less then every other year; only when acute problem).

Any adverse effects during the study period reported by the participants were registered by the research coordinators.

Intervention

The intervention used was a psychological intervention, CBT in the ACT form [12, 15], adapted to primary care settings [19, 20] and modified for the present trial. The modification included a selection of well-known ACT exercises (e.g., defusion and Bull's Eye), and was made in close collaboration with a licensed psychologist specialised in ACT and experienced in implementing ACT in primary care. Like other CBT-interventions, ACT is based on an individual case conceptualisation and a functional analysis of behaviour, and the participant and the psychologist together develop a plan for behaviour change. In Table 1 a treatment overview is provided, showing the different ACT modules.

The intervention was delivered at two general dental clinics and included two individual sessions (45 min each) with a licensed psychologist specialised in ACT (HW). To secure adherence to treatment, the psychologist in the project was regularly supervised [21]. The time between the first and the second session was 2 weeks.

Statistical analyses

Descriptive statistics used were frequencies, mean, median and standard deviation (SD). The statistical methods applied were the Chi-square test, the Mann-Whitney test for independent groups, and the Wilcoxon Signed Rank test for dependent groups. Both intention-to-treat (ITT) and per protocol (PP) analyses were performed according to the CONSORT principles [17]. The effect size according to Cohen's ES was calculated for changes over time, applying the Wilcoxon Signed Rank test using the formula $z/\sqrt{N}$, where z is the test statistic and N equals twice the number of individuals included in the respective analyses [22]. According to Cohen's criteria [23], an effect size around $0.1 =$ low effect, $0.3 =$ medium effect, and $0.5 =$ large effect. The significance level applied was 0.05. Bonferroni corrections for multiple comparisons were applied giving p-values for statistical significance of $p < 0.005$ for baseline (Table 2), and $p < 0.003$ for primary outcomes (Table 3).. The study included a blinded design with the research group and statistical analyst being blinded to which treatment was allocated to which patient.

Table 1 Treatment overview of ACT for patients with dental caries

Session 1	Session 2
Introduction	Follow-up
Brief interview	Bull's-Eye
Mindful oral health	Mindful oral health
Focused questions	Value based living
Case conceptualisation	Defusion exercises
Bull's-Eye	Plan for behavioural change and follow-up
Clarification of values	
Plan for behavioural change	

Results
Description of participants at baseline

In total, 135 individuals were included in the study, and were allocated to either intervention ($n = 67$) or control ($n = 68$). Sociodemographic and clinical characteristics of the participants are presented in Table 2. The mean age was 20 years, and the participants had a mean number of caries surfaces of 6.3 and 4.9 in the intervention and control group, respectively. The vast majority of participants experienced their oral health to be poor or fair, with 86.6% and 82.4% in the intervention and control group, respectively. About 40% in both groups rated their oral health as poor, less than 20% rated their oral health as good, and none rated it as very good. Half of the subjects were female, one third was smokers, and different ethnicities and socioeconomic positions were represented in the study group. The intervention group reported statistically significantly more Swedish-born mothers than the control group (65.7% vs. 42.6%, $p < 0.01$ (ns. after Bonferroni correction)), while the groups did not differ with regard to the other sociodemographic and clinical measures. The study groups did not differ with regard to oral health behaviour variables at baseline (Table 3).

Changes after intervention

The number of participants who received intended treatment and were analysed, as well as participant losses after randomization, are presented in Fig. 1. In the intervention group, 64 individuals received the allocated treatment and 59 of them participated in the follow-up, while 68 individuals received the control condition, and 65 of them participated in the follow-up. Per protocol analyses revealed that the intervention group improved their oral health behaviour on all four measures (Table 3): tooth-brushing ($Z = -3.43$, $p = 0.001$, effect size 0.32); flossing ($Z = -3.48$, $p = 0.0005$, effect size 0.32); toothpicks ($Z = -3.04$ $p = 0.002$, effect size 0.28); additional use of fluoride ($Z = -3.27$ $p = 0.001$, effect size 0.30). The control group improved their oral health behaviour regarding two variables: use of flossing ($Z = -2.72$, $p = 0.006$ (ns. after Bonferroni correction), effect size 0.24) and additional use of fluoride ($Z = -2.53$, $p = 0.011$ (ns. after Bonferroni correction), effect size 0.22), while no differences were found regarding tooth-brushing ($Z = -0.99$, $p = 0.320$) and toothpicks ($Z = -0.73$, $p = 0.466$).

Intention-to-treat analyses showed parallel results in that the intervention group improved their oral health behaviour on all four measures (Table 3): tooth-brushing ($Z = -3.43$, $p = 0.001$, effect size 0.30); flossing ($Z = -3.48$, $p = 0.0005$, effect size 0.30); toothpicks ($Z = -3.04$ $p = 0.002$, effect size 0.26); additional use of fluoride ($Z = -3.27$ $p = 0.001$, effect size 0.28). The control group improved their oral health behaviour over time

Table 2 Sociodemographic and clinical characteristics of participants (n = 135) allocated to Intervention or Control, at baseline

Variable	Intervention (n = 67)	Control (n = 68)	P
Age in years, Mean (SD)	20.4 (2.1)	20.8 (2.2)	ns.
Self-rated oral health, n (%)			ns.
Poor	27 (40.3)	25 (36.8)	
Fair	31 (46.3)	31 (45.6)	
Good	9 (13.4)	12 (17.6)	
Very good	0	0	
Caries, Mean (SD) Median	6.3 (5.2) 4	4.9 (3.7) 5	ns.
Dental care attendance, n (%) often	58 (86.6)	56 (82.4)	ns.
Gender, n (%) female	32 (47.8)	32 (47.1)	ns.
Smoker, n (%) smoking	23 (34.3)	24 (35.3)	ns.
Ethnicity, n (%) Swedish-born	55 (82.1)	48 (70.6)	ns.
Housing, n (%)			ns.
Rental flat	32 (47.8)	33 (48.5)	
Own flat/house	28 (41.8)	25 (36.8)	
Other	7 (10.4)	10 (14.7)	
Mother's ethnicity, n (%) Swedish-born	44 (65.7)	29 (42.6)	$p < 0.01^a$
Mother's education, n (%)			ns.
Primary	15 (22.4)	22 (32.4)	
Secondary	35 (52.2)	31 (45.6)	
University	17 (25.4)	15 (22.1)	

Chi-square (Mann-Whitney for caries), [a] Ns after Bonferroni correction

concerning two variables: use of flossing (Z = – 2.72, p = 0.006 (ns. after Bonferroni correction), effect size 0.23), and additional use of fluoride (Z = – 2.53, p = 0.011 (ns. after Bonferroni correction), effect size 0.22), while no differences were found concerning tooth-brushing (Z = – 0.99, p = 0.320) and toothpicks (Z = – 0.73, p = 0.466).

No adverse events were reported by the participants. The period of recruitment of participants to final examination at follow-up lasted between February 2013 and May 2016.

Discussion

This randomised controlled trial evaluated the effect of a brief psychological intervention (ACT) for behaviour change, delivered by a psychologist in general dental care to young adults (18–25 years of age) with dental caries. Significant positive changes with regard to oral health behaviours were found, most prominent in the intervention group compared with the control group that received standardised information. However, the hypothesis stated was only accepted in part regarding the measures of oral health behaviours (i.e., the ACT intervention improved oral health behaviours more than information alone).

There are mixed results in the literature on behavioural interventions to improve oral health behaviour in individuals with poor oral health [7, 24]. Positive effects

on tooth-brushing and interdental cleaning have been reported in studies with an RCT design including middle-aged to older individuals with periodontitis [25–27]. In the present study on young adults (18–25 years of age) with dental caries, the intervention group improved their oral health behaviour on all investigated variables (tooth-brushing, flossing, use of toothpicks and additional use of fluoride). This is a promising result. The participants in this study were all affected by severe dental caries disease, and behavioural change was necessary to halt the disease progression and to promote better oral health.

The control group also showed some improvement in oral health behaviour, although on fewer measures. There are potential general effects of being a participant in a clinical study, such as receiving extra attention from dental personnel, which may contribute to positive changes also in the control group. It is not reasonable to argue that the control condition in itself led to these changes in the control group, since the control condition consisted of the ordinary treatment-as-usual information delivered to all patients.

Previous studies on psychological interventions for behavioural change in the area of dentistry have mainly focused on interventions inspired of or based on the Motivational Interviewing technique, applied to patients with periodontitis at specialised clinics [26, 28–30].

Table 3 Oral health behaviour of the participants allocated to Intervention or Control, at baseline and follow-up, according to Per Protocol (PP) and Intention-To-Treat (ITT) analyses, respectively

Variable	Baseline				Follow-up			
	Intervention		Control		Intervention		Control	
	ITT (n = 67)	PP (n = 59)	ITT (n = 68)	PP (n = 65)	ITT (n = 67)	PP (n = 59)	ITT (n = 68)	PP (n = 65)
Tooth-brushing								
≥ 3 times/day	1 (1.5)	1 (1.7)	2 (2.9)	2 (3.1)	2 (3.0)	2 (3.4)	3 (4.4)	3 (4.6)
Twice a day	37 (55.2)	32 (54.2)	43 (63.2)	42 (64.6)	50 (74.6)	45 (76.3)	46 (67.6)	45 (69.2)
Once a day	16 (23.9)	14 (23.7)	13 (19.1)	12 (18.5)	8 (11.9)	6 (10.2)	9 (13.2)	8 (12.3)
Several times/week	8 (11.9)	7 (11.9)	9 (13.2)	8 (12.3)	6 (9.0)	5 (8.5)	9 (13.2)	8 (12.3)
Once a week	4 (6.0)	4 (6.8)	1 (1.5)	1 (1.5)	1 (1.5)	1 (1.7)	1 (1.5)	1 (1.5)
More seldom/never	1 (1.5)	1 (1.7)	0	0	0	0	0	0
Flossing								
≥ 3 times/day	0	0	0	0	2 (3.0)	2 (3.4)	2 (2.9)	2 (3.1)
Twice a day	7 (10.4)	6 (10.2)	5 (7.4)	5 (7.7)	13 (19.4)	12 (20.3)	7 (10.3)	7 (10.8)
Once a day	4 (6.0)	4 (6.8)	10 (14.7)	10 (15.4)	11 (16.4)	11 (18.6)	14 (20.6)	14 (21.5)
Several times/week	14 (20.9)	11 (18.6)	11 (16.2)	10 (15.4)	13 (19.4)	10 (16.9)	12 (17.6)	11 (16.9)
Once a week	10 (14.9)	9 (15.3)	8 (11.8)	8 (12.3)	9 (13.4)	8 (13.6)	12 (17.6)	12 (18.5)
More seldom/never	32 (47.8)	29 (49.2)	34 (50.0)	32 (49.2)	19 (28.4)	16 (27.1)	21 (30.9)	19 (29.9)
Toothpick use								
≥ 3 times/day	1 (1.5)	1 (1.7)	1 (1.5)	1 (1.5)	3 (4.5)	3 (5.1)	0	0
Twice a day	1 (1.5)	1 (1.7)	2 (2.9)	2 (3.1)	4 (6.0)	4 (6.8)	2 (2.9)	2 (3.1)
Once a day	2 (3.0)	2 (3.4)	7 (10.3)	6 (9.2)	7 (10.4)	7 (11.9)	11 (16.2)	10 (15.4)
Several times/week	6 (9.0)	6 (10.2)	7 (10.3)	7 (10.8)	5 (7.5)	5 (8.5)	6 (8.8)	6 (9.2)
Once a week	4 (6.0)	3 (5.1)	3 (4.4)	2 (3.1)	5 (7.5)	4 (6.8)	6 (8.8)	5 (7.7)
More seldom/never	53 (79.1)	46 (78.0)	48 (70.6)	47 (72.3)	43 (64.2)	36 (61.0)	43 (63.2)	42 (64.6)
Additional fluoride								
≥ 3 times/day	3 (4.5)	3 (5.1)	4 (5.9)	3 (4.6)	5 (7.5)	5 (8.5)	3 (4.4)	2 (3.1)
2 times/day	13 (19.4)	11 (18.6)	8 (11.8)	7 (10.8)	19 (28.4)	17 (28.8)	14 (20.6)	13 (20.0)
Once a day	12 (17.9)	11 (18.6)	14 (20.6)	14 (21.5)	13 (19.4)	12 (20.3)	17 (25.0)	17 (26.2)
Several times/week	10 (14.9)	8 (13.6)	13 (19.1)	13 (20.0)	16 (23.9)	14 (23.7)	18 (26.5)	18 (27.7)
Once a week	10 (14.9)	9 (15.3)	10 (14.7)	10 (15.4)	4 (6.0)	3 (5.1)	6 (8.8)	6 (9.2)
More seldom/never	19 (28.4)	17 (28.8)	19 (27.9)	18 (27.7)	10 (14.9)	8 (13.6)	10 (14.7)	9 (13.8)

Frequency n (%)

Interventions based on other theoretical models have also been presented [27, 31, 32]. This study adds important knowledge to the field by testing ACT, a theory-based psychological intervention used with promising results for various health issues in health care [13, 14] but, to our knowledge, not previously used in dentistry. With regard to ACT, one may specifically emphasize certain modules in the first session, such as the brief interview and focused questions leading to the case conceptualisation, providing information and stance for individualised interventions to increase psychological flexibility and contact with life values. However, we believe that the all-embracing model of ACT as a specific type of CBT-intervention is the most important factor for the behaviour changes accomplished.

The present study also used a multi-professional setting, where dental personnel identified eligible participants, and where the intervention was delivered by a licensed psychologist working at the same general dental clinic. Over the last decades it has become more common to include psychologists in primary care settings [33]. The same development has not taken place within dentistry, with the exception of treatment of patients with dental phobia, where psychologists are members of treatment teams in many specialised clinics [34–36].

In this paper we have discussed the effect of ACT on oral health behaviour. Other behavioural outcomes of relevance for oral health are for example tobacco use and dietary habits. Behaviour change interventions or counselling has proven effective for tobacco use cessation in adults in both general medicine and dentistry [37]. However, according to a Cochrane review [38], there is limited evidence about effective interventions (behavioural and/or medical) for smoking cessation in young people. When it comes to dietary habits, there is evidence from the field of general medicine that behaviour change or counselling could effectively change such habits [37]. Yet, in dentistry, such interventions have only had limited effect. In fact, as mentioned previously, a recent systematic review on interventions for dietary change in adult patients with dental caries found no such studies [9]. Thus, there are several knowledge gaps to address in the future.

This study has some strengths and limitations. The study used an appropriate RCT design while adhering to the standard protocol for such a design, according to the CONSORT methodology. We included a large number of participants at baseline and had a dropout rate of only 15.5% at follow-up. Moreover, the analyses included both per protocol and intention-to-treat evaluations. The study group of young adults, between the ages of 18 and 25 years, is in a period of their lives when mobility is common. Individuals move away from home, find employment or may enrol in higher education; thus, an even greater loss to follow-up was expected. The generalisability of the study is high, as the study was conducted in two general Public Dental Service clinics. In Sweden, the large majority of individuals in this age-group regularly visit Public Dental Service clinics. The participants were recruited while on their ordinary visit at the clinics, where registrations and interventions were performed. A desirable double-blind procedure was obviously not possible, due to the design and intervention tested. However, we were able to blind the research group and the statistician to which group the participants belonged. The outcome measures are self-reported only and it is therefore important to include objective clinical health measurements, such as gingivitis and caries. Even if the results are promising with regard to oral health behaviour, we need to conclude on the long-term effects of the psychological intervention, i.e. the sustainability of the results.

To the best of our knowledge, while searching the scientific literature, we have not found other RCTs testing a behavioural intervention on young adults (18–25 years of age) with high caries activity, nor do we know of a similar field study setting where a licensed psychologist has been employed within general dentistry clinics to treat young adults affected by caries disease. It may be argued that the dental professions need other professionals, such as psychologists, when treating or counselling young adults in order to alter their health behaviour related to different oral diseases. Moreover, this is particularly important considering the often high prevalence of oral diseases, the close relationship between oral diseases and health behaviour, and the fact that these diseases, in terms of etiologic fraction, are highly preventable.

Conclusions

By testing a psychological intervention (Acceptance and Commitment Therapy) on young adults (18–25 years of age) with high caries prevalence, we found an immediate positive effect with improved oral health behaviours, including more tooth-brushing, flossing, and the use of toothpicks and additional use of fluoride.

Abbreviations

ACT: Acceptance and Commitment Therapy; CBT: Cognitive Behaviour Therapy; ITT: Intention-to-treat; ns.: Non-significant; PP: Per protocol

Funding

The study was supported by grants from The Health Care Subcommittee, Region Västra Götaland, Sweden.

Acknowledgements

The research coordinators, the head of clinics and the dental personnel who contributed to identifying eligible participants are gratefully acknowledged. Licensed psychologist and ACT specialist Celia Young's role as an adviser is also gratefully acknowledged.

Authors' contributions

MH and UW planned the study, HW and JH prepared the data set, and MH is responsible for the analysis of data. All authors are responsible for drafting the manuscript and have read and approved the final manuscript.

Competing interests

The authors declare that they have no competing interests.

References

1. WHO. Sugars and dental caries. In: Technical information note. WHO/NMH/NHD/1712; 2017.
2. Petersen PE. The world Oral health report 2003: continuous improvement of oral health in the 21st century--the approach of the WHO global Oral health Programme. Community Dent Oral Epidemiol. 2003;31(Suppl 1):3–23.
3. Petersen PE. Oral health. In: International encyclopedia of public health. San Diego (CA): Academic Press; 2008. p. 677–85.
4. Guarnizo-Herreno CC, Watt RG, Pikhart H, Sheiham A, Tsakos G. Socioeconomic inequalities in oral health in different European welfare state regimes. J Epidemiol Community Health. 2013;67:728–35.

5. Guarnizo-Herreno CC, Watt RG, Pikhart H, Sheiham A, Tsakos G. Inequalities in oral impacts and welfare regimes: analysis of 21 European countries. Community Dent Oral Epidemiol. 2014;42:517–25.

6. Sabbah W, Tsakos G, Chandola T, Sheiham A, Watt RG. Social gradients in oral and general health. J Dent Res. 2007;86:992–6.

7. Werner H, Hakeberg M, Dahlstrom L, Eriksson M, Sjogren P, Strandell A, et al. Psychological interventions for poor Oral health: a systematic review. J Dent Res. 2016;95:506–14.

8. Newton JT, Asimakopoulou K. Managing oral hygiene as a risk factor for periodontal disease: a systematic review of psychological approaches to behaviour change for improved plaque control in periodontal management. J Clin Periodontol. 2015;42 Suppl 16:S36–46.

9. Al Rawahi SH, Asimakopoulou K, Newton JT. Theory based interventions for caries related sugar intake in adults: systematic review. BMC Psychol. 2017;5:25.

10. Noar SM, Zimmerman RS. Health behavior theory and cumulative knowledge regarding health behaviors: are we moving in the right direction? Health Educ Res. 2005;20:275–90.

11. Bartholomew LK, Mullen PD. Five roles for using theory and evidence in the design and testing of behavior change interventions. J Public Health Dent. 2011;71(Suppl 1):S20–33.

12. Hayes SC, Strosahl KD, Wilson KG. Acceptance and committment therapy. New York: Guilford; 1999.

13. Powers MB, MB ZVSV, Emmelkamp PM. Acceptance and commitment therapy: a meta-analytic review. Psychother Psychosom. 2009;78:73–80.

14. Ruiz FJ. Acceptance and commitment therapy versus traditional cognitive behavioral therapy: a systematic review and meta-analysis of current empirical evidence. Int J Psychol Psychol Ther. 2012;12:333–57.

15. Hayes SC, Luoma JB, Bond FW, Masuda A, Lillis J. Acceptance and commitment therapy: model, processes and outcomes. Behav Res Ther. 2006;44:1–25.

16. Pocock SJ. Clinical trials. Chichester: Wiley; 1983.

17. Moher D, Hopewell S, Schulz KF, Montori V, Gotzsche PC, Devereaux PJ, et al. CONSORT 2010 explanation and elaboration: updated guidelines for reporting parallel group randomised trials. BMJ. 2010;340:c869.

18. Pitts NB, Fyffe HE. The effect of varying diagnostic thresholds upon clinical caries data for a low prevalence group. J Dent Res. 1988;67:592–6.

19. Strosahl K, Robinson P, Gustavsson T. Brief interventions for radical change. New Harbinger: Oakland; 2012.

20. Robinson PJ, Gould DA, Strosahl KD. Real behavior change in primary care: improving patient outcomes and increasing job satisfaction. New Harbinger: Oakland, CA; 2010.

21. Borrelli B. The assessment, monitoring, and enhancement of treatment fidelity in public health clinical trials. J Public Health Dent. 2011; 71(Suppl 1):S52–63.

22. Pallant J. SPSS Survival manual. 5th ed. Berkshire, England: McGraw-Hill; 2013.

23. Cohen JW. Statistical power analysis for the behavioral sciences. Hillsdale, NJ: Lawrence Erlbaum Associates; 1988.

24. Renz A, Ide M, Newton T, Robinson PG, Smith D. Psychological interventions to improve adherence to oral hygiene instructions in adults with periodontal diseases. Cochrane Database Syst Rev. 2007;18:CD005097.

25. Jonsson B, Lindberg P, Oscarson N, Ohrn K. Improved compliance and self-care in patients with periodontitis--a randomized control trial. Int J Dent Hyg. 2006;4:77–83.

26. Jonsson B, Ohrn K, Oscarson N, Lindberg P. The effectiveness of an individually tailored oral health educational programme on oral hygiene behaviour in patients with periodontal disease: a blinded randomized-controlled clinical trial (one-year follow-up). J Clin Periodontol. 2009;36: 1025–34.

27. Kakudate N, Morita M, Sugai M, Kawanami M. Systematic cognitive behavioral approach for oral hygiene instruction: a short-term study. Patient Educ Couns. 2009;74:191–6.

28. Godard A, Dufour T, Jeanne S. Application of self-regulation theory and motivational interview for improving oral hygiene: a randomized controlled trial. J Clin Periodontol. 2011;38:1099–105.

29. Brand VS, Bray KK, MacNeill S, Catley D, Williams K. Impact of single-session motivational interviewing on clinical outcomes following periodontal maintenance therapy. Int J Dent Hyg. 2013;11:134–41.

30. Stenman J, Lundgren J, Wennstrom JL, Ericsson JS, Abrahamsson KH. A single session of motivational interviewing as an additive means to improve adherence in periodontal infection control: a randomized controlled trial. J Clin Periodontol. 2012;39:947–54.

31. Tedesco LA, Keffer MA, Davis EL, Christersson LA. Effect of a social cognitive intervention on oral health status, behavior reports, and cognitions. J Periodontol. 1992;63:567–75.

32. Little SJ, Hollis JF, Stevens VJ, Mount K, Mullooly JP, Johnson BD. Effective group behavioral intervention for older periodontal patients. J Periodontal Res. 1997;32:315–25.

33. Frank RG. Primary care psychology. Washington DC: American Psychological Association; 2003.

34. Lundgren J, Wide Boman U. Multimodal cognitive behavioural treatment. In: Öst L-G, Skaret E, editors. Cognitive behaviour therapy for dental phobia and anxiety. West Sussex UK: Wiley-Blackwell; 2013. p. 109–18.

35. Kani E, Asimakopoulou K, Daly B, Hare J, Lewis J, Scambler S, et al. Characteristics of patients attending for cognitive behavioural therapy at one UK specialist unit for dental phobia and outcomes of treatment. Br Dent J. 2015;219:501–6.

36. Agdal ML, Raadal M, Ost LG, Skaret E. Quality-of-life before and after cognitive behavioral therapy (CBT) in patients with intra-oral injection phobia. Acta Odontol Scand. 2012;70:463–70.

37. Ramseier CA, Suvan JE. Behaviour change counselling for tobacco use cessation and promotion of healthy lifestyles: a systematic review. J Clin Periodontol. 2015;42 Suppl 16:S47–58.

38. Fanshawe TR, Halliwell W, Lindson N, Aveyard P, Livingstone-Banks J, Hartmann-Boyce J. Tobacco cessation interventions for young people. Cochrane Database Syst Rev. 2017;11:CD003289.

21

The role of three interleukin 10 gene polymorphisms (− 1082 A > G, − 819 C > T,− 592 A > C) in the risk of chronic and aggressive periodontitis: a meta-analysis and trial sequential analysis

Hey Chiann Wong[1†], Yuxuan Ooi[1†], Shaju Jacob Pulikkotil[1] and Cho Naing[2,3*] (iD)

Abstract

Background: Periodontitis is a major oral health problem and it is considered as one of the reasons for tooth loss in developing and developed nations. The objective of the current review was to investigate the association between *IL10* polymorphisms − 1082 A > G (rs1800896), -819C > T (rs1800871), − 592 A > C (rs1800872) and the risk of either chronic periodontitis or aggressive periodontitis.

Methods: This is a meta- analysis study, following the preferred reporting items for systematic reviews and meta-analyses (PRISMA). Relevant studies were searched in the health related electronic databases. Methodological quality of the included studies were assessed using the Newcastle-Ottawa Scale. For individual studies, odds ratio (OR) and its 95%confidence interval (CI) were calculated to assess the strength of association between *IL10* polymorphisms (− 1082 A > G, -819C > T, − 592 A > C) and the risk of periodontitis. For pooling of the estimates across studies included, the summary OR and its 95% CIs were calculated with random-effects model. The pooled estimates were done under four genetic models such as the allelic contrast model, the recessive model, the dominant model and the additive model. Trial sequential analysis (TSA) was done for estimation of the required information size for this meta-analysis study.

Results: Sixteen studies were identified for this review. The included studies were assessed to be of moderate to good methodological quality. A significant association between polymorphism of *IL10*−1082 A > G polymorphism and the risk of chronic periodontitis in the non-Asian populations was observed only in the recessive model (OR,1.42; 95% CI:1.11, 1.8,I^2: 43%). The significant associations between − 592 A > C polymorphism and the risk of aggressive periodontitis in the non-Asian populations were observed in particular genetic models such as allele contrast (OR, 4.34; 95%CI:1.87,10.07,I^2: 65%) and recessive models (OR, 2.1; 95% CI:1.16, 3.82,I^2: 0%). The TSA plot revealed that the required information size for evidence of effect was sufficient to draw a conclusion.

Conclusions: This meta-analysis suggested that the *IL10*−1082 A > G polymorphism was associated with chronic periodontitis CP risk in non-Asians. Thus, in order to further establish the associations between *IL10* (− 819 C > T, − 592 A > C) in Asian populations, future studies should include larger sample sizes with multi-ethnic groups.

* Correspondence: cho3699@gmail.com

†Hey Chiann Wong and Ooi Yuxuan contributed equally to this work.

2Institute for Research, Development and Innovation (IRDI), International Medical University, 5700 Kuala Lumpur, Malaysia

3Division of Tropical Heath and Medicine, James Cook University, Townsville, Australia

Full list of author information is available at the end of the article

Background

Periodontitis is defined as an inflammatory disease of supporting tissues of teeth caused by specific microorganisms or groups of specific microorganisms, resulting in progressive destruction of the periodontal ligament and alveolar bone with periodontal pocket formation, gingival recession or both [1]. There are two forms of periodontitis such as chronic periodontitis (CP) and aggressive periodontitis (AP). Severe periodontitis can result in loosening of teeth, leading to occasional pain or discomfort and impaired mastication and eventual tooth loss [2]. Periodontitis is a major oral health problem and it is considered as one of the reasons for tooth loss in developing and developed nations.

Worldwide, the prevalence of CP in the general adult population was reported to be 30–35%, with approximately 10–15% diagnosed with severe CP [3] with geographic variation. For instance, the estimated prevalence of CP and severe periodontitis among general population in Malaysia was 48.5%, and 18.2% respectively [4]. According to the National Health and Nutrition Examination Survey (NHANES) 2009–2010, the prevalence of periodontitis and severe periodontitis of adults aged 30 years and above in the United States were 47.2% and 8.5%, respectively [5].

Although the presence of microorganisms is crucial for the clinical status, host response to bacteria triggers the secretion of pro-inflammatory mediators, leading to extra cellular matrix metabolism and bone resorption in periodontitis [6, 7]. Interleukin (IL)10 is an immunoregulatory cytokine and down-regulates the Th1 driven pro-inflammatory response [8]. It is produced mainly by macrophages apart from numerous other cells such as Th2 cells, dendritic cells, B-cells, monocytes, neutrophils eosinophils and mast cells [9]. Studies have shown that dysregulation of IL10 is associated with an enhanced immunopathological response to infection as well as an increased risk for the development of many autoimmune diseases [10] and infections such as tuberculosis [11]. Although about 99% of human genes are shared across the same population, variations in sequence and single nucleotide polymorphisms (SNPs) may have significant predictive relevance. Several IL10 genes implicated to affect IL10 transcription and secretion include the three biallelic polymorphisms at position – 1082, – 819 and – 592 [12, 13]. There are molecular epidemiological studies that assessed the association between IL10 and the risk of developing periodontitis. These individual studies, however, showed conflicting results. Such inconsistency of the results may be attributed to small sample size, insufficient statistical power and ethnic diversity of the population. Taken together, the objective of the current review was to investigate the association between polymorphisms of IL10–1082 A > G (rs1800896), -819C > T (rs1800871), – 592 A > C(rs1800872) and the risk of either CP or AP.

Methods

The current study followed the preferred reporting items for systematic reviews and meta- analyses (PRISMA) [14] (Additional file 1).

Study search

Relevant studies were searched in the health-related electronic databases of PubMed, EMBASE, web of science and google scholar, with the combination of the keywords with Boolean operators: "periodontitis" OR "chronic periodontitis" OR "aggressive periodontitis" AND "interleukin-10" OR "IL10" OR "-1082 A/G". OR "-819 C > T" OR "-592 A > C".

The search was limited to the studies published in English and Chinese (abstract in English) from 1968 until March 2018. The references of retrieved articles and relevant reviews were checked for any additional studies.

Inclusion criteria

Human studies of any sample size that assessed periodontitis were included, if:

i) IL10–1082 A > G (rs1800896), 592 A > C (rs1800872) and/or – 819 C > T (rs1800871) were investigated.
ii) it was case-control or nested case-control design.
iii) periodontally healthy controls were included.
iv) genotype distribution in both cases and controls were available.

CP and AP in the current analysis were as defined in the primary studies. Studies, which did not meet the inclusion criteria were excluded. Studies based on family or sibling-pairs were also excluded.

Data extraction

Three investigators (HCW, YO, CN) individually checked the titles and abstracts, and then selected the relevant full-text articles, according to the inclusion criteria. The three investigators independently extracted data, using a piloted data extraction form. The following information were collected from each study: author, publication year, country, design (e.g. hospital-based study, population-based study), the number of cases and controls, the racial descent (Asian or non-Asian), clinical types of periodontitis, genotyping method and genotype/allele distribution in both cases and controls. Any discrepancy was resolved by discussion and consensus. If allele frequency was zero, then a value of 1 was added to all allele, following Laplace approximation [15].

Methodological quality assessment

The two investigators (HCW, YO) independently assessed the methodological quality of studies, using the Newcastle-Ottawa Scale (NOS) for quality assessment [16], with necessary modifications. The scores were based on three main aspects: the selection of the study groups (maximum 4 points: whether the case definition was adequate with independent validation; whether the patients were consecutive or obviously representative series of cases; whether the controls were population-based; whether the controls were persons without history of periodontitis); the comparability of the groups (maximum 2 points: whether cases and controls were matched for age and gender; whether cases and controls were matched for region or ethnicity); and the ascertainment of exposure (maximum 3 points: whether the ascertainment of exposure was secure record; whether the same method of ascertainment was applied for cases and controls; whether the same non-response rate was reported for both groups). A total score for each study can vary from 0 (worst) to 9 (best). Studies scoring ≤4 were regarded as low quality, while a score of ≥7 was considered as a high-quality study. Any discrepancy between the two investigators was resolved by discussion and consensus.

Statistical analysis

Hardy-Weinberg Equilibrium (HWE) in the controls was tested, using the exact test for goodness-of-fit and $p > 0.05$ was regarded as consistent with HWE [17]. The strength of the association between $IL10$ (− 1082 A > G,-819 C > T, − 592 A/C) and the risk of periodontitis (CP or AP) was estimated using odds ratio (OR) and its 95% confidence interval (CIs). Heterogeneity was statistically assessed using the I^2 test. The I^2 test values describes the percentage of total variation across studies that is attributable to the heterogeneity rather than chance. I^2 values greater than 50% is considered as substantial heterogeneity [18]. For pooling of the estimates across studies included, the summary ORs and corresponding 95% CIs were calculated with random-effects model (The Der Simonian and Laird method) in the presence of between–study heterogeneity of the studies. Otherwise, fixed-effect model (the Mental-Haenszel method) was used. We estimated the pooled ORs and its 95% CIs in four genetic models: − 592 A > C the allelic contrast model (A vs C), the recessive model (AA vs CA + CC), the dominant model (AA+CA vs CC) and the additive model (AA vs CC). As for − 1082 A > G the allelic contrast model (A vs G), the recessive model (AA vs GA + GG), the dominant model (AA+GA vs GG) and the additive model (AA vs GG). As for − 819 C > T the allelic contrast model (T vs C), the recessive model (TT vs CT + CC), the dominant model (TT + CT vs CC) and

the additive model (TT vs CC) was used. Analysis was further stratified by the clinical forms of periodontitis (CP, AP) and by ethnic decent. To assess the stability of results, the sensitivity analysis was done with leave-one-out meta-analysis by sequential omission of individual studies [19]. We assessed the publication bias by visualizing funnel plots [20, 21].

Trial sequential analysis (TSA), an approach that adjust for random error risk, was done for estimation of the required information size [22]. It is classified as 'potentially spurious evidence of effect', if the cumulative Z-curve did not cross the monitoring boundaries or as 'firm evidence of effect', if the cumulative Z-curve crossed the monitoring boundaries [23].

Meta-analysis was done with RevMan 5.3 (The Cochrane collaboration, Copenhagen) and Leave-one-out meta-analysis was with *meta* package (*metabin* command) in *R* 3.4.3 software (The *R* Foundation). TSA was done with TSA version 0.9 beta (Copenhagen Trial Unit, Centre for Clinical Intervention Research, Copenhagen).

Results

Figure 1 provides a four-phase study selection process in the present meta-analysis study. A total of 132 studies were identified in the initial search. After the title and abstract screening, 29 full- text articles were retrieved. Of these, a final of 16 articles (with 1557 cases and 1447 controls) were identified for this review [24–39]. All except one study were published in English language. One study was published in Chinese language, but provided English language abstract [27]. The studies included used different criteria for diagnosis of periodontitis such as clinical criteria (44%,7 studies), 1999 classification of periodontal diseases and conditions (25%,4 studies), clinical criteria and X-ray verification (19%, 3 studies) and criteria of the American Academy of Periodontology (13%, 2 studies).

The main characteristics of the studies identified for this review are presented in Additional file 2. Summary of the 13 excluded studies [12, 40–51] are provided in Additional file 3. These 16 studies included were conducted in nine countries such as eight single studies from China [27], Germany [29], Macedonia [33], Norway [36], Peru [34], Taiwan [30], Turkey [31] and the United Kingdom [25], three studies from Iran [26, 33, 39] and six studies from Brazil [24, 28, 30, 35, 37, 38]. Of these sixteen, six studies assessed all three candidate SNPs [24, 30, 32, 36–38] in the risk of CP/AP, while thirteen and nine studies assessed − 1082 A > G, and − 819 C > T or − 592 A > C, respectively. All these studies recruited healthy controls. All, except two studies [32, 34] were consistent with HWE. All these 16 studies were with moderate to good methodological quality, based on the NOS criteria (Additional file 4).

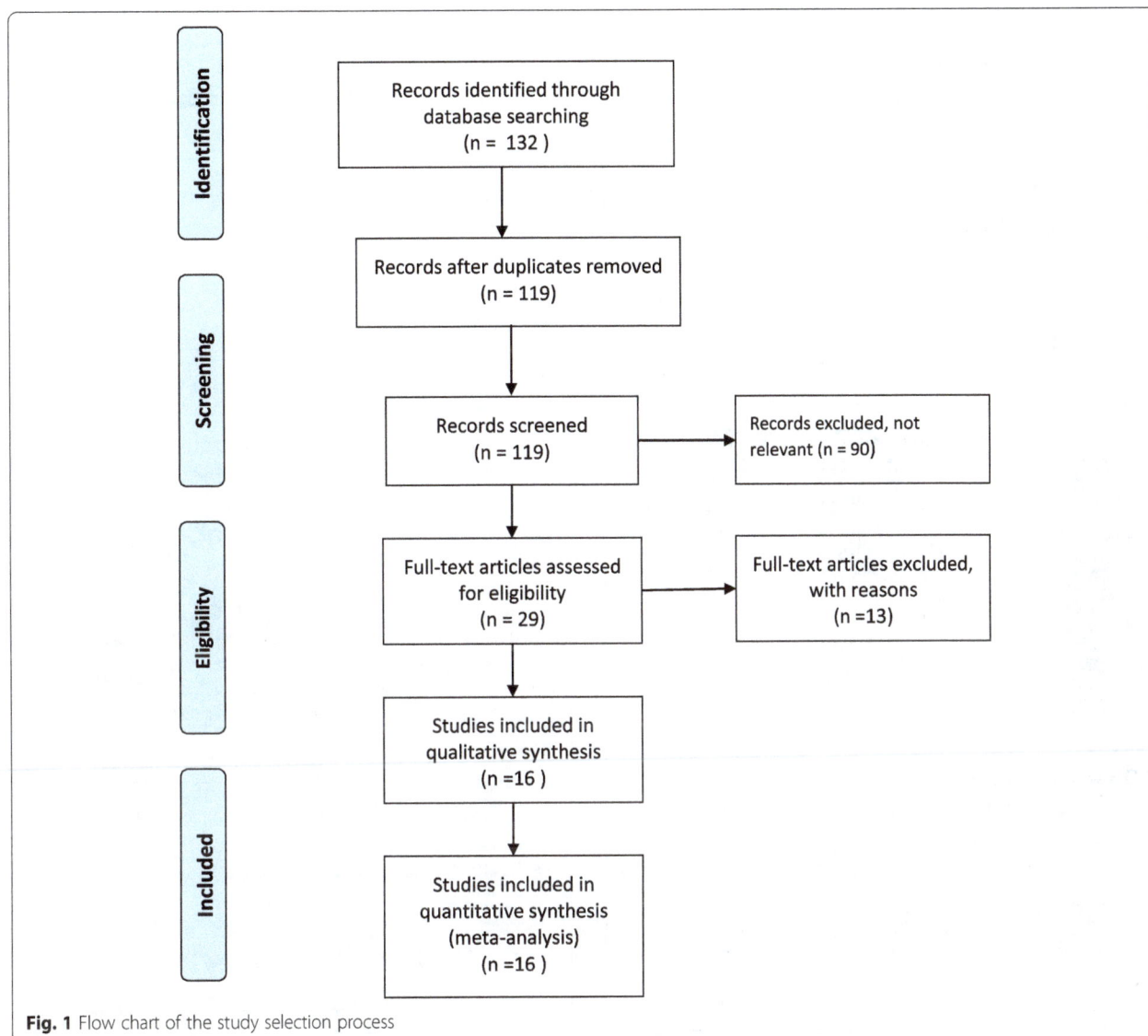

Fig. 1 Flow chart of the study selection process

Quantitative estimates

Overall, there was statistical significant associations between *IL10*–1082 A > G polymorphism and the risk of AP in a subgroup of the non-Asian population under the recessive model (OR,1.42;95% CI,1.11–1.8,I^2:43%) (Fig. 2). For *IL10*–592 A > C, only the non-Asian populations under the allele contrast model (C vs A) (OR,4.34; 95%CI:1.87–10.07, I^2:65%) and the recessive model (OR,2.1;95% CI,1.16–3.82,I^2:0%) showed significant relationship between this SNP and the risk of AP (Fig. 3). For *IL10*–819C > T, there was no significant associations between this SNP and the risk of CP/AP in any population groups under any of four genetic models (Fig. 4). Summary of the evaluation of the three candidate SNPs stratified by population groups and clinical types under four genetic models are provided in Additional file 5.

Sensitivity analysis

To assess the influence of individual data on the pooled ORs, leave-one-out meta-analysis was performed. The overall estimate of recessive model of *IL10*–1082 A > G remained statistical significance, while omitting any single study (Fig. 5). This indicates that the results are stable. This was true for all other models with the 3 candidate SNPs. As an example, a subgroup analysis stratified by diagnostic criteria was done on CP patients with – 1082 A > G under recessive model: CP patients diagnosed only by clinical criteria was significantly associated with this SNP (Additional file 6). This implied that the diagnostic criteria for CP had impact on the direction of association. Begg's and Egger's test showed no evidence of publication bias in all analyses concerning *IL10* (– 1082 A > G, – 819 C > T, 592C > A) polymorphisms. An example illustration

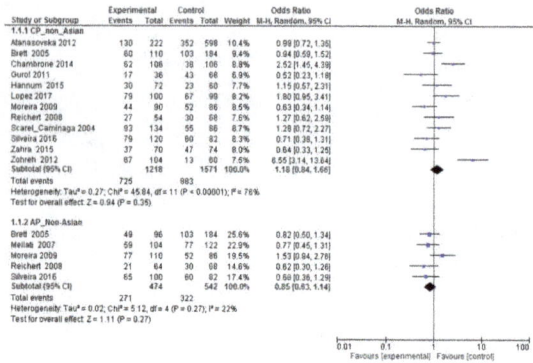

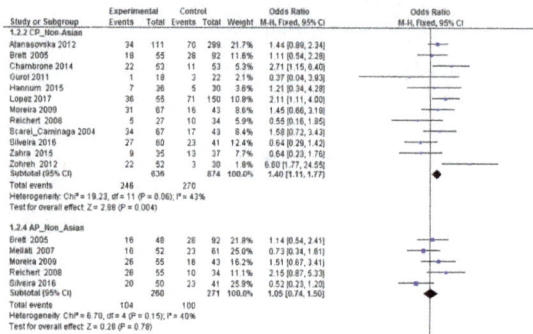

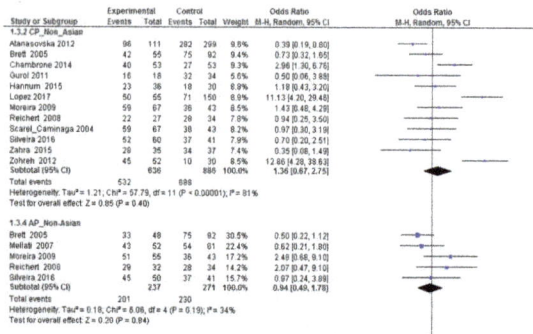

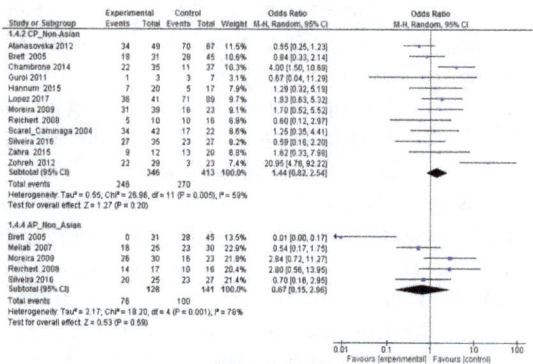

Fig. 2 Forest plot of − 1082 A > G. **a** Allele genetic model, **b** Recessive model, **c** Dominant model, **d** additive model

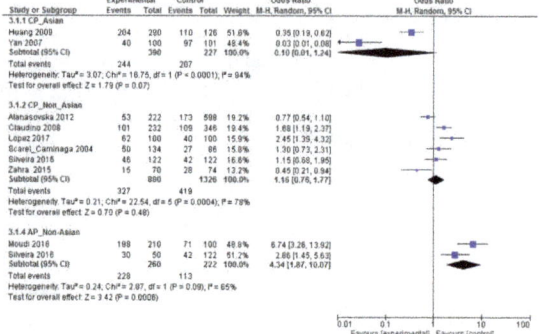

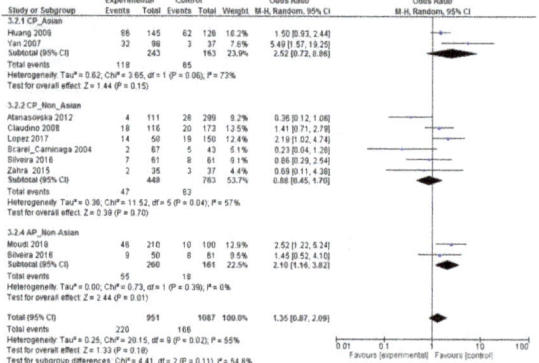

Fig. 3 Forest plot of − 592 A > C. **a** Allele genetic model, **b** Recessive model, **c** Dominant model, **d** additive model

A Allelic model (T vs C)

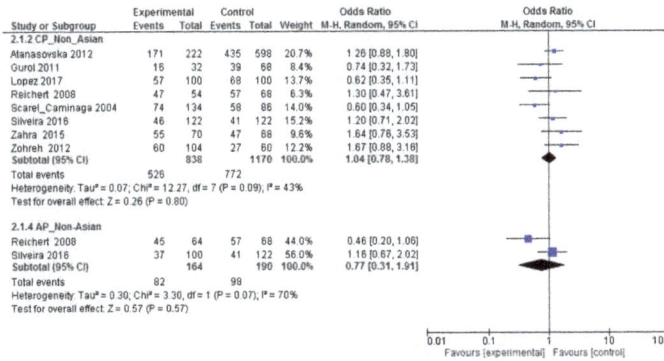

Study or Subgroup	Experimental Events	Total	Control Events	Total	Weight	Odds Ratio M-H, Random, 95% CI
2.1.2 CP_Non_Asian						
Atanasovska 2012	171	222	435	598	20.7%	1.26 [0.88, 1.80]
Gurol 2011	15	32	39	68	8.4%	0.74 [0.32, 1.73]
Lopez 2017	57	100	68	100	13.7%	0.62 [0.35, 1.11]
Reichert 2008	47	54	57	68	6.3%	1.30 [0.47, 3.61]
Scarel_Caminaga 2004	74	134	58	86	14.0%	0.60 [0.34, 1.05]
Silveira 2016	46	122	41	122	15.2%	1.20 [0.71, 2.02]
Zahra 2015	55	70	47	68	9.6%	1.64 [0.78, 3.53]
Zohreh 2012	60	104	27	60	12.2%	1.67 [0.88, 3.16]
Subtotal (95% CI)		838		1170	100.0%	1.04 [0.78, 1.38]
Total events	526		772			

Heterogeneity: Tau² = 0.07; Chi² = 12.27, df = 7 (P = 0.09); I² = 43%
Test for overall effect: Z = 0.26 (P = 0.80)

2.1.4 AP_Non_Asian						
Reichert 2008	45	64	57	88	44.0%	0.46 [0.20, 1.06]
Silveira 2016	37	100	41	122	56.0%	1.16 [0.67, 2.02]
Subtotal (95% CI)		164		190	100.0%	0.77 [0.31, 1.91]
Total events	82		98			

Heterogeneity: Tau² = 0.30; Chi² = 3.30, df = 1 (P = 0.07); I² = 70%
Test for overall effect: Z = 0.57 (P = 0.57)

B Recessive model (TT vs CT +CC)

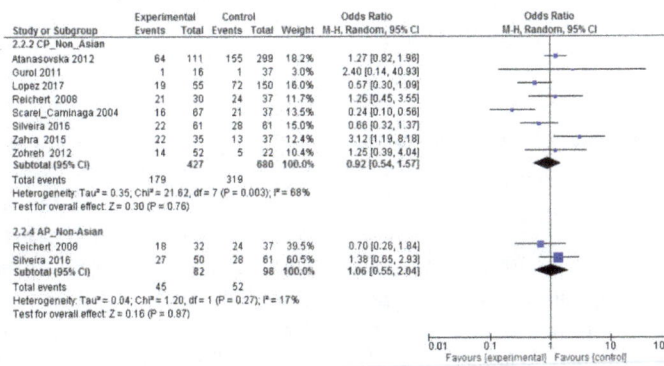

Study or Subgroup	Experimental Events	Total	Control Events	Total	Weight	Odds Ratio M-H, Random, 95% CI
2.2.2 CP_Non_Asian						
Atanasovska 2012	64	111	155	299	18.2%	1.27 [0.82, 1.96]
Gurol 2011	1	16	1	37	3.0%	2.40 [0.14, 40.93]
Lopez 2017	19	55	72	150	16.0%	0.57 [0.30, 1.09]
Reichert 2008	21	30	24	37	11.7%	1.26 [0.45, 3.55]
Scarel_Caminaga 2004	16	67	21	37	13.5%	0.24 [0.10, 0.56]
Silveira 2016	22	61	28	61	15.0%	0.66 [0.32, 1.37]
Zahra 2015	22	35	13	37	12.4%	3.12 [1.19, 8.18]
Zohreh 2012	14	52	5	22	10.4%	1.25 [0.39, 4.04]
Subtotal (95% CI)		427		680	100.0%	0.92 [0.54, 1.57]
Total events	179		319			

Heterogeneity: Tau² = 0.35; Chi² = 21.62, df = 7 (P = 0.003); I² = 68%
Test for overall effect: Z = 0.30 (P = 0.76)

2.2.4 AP_Non-Asian						
Reichert 2008	18	32	24	37	39.5%	0.70 [0.26, 1.84]
Silveira 2016	27	50	28	61	60.5%	1.38 [0.65, 2.93]
Subtotal (95% CI)		82		98	100.0%	1.06 [0.55, 2.04]
Total events	45		52			

Heterogeneity: Tau² = 0.04; Chi² = 1.20, df = 1 (P = 0.27); I² = 17%
Test for overall effect: Z = 0.16 (P = 0.87)

C Dominant model (TT+CT vs CC)

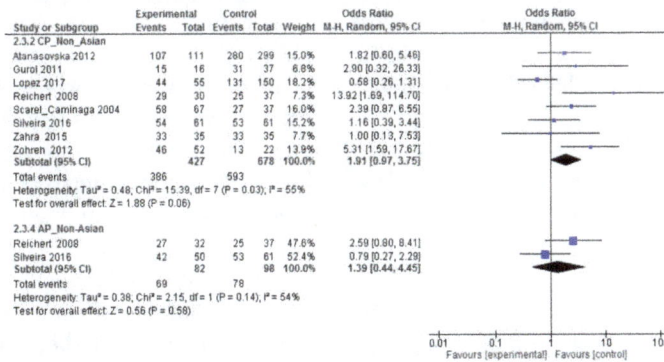

Study or Subgroup	Experimental Events	Total	Control Events	Total	Weight	Odds Ratio M-H, Random, 95% CI
2.3.2 CP_Non_Asian						
Atanasovska 2012	107	111	280	299	15.0%	1.82 [0.60, 5.46]
Gurol 2011	15	16	31	37	6.8%	2.90 [0.32, 26.33]
Lopez 2017	44	55	131	150	18.2%	0.58 [0.26, 1.31]
Reichert 2008	29	30	25	37	7.3%	13.92 [1.69, 114.70]
Scarel_Caminaga 2004	58	67	27	37	16.0%	2.39 [0.87, 6.55]
Silveira 2016	54	61	53	61	15.2%	1.16 [0.39, 3.44]
Zahra 2015	33	35	33	35	7.7%	1.00 [0.13, 7.53]
Zohreh 2012	46	52	13	22	13.9%	5.31 [1.59, 17.67]
Subtotal (95% CI)		427		678	100.0%	1.91 [0.97, 3.75]
Total events	386		593			

Heterogeneity: Tau² = 0.48; Chi² = 15.39, df = 7 (P = 0.03); I² = 55%
Test for overall effect: Z = 1.88 (P = 0.06)

2.3.4 AP_Non-Asian						
Reichert 2008	27	32	25	37	47.6%	2.59 [0.80, 8.41]
Silveira 2016	42	50	53	61	52.4%	0.79 [0.27, 2.29]
Subtotal (95% CI)		82		98	100.0%	1.39 [0.44, 4.45]
Total events	69		78			

Heterogeneity: Tau² = 0.38; Chi² = 2.15, df = 1 (P = 0.14); I² = 54%
Test for overall effect: Z = 0.56 (P = 0.58)

D Additive model (TT vs CC)

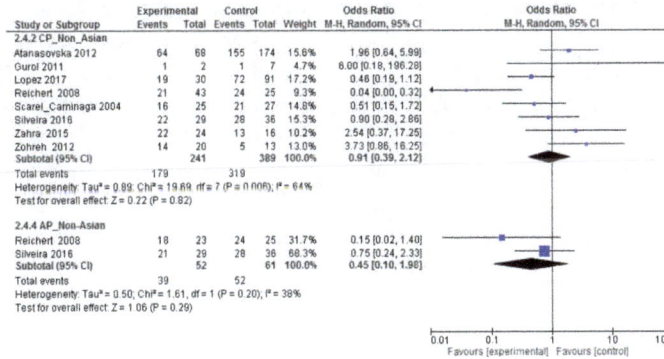

Study or Subgroup	Experimental Events	Total	Control Events	Total	Weight	Odds Ratio M-H, Random, 95% CI
2.4.2 CP_Non_Asian						
Atanasovska 2012	64	68	155	174	15.6%	1.96 [0.64, 5.99]
Gurol 2011	1	2	1	7	4.7%	6.00 [0.18, 196.28]
Lopez 2017	19	30	72	91	17.2%	0.46 [0.19, 1.12]
Reichert 2008	21	43	24	25	9.3%	0.04 [0.00, 0.32]
Scarel_Caminaga 2004	16	25	21	27	14.8%	0.51 [0.15, 1.72]
Silveira 2016	22	29	28	36	15.3%	0.90 [0.28, 2.86]
Zahra 2015	22	24	13	16	10.2%	2.54 [0.37, 17.25]
Zohreh 2012	14	20	5	13	13.0%	3.73 [0.86, 16.25]
Subtotal (95% CI)		241		389	100.0%	0.91 [0.39, 2.12]
Total events	179		319			

Heterogeneity: Tau² = 0.89; Chi² = 19.69, df = 7 (P = 0.006); I² = 64%
Test for overall effect: Z = 0.22 (P = 0.82)

2.4.4 AP_Non-Asian						
Reichert 2008	18	23	24	25	31.7%	0.15 [0.02, 1.40]
Silveira 2016	21	29	28	36	68.3%	0.75 [0.24, 2.33]
Subtotal (95% CI)		52		61	100.0%	0.45 [0.10, 1.98]
Total events	39		52			

Heterogeneity: Tau² = 0.50; Chi² = 1.61, df = 1 (P = 0.20); I² = 38%
Test for overall effect: Z = 1.06 (P = 0.29)

Fig. 4 Forest plot of − 819 C > T. **a** Allele genetic model, **b** Recessive model, **c** Dominant model, **d** additive model

Study	Experimental Events	Total	Control Events	Total	Odds Ratio	OR	95%-CI	Weight (fixed)	Weight (random)
Atanasovska 2012	34	111	70	299		1.44	[0.89; 2.34]	23.9%	15.4%
Brett 2005	18	55	28	92		1.11	[0.54; 2.28]	10.9%	10.8%
Lopes 2017	36	55	71	150		2.11	[1.11; 4.00]	13.6%	12.1%
Gurol 2011	1	18	3	22		0.37	[0.04; 3.93]	1.0%	1.7%
Chambrone 2014	22	53	11	53		2.71	[1.15; 6.40]	7.6%	8.7%
Hannum 2015	7	36	5	30		1.21	[0.34; 4.28]	3.5%	5.0%
Moreira 2009	31	67	16	43		1.45	[0.66; 3.18]	9.1%	9.8%
Reichert 2008	5	27	10	34		0.55	[0.16; 1.85]	3.8%	5.3%
Scarel-Caminaga 2004	34	67	17	43		1.58	[0.72; 3.43]	9.3%	9.9%
Silveira 2016	27	60	23	41		0.64	[0.29; 1.42]	8.8%	9.5%
Zahra 2015	9	31	13	41		0.88	[0.32; 2.44]	5.4%	7.0%
Zohreh 2012	22	52	3	30		6.60	[1.77; 24.55]	3.2%	4.7%
Fixed effect model		632		878		1.41	[1.11; 1.78]	100.0%	--
Random effects model						1.38	[1.01; 1.91]	--	100.0%

Heterogeneity: $I^2 = 38\%$, $\tau^2 = 0.1119$, $p = 0.09$

0.1   0.5 1 2   10

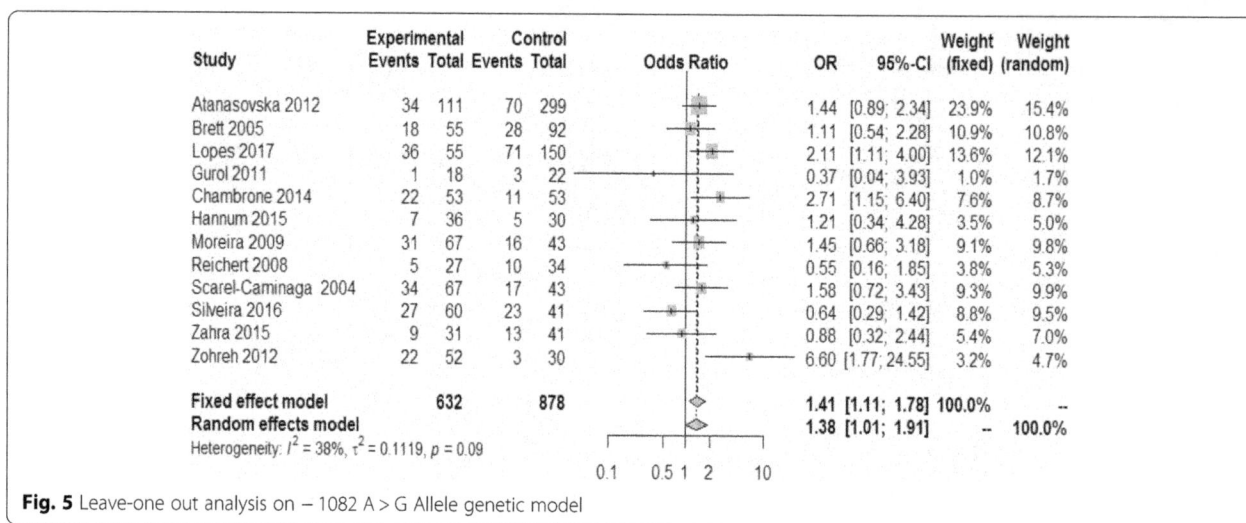

Fig. 5 Leave-one out analysis on – 1082 A > G Allele genetic model

with *IL10*–1082 A > G under dominant model is shown in Additional file 7.

TSA

We performed TSA with studies on *IL10*–1082 A > G in CP that followed HWE. We used an overall 5% risk of a type I error and 20% risk of a type II error (power of 80%). The cumulative z-curve crossed the traditional boundary and the trial sequential monitoring boundary and reached the required information size, suggesting there is no need for more evidence to establish additional study of – 1082 A > G in CP among the non-Asian population (Additional file 8).

Discussion

The current study provides evidence on the association between *IL10* (– 1082 A > G, – 819 C > T, – 592 A > C) and the risk of CP/AP, and the major observations are as follows;

i. A significant association between – 1082 A > G polymorphism and the risk of CP in the non-Asian populations was observed only in the recessive model.

ii. In subgroups with ethnicity, the significant associations between – 592 C > A polymorphism and the risk of AP in the non-Asian populations were observed in particular genetic models such as allele contrast and recessive models.

iii. The TSA plot revealed that the required information size for evidence of effect was sufficient to draw a firm conclusion.

The numbers of inflammatory leucocytes that express the anti-inflammatory IL10- cytokine are much more widely distributed than those that express the pro-inflammatory IL6- cytokine and TNF-a- cytokine

[52]. The pooled analysis of 11 studies in this review showed a significant association between -1082A > G and the risk of CP in the non-Asian population under recessive model and this estimate was stable even with sensitivity analysis. Therefore, the findings suggest a possible role of racial difference in genetic backgrounds. Genotypic differences in cytokine genes are differently inherited to ethnically different populations [24]. The lack of statistical significance in the remaining genetic models might partly be due to the relatively small sample size. This was indirectly supported by an earlier review on this SNP, which included eight studies on patients with CP had reported no significance association with -1082A > G under any of four genetic models [53]. Another meta-analysis in this field, which included nine case-control studies had also reported no significance association with -1082A > G under any genetic models [54]. In subsequent analysis of patients with AP, no significant association was found with this SNP and this also might partly be related to limited size of samples as relatively few number of studies were assessed for this clinical form.

A significant association between – 592 A > C polymorphism and the risk of AP in allele contrast and recessive model indicated the prominent role of AA in the risk development. Although environmental factors are considered to be important in the establishment of periodontitis, individuals reared or living in similar environments may manifest significantly different disease patterns [55]. The pooled results showed no significant association between – 819 C > T and the risk of CP/AP in the non-Asian population under all four genetic models could also be related to ethnical homogeneity of the studied populations [34], the limited size of samples or different in selection criteria of patients/controls. The – 819 C > T SNP lies within a DNA motif forming a putative oestrogen responsive element [56]. Hence, the dominant proportion of females or males in the primary studies was likely to affect the lack of associations in this review.

The reason why different association was observed in different SNPs remained unclear. One possible explanation is the differences in the frequencies of the polymorphisms among diverse ethnicity, which may partly give rise to heterogeneity. Moreover, the complex nature of the disease, which is the result of an interplay between immunological, microbiological and environmental factors, may be the reason for that no difference [40]. Smoking habit represents an additional factor involved in periodontal disease progression that could mask the effects of *IL10* SNPs on periodontitis outcome [44]. Additionally, gene-gene interactions along with environmental factors could also contribute to the complexity of genetic effect. Hence, variation in single genetic locus is often insufficient to predict risk of disease. For instance, there might be some extent of interaction with *IL10* (− 1082 A > G, − 819 C > T, 592 C > A) and other genes (gen-gen interaction/synergism).

It is postulated that polymorphisms in genes that codify mediators involved in the upstream positions of inflammatory-immune response pathways (such as IL-10 cytokine), which modulate a broad range of factors, may be relevant to periodontitis outcome [28, 57].

Genotypic differences in cytokine genes are differently inherited to ethnically different populations [24]. Individuals who are high producers of IL-10 cytokine might be more protected against CP due to its anti-inflammatory role. Therefore, a genetically determined increase of anti-inflammatory IL-10 cytokine would down regulate the immune response against periodontopathogenic bacteria [41, 51].

On the other side, polymorphisms in downstream genes (such as metalloproteinase and osteoclastogenesis), whose products present a narrow action in the pathways involved in periodontal tissue destruction, would play a minor role (or even do not play a significant role) in the development of periodontal diseases [28]. For the development of AP, low interleukin-10 levels lead to an enhanced release of pro-inflammatory cytokines, such as tumor necrosis factor-alpha, which have been implicated in alveolar bone loss [29, 58].

Study limitations

There are some limitations in the present study. Only two studies included in this meta-analysis (11.7%) were from the Asia population. A small sample size in the Asian population subgroup analyses may not be the representative of the population. Hence, a selection bias with geographical imbalance is a concern. Our analysis was done with the unadjusted raw data provided in the primary studies, in which patients might have some common factors

(i.e. age, gender, diets, smoking habits, diabetes). An earlier meta-analysis had highlighted that the inclusion of both smoking and non-smoking subjects in the primary studies can be an additional source of variability [54]. Stratified analysis by age group, smoking habits, oral hygiene habits or presence of comorbidity were not possible due to limited data. Hence, the findings could be confounded with these common factors. A stratification analysis on − 1082 A > G in the CP patients documented that the estimates could vary with the type of diagnosis criteria. If cases and controls have been genotyped in separate batches in the primary studies, differential misclassification of exposure is a concern. The sample sizes in most of the included studies were relatively small and were under power to detect statistically significant differences between the cases and controls. Meta-analysis, however, is a retrospective synthesis of published studies and power analysis is not applicable and type II errors are expected to be less common in a meta-analysis than in single studies [18, 19]. The manifestation of many systemic diseases which may lead to compromised host function should also be considered. For example, diabetes and rheumatoid arthritis are examples of diseases which may have a genetic component and may have enhanced periodontal breakdown as a secondary feature. In the presence of publication bias in this analysis, non-published studies and/or studies in other language might have been missed in the current review. Moreover, there might be some extent of interaction with *IL10* (− 1082 A > G, − 819 C > T, *IL10* 592 A > C) and other genes (gen-gen interaction/synergism). Hence, findings in the current meta-analysis should be interpreted with caution.

Implications

Interventions with the manipulation of anti-inflammatory cytokines have been suggested as adjuvants for treating periodontal disease. The efficacy of anti-cytokine biotherapies in patients with inflammatory diseases is a proof that blocking the effects of a cytokine can slow down the disease process [59]. Investigating the association of the *IL10* gene polymorphisms with periodontitis susceptibility may promote our understanding of its pathogenesis and explain individual differences in the risk.

Conclusions

Findings suggest that the *IL10*–1082 A > G polymorphism was associated with CP risk in non- Asians. To further establish the associations between *IL10* (819 C > T, 592 A > C), future studies with larger sample sizes and multi-ethnic sample groups more with Asian population are required.

Abbreviations

AP: Aggressive periodontitis; CI: Confidence interval; CP: Chronic periodontitis; HWE: Hardy-Weinberg Equilibrium; IL: Interleukin; OR: Odds ratio; PRISMA: Preferred reporting items for systematic reviews and meta-analyses; SNP: Single nucleotide polymorphisms; TSA: Trial sequential analysis

Acknowledgements

The authors thank the patients and researchers of the primary studies. We are grateful to the anonymous reviewers and editors for the comments provided and valuable inputs to improve the quality of manuscript. We thank our institutions for allowing us to perform this study. We are grateful to Professor Frederick Smales (IMU, Malaysia) for helping with the English editing of this manuscript.

Funding

International Medical University, Malaysia.

Authors' contributions

CN: conceptualized and designed, collected data, analysed, interpreted the results and draft and revised the manuscript, HCW and OY: participated in its design, collected data, assisted in statistical analysis, interpreted the results and helped to draft and revise the manuscript. PSJ: interpreted the results and helped to revise the manuscript. All authors approved the final manuscript for submission.

Competing interests

The authors declare that they have no competing interests.

Author details

[1]School of Dentistry, International Medical University, Kuala Lumpur, Malaysia. [2]Institute for Research, Development and Innovation (IRDI), International Medical University, 5700 Kuala Lumpur, Malaysia. [3]Division of Tropical Heath and Medicine, James Cook University, Townsville, Australia.

References

1. Newman MG, Takei H, Klokkevold PR, Carranza FA. Carranza's clinical periodontology. Elsevier Health Sciences. 11th Edn. 2011.
2. Pihlstrom BL, Michalowicz BS, Johnson NW. Periodontal diseases. Lancet. 2005;366:1809–20.
3. WHO. The WHO global oral health data bank. Geneva: World Health Organization; 2007.
4. NOHSA. National oral health survey in adults 2010. Putrajaya: OHD MOH: Oral Health Division Minitsry of Health; 2013.
5. Eke P, Dye B, Wei L, Thornton-Evans G, Genco R. Prevalence of periodontitis in adults in the United States: 2009 and 2010. J Dent Res. 2012;91:914–20.
6. Armitage GC. Development of a classification system for periodontal diseases and conditions. Ann Periodontal. 1999;4:1–6.
7. Kinane D, Hart T. Genes and gene polymorphisms associated with periodontal disease. Crit Rev Oral Biol Med. 2003;14:430–49.
8. Ouyang W, Rutz S, Crellin NK, Valdez PA, Hymowitz SG. Regulation and functions of the IL-10 family of cytokines in inflammation and disease. Annu Rev Immunol. 2011;29:71–109.
9. Moore KW, de Waal Malefyt R, Coffman RL, O'Garra A. Interleukin-10 and the interleukin-10 receptor. Annu Rev Immunol. 2001;19:683–765.
10. Iyer SS, Cheng G. Role of interleukin 10 transcriptional regulation in inflammation and autoimmune disease. Crit Rev Immunol. 2012;32:23–63.
11. Gao X, Chen J, Tong Z, Yang G, Yao Y, Xu F, et al. Interleukin-10 promoter gene polymorphisms and susceptibility to tuberculosis: a meta-analysis. PLoS One. 2015;10(6):e0127496.
12. Karhukorpi J, Laitinen T, Karttunen R, Tiilikainen AS. The functionally important IL-10 promoter polymorphism (−1082G→A) is not a major genetic regulator in recurrent spontaneous abortions. Mol Hum Reprod. 2001;7:201–3.
13. Kilpinen S, Huhtala H, Hurme M. The combination of the interleukin-1alpha (IL-1alpha-889) genotype and the interleukin-10 (IL-10 ATA) haplotype is associated with increased interleukin-10 (IL-10) plasma levels in healthy individuals. Eur Cytokine Netw. 2002;13:66–71.
14. Moher D, Liberati A, Tetzlaff J, Altman DG. Preferred reporting items for systematic reviews and meta-analyses: the PRISMA statement. Int J Surg. 2010;8:336–41.
15. Berthold VMR, Höppner BC, Klawonn F. How to intelligently make sense of real data, descriptive statistics: guide to intelligent data analysis. Germany: Springer; 2010. p. 315.
16. Wells BS GA, O'Connell D, Peterson J, Welch V, Losos MP. The Newcastle-Ottawa scale (NOS) for assessing the quality of nonrandomised studies in meta-analyses 2014 (http://www.ohri.ca/programs/clinical_epidemiology/oxford.asp). Accessed 12 July 2018.
17. Guo SW, Thompson EA. Performing the exact test of Hardy-Weinberg proportion for multiple alleles. Biometrics. 1992;48:361–72.
18. Higgins J, Thompson SG. Quantifying heterogeneity in a meta-analysis. Stat Med. 2002;21:1539–58.
19. Higgins J. Cochrane handbook for systematic reviews of interventions. Version 5.1. 0 [updated March 2011]. The Cochrane Collaboration. www.cochrane-handbook.org. Accessed 12 July 2018. 2011.
20. Egger M, Davey Smith G, Schneider M, Minder C. Bias in meta-analysis detected by a simple, graphical test. BMJ. 1997;315:629–34.
21. Sterne JA, Egger M. Funnel plots for detecting bias in meta-analysis: guidelines on choice of axis. J Clin Epidemiol. 2001;54:1046–55.
22. Thorlund K, Wetterslev J, Brok J, Imberger G, Gluud G. User manual for trial sequential analysis (TSA). Copenhagen: Copenhagen Trial Unit, Centre for Clinical Intervention Research; 2011. p. 1–115.
23. Brok J, Thorlund K, Wetterslev J, Gluud C. Apparently conclusive meta-analyses may be inconclusive - trial sequential analysis adjustment of random error risk due to repetitive testing of accumulating data in apparently conclusive neonatal meta-analyses. Int J Epidemiol. 2009;38:287–98.
24. Scarel-Caminaga RM, Trevilatto PC, Souza AP, Brito RB, Camargo LE, Line SR. Interleukin 10 gene promoter polymorphisms are associated with chronic periodontitis. J Clin Periodontol. 2004;31:443–8.
25. Brett P, Zygogianni P, Griffiths G, Tomaz M, Parkar M, D'Aiuto F, et al. Functional gene polymorphisms in aggressive and chronic periodontitis. J Dent Res. 2005;84:1149–53.
26. Mellati E, Arab HR, Tavakkol-Afshari J, Ebadian AR, Radvar M. Analysis of −1082 IL-10 gene polymorphism in Iranian patients with generalized aggressive periodontitis. Med Sci Monit. 2007;13:CR510–4.
27. Claudino M, Trombone AP, Cardoso CR, Ferreira SB Jr, Martins W Jr, Assis GF, et al. The broad effects of the functional IL-10 promoter-592 polymorphism: modulation of IL-10, TIMP-3, and OPG expression and their association with periodontal disease outcome. J Leukoc Biol. 2008;84:1565–73.
28. Reichert S, Machulla H, Klapproth J, Zimmermann U, Reichert Y, Gläser C, et al. The interleukin-10 promoter haplotype ATA is a putative risk factor for aggressive periodontitis. J Periodontal Res. 2008;43:40–7.
29. Hu K, Huang K, Ho Y, Lin Y, Ho K, Wu Y, et al. Interleukin-10 (−592 C/A) and interleukin-12B (16974 A/C) gene polymorphisms and the interleukin-10 ATA haplotype are associated with periodontitis in a Taiwanese population. J Periodontal Res. 2009;44:378–85.
30. Moreira PR, Costa JE, Gomez RS, Gollob KJ, Dutra WO. TNFA and IL10 gene polymorphisms are not associated with periodontitis in Brazilians. Open Dent J. 2009;3:184–90.
31. Gurol C, Kazazoglu E, Dabakoglu B, Korachi M. A comparative study of the role of cytokine polymorphisms interleukin-10 and tumor necrosis factor alpha in susceptibility to implant failure and chronic periodontitis. Int J Oral Maxillofac Implants. 2011;26:955–60.
32. Atanasovska-Stojanovska A, Trajkov D, Popovska M, Spiroski M. IL10 -1082, IL10 -819 and IL10 -592 polymorphisms are associated with chronic periodontitis in a Macedonian population. Hum Immunol. 2012;73:753–8.

33. Heidari Z, Hooshmand B, Hajilooi M, Kadkhodazadeh M. Study of IL-10, IL-18 polymorphisms in the sulfur agent patients with and without periodontitis. J Periodontol Implant. Dent. 2013;5:23–8.

34. Chambrone L, Ascarza A, Guerrero ME, Pannuti C, de la Rosa M, Salinas-Prieto E, et al. Association of −1082 interleukin-10 gene polymorphism in Peruvian adults with chronic periodontitis. Med Oral Patol Oral Cir Bucal. 2014;19:e569–73.

35. Hannum R, Godoy FR, da Cruz AZ, Vieira TC, Minasi LB, de Silva D, de Silva CC, et al. Lack of association between IL-10 -1082G/A polymorphism and chronic periodontal disease in adults. Genet Mol Res. 2015;14:17828–33.

36. Zahra A, Jorgensen JJ, Kristoffersen KSk AK, Zlatko D. Polymorphisms in the interleukin-10 gene and chronic periodontitis in patients with atherosclerotic and aortic aneurysmal vascular diseases. J Oral Microbiol. 2015;7:1. https://doi.org/10.3402/jom.v7.26051.

37. Silveira VR, Pigossi SC, Scarel-Caminaga RM, Cirelli JA, Rego R, Nogueira NA. Analysis of polymorphisms in interleukin 10, NOS2A, and *ESR2* genes in chronic and aggressive periodontitis. Braz Oral Res. 2016;30:e105.

38. Lopes CB, Barroso RFF, Burbano RMR, Garcia PA, Pinto PDDC, Santos NPCD, et al. Effect of ancestry on interleukin-10 haplotypes in chronic periodontitis. Front Biosci (Elite Ed). 2017;9:276–85.

39. Moudi B, Heidari Z, Mahmoudzadeh-Sagheb H, Moudi M. Analysis of interleukin-10 gene polymorphisms in patients with chronic periodontitis and healthy controls. Dent Res J. 2018;15:71–9.

40. Gonzales JR, Michel J, Diete A, Herrmann J, Bödeker R, Meyle J. Analysis of genetic polymorphisms at the interleukin-10 loci in aggressive and chronic periodontitis. J Clin Periodontol. 2002;29:816–22.

41. Babel N, Cherepnev G, Babel D, Tropmann A, Hammer M, Volk H, et al. Analysis of tumor necrosis factor-α, transforming growth factor-β, Interleukin-10, IL-6, and interferon-γ gene polymorphisms in patients with chronic periodontitis. J Periodontol. 2006;77:1978–83.

42. Sumer AP, Kara N, Keles GC, Gunes S, Koprulu H, Bagci H. Association of Interleukin-10 gene polymorphisms with severe generalized chronic periodontitis. J Periodontol. 2007;78:493–7.

43. Tervonen T, Raunio T, Knuuttila M, Karttunen R. Polymorphisms in the CD14 and IL-6 genes associated with periodontal disease. J Clin Periodontol. 2007; 34:377–83.

44. Cullinan M, Westerman B, Hamlet S, Palmer J, Faddy M, Seymour G, et al. Progression of periodontal disease and interleukin-10 gene polymorphism. J Periodontal Res. 2008;43:328–33.

45. Kobayashi T, Murasawa A, Ito S, Yamamoto K, Komatsu Y, Abe A, et al. Cytokine gene polymorphisms associated with rheumatoid arthritis and periodontitis in Japanese adults. J Periodontol. 2009;80:792–9.

46. Laine ML, Farré MA, González G, van Dijk LJ, Ham AJ, Winkel EG. Polymorphisms of the interleukin-1 gene family, oral microbial pathogens, and smoking in adult periodontitis. J Dent Res. 2001;80:1695–9.

47. Scapoli L, Girardi A, Palmieri A, et al. IL6 and IL10 are genetic susceptibility factors of periodontal disease. Dental Res J. 2012;9(Suppl 2):S197–201.

48. Crena J, Subramanian S, Victor DJ, Gnana PPS, Ramanathan A. Single nucleotide polymorphism at −1087 locus of interleukin-10 gene promoter is associated with severe chronic periodontitis in nonsmoking patients. Eur J Dent. 2015;9:387–93.

49. Pirim Gorgun E, Toker H, Korkmaz EM, Poyraz O. IL-6 and IL-10 gene polymorphisms in patients with aggressive periodontitis: effects on GCF, serum and clinic parameters. Braz. Oral Res. 2017;31.

50. Tettamanti L, Gaudio RM, Iapichino A, Mucchi D, Tagliabue A. Genetic susceptibility and periodontal disease: a retrospective study on a large Italian sample. Oral Implantol. 2017;10:20–7.

51. Toker H, Gorgun EP, Korkmaz EM, Yüce HB, Poyraz O. The effects of IL-10 gene polymorphism on serum, and gingival crevicular fluid levels of IL-6 and IL-10 in chronic periodontitis. J Appl Oral Sci. 2018;26:e20170232.

52. Lappin DF, MacLeod CP, Kerr A, Mitchell T, Kinane DF. Anti-inflammatory cytokine IL-10 and T cell cytokine profile in periodontitis granulation tissue. Clin Exp Immunol. 2001;123:294–300.

53. Zhong Q, Ding C, Wang M, Sun Y, Xu Y. Interleukin-10 gene polymorphisms and chronic/aggressive periodontitis susceptibility: a meta-analysis based on 14 case-control studies. Cytokine. 2012;60:47–54.

54. Albuquerque CM, Cortinhas AJ, Morinha FJ, Leitao JC, Viegas CA, Bastos EM. Association of the IL-10 polymorphisms and periodontitis: a meta-analysis. Mol Biol Rep. 2012;39:9319–29.

55. Townsend GC, Aldred MJ, Bartold PM. Genetic aspects of dental disorders. Aust Dent J. 1998;43:269–86.

56. Lazarus M, Hajeer AH, Turner D, Sinnott P, Worthington J, Ollier WE, et al. Genetic variation in the interleukin 10 gene promoter and systemic lupus erythematosus. J Rheumatol. 1997;24:2314–7.

57. Taylor A, Verhagen J, Blaser K, Akdis M, Akdis CA. Mechanisms of immune suppression by interleukin-10 and transforming growth factor-β: the role of T regulatory cells. Immunology. 2006;117:433–42.

58. Assuma R, Oates T, Cochran D, Amar S, Graves DT. IL-1 and TNF antagonists inhibit the inflammatory response and bone loss in experimental periodontitis. J Immunol. 1998;160:403–9.

59. Bogdanovska L, et al. Therapeutic strategies in the treatment of periodontitis. Macedonian Pharmaceutical Bulletin. 2012;58(1, 2):3–14.

Odontogenic ameloblast-associated protein (ODAM) in gingival crevicular fluid for site-specific diagnostic value of periodontitis

Hye-Kyung Lee[1], Soo Jin Kim[2], Young Ho Kim[3], Youngkyung Ko[4], Suk Ji[5]*[†] 🄳 and Joo-Cheol Park[1]*[†]

Abstract

Background: Odontogenic Ameloblast-Associated Protein (ODAM) in gingival crevicular fluid (GCF) can provide evidence of the detachment of junctional epithelium from the tooth surface by periodontitis. This study sought to investigate the ability of ODAM to reflect the severity of periodontitis at a site-specific level; thus whether there was a relationship between clinical diagnostic parameters and the value of ODAM in GCF was analyzed.

Methods: Eight periodontitis patients with various severities were enrolled, and the clinical parameters and samples of GCF were obtained from 44 to 60 sites of each subject. The ODAM concentration was quantified by enzyme-linked immunosorbent assay. Correlation analyses between clinical parameters and ODAM values and unadjusted and adjusted (linear) mixed model analyses were performed. The accuracy of ODAM to reflect sites having a probing depth (PD) ≥ 5 mm and a positive bleeding on probing (BOP) was evaluated by receiver-operating characteristic analysis.

Results: A total of 424 GCF samples were collected. The mean ODAM concentration from each patient varied from 0.2 to 1.52 ng/ml. Correlations between PD or clinical attachment level (CAL) and ODAM values were found ($p < 0.0001$). An adjusted linear mixed model showed that PD or CAL were associated with ODAM values ($p < 0.05$). The area under the curve of ODAM, which reflected sites with PD ≥ 5 mm and positive BOP, was 0.661 ($p < 0.0001$).

Conclusion: This result shows the possibility of GCF ODAM as a site-specific biomarker for periodontal tissue destruction.

Keywords: Odontogenic ameloblast-associated protein (ODAM), Periodontitis, Gingival crevicular fluid, Biomarker

Background

Periodontitis is chronic inflammation of the periodontium caused by the host's immune response to subgingival bacterial biofilm, which can lead to the irreversible destruction of connective tissue and bone. The gingival epithelium provides the first line of defense against invading bacteria, forming barriers between plaque bacteria and gingival tissue [1].

The integrity of the junctional epithelium (JE) is therefore essential for maintaining a healthy periodontium. Immunologically, the JE plays a role in protection as a physical, chemical, and immunological barrier to protect the underlying gingival connective tissue and bone from exposure to bacteria and their products [1]. It has a specialized epithelial structure that attaches the gingival soft tissue to the tooth surface consisting of an internal basal lamina and hemidesmosomes [2]. During the progress into periodontitis, JE detaches from the tooth surface and migrates apically and laterally toward the space being formed through connective tissue destruction [3, 4]. Therefore, the detachment of JE from the tooth surface is regarded as the hallmark in the progression of periodontitis.

* Correspondence: sukji@ajou.ac.kr; jcapark@snu.ac.kr
[†]Suk Ji and Joo-Cheol Park contributed equally to this work.
[5]Department of Periodontics, Institute of Oral Health Science, Ajou University School of Medicine, 164, World cup-ro, Yeongtong-gu, Suwon, South Korea
[1]Departments of Oral Histology-Developmental Biology & Dental Research Institute, School of Dentistry, Seoul National University, 101 Daehagro, Chongro-gu, Seoul 110-749, South Korea
Full list of author information is available at the end of the article

In previous study, we reported that odontogenic ameloblast-associated protein (ODAM) was extruded from the JE following the onset of JE attachment loss and was detected in gingival crevicular fluid (GCF), and proposed that ODAM could be used as a biomarker of periodontitis and peri-implantitis [5]. ODAM is a secretory calcium-binding phosphoprotein expressed by ameloblasts during the maturation stage of enamel formation, and its expression persists in the reduced enamel organ and JE of gingiva at the erupted tooth [6]. It was known that ODAM is implicated in the adhesion of epithelial cells to tooth surfaces [5, 7]. Wazen et al. recently showed that ODAM plays a role in maintaining the integrity of the JE and gingival healing using an ODAM knockout mouse model [7]. We also identified that the adhesion of the JE to the tooth surface is regulated via fibronectin/laminin-integrin-ODAM-ARHGEF5-RhoA signaling, and ODAM-mediated RhoA signaling resulted in actin filament rearrangement [5].

The diagnosis of periodontitis is currently performed using radiography and clinical measurements, such as probing depth (PD), clinical attachment level (CAL), bleeding on probing (BOP), suppuration and mobility [8]. These traditional clinical measurements not only reflect a history of periodontal disease but also help to determine prognosis, however there is an unmet need for an easily accessible test showing disease activity to diagnose periodontitis.

Extensive research has been carried out on GCF and saliva components that might serve as potential diagnostic markers for periodontitis [9, 10]. The collection of saliva is relatively simple, safe, and non-invasive, so saliva can be used as a point-of-care diagnostic tool for periodontitis [10]. However, saliva is limited in detecting disease activity at each individual tooth site, and so traditional clinical measurements should be taken to detect the tooth site affected by periodontitis, even if one subject is diagnosed with periodontitis using saliva. In this respect, the diagnosis using GCF can be useful to diagnose the disease at specific sites. GCF contains a large number of proteins and peptides liberated from the underlying tissues [9, 11, 12], so the analysis of the GCF components can reflect the disease status of individual tooth sites.

This pilot study sought to investigate the ability of ODAM to reflect the severity of periodontitis at a site-specific level. The analysis of ODAM values from single-site GCF may enable the clinician to distinguish between healthy sites and those affected by periodontitis. For this purpose, we performed a cross-section study of ODAM values in GCF as well as of corresponding clinical parameters in periodontitis patients and analyzed whether there was a relationship between clinical diagnostic parameters and the concentration of ODAM in GCF.

Methods

Patient population

Eight periodontitis patients having both sites with PD ≤ 3 mm and diseased sites with PD ≥ 4 mm were participated in this study. The study protocol was approved by the Korea University Anam Hospital, Seoul, Korea (IRB no. ED13162) and participants provided written informed consent to participate in this study. Patients with at least 25 teeth had to have at least 5 teeth having site with PD ≥ 4 mm, and had not received periodontal treatment for the last 2 years. According to the exclusion criteria, all participants had no history of systemic disease, which could influence the prognosis of periodontitis, no smoking, no untreated caries, no orthodontic appliances, were not pregnant/breast-feeding, and were not treated with medications (antibiotic, antimicrobial, and/or anti-inflammatory drugs) during the 6 months before examination and sampling.

Clinical examination and gingival crevicular fluid (GCF) collection

Panoramic X-rays and plaque index (PI) scores were recorded for all patients. Prior to measuring PD, GCF was sampled because the gingival bleeding during the measurement of PD can be sucked in GCF sampling strips. GCF samples were obtained from teeth of one quadrant that contained the teeth showing the most severe marginal bone loss on the panoramic X-ray view and the contralateral quadrant of the opposite jaw. GCF samples were obtained from four sites of each tooth (mesiobuccal, mesiolingual, distobuccal, and distolingual sites) using absorbent paper strips (ORAFLOW, Smithtown, NY, USA). Supragingival plaque on the tooth surface was carefully removed with curettes, avoiding bleeding from the gingiva, and each tooth site was gently dried for 10 s with compressed air. Paper strip was inserted carefully into the gingival sulcus/pocket until mild resistance was felt and left in place for 30 s. There was no strip that was saturated by GCF within the 30 s collection timeframe. In rare cases, the strip was saturated by saliva that was not sufficiently blocked, and those strips were discarded. Then, the strip was transferred into a microtube containing 100 μl of phosphate-buffered saline, and the microtubes were stored at − 80 °C until analyzed. Red-stained strips that were visibly contaminated with blood were discarded. After obtaining samples of GCF, clinical parameters of PD, CAL, and modified sulcus bleeding index (mSBI) [13] were recorded from the same four sites of each tooth. Therefore, a total of 428 sites were analyzed by collecting 44 to 60 recordings of clinical parameters and samples of GCF from every 11–15 teeth of each patients. For sites where GCF was not sampled, clinical parameters were also recorded at four sites per tooth, including BOP instead of mSBI.

Enzyme-linked immunosorbent assay (ELISA)

The microtubes containing the paper strip were thawed and shaken on an ELISA plate shaker for 60 min and then centrifuged at 13,200 rpm for 3 min at 4 °C. The supernatants were used for ELISA analysis. The total levels of ODAM in GCF samples were assayed using an ODAM ELISA kit according to the instructions of the manufacturer (Cusabio Biotech, Wuhan, China). The ODAM levels were calculated from standard curves and expressed as the concentration calculated from the ELISA assay itself (ng/ml per 30 s sample).The minimum detection limit was 0.002 ng/ml for ODAM.

Statistical analysis

Mean values for PD, CAL, PI and mSBI and percentages of BOP were calculated for each patient. Percentages of sites showing PD ≤ 3 mm, PD, 4–5 mm, and PD ≥ 6 mm were also calculated for each patient. Spearman's rank correlation analyses between PD, CAL, or mSBI and ODAM values were performed. The ODAM values were divided into four groups according to the degree of clinical parameters and the differences in ODAM values among groups were compared using ANOVA. Unadjusted and adjusted (linear) mixed model analysis was performed using the non-parametric test. Adjusted mixed models, adjusting the random effects of subject, and the fixed effects of age, sex, mSBI, and PI were considered to identify the linear association between PD, CAL, or mSBI and ODAM values. The accuracy of ODAM to reflect sites having a probing depth (PD) ≥ 5 mm and a positive BOP was evaluated by receiver-operating characteristic (ROC) analysis and areas under the receiver operating characteristic curve (AUC) were calculated to compare the predictive ability of the indices, and optimal cut-off values were determined using the Youden index to maximize the sum of sensitivity and specificity. On the basis of the AUC statistic, the diagnostic test can be either non-informative (AUC = 0.5), less accurate (0.5 < AUC ≤ 0.7), moderately accurate (0.7 < AUC ≤ 0.9), highly accurate (0.9 < AUC < 1), or perfect (AUC = 1) [14]. All statistical analyses were performed using SPSS version 23.0 (SPSS, Inc., Chicago, IL, USA) and MedCalc version 16.8 (MedCalc Mariakerke, Belgium). The results were considered statistically significant when p-values were less than 0.05.

Results

Characteristics of full mouth and sampled sites

Eight periodontitis patients (4 males and 4 females) with a mean age of 57 (range, 44–74) years were enrolled in this study. Table 1 presents the periodontal status of the full mouth and the selected sites for GCF sampling. Each patient had at least 18% (and up to 68.5%) of sites with a PD ≥ 4 mm, and 60% (and up to 88.7%) of sites were

BOP-positive. The percentages for sites with PD ≤ 3 mm among the sampling sites were calculated between 32.7 and 83.7% and that for sites with PD ≥ 6 mm were calculated between1.9 and 25.4%. The mean PD of the sampling sites ranged from 3.14 ± 0.13 mm (Mean ± SD) to 4.42 ± 0.27 mm in individual patients (Table 1).

Levels of ODAM in GCF

From the total of 428 GCF sites, four could not be processed properly in sampling or experimental steps, so a total 424 ODAM values in GCF were calculated from 8 subjects. In ELISA analysis, ODAM was not detected in 18.9% of the samples (80 among total 424 GCF samples) because the ODAM was below the limit of detection. In statistical analyses, these values were substituted with zero. Figure 1 illustrates the distributions of ODAM values in each individual patient. A broad range of inter-individual ODAM values was found, and the mean ODAM concentration for each periodontitis patient varied from 0.2 to 1.52 ng/ml of eluate (Fig. 1).

Associations of the ODAM values in GCF with clinical parameters

Correlations between ODAM values in GCF and clinical parameters were determined. ODAM values were significantly correlated with PD, CAL or mSBI (Table 2). The required sample size was calculated using a p value comparing PD with ODAM in GCF, the primary outcome of this study. A sample size of 193 achieves 80% power to detect a Spearman correlation of 0.214 using a two-sided hypothesis test with a significance level of 0.05. These result was based on 5000 Monte Carlo samples from the bivariate normal distribution under the alternative hypothesis [15]. When the dropout rate was considered to be 30%, the sample size was 276. Therefore, the analysis of total 424 sites was sufficient to prove the relationship between PD and the value of ODAM in GCF at site-specific level. The ODAM value according to the degree of clinical parameters was represented by a box plot, and the differences in ODAM values among groups classified by the severity of clinical parameters were analyzed by one-way ANOVA. The ODAM values showed a tendency to increase as the degree of clinical parameters increased. ODAM values were significantly different among groups divided by the severity of PD, CAL, or mSBI (PD; $p = 0.00044$, CAL; $p = 0.0001$, mSBI; $p = 0.0041$) (Fig. 2). Unadjusted and adjusted models were used to identify linear associations between PD, CAL or mSBI and ODAM in GCF. The unadjusted model showed significant linear associations between ODAM values and PD or CAL. Considering the GCF samples were collected from 44 to 60 sites from 11 to 15 teeth from each patient, the association between ODAM values in GCF and clinical parameters was analyzed

Table 1 Clinical characteristics of full mouth and GCF sampling sites

Patient code	Number of teeth	Number of sites	PD (Mean ± SD)	% of sites with PD ≤ 3 mm	% of sites with PD 4–5 mm	% of sites with PD ≥ 6 mm	CAL (Mean ± SD)	PI (Mean ± SD)	BOP %	mSBI (Mean ± SD)
Full mouth clinical data										
S1	25	100	3.12 ± 0.07	82.1	14.9	3.0	3.60 ± 0.1	0.70 ± 0.50	60.0	
S2	28	112	4.05 ± 0.13	31.5	66.2	2.3	4.77 ± 0.18	0.85 ± 0.07	87.5	
S3	28	112	4.25 ± 0.26	44.2	30.2	25.6	5.11 ± 0.3	0.40 ± 0.09	61.0	
S4	28	112	4.17 ± 0.24	48.2	42.3	9.5	4.40 ± 0.25	0.56 ± 0.07	66.7	
S5	28	112	4.56 ± 0.24	42.3	41.5	16.2	4.56 ± 0.24	0.04 ± 0.03	81.3	
S6	27	108	4.21 ± 0.22	41.3	48.5	10.2	4.75 ± 0.31	0.56 ± 0.07	78.6	
S7	25	100	3.93 ± 0.16	34.5	56.5	9.0	4.65 ± 0.22	0.24 ± 0.06	88.7	
S8	26	104	4.14 ± 0.19	46.2	40.6	13.2	4.43 ± 0.24	0.98 ± 0.07	82.1	
Clinical data of sampling sites										
S1	11	44	3.14 ± 0.13	83.7	14.0	2.3	3.51 ± 0.19	0.70 ± 0.10	67.4	1.02 ± 0.13
S2	13	52	4.16 ± 0.12	32.7	65.4	1.9	4.88 ± 0.19	0.84 ± 0.09	87.0	1.84 ± 0.13
S3	15	60	4.42 ± 0.27	45.8	28.8	25.4	5.29 ± 0.3	0.36 ± 0.07	63.0	1.17 ± 0.14
S4	14	56	4.07 ± 0.24	50.0	41.1	8.9	4.32 ± 0.24	0.54 ± 0.09	64.0	1.20 ± 0.14
S5	15	60	4.38 ± 0.22	41.7	41.7	16.7	4.38 ± 0.22	0.03 ± 0.02	80.0	1.62 ± 0.14
S6	14	56	4.16 ± 0.22	40.0	49.1	10.9	4.65 ± 0.3	0.58 ± 0.09	78.0	1.31 ± 0.12
S7	13	52	4.10 ± 0.14	33.3	58.8	7.8	4.49 ± 0.19	0.20 ± 0.06	88.0	1.47 ± 0.12
S8	12	48	3.96 ± 0.18	45.8	43.8	10.4	4.19 ± 0.23	0.96 ± 0.09	81.0	1.33 ± 0.13

PD probing depth, CAL clinical attachment level, PI plaque index, BOP bleeding on probing, mSBI modified sulcus bleeding index

using an adjusted linear mixed model adjusted within subject (as a random effect) and age, sex, plaque, and mSBI (as fixed effects). Significant associations between PD or CAL and ODAM values in GCF were also found through adjusted model (PD; $\beta = 0.087$, $p = 0.026$, CAL; $\beta = 0.090$, $p = 0.005$) (Table 3). Adjusted linear mixed model revealed that the ODAM value can be an indicator of PD or CAL. In sum, these findings suggest that raised ODAM levels in GCF can represent the degree of periodontal tissue destruction.

ROC curve analysis

The pocket with PD ≥ 5 mm is one of the most important risk indicators for periodontitis recurrence [16], therefore, the power of ODAM to reflect sites with PD ≥ 5 mm and positive BOP was evaluated by a ROC curve and the AUC. The AUC for GCF ODAM was 0.661, the 95% confidence interval was 0.613 to 0.706, and the p value was less than 0.0001 (Fig. 3). Optimal cut-off values were determined using the Youden index to maximize the sum of sensitivity and specificity. The cut-off value of 0.25 provided sensitivities of 78.18% and specificities of 45.50%.

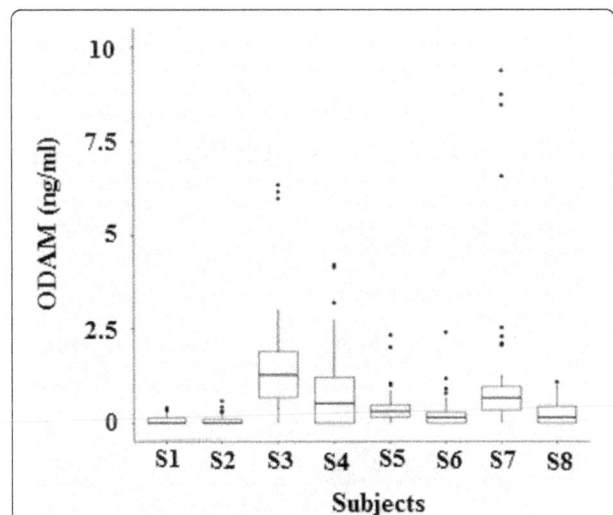

Fig. 1 Box-plots showing the distribution of ODAM values in each individual patient (S1~S8). Eight periodontitis patients were sampled, and 40–56 GCF samples were analyzed from 11 to 15 teeth from each patient. Box plots show the medians, boxes represent the 25th and 75th percentiles, and black dots represent the 10th and 90th percentiles and outlier values

Table 2 Correlation of clinical parameters with ODAM in GCF

Clinical parameters	Correlation coefficient	p-value
PD	$\rho = 0.214$	< 0.0001
CAL	$\rho = 0.232$	< 0.0001
mSBI	$\rho = 0.111$	0.0216

PD probing depth, CAL clinical attachment level, mSBI modified sulcus bleeding index

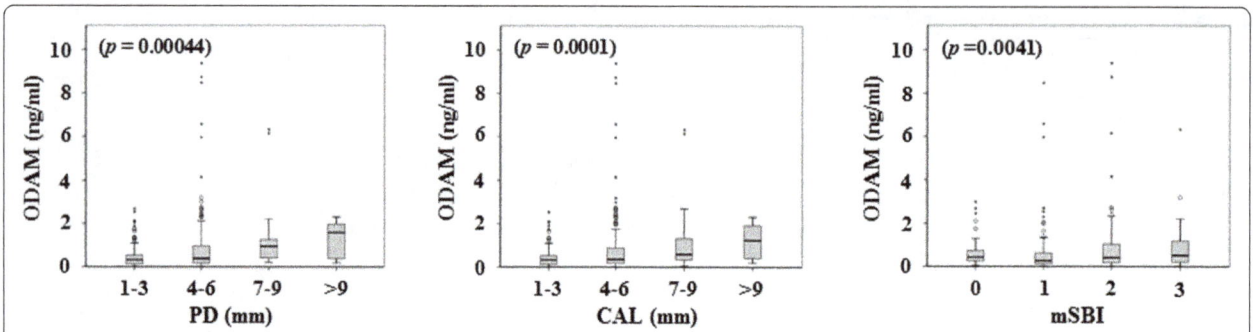

Fig. 2 The ODAM value according to the severity of clinical parameters. *p*-values indicate the differences in ODAM values among groups classified by the severity of their clinical parameters (one-way ANOVA). Box plots show medians, boxes represent the 25th and 75th percentiles, and empty dots represent the 10th and 90th percentiles. Outlier values are shown as asterisks. PD; probing depth, CAL; clinical attachment level, mSBI; modified sulcus bleeding index

Discussion

This is the first study to assess the possibility of GCF ODAM as a site-specific biomarker for periodontitis. ODAM is involved in the adhesion of the JE to the tooth surface and is released into the gingival crevice when the adhesion is broken by progress into periodontitis [5]. It was analyzed whether there was a relationship between the value of ODAM in GCF and clinical diagnostic parameters at the same sites. As a result, ODAM appears to serve as a novel site-specific biomarker of periodontitis, as demonstrated by the statistically significant association between the value of ODAM in GCF and the parameters showing the degree of periodontal tissue destruction, PD or CAL. An adjusted linear mixed model showed that the ODAM value in GCF can be an indicator of PD or CAL. Our results suggest that ODAM in GCF plays a role as a site-specific biomarker for deep pockets, although additional studies including the change of ODAM values according to treatment are needed to determine the clinical significance of GCF ODAM. Since the loss of epithelial adhesion from the tooth surface is an early event in periodontal tissue destruction, it is worth verifying the potential of ODAM in GCF as a predictive biomarker for sites that may be vulnerable to periodontal bone loss. Based on the potential of ODAM as a predictive marker for the

Table 3 Association between ODAM values in GCF and clinical parameters

Variables	Unadjusted model			Adjusted model		
	β	SE(β)	*p*-value	β	SE(β)	*p*-value
PD[a]	0.091	0.039	0.019	0.087	0.039	0.026
CAL[a]	0.092	0.032	0.004	0.090	0.032	0.005
mSBI[b]	0.055	0.062	0.374	0.043	0.063	0.503

PD probing depth, *CAL* clinical attachment level, *mSBI* modified sulcus bleeding index, adjusted linear mixed model adjusted with subject (as a random effect) and age, sex, plaque, and mSBI (as a fixed effects)[a] and age, sex, plaque(as a fixed effects)[b]

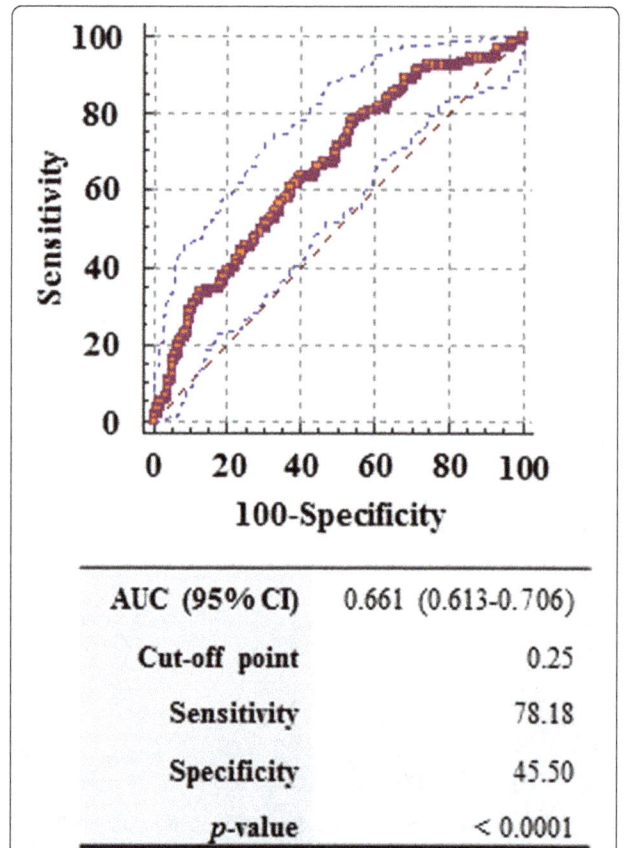

AUC (95% CI)	0.661 (0.613-0.706)
Cut-off point	0.25
Sensitivity	78.18
Specificity	45.50
p-value	< 0.0001

Fig. 3 ROC analysis of ODAM values in GCF for the reflection of sites with PD ≥ 5 mm and positive BOP. ROC analysis for GCF ODAM to reflect the sites with PD ≥ 5 mm and positive BOP were constructed and areas under the receiver operating characteristic curve (AUC) were calculated to compare the predictive ability of the indices. Optimal cut-off values were determined using the Youden index to maximize the sum of sensitivity and specificity

diagnosis of subjects (using saliva) and sites (using GCF) at risk for periodontitis, development of point-of-care diagnostic tools can help to overcome the limitations of current clinical diagnostics.

Periodontitis is developed at a site-specific level [17]. Therefore, GCF has been used as a tool for the diagnosis of periodontitis at a site-specific level because it reflects the site-specific severity of periodontitis. It contains a large number of proteins and peptides derived from underlying tissues. To date, nearly 100 different components in GCF have been reported as possible biomarkers for the progression of periodontitis [9, 12]. These include bacteria or bacterial products [18, 19], inflammatory mediators [20], host-derived enzymes and their inhibitors [21, 22] and soft and hard tissue destruction products [21, 23, 24]. Although there are many candidates, there has been no validation of factors involved in the attachment of the JE to the tooth surface. ODAM liberated from JE as a result of attachment loss can serve as an indicator of initial periodontal breakdown. Only extremely small volumes of fluid are available from a single site, so GCF requires highly sensitive techniques for quantitative analysis. In this study, ODAM was not detected in 18.9% of the samples. It is necessary to develop a highly sensitive and reliable detection tool that can detect ODAM at low concentrations through the development of a new antibody or aptamer.

The function of ODAM might be related to dentogingival attachment [5–7]. In this study, the value of ODAM in GCF was increased in deep periodontal pockets. This means that pathologic JE can also express ODAM after detachment from the tooth surface. However, in our previous study, ODAM was obviously expressed in the normal JE of healthy teeth but was absent in the pathologic pocket epithelium of diseased periodontium [5]. ODAM expression was reduced in the JE of experimental periodontitis by drugs, dextran sulfate sodium or periodontopathic bacteria (*Porphyromonas gingivalis*) compared with the sham group. Moreover, ODAM was not detected in the pocket epithelium of teeth extracted from periodontitis patients [5]. It is not readily explained that ODAM, which was not expressed or expressed at low levels in the JE of gingival biopsies from periodontitis patients, was detected at relatively high levels in the GCF from sites with deep pockets. Regarding these results, Wazen et al. noted how the level of ODAM in GCF would be maintained even though it is no longer produced by the JE [7]. Although the precise mechanism behind the expression of ODAM in periodontitis is unknown, one possibility may be that the detached JE continues to produce ODAM to maintain homeostasis for attachment to the tooth surface, and the resulting ODAM is immediately released into the pocket as soon as it is produced. Therefore, the ODAM may

not be observed in histologic specimens of periodontitis models. Since the total area occupied by the pathologic pocket epithelium capable of producing ODAM is increased in periodontitis [4], the value of ODAM can be increase in deep periodontal pockets. It is also possible that the histological examination of the expression of ODAM according to the severity of periodontitis is not sufficiently verified. In our previous study, the examination of ODAM in JE from human gingival tissue was performed on only one specimen of gingiva around teeth extracted due to periodontitis [5]. Regarding ODAM expression in the JE of periodontitis, Nakayama et al. showed that ODAM gene expression was increased in inflamed gingiva from patients with chronic periodontitis using DNA microarray [25]. Recently, they also reported that the expression of ODAM was increased not only at the early stage but also at the following stages in the inflammatory JE on gingival biopsy from an experimental periodontitis model induced by *P. gingivalis*. They also showed that the localization of ODAM was spread into the gingival epithelium in inflamed gingiva using human gingival tissues [26]. To solve these discrepancies, histological examination of the expression of ODAM according to the severity of periodontitis should be performed.

The ROC analysis and AUC calculations were used to assess the ability of the ODAM to reflect sites with $PD \geq 5$ mm and positive BOP. Pockets with a $PD \geq 5$ mm have clinical significance; when compared with $PD < 3$ mm, $PD \geq 5$ mm represented a risk factor for tooth loss [16]. Land & Tonetti divided the risk of periodontitis recurrence according to the number of pockets with a $PD \geq 5$ mm [27]. In the analysis based on total subjects, the AUC for ODAM was 0.661, and it was interpreted that the ODAM value in GCF at the least has the potential to serve as a site-specific marker of deep pockets. Additional studies are needed to overcome the low sensitivity and AUC. Considering that the concentration of ODAM in the GCF varies greatly among subjects, it is expected that more accurate cut-off points having high sensitivity and specificity will be determined through the analysis of ODAM from more periodontitis patients.

There are two distinct approaches with respect to reporting GCF mediator content and concentration: the first is to sample GCF for a fixed time period and then report the results either as ρg per 30-s sample or by using the concentration as calculated from the assay (ρg/ml per 30-s sample), and the second is to convert the concentration calculated from the assay back into a concentration based on the original GCF volume according to the Periotron data [28–30]. The second approach allows one to know the actual concentration of the mediator in the GCF; however, it can have the potential for error associated with GCF volume determination and calculation [28]. A recent review of clinical and technical considerations in the analysis of GCF mentioned that recent authors tend to sample for a fixed period of time (usually 30 s) and report according to the first option described above [28]. In this study, GCF had to be taken from 40 to 56 sites from each patient, and as it requires a lot of time to measure GCF volume, we adopted the method of reporting by a fixed time period. However, to exclude the possibility that the ODAM value is just reflecting GCF volumes in deep pockets, the relationship between the concentration of ODAM and GCF volume was analyzed from an additional 30 GCF samples collected from 6 independent patients. There was no correlation between the concentration of ODAM and GCF volume ($p = 0.750$). The correlation was analyzed using a regression model and Stata/SE 11.1.

A limitation of this study is that GCF samples were collected from sites that have the potential to affect one another in the tooth. The design of the experiments was such that GCF samples were collected from 4 sites from each tooth, and as such, the levels of ODAM in the GCF recovered from mesio (or disto)-buccal sites on a specific tooth cannot be considered to be completely independent from the levels of ODAM in the GCF recovered from the mesio (or disto)-lingual sites on the same tooth. This limitation can lead to errors when analyzing the correlation between the ODAM values in GCF and the clinical parameters. Even so, ODAM in GCF was closely associated with clinical parameters and this can indicate the possibility of ODAM being used as a site-specific marker of deep pockets. Analysis using the GCF samples obtained from completely independent sites can eliminate the related error and provide a more precise correlation. This limitation should be corrected in future studies.

The sample size was calculated that total 424 sites was sufficient to prove the correlation between PD and the value of ODAM in GCF at site-specific level, however the study has the limitation that GCF samples are collected from only 8 subjects. Moreover, the mean ODAM concentration for each periodontitis patient varied. In order to overcome the limitation and apply statistical research methods suitable for data structures, the association between ODAM values and clinical parameters was analyzed using adjusted linear mixed models adjusted with subject effect. As a result, the adjusted model showed that the ODAM value in GCF can be an indicator of PD or CAL.

Conclusion

In this cross-sectional study of periodontitis patients having simultaneously clinically healthy sites and diseased sites, levels of GCF ODAM were evaluated, and the association between the ODAM values and traditional clinical indices, including PD and CAL, were verified. It was enough to confirm the possibility of ODAM as a site-specific biomarker for periodontitis. Based on the pilot study, additional studies should be conducted on a large number of patients with various clinical severity to verify the clinical significance of GCF ODAM.

Abbreviations

AUC: Area under the curve; BOP: Bleeding on probing; CAL: Clinical attachment level; ELISA: Enzyme-linked immunosorbent assay; GCF: Gingival crevicular fluid; JE: Junctional epithelium; mSBI: Modified sulcus bleeding index; ODAM: Odontogenic Ameloblast-Associated Protein; PD: Probing depth; PI: Plaque index; ROC: Receiver-operating characteristic

Funding

This research was supported by a grant from the Korean Health Technology R&D project, Ministry of Health & Welfare, Republic of Korea (HI16C0220). The funder had no role in the design of the study and collection, analysis, and interpretation of data or in the writing of the manuscript.

Authors' contributions

HL: performing the laboratory experiments. SK: performing data statistical analysis. YHK: performing critical revision of the manuscript. YK: performing critical revision of the manuscript for important intellectual content. SJ: performing study design and drafting of manuscript. JP: performing study design and supervision of field work project coordination. All authors read and approved the final version of the manuscript.

Competing interests

The authors declare that they have no competing interests.

Author details

[1]Departments of Oral Histology-Developmental Biology & Dental Research Institute, School of Dentistry, Seoul National University, 101 Daehagro, Chongro-gu, Seoul 110-749, South Korea. [2]Office of Biostatistics, Institute of Medical Sciences, Ajou University School of Medicine, Suwon, South Korea. [3]Department of Orthodontics, Institute of Oral Health Science, Ajou University School of Medicine, Suwon, South Korea. [4]Department of Periodontics, College of Medicine, Seoul St Mary's Hospital, The Catholic University of Korea, Seoul, South Korea. [5]Department of Periodontics, Institute of Oral Health Science, Ajou University School of Medicine, 164, World cup-ro, Yeongtong-gu, Suwon, South Korea.

References

1. Ji S, Choi YS, Choi Y. Bacterial invasion and persistence: critical events in the pathogenesis of periodontitis? J Periodontal Res. 2015;50:570–85.
2. Bosshardt DD, Lang NP. The junctional epithelium: from health to disease. J Dent Res. 2005;84:9–20.
3. Pöllänen MT, Salonen JI, Uitto VJ. Structure and function of the tooth-epithelial interface in health and disease. Periodontol 2000. 2003;31:12–31.

4. Nanci A, Bosshardt DD. Structure of periodontal tissues in health and disease. Periodontol 2000. 2006;40:11–28.

5. Lee HK, Ji S, Park SJ, Choung HW, Choi Y, Lee HJ, Park SY, Park JC. Odontogenic Ameloblast-associated protein (ODAM) mediates junctional epithelium attachment to teeth via integrin-ODAM-rho guanine nucleotide exchange factor 5 (ARHGEF5)-RhoA signaling. J Biol Chem. 2015;290:14740–53.

6. Nishio C, Wazen R, Kuroda S, Moffatt P, Nanci A. Expression pattern of odontogenic ameloblast-associated and amelotin during formation and regeneration of the junctional epithelium. Eur Cell Mater. 2010;20:393–402.

7. Wazen RM, Moffatt P, Ponce KJ, Kuroda S, Nishio C, Nanci A. Inactivation of the odontogenic ameloblast-associated gene affects the integrity of the junctional epithelium and gingival healing. Eur Cell Mater. 2015;30:187–99.

8. Salvi GE, Berglundh T, Lang NP. Examination of patients. In: Lang NP, Lindhe J, editors. Clinical periodontology and implant dentistry. 6th ed. Oxford: Munksgaard; 2015. p. 559–73.

9. Barros SP, Williams R, Offenbacher S, Morelli T. Gingival crevicular fluid as a source of biomarkers for periodontitis. Periodontol 2000. 2016;70:53–64.

10. Ji S, Choi Y. Point-of-care diagnosis of periodontitis using saliva: technically feasible but still a challenge. Front Cell Infect Microbiol. 2015;5:65.

11. AlRowis R, AlMoharib HS, AlMubarak A, Bhaskardoss J, Preethanath RS, Anil S. Oral fluid-based biomarkers in periodontal disease - part 2. Gingival crevicular fluid J Int Oral Health. 2014;6:126–35.

12. Loos BG, Tjoa S. Host-derived diagnostic markers for periodontitis: do they exist in gingival crevice fluid? Periodontol 2000. 2005;39:53–72.

13. Mombelli A, van Oosten MA, Schurch E Jr, Land NP. The microbiota associated with successful or failing osseointegrated titanium implants. Oral Microbiol Immunol. 1987;2:145–51.

14. Swets JA. Measuring the accuracy of diagnostic systems. Science. 1988;240: 1285–93.

15. Kendall M, Gibbons JD. Rank correlation methods. 5th ed. New York: Oxford University Press; 1990.

16. Matuliene G, Pjetursson BE, Salvi GE, Schmidlin K, Brägger U, Zwahlen M, Lang NP. Influence of residual pockets on progression of periodontitis and tooth loss: results after 11 years of maintenance. J Clin Periodontol. 2008;35: 685–95.

17. Mineoka T, Awano S, Rikimaru T, Kurata H, Yoshida A, Ansai T, Takehara T. Site-specific development of periodontal disease is associated with increased levels of Porphyromonas gingivalis, Treponema denticola, and Tannerella forsythia in subgingival plaque. J Periodontol. 2008;79:670–6.

18. Yong X, Chen Y, Tao R, Zeng Q, Liu Z, Jiang L, Ye L, Lin X. Periodontopathogens and human β-defensin-2 expression in gingival crevicular fluid from patients with periodontal disease in Guangxi, China. J Periodontal Res. 2015;50:403–10.

19. Yakob M, Meurman JH, Sorsa T, Söder B. Treponema denticola associates with increased levels of MMP-8 and MMP-9 in gingival crevicular fluid. Oral Dis. 2013;19:694–701.

20. Zhang Q, Chen B, Zhu D, Yan F. Biomarker levels in gingival crevicular fluid of subjects with different periodontal conditions: a cross-sectional study. Arch Oral Biol. 2016;72:92–8.

21. Khongkhunthian S, Kongtawelert P, Ongchai S, Pothacharoen P, Sastraruji T, Jotikasthira D, Krisanaprakornkit S. Comparisons between two biochemical markers in evaluating periodontal disease severity: a cross-sectional study. BMC Oral Health. 2014;14:107.

22. Bildt MM, Bloemen M, Kuijpers-Jagtman AM, Von den Hoff JW. Collagenolytic fragments and active gelatinase complexes in periodontitis. J Periodontol. 2008;79:1704–11.

23. Becerik S, Afacan B, Oztürk VÖ, Atmaca H, Emingil G. Gingival crevicular fluid calprotectin, osteocalcin and cross-linked N-terminal telopeptid levels in health and different periodontal diseases. Dis Markers. 2011;31:343–52.

24. Balli U, Aydogdu A, Dede FO, Turer CC, Guven B. Gingival Crevicular fluid levels of Sclerostin, Osteoprotegerin, and receptor activator of nuclear factor-κB ligand in periodontitis. J Periodontol. 2015;86:1396–404.

25. Nakayama Y, Takai H, Matsui S, Matsumura H, Zhou L, Kato A, Ganss B, Ogata Y. Proinflammatory cytokines induce amelotin transcription in human gingival fibroblasts. J Oral Sci. 2014;56:261–8.

26. Nakayama Y, Kobayashi R, Matsui S, Matsumura H, Iwai Y, Noda K, Yamazaki M, Kurita-Ochiai T, Yoshimura A, Shinomura T, Ganss B, Ogata Y. Localization and expression pattern of amelotin, odontogenic ameloblast-associated protein and follicular dendritic cell-secreted protein in the junctional epithelium of inflamed gingiva. Odontology. 2017;105:329–37.

27. Lang NP, Tonetti MS. Periodontal risk assessment (PRA) for patients in supportive periodontal therapy (SPT). Oral health Prev Dent. 2003;1:7–16.

28. Wassall RR, Preshaw PM. Clinical and technical considerations in the analysis of gingival crevicular fluid. Periodontol 2000. 2016;70:65–79.

29. Shimada Y, Tabeta K, Sugita N, Yoshie H. Profiling biomarkers in gingival crevicular fluid using multiplex bead immunoassay. Arch Oral Biol. 2013;58: 724–30.

30. Kinney JS, Morelli T, Oh M, Braun TM, Ramseier CA, Sugai JV, Giannobile WV. Crevicular fluid biomarkers and periodontal disease progression. J Clin Periodontol. 2014;41:113–20.

An assessment of strategies to control dental caries in Aboriginal children living in rural and remote communities in New South Wales, Australia

Yvonne Dimitropoulos[1,2]*(iD), Alexander Holden[2], Kylie Gwynne[1], Michelle Irving[1,2], Norma Binge[1] and Anthony Blinkhorn[1]

Abstract

Background: A community-led oral health service for Aboriginal people in Central Northern NSW identified the need for oral health promotion, as well as dental treatment; in three remote communities with limited access to dental services. A three-stage plan based on the Precede-Proceed model was used to develop a school-based preventive oral health program. The program will be piloted in three schools over 12 months aimed at improving the oral health of local Aboriginal children.

Methods: The proposed program includes four components: daily in-school toothbrushing; distribution of free fluoride toothpaste and toothbrushes; in-school and community dental health education and the installation of refrigerated and chilled water fountains to supply a school water bottle program. Primary school children will be issued toothbrushing kits to be kept at school to facilitate daily brushing using a fluoride toothpaste under the supervision of trained teachers and/or Oral Health Aides. School children, parents and guardians will be issued free fluoride toothpaste and toothbrushes for home use at three-monthly intervals. Four dental health education sessions will be delivered to children at each school and parents/guardians at local community health centres over the 12 month pilot. Dental education will be delivered by an Oral Health Therapist and local Aboriginal Dental Assistant. The program will also facilitate the installation of refrigerated and filtered water fountain to ensure cold and filtered water is available at schools. A structured school water bottle program will encourage the consumption of water. A process evaluation will be undertaken to assess the efficiency, feasibility and effectiveness of the pilot program.

Discussion: The proposed program includes four core evidence-based components which can be implemented in rural and remote schools with a high Aboriginal population. Based on the Precede-Proceed model, this program seeks to empower the local Aboriginal community to achieve improved oral health outcomes.

Keywords: Aboriginal, Oral health promotion, Community

* Correspondence: yvonne.dimitropoulos@sydney.edu.au
Note: This protocol will use the term Aboriginal people when referring to the first people of Australia. This term is inclusive of Australian Aboriginal and Torres Strait Islander people.
[1]Poche Centre for Indigenous Health, University of Sydney, Room 223 Edward Ford Building, Sydney, New South Wales, Australia
[2]University of Sydney School of Dentistry, Mons Road, Westmead, Sydney, NSW 2145, Australia

Background

Dental caries is a serious problem for Australian Aboriginal children [1]. For example, Aboriginal children living in New South Wales (NSW) experience on average 2.64 decayed, missing or filled teeth (dmft/DMFT) due to dental caries. This is near double the dmft/DMFT rate of 1.54, experienced by non-Aboriginal children in NSW [2]. When left untreated, dental caries can cause severe pain, and negatively impact a child's quality of life, ability to concentrate at school, and capacity to eat, speak and socialize without embarrassment [3].

Improving the oral health of Aboriginal children is a priority in the Oral Health 2020: A Strategic Framework for Dental Health in NSW [4], and the NSW Aboriginal Oral Health Plan [5]. It is essential that strategies aimed at improving the oral health of Aboriginal children are sustainable, supported by the local Aboriginal community and culturally competent [6].

Culturally competent health promotion programs for Aboriginal people should be developed in consultation with Aboriginal communities and designed to meet the needs of specific communities [5]. Additionally, they should be culturally and linguistically appropriate, evidence-based, sustainable, implemented in collaboration with communities and evaluated [7]. In rural and remote communities, programs that solely rely on the input from dental professionals are often not sustainable given the general shortage of qualified professionals [4]. Therefore, prevention programs that can be delivered by the local Aboriginal community are likely to be more sustainable and suitable for the needs of that population.

In 2013, Aboriginal Elders in Central Northern NSW, identified three Aboriginal communities that had extremely limited access to dental services and needed preventive oral health care programs. Subsequently, the Poche Centre for Indigenous Health and the Centre for Oral Health Strategy were invited into these communities to work in partnership with the local Aboriginal community to introduce sustainable dental services and preventive oral health care programs for Aboriginal people in the region [8] In 2014, a community-led oral health service was established, which provides comprehensive dental treatment for Aboriginal people in Central Northern NSW. The service operates using clinicians who have relocated to the region and local Aboriginal people who have been trained and employed as dental assistants. Portable dental equipment is used to provide dental treatment to Aboriginal children and adults from schools and local community health centres. The local Aboriginal community still however, maintained the need for preventive oral health care programs to be implemented alongside dental treatment provided in schools and community health centres.

In response to the community's request for preventive oral health care programs, a three-stage plan based on the Precede-Proceed model of health program planning was used to develop a sustainable, community-led preventive oral health program (Fig. 1).

The Precede-Proceed model was used as it is a popular planning tool for population health programs [9]. It consists of a series of phases to assist researchers plan, design, implement and evaluate health programs. The first set of phases (PRECEDE) includes planned assessments to inform the design of the health program. The second set of phases (PROCEED) involves implementing a health program based on information learnt from the PRECEDE phases [10].

Guided by the Precede-Proceed model, Stage 1 included an epidemiological assessment of all Aboriginal children aged 5–12 years enrolled in local schools as well as an educational and ecological assessment of the community to determine predisposing risk factors and reinforcing and enabling factors to inform a targeted oral health program. The number of decayed, missing and filled teeth were recorded as well as baseline oral health knowledge and oral hygiene practices of children, parents/guardians, school staff and health workers.

The baseline data collected as part of Stage 1 data provided valuable planning information. The majority of children (87.5%) had untreated dental caries. The mean number of decayed primary teeth (dt) was 4.1 and the mean number of decayed permanent teeth (DT) was 0.7, indicating a clear need for dental treatment and education to prevent dental disease [11].

Ecological and educational assessment of the community identified four predisposing risk factors associated with an increased risk of developing dental caries:

1. Low levels of tooth brush ownership
2. Infrequent daily toothbrushing with a fluoride toothpaste
3. Frequent sugar consumption
4. High intake of sugar-sweetened beverages rather than drinking tap water

Based on the risk factors identified, the following oral health promotion strategies for Aboriginal children living in Central Northern NSW were developed, namely: increasing fluoride use through daily toothbrushing; ensuring safe and refreshing tap water is accessible to encourage the consumption of water rather sugar sweetened beverages; providing culturally competent oral health and nutrition education; and providing training programs to build capacity of the local Aboriginal community and existing health workforce to ensure oral health promotion is led and supported by the community.

The results of Stage 1 and proposed oral health promotion strategies were presented in a leaflet and also

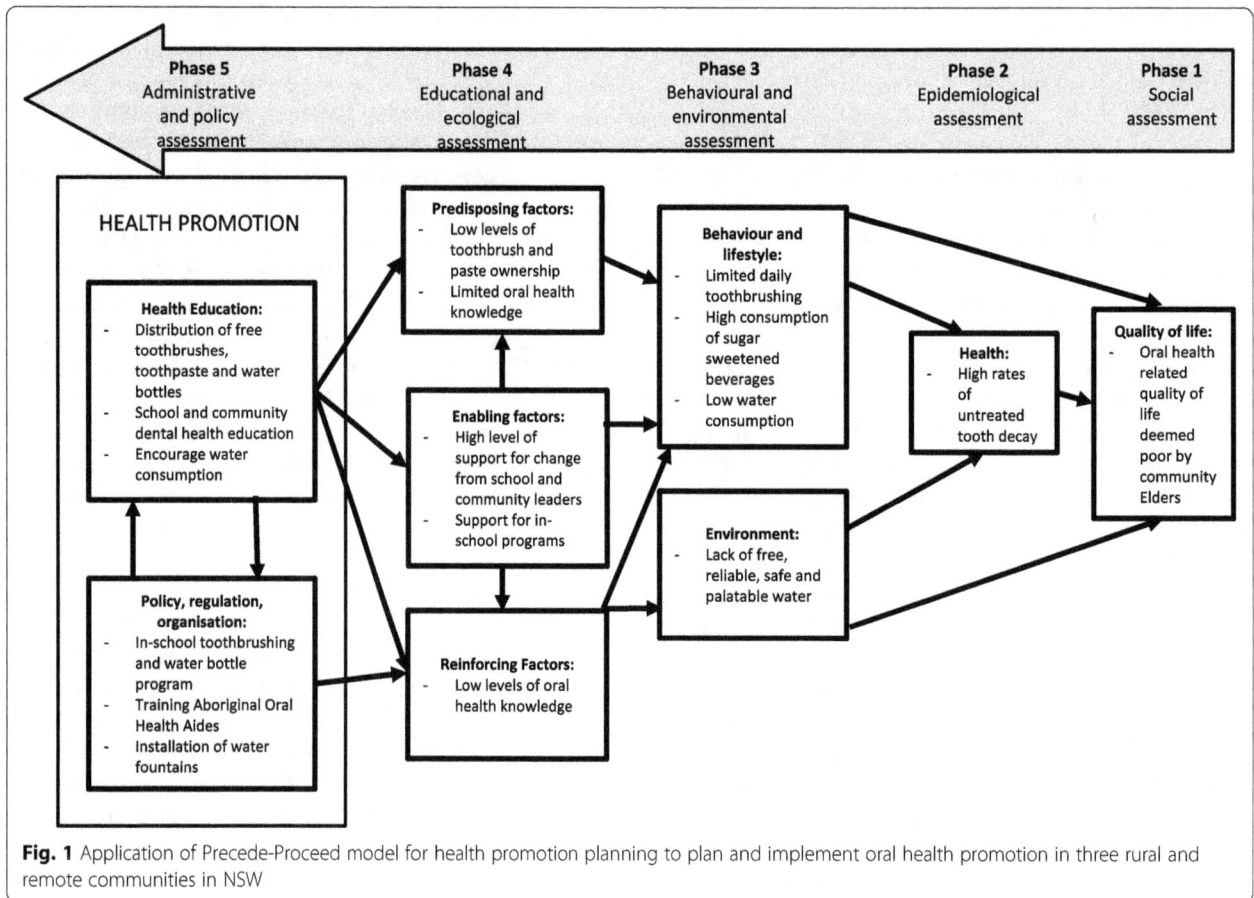

Fig. 1 Application of Precede-Proceed model for health promotion planning to plan and implement oral health promotion in three rural and remote communities in NSW

verbally reported back to the local Aboriginal people at an open community forum (locally known as a community 'yarn up') which is held to discuss local issues and events. The 'yarn up' included local Aboriginal Elders, teachers and school principals from the three local schools and representatives from the Poche Centre for Indigenous Health. The strategies were well-received at the 'yarn up' and members verbally agreed to the development of an oral health promotion program to be implemented in each of the schools in the three communities; which was later formalised in writing. This led to Stage 2 and thus the 'implementation phase' of the Precede-Proceed model.

Stage 2 involved developing a school-based oral health promotion program based on the findings of Stage 1. The program includes:

1. Daily in-school toothbrushing
2. Distribution of free fluoride toothpaste and toothbrushes to children and families
3. In-school and community dental health education
4. Installation of refrigerated and chilled water fountains to supply a school water bottle program

The four components are based on existing programs which have shown to be effective in other Aboriginal

communities [6, 12], and utilising high quality systematic reviews [13]. This study protocol describes the components of the proposed school-based program and evaluation protocol to determine the feasibility, efficiency and effectiveness of the strategies to control dental caries in Aboriginal children living in rural and remote communities in NSW.

The aim of the program is to improve the oral health of Aboriginal children by promoting daily toothbrushing using fluoride toothpaste, increasing oral health knowledge and encouraging the consumption of water to reduce the reliance on sugar-sweetened beverages.

Stage 3 will pilot the proposed program for 12 months in three schools in Central Northern NSW that enroll a high proportion of Aboriginal children. The process evaluation to be undertaken at the completion of the pilot, is based on the Precede-Proceed model for process evaluation (Phase 6) and will determine the program's feasibility, efficiency, effectiveness and overall satisfaction of the participating communities.

Methods
Daily in-school toothbrushing with a fluoride toothpaste
Daily in-school toothbrushing will be implemented in all Kindergarten to Year 6 (primary) classes in the three schools.

At the commencement of the pilot, all children enrolled in Kindergarten to Year 6 will be issued with a toothbrushing kit. This kit will be labeled for each child and kept at school for daily toothbrushing. It includes a toothbrush, 1000 ppm fluoride toothpaste and hard plastic storage case for the toothbrush and paste.

Children will brush their teeth at school once per school day under the supervision of a trained teacher and/or Oral Health Aide. The program will allow the school to choose which combination will work at their school, whether this will be the existing classroom teacher, the introduction of an Oral Health Aide or a combination of the two. This approach will be used as the program has been designed to be led and implemented by the local community. The Oral Health Aide must be a local Aboriginal person to promote a culturally safe environment for children to brush their teeth at school, this may include providing individual children with support to brush their teeth. They will be employed by the school for 1 h per day and will assist the classroom teachers to implement the program by supervising toothbrushing.. The role of an Oral Health Aide was incorporated into the design of this study as a significant barrier to in-school toothbrushing programs is the demands on a teacher's time [6]. It is based on the Children's Oral Health Initiative (COHI) in Canada which utilizes 'COHI Aides' to support oral health promotion activities and provide oral health education [14]. Teachers and Oral Health Aides will receive a NSW TAFE skillset in Infection Control (HLTIN30IC) and First Aid (HLTAID003) to ensure they can supervise in-school toothbrushing safely.

All labeled toothbrush cases will be stored in a ventilated carrier next to the sink in each classroom and a replacement toothbrushing kit will be issued to each child every three months which will coincide with the commencement of each new school term.

The following outcomes will be used during the process evaluation to measure the reach and efficiency of daily in-school toothbrushing;

- At least 70% of Aboriginal children enrolled in the school have consented to participate in the program
- 90% of children with consent to participate will brush their teeth at least 170 out of the 200 school days
- 80% of children with consent to participate are continuing to brush their teeth each day at school after six months
- Teacher support for the program both at the time of commencement and six months later is positive.

Distribution of free fluoride toothpaste and toothbrushes to communities

A strategic approach will be used in this program to distribute free fluoride toothpaste and toothbrushes to communities on a three-monthly basis to encourage the social norm of toothbrushing.

This approach will include:

- All children who participate in daily in-school toothbrushing will receive a second toothbrushing kit every three months to take home for home use
- Senior school children (Years 7–12) will receive a toothbrushing kit every three months to take home for home use
- Parents/guardians at three-monthly intervals will receive free 1000 ppm fluoride toothpaste and toothbrushes every three months during dental health education sessions.

In-school and community dental health education

Dental health education sessions will be delivered to school children and parents and guardians on a three-monthly basis over the pilot period to encourage the uptake of oral hygiene resources which will be distributed.

At the commencement of each new school term (three-monthly basis), a half-hour dental health education session will be delivered to children at each school. Therefore, a total of four sessions will be delivered at each school over the pilot period. Topics covered will be: encouraging brushing twice daily with fluoride toothpaste, restricting sugar intake and encouraging the consumption of water.

Parents/guardians will receive dental health education sessions at the local community health centre every three months (total of four sessions over 12 months). Topics will be: encouraging brushing twice a day with a fluoride toothpaste, demonstrating toothbrushing using a mouth model, restricting sugar intake and encouraging the consumption of water and information on seeking regular dental care. All education sessions will be delivered by an Oral Health Therapist and a local Aboriginal dental assistant.

Dental health knowledge and oral hygiene practices of children and parents/guardians will be collected following the completion of the pilot using the interviewer-assisted questionnaires which were used to collect baseline data in Stage 1. Results will be compared to baseline data to assess the impact of dental health education and the provision of free oral toothbrushes and toothpaste.

The following outcomes will be used during the process evaluation to measure the impact of dental health education and the provision of free oral toothbrushes and toothpaste:

- 90% of Aboriginal children have a toothbrush and toothpaste at home
- 90% of Aboriginal children brushed their teeth in the last 24 h

- 70% of parents and/or guardians are satisfied with the toothbrushing program
- 70% of parents and/or guardians assist their children to brush their teeth each night
- A 70% increase in dental health knowledge specifically relating to the importance of the primary dentition, prevention of tooth decay and the effects of giving a baby a bottle of milk to bed.

School water bottle program

The school water bottle program will ensure filtered and refrigerated water is available on school grounds to reduce the reliance on sugar-sweetened beverages brought into schools. As part of the program, each school will be offered refrigerated and filtered water fountains or refrigeration and filtration units installed to existing fountains depending on the school infrastructure. The water fountains will not remove fluoride nor provide additional fluoride to the water supply. They have been incorporated into this program to provide children with a safe, refreshing and free alternative to sugar-sweetened beverages, which are known to increase a child's risk in developing dental caries. Parents/guardians will be informed of the availability of refrigerated and filtered water at school and education regarding the effects of sugar-sweetened beverages on teeth will be delivered to school canteen staff. To encourage the consumption of water, each child will receive a free drinking water bottle to be kept at school and stored in a ventilated caddy in each classroom. Teachers will be instructed to ask children to fill their water bottle up each morning and encourage them to drink from their water bottles regularly throughout the day. Water bottles will be refilled three times per day to ensure they remain chilled.

The following outcomes will be used during the process evaluation to measure the impact and effectiveness of refrigerated and filtered water fountains:

- 70% of children drink water from the fountain every day
- 90% of children drink tap water daily
- 70% reduction of consumption of sugar-sweetened beverages on a daily basis in children aged 5–12 years
- 70% of teacher support the water fountain and water bottle program

Data collection

As part of the process evaluation (Table 1), qualitative and quantitative data will be used to evaluate the efficiency, feasibility and effectiveness of the program. A focus group will be conducted with teachers and/or Oral Health Aides who directly supervise the toothbrushing program at each school. Therefore, a total of three focus groups will be conducted. A series of pre-determined questions relating to the implementation of the program, issues encountered, and perceived benefits will be used to guide the focus group. Focus groups will be recorded and transcribed verbatim. Thematic analysis will be used to determine themes pertinent to the implementation of school based toothbrushing programs looking at the attitudes and perceptions of teachers and oral health aides to the involvement of the schools in the programs.

A daily register will be used by each school to record student participation in the brushing program. Descriptive analysis of the data will be undertaken to calculate the proportion of children who brush their teeth daily.

The use of the water fountain by the children will be recorded by a researcher on two randomly chosen days over the 12 month pilot. Teachers and students will not the purpose of the researcher's visit to minimise the possibility of altered behaviour. A record of maintenance issues for water fountains installed will also be kept to determine if the fountains are efficient.

An interviewer-assisted questionnaire will be undertaken at the completion of the pilot program with children aged 5–12 years to determine attitudes towards the fountain and changes in oral health knowledge and diet. An interviewer-assisted questionnaire will also be conducted at the completion of the pilot program with parents/guardians to determine changes in oral health knowledge. Questionnaire responses will be analysed using descriptive statistics (SPSS software, version 22 [SPSS Inc., Chicago Ill, USA]).

Discussion

Dental caries is recognised as a preventable disease [15], however, Aboriginal children continue to experience higher levels of dental caries than their non-Aboriginal peers [2]. 'Closing the gap' in Aboriginal oral health has been identified as a State and National priority [5, 16]. Developing and implementing evidence based and sustainable oral health promotion programs has been identified as an important strategy to 'Close the gap' [5, 17]. The shortages of dental professionals in rural and remote communities only reinforces the need for programs to be developed that can be delivered by the local community.

The proposed program includes four evidence-based strategies which have been well documented in international literature to prevent and reduce dental caries. While some of these strategies have been implemented and evaluated in Australian Aboriginal communities [6], Aboriginal children continue to experience near double the rate of dental caries than non-Aboriginal children. Therefore, research into the effective implementation of these strategies that can control dental caries in Aboriginal communities (such as this study) is still needed.

Table 2 Process evaluation plan for proposed oral health promotion program based on Precede-Proceed health model process evaluation

Measure	Definition	Proposed valuation method
Need	Population eligible to receive the program	• Total number of school children from three schools in Central Northern NSW eligible to participate in the program to be collected
Reach	Number of people actually exposed to the program	• Number of children participating in daily toothbrushing • Number of children using the water fountain every day
Impact	Short term effects of the program – usually health behaviour changes	• Number of children brushing every day compared to 2014 baseline data • Number of children who consume water on a regular basis compared to 2014 baseline data • Number of children who consume sugary drinks on a regular basis compared to 2014 • Oral health knowledge and oral hygiene practices of parents compared to 2014 baseline data
Effectiveness	Proportion of people intended to receive the program who successfully changed health behaviours	• Oral health knowledge of parents and oral hygiene practices compared to 2014 baseline data • Number of children brushing every day compared to 2014 baseline data • Teacher focus groups
Cost	Program expenditure	• Record of program expenditure
Efficiency	Proportion of program cost to reach	• Program expenditure over (divided by) program reach

The incorporation of fluoride into preventive oral health care programs is fundamental to ensuring programs are effective. Children who brush their teeth with fluoride toothpaste at least once daily are less likely to develop dental caries. This program proposes daily in-school toothbrushing using fluoride toothpaste for primary school students in Kindergarten to Year 6 which is to be supervised by a classroom teacher and/or Oral Health Aide. School toothbrushing programs often face staffing barriers and problems with infection control [6]. This program proposes two unique points of difference to overcome these barriers. Local Aboriginal Oral Health Aides will assist teachers supervise toothbrushing and teachers and Oral Health Aides will be offered a NSW TAFE skillset in Infection Control and First Aid to ensure they can supervise toothbrushing competently and mitigate infection control issues.

The utilisation of a local Aboriginal Oral Health Aide to supervise toothbrushing is based on the COHI in Canada which uses 'COHI Aides'. The 'COHI Aides' are Indigenous people who have been specifically trained as oral health professionals, providing dental screenings, oral health education and apply fluoride varnish to improve the oral health of Indigenous children in Canada

[14]. Aboriginal Oral Health Aides in time may become a recognised role for Aboriginal people in communities with limited access to oral health services to support the local implementation of community oral health promotion. The role of an Aboriginal Oral Health Aide could potentially include supporting local implementation of oral health promotion programs, delivering dental health education and applying fluoride varnish, similar to the role of 'COHI Aides' in Canada.

Additionally, this program includes a strategic approach to the distribution of free toothpaste and toothbrushes for home use every 3 months to all school students and parent/guardians. This aims to increase accessibility to oral hygiene implements in Aboriginal communities and encourage the social norm of toothbrushing at home.

Preventive oral health programs for Aboriginal children are more likely to be effective if they include dental health education for the wider community [6, 18]. Therefore, this program will provide three-monthly dental health education sessions for students in schools and parents/guardians at local community health centres. The dental health education delivered through this program aims to improve the oral health literacy of Aboriginal children and adults and encourage the uptake of oral hygiene implements which are to be distributed. -. The program proposes that dental health education is delivered by an Oral Health Therapist, accompanied by a local Aboriginal dental assistant to ensure the cultural competence of information given.

The frequent consumption of sugar-sweetened beverages, is associated with increased risk of developing dental caries [19].This program facilitates the installation of refrigerated and filtered water fountains in schools to ensure access to cold and filtered water at schools and reduce reliance on sugar-sweetened beverages. A structured water bottle program component which will be supervised by teachers aims to encourage the consumption of water, rather than sugar-sweetened beverages.

Genuine collaboration has been undertaken with the local Aboriginal community to ensure that these evidence-based strategies are implemented culturally competently, can be led and implemented locally and are sustainable. Oral health promotion in Aboriginal communities is often unsuccessful or ends prematurely due to unsustainable sources of funding or relying on only one individual in the community [6]. This program provides schools and communities the opportunity to work together to implement a suite of evidence-based strategies which are known to prevent and reduce dental caries in an innovative way in Aboriginal communities. This study protocol describes the implementation of four evidence based strategies in schools to improve the oral health of Aboriginal children in Central Northern NSW and may provide insight into the effective implementation of sustainable oral health promotion to reduce dental caries in Aboriginal children in NSW and Australia.These strategies include daily in-school toothbrushing, distribution of free fluoride toothpaste and toothbrushes, a school water bottle program and in-school and community dental health education.

Abbreviations

ACCHS: Aboriginal Community Controlled Health Services; COHI: Children's Oral Health Initiative; dmft/DMFT: Decayed, missing or filled teeth; NSW: New South Wales

Acknowledgements

The authors would like to thank the Poche Centre for Indigenous Health (University of Sydney), the NSW Centre for Oral Health Strategy, Armajun Health Service Aboriginal Corporation, Pius X Aboriginal Corporation, and the three participating schools for their support in this study.

Funding

This study will be funded by the Poche Centre for Indigenous Health, The University of Sydney.

Authors' contributions

YD, AH, KG, MI and AB prepared and submitted the ethics application for this study. YD, KG, MI, AB and NB were involved in the design of the study. NB provided cultural advice on the design of this study. YD, AH, KG, MI and AB were major contributors in writing the manuscript. All authors read and approved the final manuscript.

Competing interests

All authors declare they have no competing interests in the publication of this study protocol.

References

1. Jamieson L, Armfield J, Roberts-Thomson K. Oral health of aboriginal and Torres Strait islander children. Canberra: Australian institute of health and welfare; 2007. http://www.adelaide.edu.au/arcpoh/downloads/publications/reports/dental-statistics-research-series/2000-20008-atsi-children.pdf. Accessed 22 Sep 2017

2. Centre for Oral Health Strategy. The New South Wales Child Dental Health Survey 2007. Sydney: NSW Ministry of Health. p. 2009. http://www.health.nsw.gov.au/oralhealth/Publications/Child-Dental-Survey-2007.pdf. Accessed 22 Sep 2017

3. Christian B, Blinkhorn A. A review of dental caries in Australian aboriginal children: the health inequalities perspective. Rural Remote Health. 2012;12:1–11.

4. NSW Ministry of Health. Oral Health 2020: A Strategic Framework for Dental Health in NSW. North Sydney: NSW Ministry of Health; 2013. http://www.health.nsw.gov.au/oralhealth/Publications/oral-health-2020.pdf. Accessed 22 Sep 2017

5. Centre for Oral Health Strategy. NSW Aboriginal Oral Health Plan 2014–2020. Sydney: NSW Ministry of Health. p. 2014. http://www.health.nsw.gov.au/oralhealth/Publications/aboriginal-oral-health-plan.PDF. Accessed 22 Sep 2017

6. Rogers J. Evidence-based oral health promotion resource. Melbourne: Government of Victoria; 2011. https://www2.health.vic.gov.au/getfile?sc_itemid=%7b82AF49BB-860C-4F2A-A4F1-B0D4A6FE70A6%7d&title=Evidence-based%20oral%20health%20promotion%20resource%20(2011). Accessed 22 Sep 2017

7. Bainbridge R, Mc Calman J, Clifford A, Tsey K. Cultural competency in the delivery of health services for Indigenous people. Canberra: Institute of Health and Welfare; 2015.

8. Gwynne K, Irving M, McCowen D, Rambaldini B, Skinner J, Naoum S, Blinkhorn A. Developing a sustainable model of oral health care for disadvantaged aboriginal people living in rural and remote communities in NSW, using collective impact methodology. J Health Care Poor Underserved. 2016;27:46–53.

9. Ghaffarifar S, Ghofranipour F, Ahmadi F, Khoshbaten M. Barriers to effective doctor-patient relationship based on PRECEDE PROCEED model. Global J Health Sci. 2015;7:24–32.

10. Green L, Kreuter M. Health program planning: an educational and ecological approach. 4th ed. New York: McGraw-Hill; 2005.

11. Dimitropoulos Y, Gunasekera H, Blinkhorn A, Byun R, Binge N, Gwynne K, Irving M. A collaboration with local aboriginal communities in rural New South Wales, Australia to determine the oral health needs of their children and develop a community owned oral health promotion program. Rural Remote Health. 2018;18:4453.

12. Tsai C, Blinkhorn A, Irving M. Oral health Programmes in indigenous communities worldwide—lessons learned from the field: a qualitative systematic review. Community Dent Oral Epidemiol. 2017;45:389–97.

13. Marinho V, Higgins J, Logan S, Sheih A. Fluoride toothpastes for preventing dental caries in children and adolescents. Cochrane Database Syst Rev. 2003;1:CD002278. https://doi.org/10.1002/14651858.CD002278.

14. Mathu-Muju KR, McLeod J, Walker M, Chartier M, Harrison R. The Children's Oral health initiative: an intervention to address the challenges of dental caries in early childhood in Canada's first nation and Inuit communities. Canadian Journal of Public Health. 2016;107:188–93.

15. Watt R. Strategies and approaches in oral disease prevention and health promotion. Bull World Health Organ. 2005;83:711–8.

16. Oral Health Monitoring Group. Healthy Mouths, Healthy Lives: Australia's National Oral Health Plan 2015–2024. Adelaide: COAG Health Council; 2015. http://www.coaghealthcouncil.gov.au/Portals/0/Australia%27s%20National%20Oral%20Health%20Plan%202015-2024_uploaded%20170216.pdf. Accessed 22 Sept 2017.

17. Aboriginal Health & Medical Research Council. AHMRC Oral Health Position Paper: Achieving oral health equity for Aboriginal communities in NSW. Sydney: AHMRC; 2016. http://www.ahmrc.org.au/media/resources/public-health/oral-health/306-oral-health-position-paper/file.html. Accessed 22 Sep 2017.

18. Slade G, Bailie R, Roberts-Thomson K, Leach A, Raye I, Endean C, Simmons B, Morris P. Effect of health promotion and fluoride varnish on dental caries among Australian aboriginal children: results from a community-randomized controlled trial. Community Dent Oral Epidemiol. 2011;39:29–43.

24

The Oral health status of children with autism Spectrum disorder in KwaZulu-Nata, South Africa

Magandhree Naidoo[*] 🆔 and Shenuka Singh

Abstract

Background: Echoing the sentiments of the Sixty-seventh World Health Assembly of May 2014, mandating the all-inclusive and synchronized efforts for the management of autism spectrum disorder (ASD), the aim of this current study was to investigate the oral health status of children with ASD aged between 7 to 14 years in KwaZulu-Natal, South Africa.

Methods: An investigative cross-sectional quantitative design employing non-probability purposeful sampling was conducted on 149 children with ASD attending special needs schools in KwaZulu-Natal. An intra-oral examination to investigate decayed, missing and filled teeth (DMFT/dmft), gingival index (GI), and plaque index (PI), attrition and soft tissue trauma using the World Oral Health Survey Form for Children, (2013) was implemented during data collection.

Results: Average DMFT/dmft scores of 3, 42 and 0, 97 were recorded respectively. Molars dominated the decayed component of the DMFT/dmft with an average caries prevalence of (51, 7% and 40, 8%) respectively. These results displayed zero fillings indicative of unmet treatment needs. The gingival index revealed mild gingival inflammation, (46, 3%) and the plaque index demonstrated visible plaque at (43, 6%).Attrition scores revealed mild loss of dental enamel (47%). The most prevalent soft tissue trauma recorded was lip biting (37, 25%).

Conclusion: Restorative or preventative treatment measures were not evident in this study. Unmet dental needs are therefore an important concern in this population. Health care planners should develop preventive programs targeted at high risk groups such as this study population.

Keywords: Dental caries, Oral health, Plaque, Gingival inflammation, Oral care

Background

The South African Government displayed its advocacy for defending and protecting the right to health of all children aged below 18 years by ratifying the United Nations Convention on the Rights of the Child, (1989) [1]. The population with (ASD) presents with similar health problems as that of the typical population, but due to factors including poor dietary preferences; behaviors and specific aversions, this population is at a greater risk and more susceptible to developing chronic non-communicable oral health conditions [2]. The increasing prevalence of ASD coupled with this population being highlighted as one those with the greatest disease burden, has ignited an interest in their oral health concerns, which coincides with one of the global oral health goals to promote oral health within this population group [3]. ASD is a neurodevelopment disorder which presents within the first 3 years of life [4]. Typical manifestation include impaired social interactions; deficits in language acquisition; and restricted and repetitive behaviours [5]. The World Health Organisation has estimated the global prevalence of ASD to be 1:160 persons [6]. This is an average figure that however, does not include the prevalence of this condition in Sub-Saharan Africa. The scarcity of this data has been attributed to the rarity of epidemiological surveys on ASD in this geographical area [7]. Some data extracted predominantly from studies conducted at hospitals such as in South-West Nigeria documented a prevalence rate of 1:43.5; South-Eastern Nigeria, revealed a prevalence rate of 1:125; and

---
[*] Correspondence: magnaidoo@uwc.ac.za
School of Health Sciences, Discipline of Dentistry, University of KwaZulu-Natal, Westville Campus, South Africa

Uganda, documented a prevalence of 6.8:1000 [8, 9].Unfortunately due to the absence of epidemiological studies in South Africa, accurate national autism statistics in South Africa are not available. Global prevalence rates according to The World Health Organization [6] is currently being used.

There are no typical unusual oral manifestations present in individuals with ASD. However due to problematic behaviors; unusual oral habits; medications; and dietary preferences, this population appears to be at risk for the development of oral diseases [10, 11]. It has been estimated that almost 70% of individual with ASD present with self-injurious behaviours (SIB) located in the head and neck region [12]. Oral findings reported in patients with autism spectrum disorder included traumatic ulcerated lesions frequently a consequence of (SIB) such as head banging; face tapping; and gingival picking [13]. Another consequence of SIB noted in autism is auto extraction. Auto-extraction refers to the self-removal of teeth [14]. Unusual oral habits include bruxism, tongue thrusting, non-nutritive chewing on objects such as gravel, cigarette butts, or pens and repeated regurgitation [15]. The most frequently reported dental implications of bruxism in children with autism spectrum disorder include joint pain in the temporomandibular area; excessive wear of the dental enamel; and tooth avulsion [16]. Attrition has also been a consequence of a condition frequently seen in ASD called Pica. Lithophagia, a type of Pica involving the eating of grit and stones has been documented to lead to attrition and enamel wear [17]. Conditions such as over jets, spacing, Class II molar inclinations and open bites were also reportedly higher in patients with ASD [18].

Children with ASD are often cited as having certain food preferences, which includes sweets and soft foods [19]. Additionally manual dexterity required for adequate tooth brushing is often reduced in children with ASD, resulting in inadequate tooth brushing [2]. Dental care access and oral care delivery has proved to be very problematic for children with ASD. Financial costs, scarcity of medical aid coverage and the child's indifference towards dental procedures has been acknowledged as the core liabilities to oral care delivery for this population [20].

The maintenance of optimum oral care in children with ASD ought to be of significant focus, since existing oral care problems may intensify, thereby impacting the individual's overall quality of life [21]. Accordingly, an essentiality for a holistic approach to oral care in children with ASD is required [22]. However conflicting research results globally, on the oral care status of children with ASD has placed oral care interventions in this population at a crossroad [23]. Several studies have reported poor oral hygiene in children with ASD [2, 9, 24–27], whilst other research reported better oral

hygiene in participants with ASD [28–32], and comparable oral health was also recorded for this population [33, 34]. This confliction is inflated by the non-existence South African epidemiological data. Data which is vital to inform and plan preventative oral care measures is unfortunately, to the best of our knowledge, not available. Global oral health studies conducted in this population is therefore considered as a point of reference for the said study. The conflicting status of oral care in children with ASD presents a dilemma. Research is anticipatory to elucidate our understanding of ASD and oral care, specifically the oral care status of this population that will serve to inform future oral care measures and procedures.

The numerous studies conducted abroad on the ASD population have shown that children with autism spectrum disorder have either statistically higher; lower or similar caries experience when compared to those without this condition [2, 9, 24, 28, 29, 33, 34]. South African epidemiologic data on the oral care status of children with ASD is lacking. Therefore the aim of this study was to create an epidemiological oral care profile for children with ASD aged between 7 to 14 years attending special needs schools in KwaZulu-Natal, South Africa, by investigating the oral health status within the parameters of the DMFT/dmft; GI; PI; attrition and soft tissue trauma.

Methods
Study design
This study was conducted by means of a cross-sectional design, using quantitative data. In order to establish the burden of disease in a specific population, which can subsequently be used for intervention and health planning programs, data was collected at a specific time and analyzed to evaluate the oral health status of children with autism spectrum disorder.

Setting of the study
This research was undertaken in KwaZulu-Natal, one of 9 provinces in South Africa. A list from the (KwaZulu-Natal Department of Education) identified 45 special needs schools in this province. Personal communication into these 45 special needs schools revealed that only 20 of these 45 schools cater for children with ASD in KwaZulu-Natal.

Study population
Children aged between 7 to 14 years, attending identified special needs schools in KwaZulu-Natal, who were diagnosed with autism spectrum disorder according to the DSM-V criteria by a qualified professional were included in this study. The inclusion criteria also stipulated that participants would only be included after parental

consent and individual assent was obtained. The exclusion criteria included Children who presented with any other co-existing condition; with no formal diagnosis; children whose parents did not consent to the study and those who did not assent to the study were excluded from the study. This study intended to exclude children who had visited the dentist within the last 3 months of data collection to minimize any potential bias because it was anticipated that any dental intervention could potentially impact on the results of the GI scores. This exclusion was however revised and was not included as an exclusion criteria. The population size for children with ASD in KwaZulu-Natal due to the absence of existing data could not be ascertained. Data collection was subjected to the response rate from the special needs schools. At a response rate of 80, 9%, a total of 149 children with ASD were included in this study.

Data collection

Data was collected by a single researcher, an oral hygienist registered with the Health professions Council of South Africa (HPCSA), employed within the academic discipline of dentistry. The researcher was calibrated by academics involved in caries research. Calibration was performed according to the standards set out by The British Association for the Study of Community Dentistry (BASCD). During the process of data collection involving a single researcher, it is often questioned if the researcher will record and interpret a finding in the same manner when presented with the same situation twice. Intra-examiner reliability was observed by adhering to the guidelines of the World Health Organization [35] where every 5th participant was re-examined and data recorded on a separate data sheet to be compared later. Data was recorded by a registered dental therapist. The Kappa statistic were employed to ascertain intra-examiner reliability on 29 participants. A kappa value for DMFT (0,915); GI (0,920); PI (0,880); attrition (0,824) and soft tissue trauma (0,930) was reached.

Decayed, missing and filled index (DMFT/dmft); gingival index (GI); plaque index (PI); attrition; and soft tissue trauma was assessed using the world oral health survey, (2013) [36]. The Gingival Index [37] was used to assess the gingival status and to record clinical variations in the gingiva. Due to the nature of the participants, this examination was adapted to evaluate the overall gingival status by means of a visual examination. The bleeding upon probing of selected index teeth was omitted to avoid participant anxiety. Based on the visual examination, changes in color; size and shape were observed and scored. Gingiva observed with no clinical variations in color; size and shape was scored 0 and categorized as normal. Gingiva observed with slight changes in color, size and shape was scored 1 and categorized as mild

gingival inflammation. Gingiva observed with changes in color; size and shape accompanied by visible signs of bleeding was scored 2 and categorized as moderate gingival inflammation. Gingiva observed with distinctive gingival enlargement and spontaneous bleeding was scored 3 and categorized as severe gingival inflammation. Similar adaptations were made in a study on the oral health status of children with ASD in Chennai [35]. These adaptive measures were employed in the Chennai study to accommodate the characteristic behaviors of these participants. These authors have agreed that these adaptations did not show any evidence of compromise in the validity of the results.

Plaque accumulation was recorded using the plaque index [38]. Attrition and soft tissue trauma was recorded according to the categories in the (World Oral Health Survey, 2013) [39]. All infection control procedures were maintained according to the Center for Disease Control (CDC) guidelines and waste was disposed of according to the waste removal guidelines of the Health Professions Council of South Africa.

Approval to conduct this research was obtained from The Biomedical Research and Ethics Committee (BREC[1]) at The University of KwaZulu-Natal; the KwaZulu-Natal Department of Education (KZN-DOE[2]); and the KwaZulu- Natal Department of Health (KZN-DOH[3]). Consent for participation was obtained from the participating school principals; teachers; and parents of selected children. ASD has varying degrees of impairment that may impact cooperation during data collection. The designated school therapist assisted with the selection of participants based on the functioning of the child. Higher functioning children were selected by the therapist for participation in this study. Assent was obtained from the participant prior to the commencement of data collection. Provisional dates for the data collection were sent to the participating schools. This assessment was conducted in accordance with the guidelines of the World Oral Health Survey [39]. Each participant was allowed to assent to the study using a picture communication board in the presence of the teacher or teaching assistant. The facilitator/ teacher escorted the consenting participant to the mobile dental unit. A picture communication schedule, prepared using the Boardmaker Software® was used to explain the procedure to both the facilitator/teacher and the participant. The participant was seated on the dental chair. An extra-oral examination to assess the presence of any scars; lip biting; trauma to the head and neck; hands and fingers; and signs of self-injurious behaviors was conducted first. An intra-oral examination of the soft and hard tissues was conducted using disposable gloves, disposable tongue depressors for retraction and sterilize gauze. This examination assessed decayed, missing and filled teeth according to the DMFT/dmft index. Gingival inflammation; plaque accumulation; attrition; and soft tissue trauma were investigated according to categories of the World Oral health Survey, 2013. All disposable medical waste was disposed of in designated containers according to the HPCSA guidelines and returned to the oral and dental training hospital to be collected by an accredited waste removals service provider. The participants were thanked and provided with a sample toothbrush and toothpaste as a token of appreciation and escorted back to the classroom. A research assistant recorded all data.

Data was analysed using IBM SPSS version 24.0. Descriptive statistics included the use of frequency tables, cross-tabulations and means with standard deviations. Inferential statistics used the Fisher's Exact test to determine relationships between the status of teeth and factors of interest such as (gender; location and age). The Kolmogorov Smirnov test revealed that the data was not normally distributed and means companions were done using the Kruskal Wallis tests. Kappa statistics was used to determine intra-examiner reliability.

Results

A response rate of 80, 97% ($n = 149$) was recorded. The majority of participants of this study were male, (71, 1%). Most participants indicated that they live in Peri-urban geographical areas, (78%). The age distribution is reflected in Table 1.

A mean score of 3, 07 for decayed teeth (D); missing teeth (M) was 0, 39; and filled (F) 0, was recorded in the permanent dentition. An average DMFT score was recorded at 3, 42. Average caries prevalence in the permanent molars was recorded at 51, 7%; 12, 4% in the premolars; 3, 7% in the canines and in the incisors. As indicated in Table 2, an average caries prevalence of 17, 9% was recorded in the permanent dentition in this study.

A mean score for decayed (d), 0, 96; missing (m), 0, 01; and filled (f), 0 was recorded in the primary dentition. The average dmft score recorded was 0, 97. The

Table 1 Gender; Age; And Geographical Distribution of Children with ASD in KwaZulu-Natal ($n = 149$)

Gender	n (%)
Female	43 (28,9)
Male	106 (71,1)
Geographic Location	
Suburban	116 (77,9)
Rural	33 (22,1)
Age in Years	
7–8	30 (20,1)
9–10	37 (24,8)
10–11	37 (24,8)
12–14	45 (30,2)

Table 2 Caries Prevalence in Children with ASD in KwaZulu-Natal ($n = 149$)

Permanent Dentition	Prevalence of Caries (%)	Primary Dentition	Prevalence of Caries n (%)
Molars	51,65	Molars	40,8
Premolars	12,45		
Canines	3,7	Canines	21,88
Incisors	3,7	Incisors	25,45
Average Caries Prevalence	17,9	Average Caries Prevalence	29,38

caries prevalence in the primary molars was recorded at 40, 8%; canines 21, 9%; and incisors 25, 4%. The average caries experience for the primary dentition was 29, 38%.

This study also demonstrated that 16, 8% of the study participants presented with no observable dental caries, whilst 12, 8% presented with at least one decayed tooth as specified in Table 3. The prevalence of decayed teeth observed within gender, location and age is presented in Table 3. These results indicate that males were observed with more dental caries than females. The presence of decay based on location show that more caries was observed in the suburban location. Dental caries within the age category revealed high caries prevalence in the 12–14-year age group.

The assessment of the gingiva indicated that majority of the participants presented with mild gingival inflammation (46, 3%). The results of the PI in the current study as indicated in Table 4 show the following mentionable scores, namely, a film of visible plaque was recorded at 43, 6% and moderate accumulation of plaque at 42, 3%.

The results of the examination on attrition indicated that 40,9% of the participants showed no signs of dentine wear; 47,0% showed signs of loss of enamel surface characteristics; and 11,4% presented with wearing of the teeth where the dentine was just visible. There were no observations of a dentine exposure of greater than one third. The soft tissue examination indicated that the most prevalent soft tissue trauma was lip biting (37, 25%) Table 5.

Discussion

To our knowledge this is the first epidemiological study investigating the oral health status of children aged 7 to 14 years with ASD in South Africa. This condition is virtually 5 times more common amongst males than females [40]. According to this ratio, the gender representation in this study was males (71%) and females (29%). Inequality in demographic representation could be attributed to a reduced number of ASD diagnoses in the rural areas [41].

The overall caries prevalence in the permanent dentition of this study population was 85, 2%. This was significantly higher than a similar study conducted in 2011

Table 3 Decay Within Gender; Location and Age (n = 149)

Category Gender	Decay = 0	Decay = 1	Decay = 2	Decay = 3	Decay = 4	Decay = 5	Decay = 6	Decay = 7	Decay = 8	Decay = 9	Decay = 12	Total
Female	19 (23,3)	5 (11,6)	11 (25,6)	1 (2,3)	7 (16,3)	0 (0)	3 (7,0)	4 (9,3)	0 (0,9)	1 (0)	1 (2,3)	43 (28,9)
Male	15 (14,2)	14 (13,2)	19 (17,9)	7 (6,6)	32 (30,2)	3 (2,8)	9 (8,5)	1 (0,9)	5 (4,7)	1 (0,9)	0 (0)	106 (71,1)
(p < 0,05)												
Category Location	Decay = 0	Decay = 1	Decay = 2	Decay = 3	Decay = 4	Decay = 5	Decay = 6	Decay = 7	Decay = 8	Decay = 9	Decay = 12	Total
Peri-Urban	23 (19,8)	14 (12,1)	25 (21,6)	7 (6,0)	24 (20,7)	2 (1,7)	11 (9,5)	4 (3,4)	5 (4,3)	1 (0,9)	0 (0)	116 (77,9)
Rural	2 (6,1)	5 (15,2)	5 (15,2)	1 (3,0)	15 (45,5)	1(3,0)	1 (3,0)	1 (3,0)	0 (0)	1 (3,0)	1 (3,0)	33 (22,1)
(p = 0,05)												
Category Age	Decay = 0	Decay = 1	Decay = 2	Decay = 3	Decay = 4	Decay = 5	Decay = 6	Decay = 7	Decay = 8	Decay = 9	Decay = 12	Total
7–8 Years	11 (36,7)	4 (13,3)	8 (26,7)	1 (3,3)	6 (20,0)	0 (0)	0 (0)	0 (0)	0 (0)	0 (0)	0 (0)	30 (20,1)
9–10 Years	5 (13,5)	3 (8,1)	8 (21,6)	3 (8,1)	12 (32,4)	1 (2,7)	2 (5,4)	2 (5,4)	0 (0)	I (2, 7)	0 (0)	37 (24,8)
11–12 Years	5 (13,5)	5 (13,5)	9 (24,3)	2 (5,4)	8 (21,6)	1 (2,7)	4 (10,8)	1 (2,7)	1 (2,7)	0 (0)	1 (2,7)	37 (24,8)
13–14 Years	4 (8,9)	7 (15,6)	5 (11,1)	2 (4,4)	13 28,9)	1 (2,2)	6 (13,3)	2 (4,4)	4 (8,9)	1 (2,2)	0 (0)	45 (30,2)
(p = 0,05)												

[2], which reported an overall caries prevalence of 77% in children with ASD in Dubai; the statistics from the National Oral Health survey which indicated a caries prevalence of 41, 7% between 1999 and 2002 [42],; the prevalence of 30, 55% and 56,5% reported in 2014 [29] and 2015 [30], respectively. This is indicative of a greater burden of dental caries for this study population within the South African context. In 1981, the World Health Organization (WHO) and the World Dental Federation (FDI) jointly formulated goals for oral health to be achieved by the year 2000. *"By the year 2000, the global average for dental caries was to be no more than 3 DMFT at 12 years of age."* [36]This study 17 years later, with an average DMFT of 3, 42 is above the global average, indicating that oral health goals were not met for this study population.

The mean DMFT score recorded in the current study when compared to previous DMFT scores for South African studies shows that it is lower than the mean DMFT recorded in Durban in 1988; same as that recorded in Durban in 2002 [38], but significantly higher than the study

in Venda, South Africa [28].When compared to DMFT scores on studies conducted abroad with Children with ASD [2, 9, 24, 28–30, 34], the current DMFT scores are higher, except for the study conducted in 2014 [17]. The DMFT of the current study indicates high caries prevalence in the permanent dentition of children with ASD in KwaZulu-Natal when compared to both South African studies and studies conducted abroad. These results support previous studies that the burden of dental caries in the permanent dentition of children with ASD is of concern [28]. This may be due to the presence of more permanent teeth in the oral cavity as the child's age increases.

This study also demonstrated that both maxillary and mandibular molars (51, 7%) presented as the major contributors to the decayed component of the DMFT. Previous reports have indicated the preference for soft and sugary foods, further compounded by the pouching of food at the back of the oral cavity, rather than swallowing it, to be accountable for the high prevalence of caries in the molar region of children with ASD [43]. Oral care practices at home and the frequency of brushing have

Table 4 Adapted Gingival Index and Plaque Index [38] of children with Autism spectrum Disorder in KwaZulu- Natal (n = 149)

Gingival Status	Average Gingival Index Score n (%)	Plaque Index	Plaque Index n (%)
Healthy Gingiva	6 (4)	No plaque	14 (9,4)
Mild Gingival Inflammation	69 (46,3)	A film of visible plaque after the use of a disclosing agent or probe.	65 (43,6)
Moderate Gingival Inflammation	66 (44,3)	Moderate accumulation of plaque on more than one third of the tooth surface, Can be seen with the naked eye.	63 (42,3)
Severe Gingival Inflammation	8 (5,4)	Accumulation of plaque on more than two thirds of the tooth surface. Presence of calculus.	7 (4,7)
Total	149 (100)	Total	149 (100)

Table 5 Attrition in Children with Autism spectrum Disorder in KwaZulu-Natal ($n = 149$)

Description of Dentition	Average Attrition Score (%)
No tooth loss (no wear into dentine)	40,9
Loss of enamel surface characteristic	47,0
Tooth loss (with dentine just visible)	11,4
Enamel loss exposing greater than 1/3 of dentine.	0,0
Total	100

also contributed to caries levels in children with ASD [44]. Increased caries noted in this study population might also be as a result of challenges faced by parents during oral care routines [45], and manual dexterity required for adequate tooth brushing resulting in poor and unsatisfactory plaque control and removal [2].

The dmft recorded for this study is lower than the mean dmft score of the recent study, conducted in KwaZulu-Natal [31]. However important to note is that fact that despite a low dmft index, once again the major contributors to the decay component in the primary dentition was the molars (40, 8%). This further supports findings of the pouching of food at the back of the mouth for extended periods of time as a significant contributing factor to dental caries in this population [41].

The decayed teeth recorded in both the permanent and primary dentition in this study were all untreated, highlighting unmet dental needs amongst children with ASD [46]. The mean filled component for the DMFT/dmft was recorded as, 0 in this study. This supports previously reported studies of unmet dental needs, poor access to restorative dentistry, poor preventive care or an aversion to dental treatment in children with ASD [47]. Dental care access and oral care delivery has proved to be very problematic for children with ASD. Unmet dental needs within the South African context may be as a result of core liabilities such as financial costs and scarcity of medical aid coverage for this population [12].

This study showed that 16, 8% of children with ASD presented with no dental caries and 12, 7% presented with at least one decayed tooth. This can be attributed to families and caregivers monitoring dietary intake, thereby limiting the consumption of cariogenic foods. Moreover, efficient supervision of parents during home oral care practices has contributed to children with ASD having a low or zero caries prevalence [48]. This emphasizes the need for inclusion of family members and caregivers during the planning of oral care programs for children with ASD. The distinctive obsession with certain low carbohydrate diets have also impacted dental caries positively by reducing the risk to dental caries [39].

This study consisted of 106 males and 43 females, revealing a male-female ratio of 2.5:1, which was undeviating from former a study reporting a male gender bias in ASD [49]. A Chi square test was performed to determine whether there was a statistically significant relationship between the prevalence of dental caries and gender. The p-value between *"gender"* and *"dental caries"* is 0.049 ($p < 0.05$). Significantly more males exhibited dental caries than females. This finding was contradictory to findings that demonstrated that females exhibited higher caries prevalence than males [20, 41]. These results were however consistent with findings in a study in Chennai that indicated higher prevalence of caries in males with ASD [35].

Females clinically diagnosed with ASD are most likely to be at the advanced end of the IQ spectrum [50, 51]. Furthermore, females with ASD that have an "average" IQ demonstrate amplified functional attributes compared to their male counterparts [52]. This may account for better oral care practices amongst females, thereby exhibiting better oral hygiene and fewer caries. The results of caries prevalence within gender in this study may also be attributed to the sample size.

The p-value between *"age"* and *"dental caries"*, ($p = 0.05$), indicated a significant relationship between *"age"* and *"dental caries"*. The prevalence of caries recorded in this study was predominantly in the 12 to 14 year age category (30, 2%). This finding is in line with the findings of an almost doubled DMFT score for the 12 to 15 year age in Venda, South Africa [28]. The results of this study are also similar to the report showing that the 12 to 15 year age group was in great need of preventative and restorative dental services in South Africa [33]. An increase in age is accompanied by an increase in the number of permanent teeth present in the oral cavity. The finding of an increased prevalence of caries in this age group may be attributed to the increased number of permanent teeth present. Preventative oral health programs targeted at this specific age group should be tailored to include fissure sealants on all newly erupted molars. Fissure sealants have been demonstrated as an efficient dental caries preventative measure [53]. Assistance provided by family members during oral care practices also tend to become more challenging as the child ages and this has impacted the oral care status and the prevalence of dental caries [18]. Besides this being the age during which permanent molars replace deciduous premolars, it is also the age at which adolescence emerges and the child tends to declare independence requiring less family assistance and supervision during oral care routines. Oral care program should also include practices to assist this newly found independence in this specific age group.

An investigation into the prevalence of dental caries and geographical location indicated that participants located in the peri-urban area presented with a higher prevalence of dental caries than those in the rural areas. Similar results were obtained in 2014 [28]. Due to affordability and socioeconomic implication, access to sugar and sugar containing foods are limited in rural areas, accounting for the low caries prevalence in these areas [54].

The data analysis indicates an overall prevalence of gingival inflammation of 94%. A high prevalence of mild gingival inflammation was recorded (46, 3%). Some of the challenges for optimal gingival status include behaviors in the dental office and at home, oral care practices; insufficient manual dexterity and deficient oral hygiene knowledge [2, 36]. Research has indicated that reduced upper limb fine motor coordination tends to produce challenges for the maintenance of optimum oral hygiene in children with ASD, thus increasing the probability of gingival inflammation [18]. Furthermore the frequently consumed psychotropic medication has also impacted the gingival status in ASD due to its side effects such as gingival hyperplasia [55].

The plaque index scores indicate that most of the children presented with either a film of visible plaque or moderate plaque accumulation. This finding is in agreement with previous findings [2, 13, 16, 17], which recorded poor oral hygiene in children with ASD as result of plaque accumulation. Rearing a child with ASD is an overwhelming experience for all involved, frequently resulting in stressful situations. In an attempt to minimize these stressful situations, adaptations are made to the child's routines. This leads to interferences in the oral health care regimen [56]. Children with ASD often do not practice proper oral care routines due to an aversion to the presence of a toothbrush in their mouth and a dislike of the taste and texture of toothpaste. Consequently they tend to brush their teeth less frequently than children without ASD [36].

Attrition scores (47%) in the mild category were noteworthy in this study. Bruxism, a form of vigorous grinding of teeth has being reported as one of the sleep problems frequently experienced by children with ASD [57]. Reports indicate a higher prevalence of bruxism in children with special needs resulting in extreme dental wear, avulsion of teeth and temporomandibular joint pain [16].

Soft tissue trauma in the head and neck region was found in 68, 5% of the study participants. This is in agreement with past reports that almost 70% of autistic individuals present with self-injurious behaviours located in the head and neck region [9]. Of the 68, 5% that presented with soft tissue trauma, lip biting (37, 25%) was the most prevalent. The high prevalence of lip biting in this study may also be due to the distorted pain tolerance that has been noted in children with ASD [21].

Clinical relevance
Optimum oral health is an essential component to the overall maintenance of optimum general health for children with ASD. This vulnerable special needs population has

been posited as *"at risk"* for the development of non-communicable dental diseases such as dental caries, a condition that is very prevalent amongst these children. The expansive knowledge of dental caries and the preventative measures available, renders the effective prevention of dental caries a reasonably manageable objective. Research findings will henceforth serve to inform the development and implementation of applicable and efficient oral health preventative programs. These programs will not only serve to address identified areas in the research findings but also attempt to moderate the access to care and minimize oral health care inequalities as identified in unmet dental needs in this study population. The findings of this study will also serve as an important data source during the creating, assimilating, evolving, and implementing of community preventative oral care programs for children with ASD.

Conclusion
The results of this study indicate that the children aged between 7 to 14 years with ASD in KwaZulu-Natal, displayed an average DMFT of 3, 42. The molars presented as significant contributors to the DMFT/dmft recorded in this study. Furthermore all of the carious lesions recorded were untreated. There was no evidence of any restorative or preventative treatment measures. Unmet dental needs are therefore an important concern in this population. Mild gingival inflammation and evidence of the presence of moderate plaque accumulation further emphasize the need for preventive intervention in this study population. Health care planners should develop preventive programs that are targeted at caries prevention; oral care practices and oral care education to address the various oral care challenges in ASD.

Abbreviations
ASD: Autism spectrum disorder; DOE: Department of Education; DOH: Department of Health; IBM SPSS: SPSS Statistics is a software package used for logical batched and non-batched statistical analysis. Long produced by SPSS Inc., it was acquired by IBM in 2009. The current versions are officially named IBM SPSS Statistics; KZN: KwaZulu-Natal; SIB: Self-injurious behaviors; WHO: World Health Organization

Acknowledgements
1. University of Kwa-Zulu Natal, South Africa and Professor Shenuka Singh for her role as a supervisor.
2. Mrs. L. Reddy; Miss S.Kanniapen; and Mr. D. Singh for their roles as a research assistant; data capture and statistician.
3. Colgate-Palmolive (Pty) Ltd. - South Africa for the use of the mobile dental unit and dental traders in South Africa for the provision of samples.

Funding
This study was funded by:

1) College of Health Sciences Scholarship (CHS Scholarship – UKZN, 8829859)
2) International Federation of Dental Hygienists (IFDH Research Grant - 7004160165085)

Authors' contributions

Mrs. MN: Coordination of the research project, Obtaining consents and assents, the dental examination procedure, training of research assistant, data entry and analysis and writing of the manuscript. Prof. SS: Review of the manuscripts and supervision of the research project. All authors read and approved the final manuscript.

Competing interests

The authors declare that they have no competing interests.

References

1. The United Nations. Convention on the Rights of the Child. Treaty Series. 1989;1577:3.
2. Jaber MA. Dental caries experience, oral health status and treatment needs of dental patients with autism. J Appl Oral Sci. 2011;19(3):212–7. https://doi.org/10.1590/s1678-77572011000300006.
3. World Health Organization. World health report .Shaping the future. Geneva: World Health Organization; 2003.
4. Schwartz, A. Causes. Etiology and biochemical abnormalities of autism. Chapter I. 2004; http://www.springboard4health.com/notebook/health_autism.html.
5. American Psychiatric Association. Diagnostic and statistical manual of mental disorders (5th Ed). Arlington: American Psychiatric Publishing; 2013.
6. WHO, World Health Organisation. Autism spectrum disorders & other developmental disorders. Geneva: From Raising Awareness to Building Capacity; 2013.
7. Franz L, Chambers N, von Isenburg M, de Vries PJ. Autism spectrum disorder in sub-Saharan Africa: a comprehensive scoping review. Autism Res. 2017;10:723–49. https://doi.org/10.1002/aur.1766.
8. Lagunju IA, Bella-Awusah TT, Omigbodun OO. Autistic disorder in Nigeria: profile and challenges to management. Epilepsy Behav. 2014;39:126–9.
9. Kakooza-Mwesige A, Ssebyala K, Karamagi C, Kiguli S, Smith K, Anderson MC, et al. Adaptation of the "ten questions" to screen for autism and other neurodevelopmental disorders in Uganda. Autism. 2014;18:447–57.
10. Klein U, Nowak A. Characteristics of patients withautistic disorder (AD) presenting for dental treatment: A Surreyand chart review. Spec Care Dent. 1999;19(5):200–7.
11. Dávila JM, Jensen OE. Behavioural and pharmacological dental management of a patient with autism. Spec Care Dentist. 1988;8:58–60.
12. Medina AC, Sogbe R, Gómez-Rey AM, Mata M. Factitial oral lesions in an autistic paediatric patient. Int J Paediatr Dent. 2003;13:130–7.
13. Ravel D. Dental Management of Children with autism: Pediatric Dental Health; 2005.
14. Keles S, Dogusal G, Sönmez I. Autoextraction of Permanent Incisors and Self-Inflicted Orodental Trauma in a Severely Burned Child, Case Reports in Dentistry. Hindawi Publishing Corporation; 2015. p. 425251. https://doi.org/10.1155/2015/425251.
15. Nagendra J, Jayachandra S. Autism spectrum disorders: dental treatment considerations. J Int Dent Med Res. 2012;5(2):118–21.
16. Monroy PG, Da Fonseca MA. The use of botulinum toxin a in the treatment of severe bruxism in a patient with autism. Spec Care Dentist. 2006;26:37–9.
17. Bhargava S, Motwani MB, Patni V. Oral Implications of Eating Disorder: A Review. Arch Orofac Sci. 2013;8(1):1–8 ISSN 1823:8602.
18. Luppanapornlarp S, et al. Periodontal status and orthodontic treatment need of autistic children. World J Orthod. 2010;11(3):256–61.
19. Cermak SA, Curtin C, Bandini LG. Food selectivity and sensory sensitivity in children with autism Spectrum disorders. J Am Diet Assoc. 2010;110(2):238–46. https://doi.org/10.1016/j.jada.2009.10.032.
20. Lai B, Milano M, Roberts MW, Hooper SR. Unmet dental needs and barriers to dental care among children with autism spectrum disorders. J Autism Dev Disord. 2012;42(12):94–303.
21. Richa YR, Puranik MP. Oral health status and parental perception of child oral healthrelated quality-of-life of children with autism in Bangalore, India. J Indian Soc Pedod Prev Dent. 2014;32:135–9.
22. Norderyd J, Klingberg G, Faulks D, Granlund M. Specialised dental care for children with complex disabilities focusing on child's functioning and need for general anaesthesia. Disabil Rehabil. 2017;39(24):2484–91. https://doi.org/10.1080/09638288.2016.1236406.
23. Blomqvist M, Bejerot S, Dahllöf G. A cross-sectional study on oral health and dental care in intellectually able adults with autism spectrum disorder. BMC Oral Health. 2015;15(1):81.
24. Vishnu Rekha C, Arangannal P, Shahed H. Oral health status of children with autistic disorder in Chennai. Eur Arch Paediatr Dent. 2012;13:126–31.
25. Al-Maweri S, et al. Oral lesions and dental status of autistic children in Yemen: a case-control study. J Int Soc Prev Community Dent. 2014;4(3):199–203. https://doi.org/10.4103/2231-0762.149040.
26. Goncalves LTYR, Goncalves FYYR, Nogueira BML, Fonseca RRS, DE Menezes SAF, DA Silva E Souza PAR, Menezes TOA. Conditions for oral health in patients with autism. Int J Odontostomat. 2016;10(1):93–7.
27. Morales-Chávez MC. Oral health assessment of a Group of Children with autism disorder. J Clin Pediatr Dent. 2017;41(2):147–9.
28. Namal N, Vehit H, Koksal S. Do autistic children have higher levels of caries? A cross-sectional study in Turkish children. J Indian Soc Pedod Prev Dent. 2007;25(2):97–102. https://doi.org/10.4103/0970-4388.33457.
29. Loo CY, Graham RM, Hughes CV. The caries experience and behavior of dental patients with autism Spectrum disorder. J Am Dent Assoc. 2008;139(11):1518–24. https://doi.org/10.14219/jada.archive.2008.0078.
30. Subramaniam P, Gupta M. Oral health status of autistic children in India. J Clin Pediatr Dent. 2011;36(1):43–4.
31. Du, Y., Yiu, C., King, N., Wong, V., & Pj McGrath, C. (2014). Oral health among preschool Children with autism spectrum disorders: A case-control study. Autism. 2014;19(6):746–751.
32. Fakroon S, Arheiam A, Omar S. Dental caries experience and periodontal treatment needs of children with autistic spectrum disorder. Eur Arch Paediatr Dent. 2015;16:205.
33. Sverd J, Montero G, Gurevich N. Brief report: cases for an association between Tourette syndrome, autistic disorder, and schizophrenia-like disorder. J Autism Dev Disord. 1993;23(2):407–13.
34. Bayat-Movahed S, Samadzadeh H, Ziyarati L, Memary N, Khosravi R, Sadr-Eshkevari PS. Oral health of Iranian children in 2004: a national pathfinder survey of dental caries and treatment needs. East Mediterr Health J. 2011;17(3):243–9.
35. World Health Organization. Oral health surveys: basic methods. 5th ed. Geneva: World Health Organization; 2013.
36. WHO Expert Committee on Disability Prevention and Rehabilitation & World Health Organization. Disability prevention and rehabilitation: report of the WHO Expert Committee on Disability Prevention and Rehabilitation [meeting held in Geneva from 17 to 23 February 1981: Geneva.
37. Loe H, Silness J. Periodontal disease in pregnancy I. prevalence and severity. Acta Odontol Scand. 1963;21:533–51.
38. Silness J, Loe H. Correlation between oral hygiene and periodontal condition. ActaOdontol Scand. 1964;22:121–35.
39. Kopel HM. The autistic child in dental practice. ASDC J Dent Child. 1977;44:302–9.
40. Dworzynski K, Ronald A, Bolton P, Happé F. How different are girls and boys above and below the diagnostic threshold for autism Spectrum disorders? J Am Acad Child Adolesc Psychiatry. 2012;51(8):788–97.
41. Robinson EB, Lichtenstein P, Anckarsater H, Happe F, Ronald A. Examining and interpreting the female protective effect against autistic behaviour. Proc Natl Acad Sci U S A. 2013;110(13):5258–62.
42. van Wyk C, van Wyk PJ. Trends in dental caries prevalence, severity and unmet treatment need levels in South Africa between 1983 and 2002. SADJ 2010; 65(7):310, 2–4.
43. Murshid EZ. Diet, oral hygiene practices and dental health in autistic children in Riyadh, Saudi Arabia. Oral Health Dent Manag. 2014;13:91–6.

44. Dominguez-Rojas V, Astasio-Arbiza P, Ortega-Molina P, Gordillo-Florencio E, Garcio-Nunez JA, Boscones-Martinez A. Analysis of several risks factors involved in dental caries through multiple logistic regressions. Int Dent J. 1993;43:149–56.
45. Stein LI, Polido JC, Najera SO, Cerrnak SA. Oral care experiences and challenges in children with autism spectrum disorders. Pediatr Dent. 2012;34(5):387–91.
46. McKinney CM, Nelson T, Scott JM, Heaton LJ, Vaughn MG, Lewis CW. Predictors of unmet dental need in children with autism spectrum disorder: results from a national sample. Acad Pediatr. 2014;14(6):624–31.
47. Mala D, Brearley ML, Hanny C. A study of the dental treatment needs of children with disabilities in Melbourne, Australia. Aust Dent J. 2001;46(1):41–50.
48. Kalyoncu IÖ, Tanboga I. Oral health status of children with autistic Spectrum disorder compared with non-authentic peers. Iran J Public Health. 2017; 46(11):1591–3.
49. Kim YS, Leventhal BL, Koh YJ. Prevalence of autism spectrum disorders in a total population sample. Am J Psychiatry. 2011;168(9):904–12.
50. Frazier TW, Georgiades S, Bishop SL, Hardan AY. Behavioural and cognitive characteristics of females and males with autism in the Simons simplex collection. J Am Acad Child Adolesc Psychiatry. 2014;53:329–40.
51. Gamsiz ED, Viscidi EW, Frederick AM, Nagpal S, Sanders SJ, Murtha MT, et al. Intellectual disability is associated with increased runs of homozygosity in simplex autism. Am J Hum Genet. 2013;93:103–9.
52. Head AM, McGillivray JA, Stokes MA. Gender differences in emotionality and sociability in children with autism spectrum disorders. Mol Autism. 2014;5:19.
53. Weintraub JA, Stearns SC, Rosier RG, Huang CC. Treatment outcomes and costs of dental sealants among children enrolled in Medicaid. Am J Public Health. 2001;91(11):1877–81.
54. Sheiham A, Watt RG. The common risk factor approach: a rational basis for promoting oral health. Community Dent Oral Epidemiol. 2000;28(6):399–406. https://doi.org/10.1034/j.1600-0528.2000.028006399.x.
55. Friedlander, A.H., Yagiela, J.A., Paterno, V.I., & Mahler, M.E. The pathophysiology, medical management, and dental implications of autism. J Calif Dent Assoc 2003; 31:681-2, 684, 686.
56. Twoy R, Connolly PM, Novak JM. Coping strategies used by parents of children with autism. J Am Acad Nurse Pract. 2007;19:251–60.
57. Gail Williams P, Sears LL, Allard A. Sleep problems in children with autism. J Sleep Res. 2004;13(3):265–8.

25

Factors associated with future dental care utilization among low-income smokers overdue for dental visits

Paula R. Blasi[1]* (ID), Chloe Krakauer[2], Melissa L. Anderson[1], Jennifer Nelson[1], Terry Bush[3], Sheryl L. Catz[4] and Jennifer B. McClure[1]

Abstract

Background: Smokers are at increased risk of oral disease. While routine dental care can help prevent and treat oral health problems, smokers have far lower rates of dental care utilization compared with non-smokers. We sought to better understand which factors may facilitate or hinder dental care utilization among low-income smokers participating in a randomized intervention trial in order to inform future intervention planning.

Methods: This is a secondary analysis of data collected between 2015 and 2017 as part of the OralHealth4Life trial. Participants were eligible callers to the Louisiana, Nebraska, and Oregon state tobacco quitlines who had no dental appointment in the prior or upcoming six months. We examined the association between participants' baseline characteristics and their receiving professional dental care between baseline and the 6-month follow-up survey.

Results: Participants were racially diverse (42% non-White) and two-thirds had an annual household income under $20,000. Most (86.7%) had not had a dental cleaning in more than one year. Commonly cited barriers to dental care included cost (83.7%) and no dental insurance (78.1%). Those with dental insurance were more likely to see a dentist at follow-up (RR 1.66). Similarly, those reporting a dental insurance barrier to care were less likely to see a dentist at follow-up (RR 0.69); however, there was no significant utilization difference between those reporting a cost barrier vs. those who did not. After controlling for these financial factors, the following baseline characteristics were significantly associated with a higher likelihood of dental care utilization at 6 months: higher motivation (RR 2.16) and self-efficacy (RR 1.80) to visit the dentist, having a disability (RR 1.63), having a higher education level (RR 1.52), and having perceived gum disease (RR 1.49). Factors significantly associated with a lower likelihood of dental care utilization included being married (RR 0.68) and not having a last dental cleaning within the past year (RR 0.47).

Conclusions: Our findings provide important insight into factors that may facilitate or deter use of professional dental care among low-income smokers. This information could inform the development of future interventions to promote dental care utilization.

Keywords: Oral health, Oral health care, Dental care, Smoking, Tobacco, Dental insurance, Access to dental care, Dental care barriers, Motivation, Self-efficacy

* Correspondence: Paula.R.Blasi@kp.org
[1]Kaiser Permanente Washington Health Research Institute, 1730 Minor Ave, Suite 1600, Seattle, WA 98101, USA
Full list of author information is available at the end of the article

Background

Oral health is an important component of overall health and well-being [1]. However, many population groups face a disproportionate burden of oral health problems. Low-income individuals, those with limited education, non-White racial and ethnic groups, and smokers all face higher rates of oral disease than the general population [1–4]. Smokers are a particularly high-risk group because tobacco use is a risk factor for periodontal disease, tooth loss, and oral and pharyngeal cancers [1]. Moreover, smokers are about twice as likely as non-smokers to have not seen a dentist in more than 5 years or to have never seen one [5, 6].

Promoting and facilitating regular dental visits is one strategy to address oral health disparities, as routine dental care can help prevent and treat oral disease [7, 8]. For smokers, routine dental visits may even lessen the negative effects of smoking on oral health because dental providers can evaluate smokers' oral health, check for early signs of oral and pharyngeal cancers, [6] clean their teeth, and counsel them about oral hygiene behaviors such as brushing and flossing [9]. However, despite the potential benefits of dental visits for smokers [6, 9], there is little research on best practices for improving dental care utilization among this high-risk population.

To address this knowledge gap, we sought to promote dental care utilization among smokers calling state-funded tobacco quitlines. State quitlines offer free phone-based counseling and other assistance to support callers in quitting smoking [10]. Quitline callers include many populations facing oral health disparities, including low-income individuals, those with limited education, and racial or ethnic groups known to have higher rates of oral disease and lower oral cancer survival rates [11, 12]. Quitline callers also have low rates of dental care utilization, [13] and both quitline callers and quitline providers support the idea of integrating oral health promotion content into quitlines [10, 13, 14]. In addition, smokers who call tobacco quitlines presumably are already interested in behavior change, and therefore may be receptive to interventions to promote dental care.

Together with the quitlines and a team of behavioral scientists and oral health experts, we designed an intervention (OralHealth4Life, or OH4L) to encourage dental care utilization among smokers who are overdue for dental visits. The intervention included oral health counseling from quitline coaches, referral information for local low-cost dental providers, and other motivational and educational content. However, the OH4L intervention did not increase dental care utilization compared to usual quitline care in a randomized controlled trial. About 18% of both the intervention and control groups reported seeing a dentist during the 6

months following study enrollment [15]. This finding suggests that smokers, particularly those who are more socio-economically disadvantaged and have multiple barriers to care, may require a different type of intervention to increase their use of professional dental care.

There is little existing research on predictors of future dental visits among low-income smokers or on strategies for increasing dental care utilization among low-income smokers who are overdue for dental care. According to Andersen's Behavioral Model of Health Services Use, predictors of health care utilization include predisposing factors (such as demographic characteristics and health beliefs), enabling factors (such as financial resources and access to health insurance), and the need for health services [16, 17]. Thus, the goal of the current analysis was to better understand which potential predisposing and enabling factors may facilitate or hinder future dental care utilization among smokers who are overdue for dental care. Based on prior research, we anticipated that lacking dental insurance, self-reporting dental insurance as a barrier, and self-reporting cost as a barrier would be associated with a lower likelihood of seeing a dentist, as previous research shows that a lack of dental insurance and cost are the most commonly cited reasons for forgoing needed dental care [5, 18–20]. Therefore, a primary aim of this analysis was to assess the influence of additional factors on dental care utilization, after accounting for these financial barriers. Based on prior research, we hypothesized that individuals with lower incomes, those with lower education levels, and those living in rural areas would be less likely to see a dentist [6, 21–23]. Based on common health promotion theories and supporting research, we also hypothesized that individuals with higher levels of motivation and self-efficacy for seeing a dentist would be more likely to do so [24–29]. Ultimately, this work seeks to provide important insight into which smokers are more or less likely to see dental care providers, which in turn, could help public health professionals and policymakers design more effective interventions for these individuals in the future.

Methods

Overview

This is a secondary analysis of data collected between June 2015 and March 2017 as part of the OH4L trial. Since the main trial did not find a significant treatment effect, we combined intervention groups for this cohort data analysis. Additional trial details can be found in the published protocol, [30] at Clinical-Trials.gov (NCT02347124), and in the results from the main trial [15]. The Kaiser Permanente Washington Institutional Review Board approved this study.

Participants

Callers to the Oregon (OR), Nebraska (NE), and Louisiana (LA) state tobacco quitlines were invited to be screened for eligibility following registration for services. Callers were eligible to be screened if they were age 18 or older, could read and speak in English, smoked at least 5 cigarettes daily, were ready to quit smoking, and were eligible for their state's multi-call quitline program. To be eligible for the study, participants also had to have at least some of their natural teeth, no dental appointment in the prior or upcoming 6 months, an interest in improving their oral health, access to the internet, and the ability to receive text messages. We excluded individuals who were incarcerated, were receiving inpatient substance abuse treatment, had significant cognitive impairment or psychosis, were unable to read small text, had plans to move in the next 6 months, or had a household member enrolled in the study.

Consent, enrollment, and baseline data collection

Eligible callers provided verbal consent, completed the baseline assessment, and were randomized to the control or intervention arm. Randomization was stratified by participants' dental insurance (yes vs. no/unsure) and quitline (LA, NE, or OR).

Intervention

Intervention details are available in the published protocol [30]. Briefly, the control group received the standard quitline program, which included 4 to 5 calls with a quitline coach and mailed and online smoking cessation content. Controls also received an attention-matched text messaging intervention focused on generic health promotion tips, excluding smoking cessation or oral health. The experimental group received the standard quitline program plus additional scripted oral health counseling during each quitline call, mailed and online oral health promotion materials, and text messages focused on oral health promotion. The oral health counseling and materials discussed the benefits of oral health care and provided referral information for local low-cost dental providers. To prevent treatment contamination, different quitline counselors treated control and experimental participants. Finally, experimental participants each received a toothbrush, dental floss, and xylitol gum.

Assessment measures

Demographic data included age, gender, race/ethnicity, state of residence (LA, NE or OR), education, income, disability status, and marital status (single vs. married or living as married). Geographic classification was assessed using the U.S. Department of Agriculture's rural-urban commuting area (RUCA) codes, [31] based on participant street address. We followed previously used definitions [32] of "urban" as RUCA code 1, "suburban" as RUCA codes 2–6, and "rural" as RUCA codes 7–10.

Oral health-related assessments were self-reported and included standardized items from the 2011–2012 National Health and Nutrition Examination Survey (NHANES), [33] the 2008 National Health Interview Survey (NHIS), [34] and the 2008 Behavioral Risk Factor Surveillance System (BRFSS) [35]. Participants reported whether they thought they had gum disease (yes/no) after being informed that symptoms of gum disease included loose teeth or swollen, receding, sore, or infected gums. Responses of "I don't know" were coded as not having gum disease. Dental insurance status was assessed by asking participants whether they had dental insurance (yes/no, with responses of "I don't know" coded as not having dental insurance). Participants also reported length of time since their last dental cleaning (ranging from "in the last 6 months" to "never" on a six-point Likert scale.)

In addition, perceived barriers to dental care were assessed by asking participants to rate the extent to which they believed each of 11 common barriers – such as cost or no dental insurance – affected their ability to seek dental care. Participants rated each barrier on a five-point Likert scale ranging from 1 ("definitely not true") to 5 ("definitely true") to indicate the extent to which they perceived that factor as affecting their ability to see a dentist. For our analysis and for ease of interpretation, we grouped similar barriers into the following categories: access (unable to find a dentist, too difficult to get to the clinic), psychological (fear or nervousness, dislike going to the dentist), and prioritization (mean to go but put it off, other health concerns are more important, have no problems with teeth or gums, don't have time, do not think of it). We reported the cost barrier and no dental insurance barrier separately, as existing literature suggests these barriers affect rates of dental care utilization [5, 18–20]. If a participant rated any individual barrier or barrier in a category as present (rating of 4 or 5), we deemed that individual barrier or category of barrier to be present for that participant. It was possible for participants to report cost or a lack of dental insurance as perceived barriers to dental care, even if they also reported having dental insurance. This situation might arise if a participant had dental insurance that covered few services or involved high premiums and copayments.

Participants rated their motivation and self-efficacy to see a dentist in the next 6 months on a five-point Likert scale ranging from 1 ("not at all motivated/confident") to 5 ("very motivated/confident"). We deemed ratings of

4 and 5 as "high" motivation or self-efficacy and ratings of 3 or lower as "low" motivation or self-efficacy.

For this analysis, the primary outcome measure was receipt of professional dental care between study enrollment and the 6-month follow-up survey. Receipt of professional dental care was self-reported using an item from the 2012 NHIS, which assessed time since last seeing a dentist, orthodontist, oral surgeon, or dental hygienist [36]. We defined utilization as reporting a dental visit in the prior 6 months at the 2-month or 6-month follow-up survey. Since we excluded individuals from the study who had seen a dentist in the prior 6 months at enrollment, any dental visits reported during the study period represent post-enrollment care. To encourage accurate reporting, we used a modified bogus pipeline methodology [30] which asked participants to provide the contact details for the dental provider they visited. Participants were aware they would be asked for this information if they reported seeing a dental provider during the study period. More than 90% of participants who reported seeing a dentist at 6 months provided contact information for their provider [15].

Analysis

In the original randomized trial, dental care utilization did not differ significantly by treatment arm at 6-month follow-up, [15] thus we pooled all participants in the current analysis. We used descriptive statistics to characterize the demographic and oral health characteristics of study participants and their baseline barriers to seeing a dental provider.

Our primary analytic goal was to explore the effects of multiple baseline characteristics of interest (e.g., motivation to see a dentist and timing of last dental cleaning) on dental care utilization after accounting for a priori identified financial variables (dental insurance status, dental insurance barrier, cost barrier) and important potential confounders (age, gender, and state) of these associations. As a preliminary step to first understand the influence of each financial barrier previously shown to be associated with dental care utilization (dental insurance status, a dental insurance barrier, and a cost barrier), [5, 18–20] we estimated the relative risk (RR) of dental care receipt within 6 months of follow-up (yes/no) using a separate, unadjusted loglinear regression model with robust standard errors for each financial factor (i.e., using single variable adjusted models). We used this same approach to assess the unadjusted association between receipt of dental care and each potential demographic confounder (age, gender, and state).

Then, to assess the independent effect of each baseline characteristic on future dental care utilization above-and-beyond these financial factors and potential

confounders, we used a 2-step process. In step 1, we calculated the RR of seeing a dentist at any time between baseline and the 6-month follow-up for each baseline characteristic of interest using a separate loglinear regression model with robust standard errors. Each model was adjusted for the a priori financial and demographic factors described above (dental insurance status, dental insurance barrier, cost barrier, age, gender, and state). Analyses were limited to participants providing baseline data for each item of interest.

In step 2, we fit one multivariable adjusted loglinear regression model with robust standard errors that included the a priori financial and demographic factors plus all the baseline characteristics found in step 1 to be associated with dental care utilization at the $p \leq 0.10$ level.

We report 95% confidence intervals for each RR estimate and p-values for Wald tests. All confidence intervals and tests use robust standard errors and all analytic results were produced using the *geepack* package in R [37–39].

As a sensitivity analysis, we repeated both step 1 and step 2, limiting the analytic sample to individuals who had not had a dental cleaning in the past year at baseline. The rationale for this analysis was that this subgroup may be more hesitant to seek dental care, and therefore may have different baseline characteristics associated with seeking care.

Results

Baseline demographic characteristics

Our final analytic sample consisted of 718 participants from Louisiana (73%), Nebraska (13%) and Oregon (13%) (Table 1). Most participants (59.7%) smoked 21 or more cigarettes per day. Nearly two-thirds had an annual household income under $20,000, and 55.0% had a high school education or less. Participants were racially diverse (58.4% White, 29.1% Black, and 12.5% other or multiple races), and most (87.6%) lived in an urban or suburban area. Nearly all participants were younger than age 65 (mean age 44.3; standard deviation 12.2), and 61.8% were female. Our sample was representative of typical state quitline callers, with the exception that a higher proportion of study participants were non-White [40]. Baseline characteristics by state are presented in Table 1.

Baseline oral health-related characteristics and self-reported barriers

At baseline, most participants (86.8%) had not had a dental cleaning in more than 1 year (Table 1) and 41.7% had not had one in more than 5 years or had never had one (data not shown). Most participants reported high levels of motivation (81.3%) and self-efficacy (67.0%) for visiting

Table 1 Baseline demographic characteristics of tobacco quitline callers in OH4L study by state of residence, $n = 718$

		Louisiana N = 527 N (%)	Nebraska N = 95 N (%)	Oregon N = 96 N (%)	Overall N = 718 N (%)
Age categories	18–44	237 (45.1)	45 (48.4)	53 (55.2)	335 (46.9)
	45–64	271 (51.5)	45 (48.4)	35 (36.5)	351 (49.1)
	65 or older	18 (3.4)	3 (3.2)	8 (8.3)	29 (4.1)
Cigarettes per day	10 or few	51 (9.7)	9 (9.5)	10 (10.5)	70 (9.8)
	11 to 20	149 (28.4)	36 (37.9)	33 (34.7)	218 (30.5)
	21 or more	324 (61.8)	50 (52.6)	52 (54.7)	426 (59.7)
Gender	Male	195 (37.1)	30 (31.6)	49 (51.0)	274 (38.2)
	Female	331 (62.9)	65 (68.4)	47 (49.0)	443 (61.8)
Marital status	Single	303 (58.0)	54 (56.8)	57 (60.0)	414 (58.1)
	Married or living as married	219 (42.0)	41 (43.2)	38 (40.0)	298 (41.9)
Hispanic/Latino	Not Hispanic or Latino	508 (97.3)	93 (97.9)	90 (94.7)	691 (97.1)
	Hispanic or Latino	14 (2.7)	2 (2.1)	5 (5.3)	21 (2.9)
Race/ethnicity	White	260 (49.5)	80 (84.2)	77 (81.9)	417 (58.4)
	Black	201 (38.3)	6 (6.3)	1 (1.1)	208 (29.1)
	Other or multi-racial	64 (12.2)	9 (9.5)	16 (17.0)	89 (12.5)
Geographic classification	Rural	51 (9.7)	27 (28.4)	11 (11.5)	89 (12.4)
	Suburban	140 (26.6)	22 (23.2)	26 (27.1)	188 (26.2)
	Urban	336 (63.8)	46 (48.4)	59 (61.5)	441 (61.4)
Education	GED, HS Degree, or less	307 (59.3)	42 (44.2)	40 (42.6)	389 (55.0)
	At least some college, technical, or trade school	211 (40.7)	53 (55.8)	54 (57.4)	318 (45.0)
Currently employed	Not employed	274 (52.1)	60 (63.2)	51 (53.1)	385 (53.7)
	Employed	252 (47.9)	35 (36.8)	45 (46.9)	332 (46.3)
Living with a disability	No disability	387 (74.0)	57 (60.6)	68 (71.6)	512 (71.9)
	Disability	136 (26.0)	37 (39.4)	27 (28.4)	200 (28.1)
Annual household income	Less than $20,000	310 (61.6)	69 (74.2)	51 (54.3)	430 (62.3)
	More than $20,000	193 (38.4)	24 (25.8)	43 (45.7)	260 (37.7)
Dental insurance status	No dental insurance	390 (74.0)	43 (45.3)	50 (52.1)	483 (67.3)
	Dental insurance	137 (26.0)	52 (54.7)	46 (47.9)	235 (32.7)
Last dental cleaning	Less than 1 year	65 (12.4)	13 (13.8)	16 (16.8)	94 (13.2)
	Over 1 year ago or never	459 (87.6)	81 (86.2)	79 (83.2)	619 (86.8)
Perceived gum disease	No perceived gum disease	322 (61.1)	56 (58.9)	50 (52.1)	428 (59.6)
	Perceived gum disease	205 (38.9)	39 (41.1)	46 (47.9)	290 (40.4)
Motivation to see dentist in next 6 months	Low motivation	88 (16.7)	21 (22.1)	25 (26.0)	134 (18.7)
	High motivation	439 (83.3)	74 (77.9)	71 (74.0)	584 (81.3)
Self-efficacy to see dentist in next 6 months	Low self-efficacy	168 (31.9)	30 (31.6)	39 (40.6)	237 (33.0)
	High self-efficacy	359 (68.1)	65 (68.4)	57 (59.4)	481 (67.0)
Dental insurance barrier	No such barrier	88 (16.8%)	42 (44.2%)	27 (28.1%)	157 (21.9%)
	Dental insurance barrier	437 (83.2%)	53 (55.8%)	69 (71.9%)	559 (78.1%)
Cost barrier	No such barrier	74 (14.1%)	23 (24.5%)	20 (20.8%)	117 (16.3%)
	Cost barrier	452 (85.9%)	71 (75.5%)	76 (79.2%)	599 (83.7%)
Psychological barriers[a]	No such barriers	247 (46.9)	35 (36.8)	46 (47.9)	328 (45.7)
	Psychological barriers	280 (53.1)	60 (63.2)	50 (52.1)	390 (54.3)

Table 1 Baseline demographic characteristics of tobacco quitline callers in OH4L study by state of residence, *n* = 718 *(Continued)*

		Louisiana N = 527 N (%)	Nebraska N = 95 N (%)	Oregon N = 96 N (%)	Overall N = 718 N (%)
Prioritization barriers[a]	No such barriers	128 (24.3%)	19 (20.0%)	29 (30.2%)	176 (24.5%)
	Prioritization barriers	399 (75.7%)	76 (80.0%)	67 (69.8%)	542 (75.5%)
Access barriers[a]	No such barriers	349 (66.2%)	66 (69.5%)	66 (68.8%)	481 (67.0%)
	Access barriers	178 (33.8%)	29 (30.5%)	30 (31.2%)	237 (33.0%)

Missing values: Age (3); Cigarettes per day (4); Gender (1); Marital status (6); Hispanic/Latino (6); Race/ethnicity (4); Education (11); Currently employed (1); Living with a disability (6); Annual household income (28); Last dental cleaning (5)
[a]For our analysis and for ease of interpretation, we grouped similar barriers into the following categories: access (unable to find a dentist, too difficult to get to the clinic), psychological (fear or nervousness, dislike going to the dentist), and prioritization (mean to go but put it off, other health concerns are more important, have no problems with teeth or gums, don't have time, do not think of it)

a dentist in the next six months. Only about one-third of participants reported having dental insurance, 83.7% cited cost as a barrier to obtaining dental care, and 78.1% cited a dental insurance barrier. Many participants (75.5%) reported one or more prioritization barriers, such as meaning to go but putting it off, or viewing other health concerns as more important. About half of participants (54.3%) reported psychological barriers, which included fear or nervousness and disliking dental visits. Only about one-third (33.0%) of participants reported access-related barriers, such as an inability to find a dentist or difficulty getting to the office or clinic.

Association of financial barriers and potential demographic confounders with dental care utilization

When we examined each of our a priori identified financial and demographic factors (dental insurance status, dental insurance barrier, cost barrier, age, gender, and state), we found no association between dental care utilization at 6-month follow-up and either age, gender, or state (Table 2). Consistent with prior research, dental insurance status and perceived dental insurance barriers were associated with receipt of dental care. Participants with dental insurance were more likely to have seen a dentist by 6-month follow-up than those without (RR 1.66 [95% CI 1.22–2.26]). Participants who reported having a dental insurance barrier to care were less likely to have seen a dentist compared with those who did not report this barrier (RR 0.69 [95% CI 0.50–0.97]). Of those who reported cost as a barrier to dental care, 17.5% had seen a dentist compared with 23.1% of those who did not report this barrier; however, the cost barrier was not significantly associated with dental care utilization (RR 0.76 [95% CI 0.52–1.10]).

Associations between baseline characteristics of interest and dental care utilization

In the single variable adjusted models (Table 3), we found that factors significantly associated with a higher likelihood of dental care utilization at followup included having high levels of motivation to see the dentist (RR 2.86 [95% CI 1.55–5.29]) and high self-efficacy for seeing

Table 2 Association of a priori identified financial and demographic confounders with dental utilization by 6-month follow-up

		Use of Dental Care, %	Unadjusted RR (95% CI)	p-value
Age	18 to 44	16.7	1 (ref)	0.661
	45 to 64	19.4	1.16 (0.84–1.60)	
	65 or older	17.2	1.03 (0.45–2.37)	
Gender	Male	17.2	1 (ref)	0.496
	Female	19.2	1.12 (0.81–1.55)	
State	Louisiana	16.5	1 (ref)	0.090
	Nebraska	24.2	1.47 (0.98–2.20)	
	Oregon	22.9	1.39 (0.92–2.10)	
Dental insurance status	No dental insurance	15.1	1 (ref)	**0.001**
	Dental insurance	25.1	1.66 (1.22–2.26)	
Dental insurance barrier	No such barrier	24.2	1 (ref)	**0.030**
	Dental insurance barrier	16.8	0.69 (0.50–0.97)	
Cost barrier	No such barrier	23.1	1 (ref)	0.144
	Cost barrier	17.5	0.76 (0.52–1.10)	

Note Bolded text indicates associations that are significant at the *p* < 0.05 level

Table 3 Associations between baseline characteristics and dental utilization by 6-month follow-up in single variable adjusted models[a]

		Use of Dental Care, %	Adjusted RR (95% CI)[a]	p-value
Marital status	Single	21.0	1 (ref)	**0.023**
	Married or living as married	14.4	0.68 (0.48–0.95)	
Education	GED, HS Degree, or less	14.4	1 (ref)	**0.004**
	At least some college, technical, or trade school	23.9	1.63 (1.17–2.26)	
Living with a disability (employed & unemployed)	No disability	15.2	1 (ref)	**0.005**
	Disability	26.5	1.65 (1.17–2.32)	
Last dental cleaning	Less than 1 year	36.2	1 (ref)	**< 0.001**
	Over 1 year ago or never	15.7	0.47 (0.33–0.67)	
Perceived gum disease	No perceived gum disease	15.8	1 (ref)	0.066
	Perceived gum disease	22.1	1.35 (0.98–1.85)	
Motivation to see dentist in next 6 months	Low motivation	7.5	1 (ref)	**0.001**
	High motivation	20.9	2.86 (1.55–5.29)	
Self-efficacy to see dentist in next 6 months	Low self-efficacy	9.7	1 (ref)	**< 0.001**
	High self-efficacy	22.7	2.26 (1.46–3.49)	
Cigarettes per day	10 or fewer	20	1 (ref)	0.95
	11 to 20	19.3	0.92 (0.54–1.58)	
	21 or more	17.8	0.93 (0.56–1.55)	
Hispanic/Latino	Not Hispanic or Latino	18.7	1 (ref)	0.35
	Hispanic or Latino	9.5	0.52 (0.13–2.07)	
Race/ethnicity	White	20.1	1 (ref)	0.21
	Black	16.8	0.92 (0.62–1.36)	
	Other or multi-racial	10.1	0.56 (0.29–1.07)	
Geographic classification	Rural	21.3	1 (ref)	0.73
	Suburban	19.7	0.10 (0.61–1.6)	
	Urban	17.2	0.88 (0.56–1.39)	
Currently employed	Not employed	19	1 (ref)	0.72
	Employed	17.5	0.94 (0.68–1.30)	
Annual household income	Less than 20 K	19.5	1 (ref)	0.25
	Over 20 K	16.5	0.82 (0.58–1.15)	
Psychological barriers	No such barriers	19.2	1 (ref)	0.31
	Psychological barriers	17.7	0.85 (0.61–1.17)	
Prioritization barriers	No such barriers	15.9	1 (ref)	0.61
	Prioritization barriers	19.2	1.11 (0.75–1.63)	
Access barriers	No such barriers	18.3	1 (ref)	0.99
	Access barriers	18.6	1.00 (0.72–1.38)	

Bolded text indicates associations that are significant at the p < 0.05 level
[a]A separate model assesses each baseline characteristic of interest one at a time. All models are adjusted for a priori identified financial variables (dental insurance status, dental insurance barrier, cost barrier) and potential confounders (age, gender, and state). All p-values are global p-values

the dentist (RR 2.26 [95% CI 1.46–3.49]). Participants with a disability were more likely to see a dentist than those without a disability (RR 1.65 [95% CI 1.17–2.32]), and those who had at least some college education were more likely to see a dentist compared with those who had a high school education or less (RR 1.63 [95% CI 1.17–2.26]). Factors significantly associated with a lower

likelihood of dental care utilization at followup including being married (RR 0.68 [95% CI 0.48–0.95]), and not having received a dental cleaning in more than 1 year (RR 0.47 [95% CI 0.33–0.67]).

All associations that were significant in our single variable models (Table 3) remained significant in our multivariable model (Table 4), though RR estimates were

Table 4 Associations between baseline characteristics and dental utilization by 6-month follow-up in multivariable adjusted model[a]

		Use of Dental Care, %	Adjusted RR (95% CI)[a]	p-value
Age	18 to 44	16.7	1 (ref)	0.96
	45 to 64	19.4	0.97 (0.69–1.38)	
	65 or older	17.2	0.89 (0.39–2.03)	
Gender	Male	17.2	1 (ref)	0.83
	Female	19.2	0.97 (0.70–1.33)	
State	Louisiana	16.5	1 (ref)	0.45
	Nebraska	24.2	1.14 (0.75–1.75)	
	Oregon	22.9	1.30 (0.86–1.96)	
Dental insurance status	No dental insurance	15.1	1 (ref)	0.33
	Dental insurance	25.1	1.20 (0.84–1.73)	
Dental insurance barrier	No such barrier	24.2	1 (ref)	0.61
	Dental insurance barrier	16.8	0.90 (0.60–1.35)	
Cost barrier	No such barrier	23.1	1 (ref)	0.88
	Cost barrier	17.5	0.97 (0.64–1.46)	
Marital status	Single	21.0	1 (ref)	**0.02**
	Married or living as married	14.4	0.67 (0.48–0.94)	
Education	GED, HS Degree, or less	14.4	1 (ref)	**0.013**
	At least some college, technical, or trade school	23.9	1.52 (1.09–2.12)	
Living with a disability (employed & unemployed)	No disability	15.2	1 (ref)	**0.004**
	Disability	26.5	1.63 (1.17–2.27)	
Last dental cleaning	Less than 1 year	36.2	1 (ref)	**< 0.001**
	Over 1 year ago or never	15.7	0.52 (0.37–0.72)	
Perceived gum disease	No perceived gum disease	15.8	1 (ref)	**0.014**
	Perceived gum disease	22.1	1.49 (1.09–2.05)	
Motivation to see dentist in next 6 months	Low motivation	7.5	1 (ref)	**0.029**
	High motivation	20.9	2.16 (1.08–4.32)	
Self-efficacy to see dentist in next 6 months	Low self-efficacy	9.7	1 (ref)	**0.019**
	High self-efficacy	22.7	1.80 (1.10–2.93)	

Bolded text indicates associations that are significant at the $p < 0.05$ level
[a]Includes our a priori identified covariates (cost barrier, dental insurance barrier, having dental insurance [yes/no], gender, age, and state), as well as each variable found to be significant at the $p \le 0.10$ level in the single variable models (step 1). All p-values are global p-values

somewhat attenuated (RRs 2.16 for motivation, 1.80 for self-efficacy, 0.52 for having a recent dental cleaning, 1.52 for having a higher education level, 0.67 for being married, and 1.63 for living with a disability). The association between perceived gum disease and dental care utilization was near-significant in our single variable models (RR 1.35 [95% CI 0.98–1.85]) and became significant with multivariable adjustment (RR 1.49 [95% CI, 1.09–2.05]).

Age, gender, and state all remained unassociated with dental care utilization in the multivariable model. Contrary to our expectations, we found little to no association in the multivariable model between dental care utilization and any financial factors, including dental insurance status (RR 1.20 [95% CI, 0.84–1.73]), self-reported dental insurance barriers (RR 0.90 [95% CI, 0.60–1.35]), or self-reported cost barriers (RR 0.97 [95% CI, 0.64–1.46]).

Post-hoc sensitivity and exploratory analyses

In sensitivity analyses conducted among individuals whose last dental cleaning was more than 1 year ago ($n = 459$), the single variable adjusted model results mirrored the full cohort analysis, with no change in the significance of any variables nor the direction of association for any significant variables (data not shown). In the multivariable adjusted model, the estimated associations were also generally in the same direction and of similar magnitude as found in the broader sample, but due to reduced power, many associations were no longer significant in this subgroup (data not shown).

We also conducted exploratory analyses to further examine our unexpected findings that being single and having a disability were associated with receipt of dental care at follow-up. For this analysis, we compared other baseline characteristics between single vs. married participants as well as between participants with a disability vs. those without. We found that a higher proportion of single participants had completed at least some college (48.3% compared to 39.9% among married participants). We also found that a much higher percentage of individuals living with a disability were unemployed (92.0% vs. 38.5% for those without a disability), and that Nebraska had a higher proportion of participants with a disability (39.4%) compared with Oregon (28.4%) and Louisiana (26.0%). However, as shown in the multivariable findings, adjusting for education status and state did not change the significance of the association between either disability status or marital status and dental care utilization.

Discussion

Smokers, particularly those who are low-income or uninsured, are an important target group for promoting dental care utilization. To better inform future efforts to promote dental visits in this high-risk group, we examined baseline factors associated with future dental care among participants in the OH4L trial. We found that significant predictors of future dental care included being single, not reporting dental insurance as a barrier to care, and having dental insurance, high levels of motivation and self-efficacy to visit the dentist, a disability, a higher education level, perceived gum disease, and a dental cleaning within the past year.

Our finding that having dental insurance was associated with a greater likelihood of seeking future dental care was consistent with research from other countries, including studies from Korea [41] and Finland [42] showing an increase in dental visit attendance after a nationwide expansion in public dental insurance coverage. In the U.S., only about 7% of adults have public dental insurance (provided through Medicaid) and about 60% have private dental insurance, usually obtained through their employer or on the individual insurance market [43]. About 33% of U.S. residents – and about 67% of our study sample – have no dental insurance and therefore bear the cost burden of dental care [43]. In our analysis, we found lower rates of dental care utilization among study participants who reported cost as a barrier

to dental care, although this association was not significant. Together, these findings about cost and dental insurance support the notion that financial factors may represent important barriers to accessing dental care, a finding that is consistent with prior research [5, 18–20].

However, we found these financial barriers were no longer significantly associated with the likelihood of seeking dental services after adjusting for other baseline variables. This unexpected finding contrasts with prior research, and suggests financial barriers do little to alter the likelihood of seeking professional dental care after adjusting for other personal characteristics, such as having high levels of motivation and self-efficacy to visit the dentist, perceived gum disease, a more recent dental cleaning, a higher education level, being single, and having a disability.

There are several possible explanations for the discrepancies between prior research and our findings regarding the role of financial factors as barriers to dental care. Most prior studies were conducted among nationally or regionally representative samples of civilian non-institutionalized populations, [18–20] which in some cases were stratified by smoking status [5]. In contrast, our sample consisted exclusively of smokers from Louisiana, Nebraska, and Oregon, most of whom were very low-income. Therefore, the factors that influence dental care utilization among these smokers in our three states might differ from those that influence utilization among a population with a greater diversity of income levels. In addition, most prior studies were cross-sectional analyses that provided the frequencies of participants' self-reported reasons for forgoing needed dental care without adjusting for other personal characteristics, [5, 19, 20] or assessed the likelihood of different outcomes, such as lack of care for known dental problems [18]. In contrast, our prospective, longitudinal analysis offers insight into the characteristics associated with an increased likelihood of transitioning from being a non-utilizer to a utilizer of dental services, which may involve different influences.

We undertook this analysis to explore factors that might be hindering or facilitating dental visits among high-risk smokers to inform future intervention development. In contrast to our expectations, neither income level nor geographic classification (urban, suburban, rural) were significantly associated with future dental care utilization; however, the former may reflect the lack of economic diversity in our sample. Two-thirds had annual household incomes below $20,000, and less than 5% had annual household incomes over $60,000 [15]. Other factors not associated with future dental care utilization included psychological barriers such as fear or nervousness, access-related barriers such as difficulty finding a dentist, and prioritization barriers such as viewing other health concerns as more important. We initially expected these factors to play a role in dental utilization, and in fact, the OH4L intervention sought to address these issues through a combination of cognitive behavioral counseling, oral health education, and referrals to local low-cost dental providers. However, our comprehensive, multi-modal intervention had no effect on future dental care [15]. Taken together, the results of our randomized trial and the findings from this secondary analysis suggest income, geographic classification, and perceived barriers may be less important drivers of future dental care among low-income smokers than one's motivation to see a dentist or confidence in one's ability to see the dentist.

Since higher levels of motivation and self-efficacy to visit the dentist were associated with a greater likelihood of future dental care utilization, we recommend future interventions specifically seek to build individuals' motivation and self-efficacy to visit the dentist, independent of their concerns about cost. In addition, our finding that people with perceived gum disease were more likely to see a dental provider suggests future interventions should educate smokers about their gum health and oral disease risk while simultaneously fostering their self-efficacy and motivation to see a dental provider. Based on evidence that gain-framed health risk messaging is more persuasive than loss-framed messaging for oral hygiene behaviors, [44–46] we recommend that such an intervention emphasize the positive benefits of seeing a dentist, as opposed to the health consequences of neglecting this care.

Other significant correlates of future dental care included having a higher education level, being single, and having a disability. While the association between dental care utilization and education aligns with prior research, [22] our findings on marital status and disability status were unexpected. Our exploratory analysis found that single participants generally had higher levels of education than married participants; however, adjusting for education level did not impact the significance of the association between marital status and seeking dental care. In addition, participants with a disability were more likely to report being unemployed than participants without a disability, so it is possible that participants with a disability had more free time to visit the dentist. Nebraska also had a higher proportion of participants with a disability compared with Oregon and Louisiana. However, neither employment status nor state were significantly associated with future dental care use in any of our analyses, suggesting the association between disability status and dental care utilization may be complex and not easily explained by our current analyses or available data.

Overall, our findings highlight the difficulty of increasing dental care utilization among high-risk, low-income smokers and the need for additional research to improve our understanding of how to best support tobacco users in obtaining dental care. For example, future studies could interview smokers about what they would need to schedule, attend, and maintain routine dental visits. Such interviews might uncover factors that were not explored in our present analysis but could play a role in supporting dental visit attendance, such as assistance with appointment scheduling, appointment reminders, or childcare during visits.

Strengths and limitations

This study has several strengths, including its longitudinal, population-based design that allowed us to follow individuals who transitioned from being non-utilizers to utilizers of dental care. It includes a diverse population of smokers interested in quitting (42% non-White) and a high proportion of very low-income smokers. These are priority populations for intervention because of their high risk of oral disease and low rates of dental care utilization, however, they also face substantial barriers to obtaining dental care. Therefore, understanding the characteristics of participants who transitioned from non-utilizers to utilizers of dental care offers valuable insight for future efforts to facilitate dental care utilization among similar high-risk groups.

This study also has certain limitations. Our sample consisted of a low-income population of smokers from Louisiana, Nebraska, and Oregon who were overdue for dental visits, and our findings may not be generalizable to higher-income smokers, those from other regions or countries, those who visit a dentist regularly, or smokers who have not contacted a quitline for help with tobacco cessation. As a condition of enrollment, participants had to be interested in improving their oral health. As such, the results may not generalize to persons with no interest in improving their oral health. All participant data was based on self-report, and thus subject to bias and misreporting. However, for our main outcome of dental care utilization, our methodology was designed to deter misreporting by requiring a provider name. Since more than 90% of participants provided this information with an understanding that we may also ask their permission to contact their provider to verify the accuracy of their report, we have great confidence in the veracity of this self-reported data.

Conclusions

Low-income smokers are at high risk for oral disease and are a priority group for oral health intervention. The findings from our randomized trial underscore the difficulty of increasing dental care utilization among this population, but the current analysis provides useful insight into those who are more or less likely to seek dental care. This information can inform the design of future oral health promotion programs either by helping public health officials target those at greatest risk for not seeking dental care (e.g., smokers with lower education levels) or by suggesting potential targets for future behavioral interventions (e.g., perceived disease risk, self-efficacy, motivation). Future research should evaluate whether interventions that target these individuals and address these factors can increase dental care utilization among low-income individuals, particularly smokers.

Abbreviations
BRFSS: Behavioral Risk Factor Surveillance System; LA: Louisiana; NE: Nebraska; NHANES: National Health and Nutrition Examination Survey; NHIS: National Health Interview Survey; OH4L: OralHealth4Life; OR: Oregon; RR: Relative risk; RUCA: Rural-Urban Commuting Area

Acknowledgements
We would like to thank study team members at KPWHRI and Optum who made this work possible. At KPWHRI this included Ella Thompson, the Survey Research Program, Ellen Schartz, Mary Shea, Eric Baldwin, Andrew Baer, DT Tran, Deborah King, and Zoe Bermet. At Optum this included Erica Salmon, Mark Campbell, and Mona Deprey. We are also grateful to the Louisiana Campaign for Tobacco-Free Living and the Louisiana Department of Health, Well-Ahead Louisiana; the Oregon Health Authority, Public Health Division, Tobacco Prevention and Education Program; and the Tobacco Free Nebraska, Public Health Division, Nebraska Department of Health of Human Services for supporting this research. Finally, we thank Dr. Dolphine Oda, DDS, MSc; Dr. Johnny Wang, DDS, MPH, MS; and Dr. Helga Ding, DDS, MBA, MHA for consulting on the development of the Oral Health 4 Life intervention.

Funding
This research was supported by the National Institute of Dental and Craniofacial Research (NIDCR; grant U01DE024462).

Authors' contributions
PB led the conceptualization and writing of this manuscript. CK conducted data analyses and wrote sections of the methods. MA and JL oversaw the implementation of the analytic plan. TB oversaw study activities at the Optum Center for Wellbeing Research. SC assisted in intervention development and fidelity oversight. JM conceptualized the study, secured research funding, and oversaw intervention development. All authors interpreted the data, provided input on manuscript drafts, and approved the final manuscript.

Competing interests
The authors declare that they have no competing interests.

Author details
[1]Kaiser Permanente Washington Health Research Institute, 1730 Minor Ave, Suite 1600, Seattle, WA 98101, USA. [2]Department of Biostatistics, University of Washington, F-600, Health Sciences Building 1705 NE Pacific Street, Seattle, WA 98195, USA. [3]Optum Center for Wellbeing Research, 999 3rd Ave., Suite 2000, Seattle, Washington 98104, USA. [4]Betty Irene Moore School of Nursing, University of California-Davis, 2450 48th Street, Suite 2600, Sacramento, CA 95817, USA.

References
1. U.S. Department of Health and Human Services. Oral Health in America: A Report of Surgeon General. Rockville, MD: U.S. Department of Health and Human Services, National Institute of Dental and Craniofacial Research, National Institutes of Health; 2000.
2. Eke PI, Dye BA, Wei L, Slade GD, Thornton-Evans GO, Borgnakke WS, Taylor GW, Page RC, Beck JD, Genco RJ. Update on prevalence of periodontitis in adults in the United States: NHANES 2009 to 2012. J Periodontol. 2015;86(5): 611–22.
3. SEER Cancer statistics review, 1975–2015. https://seer.cancer.gov/csr/1975_2015/.
4. Drury TF, Garcia I, Adesanya M. Socioeconomic disparities in adult oral health in the United States. Ann N Y Acad Sci. 1999;896:322–4.
5. Bloom B, Adams PF, Cohen RA, Simile C. Smoking and Oral health in dentate adults aged 18–64. NCHS data brief, no 85. Hyattsville, MD: Centers for Disease Control and Prevention, National Center for Health Statistics; 2012.
6. Drilea SK, Reid BC, Li CH, Hyman JJ, Manski RJ. Dental visits among smoking and nonsmoking US adults in 2000. Am J Health Behav. 2005;29(5):462–71.
7. Vujicic M, Nasseh K. A decade in dental care utilization among adults and children (2001-2010). Health Serv Res. 2014;49(2):460–80.
8. Institute of Medicine. Advancing Oral health in America. Washington, DC: the National Academies Press; 2011.
9. Emanuel AS, Parish A, Logan HL, Dodd VJ, Zheng D, Guo Y. Dental visits mediate the impact of smoking on Oral health. Am J Health Behav. 2018; 42(1):59–68.
10. McClure JB, Riggs K, St John J, Catz SL. [more] evidence to support oral health promotion services targeted to smokers calling tobacco quitlines in the United States. BMC Public Health. 2013;13:336.
11. Results from the 2016 NAQC Annual Survey of Quitlines [https://www.naquitline.org/page/2016Survey].
12. Disparities in Oral Health [https://www.cdc.gov/oralhealth/oral_health_disparities/index.htm].
13. McClure JB, Riggs KR, St John J, Cerutti B, Zbikowski S. Understanding oral health promotion needs and opportunities of tobacco quitline callers. Public Health Rep (Washington, DC: 1974). 2012;127(4):401–6.
14. McClure JB. Leveraging the US tobacco quitline infrastructure to promote oral health: feedback from key stakeholders. Prev Med. 2014;60:134–5.
15. McClure JB, Bush T, Anderson ML, Blasi P, Thompson E, Nelson J, Catz SL. Oral health promotion and smoking cessation program delivered via tobacco Quitlines: the Oral health 4 life trial. Am J Public Health. 2018:e1–7.
16. Andersen R. Families' use of health services: a behavioral model of predisposing, enabling and need components [dissertation]. West Lafayette, IN: Purdue University; 1968.
17. Andersen R, Davidson P. Improving access to care in America: individual and contextual indicators. In: Andersen R, Rice T, Kominski E, editors. Changing the US health care system: key issues in Health services, policy, and management. San Francisco: Jossey-Bass; 2001. p. 3–30.
18. Malecki K, Wisk LE, Walsh M, McWilliams C, Eggers S, Olson M. Oral health equity and unmet dental care needs in a population-based sample: findings from the survey of the health of Wisconsin. Am J Public Health. 2015; 105(Suppl 3):S466–74.
19. Wall T, Nasseh K, Vujicic M. Most important barriers to dental care are financial, not supply related. Health policy institute brief. In. Chicago: American Dental Association; 2014.
20. Vujicic M, Buchmueller T, Klein R. Dental care presents the highest level of financial barriers, compared to other types of health care services. Health Aff (Millwood). 2016;35(12):2176–82.
21. Doescher M, Keppel G. Dentist supply, dental care utilization, and Oral health among rural and urban U.S. residents. In: final report #135. Seattle, WA: WWAMI Rural Health Research Center, University of Washington; 2015.
22. Reda SF, Reda SM, Thomson WM, Schwendicke F. Inequality in utilization of dental services: a systematic review and meta-analysis. Am J Public Health. 2018;108(2):e1–7.
23. Zhang Y. Racial/ethnic disparity in utilization of general dental care services among US adults: medical expenditure panel survey 2012. J Racial Ethn Health Disparities. 2016;3(4):565–72.
24. Bandura A. Self-efficacy: toward a unifying theory of behavioral change. Psychol Rev. 1977;84(2):191.
25. Hollister MC, Anema MG. Health behavior models and oral health: a review. J Dent Hyg. 2004;78(3):6.

26. Rosenstock IM. The health belief model and preventive health behavior. Health Educ Monogr. 1974;2(4):354–86.

27. Becker MH. The health belief model and personal health behavior. Health Educ Monogr. 1974;2:324–73.

28. Kakudate N, Morita M, Kawanami M. Oral health care-specific self-efficacy assessment predicts patient completion of periodontal treatment: a pilot cohort study. J Periodontol. 2008;79(6):1041–7.

29. Woelber JP, Bienas H, Fabry G, Silbernagel W, Giesler M, Tennert C, Stampf S, Ratka-Kruger P, Hellwig E. Oral hygiene-related self-efficacy as a predictor of oral hygiene behaviour: a prospective cohort study. J Clin Periodontol. 2015;42(2):142–9.

30. McClure JB, Blasi PR, Cook A, Bush T, Fishman P, Nelson J, Anderson ML, Catz SL. Oral health 4 life: design and methods of a semi-pragmatic randomized trial to promote oral health care and smoking abstinence among tobacco quitline callers. Contemp Clin Trials. 2017;57:90–7.

31. Rural-Urban Commuting Area Codes [https://www.ers.usda.gov/data-products/rural-urban-commuting-area-codes/].

32. Weeks WB, Kazis LE, Shen Y, Cong Z, Ren XS, Miller D, Lee A, Perlin JB. Differences in health-related quality of life in rural and urban veterans. Am J Public Health. 2004;94(10):1762–7.

33. National Health and Nutrition Examination Survey, 2011-2012 Survey Questionnaires [https://wwwn.cdc.gov/nchs/nhanes/continuousnhanes/questionnaires.aspx?BeginYear=2011].

34. National Health Interview Survey 2008 [https://www.cdc.gov/nchs/nhis/data-questionnaires-documentation.htm].

35. Behavioral Risk Factor Surveillance System 2008 [https://www.cdc.gov/brfss/annual_data/2008/2008_multiple.html].

36. NHIS Data, Questionnaires, and Related Documentation [https://www.cdc.gov/nchs/nhis/data-questionnaires-documentation.htm].

37. Højsgaard S, Halekoh U, Yan J. The R Package geepack for Generalized Estimating Equations. J Stat Softw. 2005;15(2):11.

38. Yan J, Fine J. Estimating equations for association structures. Stat Med. 2004;23(6):859–74 discussion 875–857,879–880.

39. Yan J: geepack: Yet Another Package for Generalized Estimating Equations. R-News 2002, 2/3:12--14.

40. Nash CM, Vickerman KA, Kellogg ES, Zbikowski SM. Utilization of a web-based vs integrated phone/web cessation program among 140,000 tobacco users: an evaluation across 10 free state quitlines. J Med Internet Res. 2015;17(2):e36.

41. Park HJ, Lee JH, Park S, Kim TI. Changes in dental care access upon health care benefit expansion to include scaling. J Periodontal Implant Sci. 2016;46(6):405–14.

42. Linden J, Josefsson K, Widstrom E. Frequency of visits and examinations in the public dental Service in Finland - a retrospective analysis, 2001-2013. BMC Oral Health. 2017;17(1):138.

43. Dental Benefits Coverage in the U.S. [https://www.ada.org/~/media/ADA/Science%20and%20Research/HPI/Files/HPIgraphic_1117_3.pdf?la=en].

44. Brick C, McCully SN, Updegraff JA, Ehret PJ, Areguin MA, Sherman DK. Impact of cultural exposure and message framing on Oral health behavior: exploring the role of message memory. Med Decis Mak. 2016;36(7):834–43.

45. Sherman DK, Updegraff JA, Mann T. Improving oral health behavior: a social psychological approach. J Am Dent Assoc (1939). 2008;139(10):1382–7.

46. Rothman AJ, Salovey P. Shaping perceptions to motivate healthy behavior: the role of message framing. Psychol Bull. 1997;121(1):3–19.

Assessment of the effect of the corticotomy-assisted orthodontic treatment on the maxillary periodontal tissue in patients with malocclusions with transverse maxillary deficiency

Magdalena Sulewska[1], Ewa Duraj[1], Beata Bugała-Musiatowicz[2], Emilia Waszkiewicz-Sewastianik[3], Robert Milewski[4], Jan K. Pietruski[3], Eugeniusz Sajewicz[5] and Małgorzata Pietruska[1,3]* (iD)

Abstract

Background: The aim of the study was to assess the effect of corticotomy–assisted orthodontic treatment on soft tissue clinical parameters in patients with malocclusions with transverse maxillary deficiency.

Methods: The study included 20 generally healthy adult individuals with malocclusion, who underwent a corticotomy-assisted orthodontic treatment in maxilla. During the corticotomy performed after full-thickness flap elevation, only the buccal cortical plate was cut with the use of OTS-7, OTS7–4, OTS7-3 ultrasound tips of the piezosurgery device (Mectron s. p. a., Italy). A clinical examination was performed prior to the corticotomy procedure, then repeated – 3, 6, 9 and 12 months after the procedure. The following parameters were assessed: FMPI (full mouth plaque index), FMBOP (full mouth bleading on probing), PD (probing depth), CAL (clinical attachment level), GR (gingival recession height), RW (recession width), PH (papilla height), PW (papilla width), BS (bone sounding), biotype and KT.

Results: There was a statistically significant reduction in PD (mean difference: 0.06; 95% CI: − 0.33, − 0.18), CAL (mean difference: 0.07; 95% CI: − 0.33, − 0.19), PH (mean difference: 0.26; 95% CI: − 0.47, 0.05) and BS (mean difference: 0.13; 95% CI: − 0.41, − 0.14) after the treatment. Statistically significant changes were also noted in relation to KT (mean difference: 0.17; 95% CI: − 0.07, 0.27) and biotype (mean difference: 0.07; 95% CI: 0.26, 0.39), which thickness increased significantly after the treatment. No statistically significant differences were observed in GR, RW and PW.

Conclusions: The corticotomy–assisted orthodontic treatment did not jeopardize the periodontal clinical status in maxilla. There is a need for further studies on a larger number of patient to compare the clinical findings with a control group as well as in patients with conventional orthodontic treatment in a longer follow-up time to find out more about the post-treatment periodontal tissue changes and stability.

Keywords: Corticotomy, Orthodontics, Periodontics, Malocclusion

* Correspondence: mpietruska@wp.pl
[1]Department of Periodontal and Oral Mucosa Diseases, Medical University of Białystok, ul. Waszyngtona 13, 15-269 Białystok, Poland
[3]Dental Practice, ul. Waszyngtona 1/34, 15-269 Białystok, Poland
Full list of author information is available at the end of the article

Background

The introduction of corticotomy-assisted orthodontics provided new solutions to some limitations in orthodontic treatment [1]. Corticotomy-assisted orthodontics induces a state of increased tissue turnover and transient osteopenia, followed by a faster rate of orthodontic tooth movement [2]. The corticotomy technique has several advantages, including faster tooth movement, shorter treatment time, safer expansion of constricted arches, enhanced post-orthodontic treatment stability, and an extended envelope of tooth movement [2–4].

The accelerated tooth movement technique was described for the first time by Köle [5]. The method involved the formation of bone blocks by means of vertical inter-root corticotomy from the vestibular and lingual side as well as supra-apical osteotomy, which allowed for quicker movement of bony blocks along with the teeth without any potential adverse consequences for the periodontium. In 1990, Gantes et al. [6] used Köle's modified technique, in which osteotomy was replaced by horizontal corticotomy, and concluded that the corticotomy procedure caused minimal changes in the periodontal attachment apparatus and allowed for a reduction in treatment duration of up to 50%. Wilcko et al. [7] described the periodontally accelerated osteogenic orthodontics (PAOO) technique. This new surgical technique included buccal and lingual full-thickness flaps, selective partial decortication of the cortical plates, and concomitant bone grafting. In a subsequent study Wilcko and co-workers found that orthodontic movement is not a simple repositioning of single tooth-bone units, but is a cascade of physiological events leading to bone healing [8–10]. This process, called by Frost [11] the regional accelerated phenomenon (RAP), and described in the periodontal literature by Yaffe et al. [12], assumes that healing is a complex physiologic process with dominating features involving accelerated bone turnover and decreases in regional bone densities. RAP is not a separate healing event, but it can expedite hard and soft tissue healing stages two- to tenfold [2, 13]. After corticotomy, demineralization occurs in the alveolar bone and the remaining collagenous matrix of bone is transported with the tooth during its movement [2]. The matrix then remineralizes after the orthodontic movement [7, 8]. Computerized tomography imaging, animal studies, and histological evaluation support the hypothesis of reversible osteopenia that is responsible for rapid tooth movement in corticotomy-assisted orthodontics [9, 14, 15]. In 2007, Vercellotti and Podesta [16] reported a microsurgical technique in which cuts are made around each tooth root with only one full thickness flap on the side corresponding to the direction of dental movement. In this monocortical tooth dislocation and ligament distraction technique (MTDLD) dental movement occurs via dislocation of the root and cortical bone together, without

periodontal ligament compression and bone resorption. Then in 2009 Dibart et al. [17] proposed, minimally invasive technique combining microincisions with selective tunneling and piezoelectric incisions between roots with consecutive hard- or soft-tissues grafting.

The literature gathers the evidence of successful corticotomy as an aid to orthodontic treatment and doesn't report it's negative effects, however, there is lack of a detailed analysis of the changes that occur in the periodontal tissues during and after treatment [2, 7–9, 18–22]. That is why the aim of this study was to assess the effects of the corticotomy-assisted orthodontic treatment on clinical status of soft tissues in patients with malocclusion.

Methods

The study included 20 generally healthy adult individuals (10 female and 10 male) aged 19 to 35 with Class I and II malocclusion which a common feature was transverse maxillary deficiency.

A full aesthetic, functional and orthodontic analysis was done prior to the treatment. A periodontal examination was conducted along with photographic and radiographic documentation including orthopanthomogram, cephalometric x-ray as well as cone beam computed tomography. The patients were told about the advantages, disadvantages and risk involved in the corticotomy-assisted orthodontic treatment. All the patients gave their written informed consent for treatment and participation in the study. The study was carried out in accordance with the Helsinki Declaration of 1975, as revised in 2000, and was reviewed and approved by the local ethical committee (Ethics Committee Nr.: R-I-002/344/2011).

Inclusion criteria

Voluntary participation; Legal adult (> 18 years old); Non-smoking; Generally healthy; Malocclusion with transverse maxillary deficiency; Indications for upper arch expansion during treatment; Good oral hygiene and motivation at screening quantified as: FMPI (full mouth plaque index) < 20%, FMBOP (full mouth bleading on probing) < 20%.

Exclusion criteria

Periodontal disease; Oral mucosa lesions; Bisphosphonate and long-term corticosteroid therapy; Current therapy with: anti-epileptic drugs, contraceptives, estrogen, antihistamine drugs, calcitonin, vitamin D; Alcohol and/or drug addiction; Presence of periapical endo-perio lesions; Severe gingival recession; Pregnancy, breast feeding; Previous orthodontic treatment; Previous root resorption; Inability to commit to one-year follow-up.

Surgical procedure

One day prior to the surgery thin arch self-ligating brackets (System Damon, Ormco, Orange, CA, USA) were bonded without placing the archwire. Amoxicillin at a dose of 1 g and ibuprofen at a dose of 200 mg were administered before the surgical procedure. The surgery was done in maxilla under local anesthesia with 4% articaine (Ubistesin forte, 3 M ESPE, USA). The mucoperiosteal flap was elevated up to the point above the apical parts of roots following modified papilla preservation technique as well as performing vertical releasing incisions [23]. Then osteotomy of the buccal cortical plate of the alveolar process was performed by using OTS7, OTS7-4, OTS7-3 ultrasound tips of the piezosurgery device (Mectron s. p. a., Italy). The extension of the osteotomy was determined by the mesio-distal dimension of the teeth roots as well as by the position of the apexes of roots. In order to avoid interproximal bone picks resorption, the vertical cuts ended 5 mm apically from the crest and then Y-shape spread towards the neighboring teeth. The horizontal corticotomy was performed approximately 2–4 mm apically above the root apexes. The depth of the cuts was limited to the thickness of the cortical plate. The repositioned flap was sutured with non-resorbable monofilament 5.0 and 6.0 sutures (Resolon, Resorba Medical GmbH, Germany). Amoxicillin 1 g 2×/day for 7 days, ibuprofen 200 mg 3×/day, mouth rinsing with chlorhexidine (0.10% Eludril, Pierre Fabre Sante, France) 2×/day were prescribed and gentle tooth brushing in the surgical area for two weeks was recommended to the patients. The supragingival plaque was cleaned out 7 and 14 days after the surgery. The sutures were removed 14 days post-op.

Orthodontic treatment
Subsequently after the corticotomy, initial orthodontic wires (0.012 or 0.014 Cooper Ni-Ti) were placed (Ormco, Orange, CA, USA). The follow-ups were performed every 2 weeks for the first three months of treatment, then every 4–6 weeks. The arches were fully leveled and aligned by using increasing sizes of nickel-titanium alloy archwires. The subsequent stages of treatment involved the use of: 0.018 Cooper Ni-Ti wires, replaced with rectangular ones. The therapy was completed with 0.019 × 0.025 steel archwires. The total time of treatment in both jaws took 9 to 12 months. Once the treatment was completed, a permanent retainer was bonded to the lower incisors and canines, while a removable retainer was provided for the upper arch.

Clinical examination
The clinical examination was performed in maxilla prior to the treatment, then 3, 6, 9 and 12 months after the surgery in accordance with the established protocol. The measurements were done using a manual PCP UNC 15 periodontal probe (Hu-Friedy, Chicago, IL, USA) by one calibrated investigator. The total number of examined teeth was 159. The clinical status of the surgical sites

was photographically documented during the subsequent appointments.

The following clinical parameters were evaluated: FMPI (full mouth plaque index), FMBOP (full mouth bleading on probing), PD (probing depth), CAL (clinical attachment level), GR (gingival recession height), RW (recession width), PH (papilla height), PW (papilla width), BS (bone sounding), biotype and KT (keratinized tissue).

Clinical parameters were assesed as follows:

PD (probing depth) and CAL (clinical attachment level) - at six points for each tooth,
GR (gingival recession, height) - measured at mid-buccal aspect of the tooth from the CEJ to the most apical extension of gingival margin,
RW (recession width) – mesio-distal dimention of denudated root surface measured at CEJ level,
PH (papilla height) - measured on the midline of papilla from PW level to the tip of papilla,
PW (papilla width) - measured at the level of CEJ of adjacent teeth,
BS (bone sounding) - distance from the gingival margin to the the alveolar crest, measured using a periodontal probe under anesthesia, on the interproximal surfaces of teeth,
biotype - gingival thickness - measured under anesthesia at mid-facial aspect of the tooth on a long axis 1 mm apicaly fom the bottom of the sulcus with the use of K-file 25 ISO with a silicone marker,
KT (keratinized tissue) - measured from the most apical point of gingival margin to the mucogingival junction.

All measurements were rounded to the nearest 0.5 mm.

Statistical analysis
All continous variables were tested for normal distribtion by the Kolmogorov–Smirnov test, with Lilliefors corretion and Shapiro-Wilk test. Normal distribution of the quantitative variables was not found. The Friedman ANOVA non-parametric test was used for multiple comparisons to compare more than two related variables. 95% coinfidence intervals were also calculated for differences between baseline and 12 months post-op. Statistical significance was determined at $p < 0.05$. All calculations were performed using Statistica 10.0 software (StatSoft, USA).

Results
FMPI and FMBOP remained at similar levels throughout the treatment with a tendency to decrease during retention (Table 1). There was a statistically significant reduction in mean PD and CAL after corticotomy-assisted orthodontic treatment as compared with the baseline. PD

Table 1 Full mouth plaque index (FMPI) and full mouth bleeding on probing (FMBOP) before and after orthodontic treatment

Parameter	[%]	Time of observation [months]		Difference between baseline and 12 months post-op	p-value (Friedman ANOVA)	Mean diff. (95% CI) between baseline and 12 months post-op
FMPI	x ± SD	Baseline	17.33 ± 2.11	−0.35%	p = 0.28	0.86 (−1.29, 0.43)
		3	19.28 ± 2.52			
		6	20.13 ± 2.11			
		9	19.37 ± 2.17			
		12	16.90 ± 2.25			
FMBOP	x ± SD	Baseline	13.44 ± 1.87	−0.20%	p = 0.30	0.43 (−0.63, 0.23)
		3	15.07 ± 1.78			
		6	17.15 ± 1.80			
		9	15.79 ± 1.75			
		12	13.24 ± 1.75			

x ± SD mean values and standard deviation
Mean diff. mean difference
CI Confidence interval

values decreased from 2.74 ± 0.57 mm to 2.48 ± 0.51 mm and CAL values decreased from 2.75 ± 0.57 mm to 2.49 ± 0.51 mm respectively. Mean pre- and post-treatment PD and CAL values are shown in Table 2.

There was also a statistically significant reduction in papilla height and bone sounding after the treatment. Reduced papilla height (PH) was reflected in the bone sounding (BS) value, which decreased by 0.27 mm post-treatment (Tables 2 and 3).

Miller Class I gingival recessions were found in 12 (7.55%) out of a total 159 assessed teeth. The mean pre-treatment recession height was 0.13 ± 0.47 mm, which decreased to 0.07 ± 0.32 mm after treatment completion, while recession width decreased from 0.21 ± 0.75 mm to 0.10 ± 0.49 mm. No new recessions developed despite the vestibular tooth movement. Out of 12 cases of recession observed before treatment, 5 disappeared, 4 remained unchanged and in 3 GR decreased by 1 mm (Table 3).

Table 2 Probing depth (PD), clinical attachment level (CAL), bone sounding (BS) before and during subsequent follow-up assessments

Parameter	[mm]	Time of observation [months]		Difference between baseline and 12 months post-op	p-value (Friedman ANOVA)	Mean diff. (95% CI) between baseline and 12 months post-op
PD	x ± SD	Baseline	2.74 ± 0.57	− 0.26 mm	p < 0.001	0.07 (− 0.33, − 0.18)
		3	2.54 ± 0.64			
		6	2.58 ± 0.55			
		9	2.62 ± 0.57			
		12	2.48 ± 0.51			
CAL	x ± SD	Baseline	2.75 ± 0.57	−0.26 mm	p < 0.001	0.07 (− 0.33, − 0.19)
		3	2.55 ± 0.64			
		6	2.59 ± 0.55			
		9	2.61 ± 0.58			
		12	2.49 ± 0.51			
BS	x ± SD	Baseline	4.76 ± 0.94	−0.27 mm	p < 0.001	0.13 (−0.41, − 0.14)
		3	4.65 ± 0.84			
		6	4.82 ± 0.82			
		9	4.65 ± 0.88			
		12	4.49 ± 0.77			

x ± SD mean values and standard deviation
Mean diff. mean difference
CI Coinfidence interval

Table 3 Biotype, papilla width (PW), papilla height (PH), gingival recession (GR), recession width (RW) and keratinized tissue (KT) before and after orthodontic treatment

Parameter	[mm]	Time of observation [months]		Difference between baseline and 12 months post-op	p-value (Friedman ANOVA)	Mean diff. (95% CI) between baseline and 12 months post-op
Biotype	x ± SD	Baseline	1.71 ± 0.52	+ 0.32 mm	$p < 0.0001$	0.07 (0.26, 0.39)
		3	1.95 ± 0.54			
		6	1.89 ± 0.56			
		9	1.94 ± 0.59			
		12	2.03 ± 0.47			
PW	x ± SD	Baseline	3.75 ± 0.92	−0.21 mm	NS	0.29 (−1.11, −0.53)
		3	3.60 ± 1.17			
		6	3.77 ± 0.95			
		9	3.80 ± 1.13			
		12	3.54 ± 1.50			
PH	x ± SD	Baseline	4.82 ± 1.16	−0.82 mm	$p < 0.0001$	0.26 (− 0.47, 0.05)
		3	4.16 ± 1.23			
		6	4.52 ± 0.85			
		9	4.51 ± 1.14			
		12	4.00 ± 1.60			
GR	x ± SD	Baseline	0.13 ± 0.47	−0.06 mm	NS	0.05 (−0.11, −0.01)
		3	0.09 ± 0.39			
		6	0.08 ± 0.34			
		9	0.09 ± 0.36			
		12	0.07 ± 0.32			
RW	x ± SD	Baseline	0.21 ± 0.75	−0.11 mm	NS	0.08 (−0.20, −0.03)
		3	0.17 ± 0.65			
		6	0.16 ± 0.66			
		9	0.14 ± 0.61			
		12	0.10 ± 0.49			
KT	x ± SD	Baseline	5.02 ± 1.79	−0.10 mm	$p = 0.0039$	0.17 (−0.07, 0.27)
		3	5.21 ± 1.65			
		6	5.08 ± 1.75			
		9	5.12 ± 1.83			
		12	5.12 ± 1.78			

x ± SD mean values and standard deviation
Mean diff. mean difference
CI Coinfidence interval

Figures 1, 2 and 3 show photographic documentation of selected case treatment.

A statistically significant increase was noted in relation to the biotype. Its thickness values rose 3 months post-op (from 1.71 ± 0.52 mm to 1.95 ± 0.54 mm), then decreased 6 months post-op as compared with the 3-month-post-op examinations; then it increased again reaching the maximum mean value (2.03 ± 0.47 mm) in twelfth month, i.e. at the end of the treatment (Table 3). The KT values also increased significantly during the course of the treatment. Its mean value at baseline was 5.02 ± 1.79 mm and rose to 5.12 ± 1.78 mm at the treatment completion (Table 3). No statistically significant differences were observed in GR, RW and PW (Table 3).

Discussion

The aim of presented study was detailed clinical evaluation of periodontal tissues in adult patients after corticotomy-assisted orthodontic treatment. The results of the study have demonstrated lack of negative influence of the treatment on the periodontal status confirmed by significant reduction in PD and CAL (of 0.26 mm) as well as BS (of 0.27 mm) after treatment. In the available literature Gantes et al. [6], Charavet et al. [24] and Cassetta et al. [25]

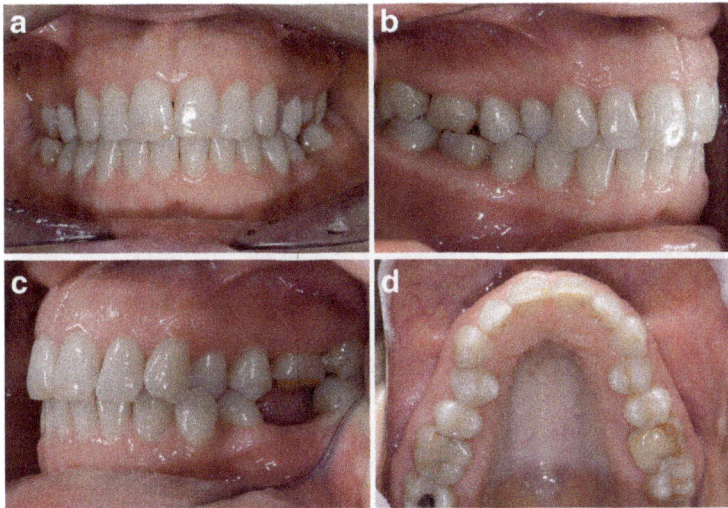

Fig. 1 a-d. The status before the orthodontic treatment - bilateral crossbite

examined periodontal tissues response to corticotomy-assisted orthodontic treatment. Gantes et al. [6] assessed periodontal parameters - PI, PD, CAL and concluded that corticotomy procedure caused minimal changes in the periodontal attachment apparatus. However, the authors did not provide specific values for periodontal parameters and the study group consisted of only 5 people. Charavet et al. [24] conducted randomized controlled study in the group of 24 adult patients with mild overcrowdings who were randomly allocated to a control group that was treated with conventional orthodontics or a test group that received piezo assisted orthodontics. In both groups, periodontal parameters: PD, PI, papilla bleeding index and recession depth remained unchanged between the baseline and treatment completion time points. Analyze of recession depth in particular cases revealed that recession depth increased only in 3 patients - 2 from the control group and 1 from the test group. This observation is even more interesting because the mean value of the recession depth in the control group was substantially lower than in the test group (2.5 ± 2.3 mm vs 5.7 ± 7.6 mm). In our study, in none of patients new recessions developed despite that orthodontic

vestibular movement of teeth was performed. Additionally, 5 of 12 of existing recessions disappeared and 3 reduced of 1 mm. Nevertheless, such changes in the recessions parameters, decrease in the mean values of GR as well as gingival width (respectively 0.06 mm and 0.11 mm) were not statistically significant. Findings of our research may confirm the hypothesis that the potential to increase the post-cortycotomy alveolar volume and cover vital root surfaces can result in repairing pre-existing alveolar dehiscences over the root prominences and lessen a risk of forming new ones, which can contribute to gingival recession [6]. Cassetta et al. [25, 26] assesed modified gingival index (mGI) and probing pocket depth (PPD) before and at the end of the orthodontic treatment assisted with minimally invasive coricotomy performed with the use of printed CAD/CAM surgical guide. The authors didn't show significant changes in the values of the tested parameters before and after treatment. The mean mGI value at baseline was 0.15 whereas post-op - 0.10. The mean PPD values at baseline and post-op were 1.93 mm and 1.68 mm respectively. The above data showed that both, corticotomy after full-thickness flap elevation and the minimally invasive

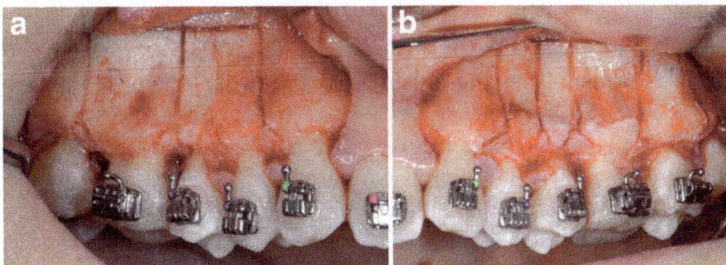

Fig. 2 a-b. A corticotomy in the area of upper premolars and molars. Incision of the cortical plate in the interdental spaces and above the apexes of the teeth

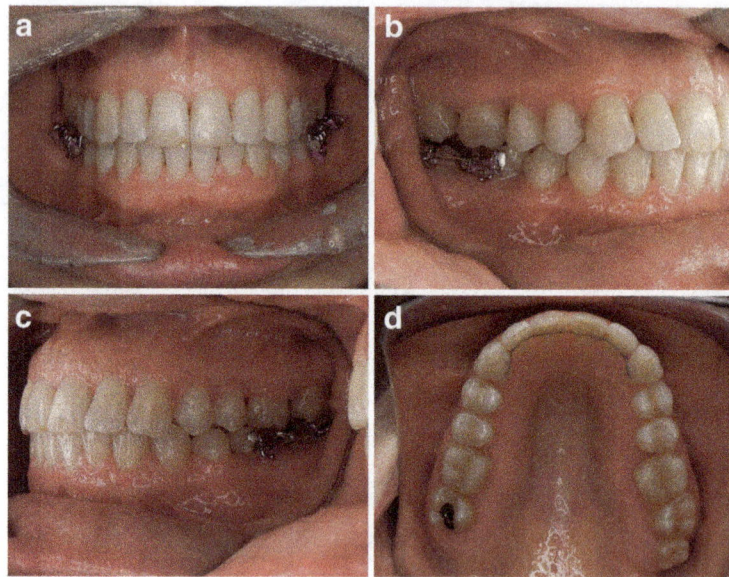

Fig. 3 a-d. The status imediately after orthodontic treatment completion (missing two lower first molars temporarily restored, partial orthodontic appliance left till the moment of the definitive restoration delivery). There are no adverse changes in the position of the gingival margin after labial tooth movement

flapless corticotomy do not adversely affect the status of periodontal tissues. Flapless corticotomy brings also additional benefits - significantly less trauma to the patient and reduced time of the surgery [25, 26].

From the clinical point of view any labial tooth movement should be preceded by a careful examination of the dimensions of the tissue which covers the teeth to be moved. As long as a tooth can be moved within the envelope of the alveolar process, the risk of harmful side-effects on the gingival tissue is minimal, irrespective of the thickness of the soft tissue [27]. If, however, there is danger of alveolar bone dehiscences, thickness of the covering soft tissue must be considered to be a factor leading to gingival recession, both during and after the therapy. Thin gingiva may also serve as a locus minoris resistentiae for gingival recession in the presence of bacterial plaque [28]. Our observations show that the model of corticotomy-facilitated orthodontic treatment may have favourable impact on soft tissue parameters. We have observed a statistically significant increase of KT of 0.1 mm and tissue thickness of 0.32 mm after the treatment. Biotype thickening as well as decrease of the number and dimension of recessions after the treatment suggest that alterations in hard and soft tissues after corticotomy may protect soft tissues position during the teeth movement toward labial direction. Similar findings achieved Liou and Huang [29], who concluded that the periodontal ligament could be rapidly distracted without complications after corticotomy and this technique could be used to generate new bone growth and keratinized gingiva. It seems that this favorable reaction

for treatment is due to RAP, which according to Yaffe et al. [12] is essentially a temporary stage of localized soft- and hard tissues remodeling in the process of bringing the surgical site to a normal state and usually takes about four months to heal [30]. It is also possible that the optimistic results obtained are due to the use of piezosurgery device. Dibart el al. [31] has shown that although all corticotomy procedures involve physical injury to the bone, the clinical outcomes may depend on the instrument used. Using an ex vivo calvarial bone organ culture model system, the authors evaluated the biologic response of bone to different corticotomies. Bone injuries were generated in neonatal mice using a piezoelectric knife, a bur, and a handheld screw device. It was demonstrated that the piezoelectric knife led to the most extensive impact in both bone resorption and formation models. Farid et al. [32] arrived at the opposite conclusions whose purpose of the research was to evaluate corticotomy-facilitated orthodontics using piezosurgery versus conventional rotary instruments in mongrel dogs. A statistically significantly higher mean amount of tooth movement (1.6 times faster) for conventional rotary instrument versus the piezosurgery corticotomy technique was observed at all time intervals. Notwithstanding the above controversies, there are other advantages of piezosurgery, i.e. permitting a selective cut of mineralized tissue while preserving soft tissues. Moreover, the major advantages of this technique include high precision, curvilinear design of the osteotomy, less trauma to soft tissues, preservation of neurological and vascular structures, reduced hemorrhage, minimal thermal damage to the bone, as well as overall improvement of healing [33]. However, taking into account the oral health-related quality of life - OHIP-14 (which represents: functional limitation, physical pain, psychological discormfort, physical disability, psychological disability, social disability, and handicap) corticotomy with the use of bur or piezoelectric knife do not differ significantly [34].

As post-corticotomy tooth movement does not have negative effects on the periodontium, our results may also suggest, that there is no need for additional bone augmentation although some authors recommend bone grafting in the area where expansion of the alveolar bone is needed [9, 10, 12]. All the more that Nowzari et al. [13] pointed out that an optimal quantity of bone graft has not been determined yet and more clinical research should be undertaken to do so. Significant confirmation of such suggestion is study done by Chavret et al. [24] in which minimally invasive corticotomy technique - piezocision without hard and soft tissue augmentation was used. No significant increases in dehiscence or fenestration were observed. Additionally, the thickness of the buccal alveolar plate and the bucco-lingual dimensions of the alveolar crest did not significantly change from baseline to the completion of treatment.

The last aspect of our research was the evaluation of interdental papillae. In opposition to other authors who haven't observed papillae height reduction after osteotomy accelerated orthodontics, we have noticed a statistically significant reduction in papillae height that was also reflected in the bone sounding values [35]. Indeed, mean PH value decreased of 0.82 mm comparing to baseline but it cannot be directly related to corticotomy procedure but rather as the effect of the teeth position changes [36]. Within the course of orthodontic treatment arches were extended, crowded teeth were aligned and unrotated if needed. Alterations of teeth position and arches shape cause papillae remodeling including changes in the distance between papilla tip and interproximal contact point. Considering the fact that the papillae height is influenced by many factors (distance between bone level and approximal contact point, distance between roots at the bone level and divergent roots position), it is not possible to explicitly refer to changes in their height after treatment [36–38]. That is why in our opinion reduction of PH parameter cannot be unequivocally considered as deterioration in interproximal papillae condition.

Summarizing all above data, it should be underlined that the results presented in this article included entire estimation of clinical soft tissues parameters which, according to our knowledge, have not been presented in the literature yet. It was shown up that there was a statistically significant reduction in PD, CAL and BS after the treatment. Statistically significant changes were also noted considering KT and biotype, which increased significantly after utilization of the corticotomy-assisted orthodontic treatment. Therefore, the achieved findings may suggest protective role of corticotomy on soft tissues condition in the course of orthodontic treatment. However, the presented study is burdened with a limitation resulting from the lack of a control group in which patients were treated orthodontically without additional corticotomy. In future studies it would be also helpful to analyze CBCT images to assess the changes in the bone morphology following the piesosurgery-assisted orthodontics.

Conclusion

The corticotomy–assisted orthodontic treatment does not jeopardize a periodontal clinical status. Since the currently available literature misses detailed studies on the periodontal changes which occur after the procedure, there is a need to continue studies on a larger number of cases with a control group and a longer follow-up time to find out about the post-treatment periodontal tissue changes and stability.

Abbreviations
BS: Bone sounding; CAL: Clinical attachment level; CEJ: Cemento-enamel junction; FMBOP: Full mouth bleading on probing; FMPI: Full mouth plaque index; GR: Gingival recession height; KT: Keratinized tissue; MTDLD: Monocortical tooth dislocation and ligament distraction; PAOO: Periodontally accelerated osteogenic orthodontics; PD: Probing depth; PH: Papilla height; PW: Papilla width; RAP: Regional accelerated phenomenon; RW: Recession width

Funding
The study was supported by Medical University of Białystok.

Authors' contributions
MS - data collection, the manuscript draft. ED - surgical treatment. BBM - orthodontic treatment. EWS - orthodontic treatment. RM - statistical analyses. JP - the study supervision, data interpretation, final manuscript approval. ES - statistical analyses. MP - the study design and supervision, data interpretation, final manuscript approval. All authors read and approved the final manuscript.

Competing interests
The authors declare that they have no competing interests.

Author details
[1]Department of Periodontal and Oral Mucosa Diseases, Medical University of Białystok, ul. Waszyngtona 13, 15-269 Białystok, Poland. [2]Dental Practice, ul. Żeromskiego 1A/1U, 15-349 Białystok, Poland. [3]Dental Practice, ul. Waszyngtona 1/34, 15-269 Białystok, Poland. [4]Department of Statistics and Medical Informatics, Medical University of Białystok, ul. Szpitalna 37, 15-295 Białystok, Poland. [5]Department of Biocybernetics and Biomedical Ingeenering, Białystok University of Technology, ul. Wiejska 45c, 15-351 Białystok, Poland.

References

1. Patel N. Corticotomy assisted orthodontic: a review of surgical technique and literature. OA Dentistry. 2014;2(1):1–18.
2. Hassan AH, Al-Fraidi AA, Al-Saeed SH. Corticotomy-assisted orthodontic treatment: review. Open Dent J. 2010;4(4):159–64.
3. Oliveira DD, Oliveira BF, Soares RV. Alveolar corticotomies in orthodontics: indications and effects on tooth movement. Dental Press J Orthod. 2010; 15(4):144–57.
4. Buschang PH, Phillip M, Campbell PM, Ruso S. Accelerating tooth movement with Corticotomies: is it possible and desirable? Semin Orthod. 2012;18(4):286–94.
5. Köle H. Surgical operations on the alveolar ridge to correct occlusal abnormalities. Oral Surg Oral Med Oral Pathol. 1959;12(5):515–29.
6. Gantes B, Rathbun E, Anholm M. Effects on the periodontium following corticotomy-facilitated orthodontics. Case reports. J Periodontol. 1990;61(4):234–8.
7. Wilcko WM, Wilcko TM, Bouquot JE, Ferguson DJ. Rapid orthodontics with alveolar reshaping: two case reports of decrowding. Int J Periodontics Restorative Dent. 2001;21(1):9–19.
8. Wilcko MT, Wilcko WM, Bissada NF. An evidence based analysis of periodontally accelerated orthodontic and osteogenic techniques: a synthesis of scientific perspectives. Semin Orthod. 2008;14:305–16.
9. Wilcko MT, Wilcko WM, Pulver JJ, Bissada NF, Bouquot JE. Accelerated osteogenic orthodontics technique: a 1-stage surggically facilitated rapid orthodontic technique with alveolar augmentation. J Oral Maxillofac Surg. 2009;67(10):2149–59.
10. Murphy KG, Wilcko MT, Wilcko WM, Ferguson DJ. Periodontal accelerated Osteogenic orthodontics: a description of the surgical technique. J Oral Maxillofac Surg. 2009;67(10):2160–6.
11. Frost HM. The regional accelerator phenomenon: a review. Henry Ford Hosp Med J. 1983;31(1):3–9.
12. Yaffe A, Fine N, Binderman I. Regional accelerated phenomenon in the mandible following mucoperiosteal flap surgery. J Periodontol. 1994;65(1):79–83.
13. Nowzari H, Yorita FK, Chang HC. Periodontally accelerated osteogenic orthodontics combined with autogenous bone grafting. Compend Contin Educ Dent. 2008;29(4):200–6.
14. Sebaoun JD, Kantarci A, Turner JW, Carvalho RS, Van Dyke TE, Ferguson DJ. Modeling of trabecular bone and lamina dura following selective alveolar decortication in rats. J Periodontol. 2008;79(9):1679–88.
15. Lee W, Karapetyan G, Moats R, Yamashita DD, Moon HB, Ferguson DJ, Yen S. Corticotomy-/osteotomy-assisted tooth movement microCTs differ. J Dent Res. 2008;87(9):861–7.
16. Vercellotti T, Podesta A. Orthodontic microsurgery: a new surgically guided technique for dental movement. Int J Periodontics Restorative Dent. 2007;27(4):325–31.
17. Dibart S, Sebaoun JD, Surmenian J. Piezocision: a minimally invasive, periodontally accelerated orthodontic tooth movement procedure. Compend Contin Educ Dent. 2009;30(6):342 -4, 346, 348-50.
18. Nazarov AD, Ferguson DJ, Wilcko WM, Wilcko MT. Improved orthodontic retention following corticotomy using ABO objective grading system. J Dent Res. 2004;83:2644.
19. Fischer TJ. Orthodontic treatment acceleration with corticotomy assisted exposure of palatally impacted canines. Angle Orthod. 2007;77(3):417–20.
20. Mostafa YA, Mohamed Salah Fayed M, Mehanni S, ElBokle NN, Heider AM. Comparison of corticotomy-facilitated vs standard tooth-movement techniques in dogs with miniscrews as anchor units. Am J Orthod Dentofac Orthop. 2009;136(4):570–7.
21. Dorfman HS, Turvey TA. Alterations in osseous crestal height following interdental osteotomies. Oral Surg Oral Med Oral Pathol. 1979;48(2):120–5.
22. Kwon HJ, Pihlstrom B, Waite DE. Effects on the periodontium of vertical bone cutting for segmental osteotomy. J Oral Maxillofac Surg. 1985;43(12):952–5.
23. Cortellini P, Pini Prato G, Tonetti MS. The modified papilla preservation technique. A new surgical approach for interproximal regenerative procedures. J Periodontol. 1995;66(4):261–6.
24. Charavet C, Lecloux G, Bruwier A, Rompen E, Maes N, Limme N, Lambert F. Localized piezoelectric alveolar decortication for orthodontic treatment in adults: A randomized controlled trial. J Dent Res. 2016;95(9):1003–9.
25. Cassetta M, Giansanti M, Di Mambro A, Calasso S, Barbato E. Minimally invasive corticotomy in orthodontics using a three-dimensional printed CAD/CAM surgical guide. Int J Oral Maxillofac Surg. 2016;45:1059–64.
26. Cassetta M, Pandolfi S, Giansanti M. Minimally invasive corticotomy in orthodontics: a new technique using a CAD/CAM surgical template. Int J Oral Maxillofac Surg. 2015;44:830–3.
27. Borzabadi-Farahani A. A review of the oral health-related evidence that supports the orthodontic treatment need indices. Prog Orthod. 2012;13(3):314–25.
28. Wennström JL, Lindhe J, Sinclair F. Some periodontal tissue reactions to orthodontic tooth movement in monkeys. J Clin Periodontol. 1987;14(3):121–9.
29. Liou EJ, Huang CS. Rapid canine retraction through distraction of the periodontal ligament. Am J Orthod Dentofac Orthop. 1998;114(4):372–82.
30. Abbas IT, Moutamed GM. Acceleration of orthodontic tooth movement by alveolar corticotomy using piezosurgery. J Am Sci. 2012;8(2):13–9.
31. Dibart S, Alasmari A, Zanni O, Salih E. Effect of Corticotomies with different instruments on cranial bone biology using an ex vivo Calvarial bone organ culture model system. Int J Periodontics Restorative Dent. 2016;36(suppl):123–36.
32. Farid KA, Mostafa YA, Kaddah MA, El-Sharaby FA. Corticotomy-facilitated orthodontics using piezosurgery versus rotary instruments: an experimental study. J Int Acad Periodontol. 2014;16(4):103–8.
33. Hennet P. Piezoelectric bone surgery: a review of the literature and potential applications in veterinary oromaxillofacial surgery. Front Vet Sci. 2015;2:1–7. https://doi.org/10.3389/fvets.2015.00008.
34. Cassetta M, Di Carlo S, Giansanti M, Pompa V, Pompa G, Barbato E. The impact of osteotomy technique for corticotomy-assisted orthodontic treatment (CAOT) on oral health-related quality of life. Eur Rev Med Pharmacol Sci. 2012;16:1735–40.
35. Bertossi D, Vercellotti T, Podesta A, Nocini PF. Orthodontic microsurgery for rapid dental repositioning in dental malpositions. J Oral Maxillofac Surg. 2011;69(3):747–53.
36. Cho HS, Jang HS, Kim DK, Park JC, Kim HJ, Choi SH, Kim CK, Kim BO. The effects of interproximal distance between roots on the existence of interdental papillae according to the distance from the contact point to the alveolar crest. J Periodontol. 2006;77:1651–7.
37. Sharma AA, Park JH. Esthetic considerations in interdental papilla: remediation and regeneration. J Esthet Restor Dent. 2010;22:18–30.
38. Martegani P, Silvestri M, Mascarello F, Scipioni T, Ghezzi C, Rota C, Cattaneo V, Kim BO. Morphometric study of the interproximal unit in the esthetic region to correlate anatomic variables affecting the aspect of soft tissue embrasure space. J Periodontol. 2007;78:2260–5.

27

Oral health and health-related quality of life in HIV patients

Vinicius da Costa Vieira[1], Liliane Lins[1*] ⬤, Viviane Almeida Sarmento[2], Eduardo Martins Netto[3] and Carlos Brites[3]

Abstract

Background: Oral health care may improve the health-related quality of life (HRQoL) of HIV/AIDS patients. We aimed to evaluate oral health and HRQoL of HIV/AIDS patients using antiretroviral therapy.

Methods: A cross-sectional study included 120 HIV-infected patients, aged ≥18 years, from February, 2016 to September, 2017. The 36-Item Short Form Health Survey (SF-36) was used to evaluate the HRQoL. We assessed dental caries status using the Decayed, Missing and Filled Teeth (DMFT) index. Information about demographic, socioeconomic status, depression, and other comorbidities were collected. All patients with depression had a medical diagnosis. Comorbidities were defined as medical diagnoses of arterial hypertension, type-2 diabetes, tuberculosis, syphilis, cardiopathy, chronic renal failure, lymphoma, HCV infection, HBV infection and fatty liver disease. Independent t-tests were used to compare differences between mean levels of HRQoL, age, and DMFT and its components according to groups of sex, comorbidities and depression. Simple linear regression was used to analyze the relationship between the Mental Component Summary (MCS) and DMFT, and a multiple regression equation investigated depression, age, MCS, and comorbidities as predictors of DMFT.

Results: The mean DMFT index was 12.4 ± 8.2. A linear regression equation estimated a significant ($p = 0.022$) decrease of 0.25 unit (%) in MCS for each unit increase in DMFT. Among depressed patients, a significant ($p = 0.008$) decrease of 0.67% in MCS for each unity increase in DMFT was estimated. Depressed patients showed worse oral health indicators (DFMT index; $p \leq 0.001$; and mean Missing Teeth; $p \leq 0.052$) and lower HRQoL domains than non-depressed patients. DMFT remained associated with depression ($P < 0.005$) after controlling for age, MCS, and comorbidities.

Conclusions: We found association between poorer oral health (higher DMFT index) and lower Mental Health Component Summary in HIV-infected patients with depression. Patients with depression deserve especial attention to their HRQoL and oral care.

Keywords: Health-related quality of life, Oral health, Depression, HIV

Background

The proper use of antiretroviral therapy (ART) has extended the life expectancy of people living with HIV/AIDS [1]. In consequence, several health-related outcomes have been observed, that contributed to a higher frequency of chronic comorbidities [2–4], depression and depressive symptoms [5, 6] that lead to a poorer health-related quality of life (HRQoL) [3, 6–8] and increases the risk of low adherence to ART [9]. Assessing depression symptoms before initiating ART may be effective to improve adherence and characterize the health-related quality of life of these patients [10]. The assessment of the health-related quality of life became an integral part of HIV/AIDS patients' follow-up [4].

In the past, detection of oral health lesions were often useful in the clinical diagnosis of HIV/AIDS infection, particularly among immunosuppressed patients [11]. There is no consensus about the association of poor oral health, particularly measured by DMFT index, with HIV infection. Some reports have shown greater risk for development of dental caries in HIV patients during antiretroviral drugs treatment [12, 13]. Another study reported a decrease in the incidence of dental caries following

* Correspondence: liliane.lins@ufba.br
[1]School of Medicine, Federal University of Bahia, Praça XV de Novembro, Largo do Terreiro de Jesus s/n, Salvador, Bahia CEP 400260-10, Brazil
Full list of author information is available at the end of the article

antiretroviral therapy [14]. A study among HIV-positive patients reported higher levels of immune activation markers HLA-DR and CD38 expressions in the peripheral blood when oral lesions were present [15], suggesting that oral health may significantly impact the immune response of HIV patients, including those under suppressive ART. However, HLA-DR and CD38 levels did not vary substantially according to the DMFT index.

Oral health care may improve the HRQoL of HIV/AIDS patients. A study in HIV patients has reported higher DMFT index associated with poorer Oral Health–Related Quality of Life [16]. However, this study did not investigate the association between DMFT index and the SF-36 domain scores. The SF-36 questionnaire is a widely used instrument to evaluate HRQoL, based on two different constructs, the Physical Component and the Mental Component [17]. This study aimed to evaluate the oral health and HRQoL of HIV/AIDS patients in use of ART.

Methods
Study design and participants
This is a cross-sectional study of HIV-infected patients, aged 18 years or more, consecutively recruited at the HIV Clinic of the University Hospital Professor Edgard Santos, Federal University of Bahia, Salvador, Bahia, Brazil, between February 2016 and September 2017. We excluded from the study patients unable to communicate or who had difficulty to understand SF-36 questionnaire.

Assessment
Information about demographic, socioeconomic status, clinical history, HIV-1 RNA plasma viral load and CD4/CD8 cells count were collected from each patient during medical examination, using a structured questionnaire. The 36-Item Short Form Health Survey (SF-36) was used to evaluate the HRQoL[17]. We used the SF-36 as recommended by QualityMetric Incorporated [17] to generate eight domains - physical functioning (PF), role limitations due to physical problems (RP), bodily pain (BP), general health perceptions (GH), vitality (VT), social functioning (SF), role limitations due to emotional problems (RE) and mental health (MH). The raw score of these domains varies from 0 to 100, where 100 represents the best HRQoL. SF-36 scores were normalized, assuming a mean of 50 and a standard deviation of 10, taking the general population of the USA as standard. The normalized domains were aggregated into either Physical Component Summary (PCS) or Mental Component Summary (MCS) [17]. Our study was licensed by Quality-Metric Health Outcomes™ under number QM025905.

We used the World Health Organization and the European Association of Dental Public Health criteria for oral health status evaluation [18, 19]. We measured clinical attachment loss, probing pocket depth and tooth mobility to evaluate periodontal disease. The number of Decayed, Missing and Filled Teeth were determined. Cariogenic diet was accessed using open *questions in the structured questionnaire*. The same researcher has evaluated all patients. The *intrarater* reliability (k = 0.67) was substantially satisfactory, as measured by the Kappa statistics [20]. Stimulated salivary flow measured less than 1 mL/min was considered as reduced [21].

Statistical analysis
Health-related quality of life (HRQoL) [17] and the number of Decayed, Missing and Filled Teeth (DMFT index) [18] were considered as dependent variables. Independent t-tests were used to compare differences between mean levels of HRQoL, age, and DMFT and its components according to groups of sex, comorbidities and depression. Simple linear regression technique was used to analyze the relationship between MCS and DMFT, and a multiple regression equation investigated age, depression, MCS, and comorbidities as predictors of DMFT. All patients with depression had a medical diagnosis. Comorbidities were defined as medical diagnoses of arterial hypertension, type-2 diabetes, tuberculosis, syphilis, cardiopathy, chronic renal failure, lymphoma, HCV infection, HBV infection and fatty liver disease. Data were analyzed by using the Statistical Package for the Social Sciences 18 (SPSS).

Ethical procedures
The study was approved by the Ethics Review Board of University Hospital Professor Edgard Santos, Federal University of Bahia under the Certificate of Presentation of Ethical Appreciation (CPEA 57172216.2.0000.0049) in accordance with the Declaration of Helsinki 2013 and the National Council Resolution 466/12 and. All participants were informed and signed a consent form approved by the Ethics Board.

Results
The study enrolled 120 patients (64 males; 56 females). Age ranged from 20 to 72 years, and the mean (±SD) was 44.9 ± 11.7 years. Most were Mulatto (57.5%) or Black (24.2%) and were not in a stable relationship (73.3%). Thirty-six (30.0%) of the patients had elementary schooling level (four or less years); 70.8% were non-smokers; 65.0% consumed alcohol, and 28 (23.3%) had diagnosis of depression.

Arterial hypertension was present in 22 (18.3%) patients, type-2 diabetes in seven (5.8%), tuberculosis in eight (6.7%), syphilis in six (5.0%), cardiopathy in four (3.3%), chronic renal failure in two (3.5%) and lymphoma in one (0.8%). Of the patients with hepatic comorbidities, five (4.2%) had HCV, three (2.5%) HBV and three (2.5%) had fatty liver disease. Periodontitis and gingivitis

Table 1 Demographic and clinical characteristics of 120 HIV-infected patients, Salvador, Bahia, 2017

Demographic and clinical characteristic	
Age, mean SD	44.9 ± 11.7
Sex N (%)	
Male	64 (53.3)
Female	56 (46.7)
Marital status N (%)	
Single	88 (73.3)
Married/stable relationship	32 (26.7)
Ethnicity N (%)	
Caucasian	22 (18.3)
Mulatto	69 (57.5)
Black	29 (24.2)
Educational status N (%)	
Elementary	36 (30.0)
High School	66 (55.0)
College	18 (15.0)
Alcohol consumption N (%)	
Yes	78 (65.0)
No	42 (35.0)
Smoking status N (%)	
Non Smoker	85 (70.8)
Smoker	35 (29.2)
Comorbidities N (%)	
Yes	62 (51.7)
No	58 (48.3)
Depression N (%)	
Yes	28 (23.3)
No	92 (76.7)
Daily dental brushing N (%)	
≥ 3 times	58 (48.3)
< 3 times	62 (51.7)
Dental floss use N (%)	
Yes	51 (42.5)
No	69 (67.5)
Cariogenic diet N (%)	
Yes	65 (54.2)
No	55 (45.8)
Edentulism N (%)	
Dentate	112 (93.3)
Edentulous	8 (6.7)
Periodontal disease	
Periodontitis	52 (46.4)
Gingivitis	47 (42.0)
No periodontal disease	13 (11.6)

Table 1 Demographic and clinical characteristics of 120 HIV-infected patients, Salvador, Bahia, 2017 *(Continued)*

Demographic and clinical characteristic	
DMFT, mean SD	12.4 ± 8.2
Decayed, mean SD	1.1 ± 1.9
Missing, mean SD	7.9 ± 8.7
Filled, mean SD	3.4 ± 4.0
CD4 cells/mm3, mean SD	656 ± 363
CD8 cells/mm3, mean SD	1008 ± 486
CD4/CD8 ratio	0.75 ± 0.44
Viral Load, mean SD[a]	35,245 ± 135,993
Viral Load, geometric mean SD[a]	309.3 */÷ 17.1

[a]Only patients with viral loads > zero

were found in 52 (46.4%) and 47 (42.0%) of dentate patients, respectively. Twenty-four patients (20.0%) had reduced salivary flow; and the mean DMFT index was 12.4 ± 8.2 (1.1 ± 1.9 decayed teeth; 7.9 ± 8.7 missing teeth and 3.4 ± 4.0 filled teeth). Eighty patients (66.7%) had CD4 counts equal or greater than 500 cells/mm3 and 75 (62.5%) had undetectable viral load (Table 1).

Patients with comorbidities were older (47.2 ± 11.0 vs. 42.4 ± 11.9; $P = 0.026$), and presented higher mean DMFT (14.0 ± 7.9 vs. 10.7 ± 8.2; $P = 0.026$). All SF-36 normalized mean scores were systematically lower in patients with comorbidities. Among patients with comorbidities, means of all SF-36 domains were significantly lower ($P < 0.05$), except for MH (Table 2). Women showed SF-36 scores systematically lower than men in all domains, and means of RP (0.006), BP (0.016), VT (0.044), MH (0.001) and MCS (0.013) were significantly lower. Compared to males, females presented higher mean DMFT ($P < 0.001$) and mean Missing Teeth indexes ($P < 0.033$) (Table 3).

A linear regression equation estimated a significant ($p = 0.022$) decrease of 0.25 unit (%) in MCS for each unit increase in DMFT. Among depressed patients, a significant ($p = 0.008$) decrease of 0.67% in MCS for each unity increase in DMFT was estimated. (Fig. 1 and Table 4). Depressed patients showed worse oral health indicators (DFMT index; $p \leq 0.001$ and mean Missing Teeth; $p \leq 0.052$) and lower HRQoL domains than those without depressive symptoms. DMFT remained associated with depression ($P < 0.005$) after controlling for age, MCS, and comorbidities.

Discussion

Depression is the most common prevalent neuropsychiatric symptom in HIV-1 patients [5]. According to our results, patients with depression had higher mean of missing teeth than patients without depression ($P \leq 0.052$). A linear regression equation predicted a significant ($P < 0.008$) decrease of 0.67 unit (%) in MCS for each unit of DMFT

Table 2 Mean and Standard Deviations of characteristics (Age, Oral Health Profile, and Health-related Quality of Life) of 120 patients according to comorbidities, Salvador, Bahia, Brazil, 2017

Characteristics	With Comorbidity (N = 62)	Without Comorbidity (N = 58)	Mean Difference	P≤*
Age	47.2 ± 11.0	42.4 ± 11.9	4.8	0.026
DMFT Index	14.0 ± 7.9	10.7 ± 8.2	3.3	0.026
Decayed	1.2 ± 1.6	1.2 ± 2.2	0.0	0.652
Missing	9.2 ± 8.5	6.4 ± 8.7	2.8	0.072
Filled	3.7 ± 4.4	3.1 ± 3.4	0.6	0.377
Physical Functioning (PF)	48.9 ± 9.8	54.8 ± 4.9	−5.9	0.001
Role Physical (RP)	40.6 ± 9.6	45.3 ± 8.7	− 4.7	0.006
Bodily Pain (BP)	46.4 ± 11.8	52.5 ± 9.3	− 6.1	0.002
General Health (GH)	48.5 ± 10.9	54.1 ± 9.9	−5.6	0.004
Vitality (VT)	52.1 ± 10.8	56.1 ± 8.9	− 4.0	0.030
Social Functioning (SF)	47.5 ± 12.1	52.2 ± 8.1	− 4.7	0.014
Role Emotional (RE)	35.4 ± 11.2	42.2 ± 9.0	− 6.8	0.001
Mental Health (MH)	46.9 ± 12.8	50.3 ± 9.2	−3.4	0.099
Physical Component Summary (PCS)	48.3 ± 8.6	53.8 ± 6.9	−5.5	0.001
Mental Component Summary (MCS)	43.8 ± 10.8	48.0 ± 8.2	−5.2	0.019

*Independent Sample Student-t Test

among patients with depression. Depression can decrease the likelihood of using oral health services, and is associated with teeth loss [22].

In this study, patients with HIV had a mean DMFT of 12.4. DMFT mean in patients with HIV varies around the world, ranging from 8.7 in Australia [23], to 16.9 in Portugal [24]. In Brazil, DMFT means of 16.9, 17.64 and 18.8 have been reported [25–27]. These differences in DMFT means can be attributed to hygienic behavioral, access to dental services and socioeconomic status [28, 29].

A multivariate linear regression identified age ($P < 0.001$) and depression ($P < 0.004$) as good and independent predictors of DMFT, even after adjusting for mental health and comorbidities. Correlation between age and the mean DMFT index have also been reported not only in HIV/AIDS patients [28], but also in non-HIV/AIDS patients [30]. Older age is associated with greater frequency of dental extraction due to caries, periodontal disease, and presence of comorbidities such as diabetes, hypertension or hyperlipidemia [30].

Table 3 Mean and Standard Deviations of Oral Health Profile and Health-related Quality of Life indicators of 120 patients according to sex, Salvador, Bahia, Brazil, 2017

Indicator	Male (N = 64)	Female (N = 56)	Mean Difference	P≤*
DMFT Index- mean (SD)	10.1 ± 8.0	15.1 ± 7.8	−5.0	0.001
Decayed- mean (SD)	0.8 ± 1.4	1.5 ± 2.4	− 0.7	0.065
Missing- mean (SD)	6.3 ± 7.8	9.7 ± 9.3	−3.4	0.033
Filled- mean (SD)	3.0 ± 3.5	3.9 ± 4.4	−0.9	0.229
Physical Functioning (PF)	53.0 ± 7.6	50.4 ± 9.0	2.6	0.089
Role Physical (RP)	45.1 ± 8.2	40.3 ± 10.2	4.8	0.006
Bodily Pain (BP)	51.6 ± 10.0	46.8 ± 11.7	4.8	0.016
General Health (GH)	52.3 ± 10.3	50.0 ± 11.3	2.3	0.236
Vitality (VT)	55.8 ± 10.2	52.1 ± 9.7	3.7	0.044
Social Functioning (SF)	50.9 ± 9.3	48.6 ± 11.9	2.3	0.236
Role Emotional (RE)	39.7 ± 10.7	37.5 ± 10.8	2.2	0.247
Mental Health (MH)	52.1 ± 8.6	44.6 ± 12.7	7.5	0.001
Physical Component Summary (PCS)	52.3 ± 7.2	49.4 ± 9.2	2.9	0.057
Mental Component Summary (MCS)	47.9 ± 8.6	43.4 ± 10.6	4.5	0.013

*Independent Sample Student-t Test

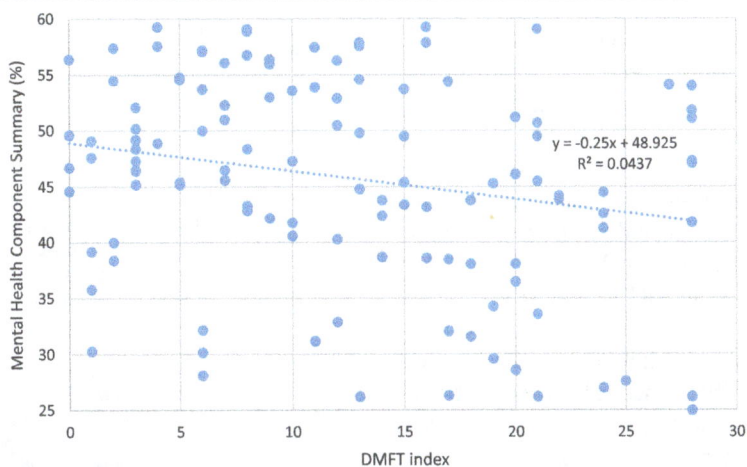

Fig. 1 Association between Mental Health Component Summary and DMFT index in 120-HIV-infected patients

In our study, women had systematically lower mean scores of SF-36 domains, lower MCS ($P < 0.013$) and PCS ($P < 0.057$). Our data are according to a previous study that reported females have significant lower MCS score, but not PCS [31]. Our male patients presented significantly lower mean of missing teeth than the females, differing of the results reported by in an Iranian study [28].

In a meta-analysis with 42,366 patients, from 111 studies, the prevalence of depressive symptoms ranged from 12.8 to 78.0% in HIV/AIDS patients using ART [9]. In our patients, the prevalence of depression was 23.3%, which is in accordance with the mentioned meta-analysis. The actual diagnosis of depression, as well as its previous history, have been associated with poorer HRQoL in HIV-infected patients [32]. The group with confirmed diagnosis of depression exhibited significantly lower means in all SF-36 domains and in physical and mental summary components. As expected, depression was more associated with mental health domains. The presence of major depressive disorders along patient's life is correlated with both Physical and Mental summary scores of HRQoL [2]. Depression may also be associated with sleep disorders and appetite decrease [8].

HIV-infected patients aged 50 years or older may have multiple comorbidities and risk for cardiovascular and renal diseases [4]. In our study, at least one comorbidity was present in 51.7% of the IHV-patients. Patients without comorbidities presented lower mean DMFT. Patients with comorbidity were 4.8 years older than those without

Table 4 Mean and Standard Deviations characteristics (Oral Health Profile and Health-related Quality of Life) of 120 patients according to depression, Salvador, Bahia, Brazil, 2017

Characteristics	Depressed ($N = 28$)	Nondepressed ($N = 92$)	Mean Difference	P≤*
DMFT Index- mean (SD)	16.9 ± 6.5	11.1 ± 8.2	5.8	0.001
Decayed- mean (SD)	1.5 ± 2.0	1.0 ± 1.9	0.5	0.217
Missing- mean (SD)	10.6 ± 8.4	7.0 ± 8.6	3.6	0.052
Filled- mean (SD)	4.8 ± 4.8	3.0 ± 3.6	1.8	0.083
Physical Functioning (PF)	48.0 ± 9.3	52.9 ± 7.7	− 4.9	0.006
Role Physical (RP)	36.6 ± 10.9	44.8 ± 8.1	−8.2	0.001
Bodily Pain (BP)	43.3 ± 11.4	51.2 ± 10.4	−7.9	0.001
General Health (GH)	47.0 ± 13.2	52.5 ± 9.7	− 5.5	0.050
Vitality (VT)	49.2 ± 9.1	55.5 ± 10.0	− 6.3	0.003
Social Functioning (SF)	44.1 ± 13.0	51.6 ± 9.2	−7.5	0.008
Role Emotional (RE)	29.2 ± 10.8	41.6 ± 9.0	−12.4	0.001
Mental Health (MH)	39.9 ± 13.6	51.2 ± 9.1	− 11.3	0.001
Physical Component Summary (PCS)	47.8 ± 9.1	51.9 ± 7.8	−4.1	0.021
Mental Component Summary (MCS)	37.1 ± 8.8	48.5 ± 8.5	−11.4	0.001

*Independent Sample Student-t Test

comorbidities, what may partially explain the worse mean DMFT. The group with comorbidities also presented lower means of PCS and MCS scores. The negative effect of comorbidities, specifically on the physical domains of HRQoL, has been also reported [2]. On the other hand, our patients were in use of ART for at least one year, so we can assume that they had enough time to get benefits from this medical treatment, including in their HRQoL. Improvements in physical and mental aspects of HRQoL were reported in patients using ART for one year [31].

Our study has some limitations. First, we used a cross-sectional design that have inherent methodological limitations, like the difficulty to establish the correct temporal sequence of exposure and effect. Our patients were recruited from a single reference center for HIV-infected patients. We did not take the exposure duration to ART into consideration in our analysis. The results of some clinical data were obtained from medical records. We did not have an HIV-uninfected population to compare the frequency of comorbidities. However, this is a well characterized sample that was large enough to provide insights on significant associations between oral health and HRQoL, a field with scarce data, especially in less-developed settings.

Conclusions

In conclusion, this study found associations between poor oral health (high DMFT index) and Mental Health Component Summary in HIV-infected patients with depression. Lower health-related quality of life and poorer oral health were observed in patients with comorbidities. These findings reinforce that patients with depression should deserve especial attention to their HRQoL and oral care.

Authors' contributions
We declare that all authors included in this paper fulfill authorship criteria. LL, VAS, EMN and CB have worked in the conception and design of the study; VCV and VAS have worked on data collection. LL, EMN and CB have performed statistical data analyses and interpretation. LL and VCV have written the article. All authors have critically reviewed the manuscript and approved its last version for publication.

Competing interests
The authors declare that they have no competing interests.

Author details
[1]School of Medicine, Federal University of Bahia, Praça XV de Novembro, Largo do Terreiro de Jesus s/n, Salvador, Bahia CEP 400260-10, Brazil. [2]School of Dentstry, Federal University of Bahia, Salvador, Bahia, Brazil. [3]Research Laboratory of Infectious Diseases, Edgard Santos Federal University Hospital, Salvador, Bahia, Brazil.

References

1. Brites-Alves C, Netto EM, Brites C. Coinfection by hepatitis C is strongly associated with abnormal CD4+/CD8+ ratio in HIV patients under stable ART in Salvador. Brazil J Immunol Res. 2015;2015:174215.
2. Rodriguez-Penney AT, Iudicello JE, Riggs PK, Doyle K, Ellis RJ, Letendre SL, Grant I, Woods SP. Group HIVNRPH: co-morbidities in persons infected with HIV: increased burden with older age and negative effects on health-related quality of life. AIDS Patient Care STDs. 2013;27:5–16.
3. Jia HG, Uphold CR, Zheng Y, Wu S, Chen GJ, Findley K, Duncan PW. A further investigation of health-related quality of life over time among men with HIV infection in the HAART era. Qual Life Res. 2007;16:961–8.
4. Wu P-Y, Chen M-Y, Hsieh S-M, Sun H-Y, Tsai M-S, et al. Comorbidities among the HIV-Infected Patients Aged 40 Years or Older in Taiwan. PLoS ONE. 2014;9(8):e104945.
5. Betancur MN, Lins L, Oliveira IR, Brites C. Quality of life, anxiety and depression in patients with HIV/AIDS who present poor adherence to antiretroviral therapy: a cross-sectional study in Salvador, Brazil. Braz J Infect Dis. 2017;21(5):507–14. https://doi.org/10.1016/j.bjid.2017.04.004. Epub 2017 May 21
6. Ngum PA, Fon PN, Ngu RC, Verla VS, Luma HN. Depression among HIV/AIDS patients on highly active antiretroviral therapy in the southwest regional hospitals of Cameroon: a cross sectional study. Neurol Ther. 2017;6:103–14.
7. Liu CL, Ostrow D, Detels R, Hu Z, Johnson L, Kingsley L, Jacobson LP. Impacts of HIV infection and HAART use on quality of life. Qual Life Res. 2006;15:941–9.
8. Degroote S, Vogelaers D, Vandijck DM. What determines health-related quality of lifemong people living with HIV: an updated review of the literature. Arch Public Health. 2014;72:40.
9. Uthman OA, Magidson JF, Safren SA, Nachega JB. Depression and adherence to antiretroviral therapy in low-, middle- and high-income countries: a systematic review and meta-analysis. Curr HIV/AIDS Rep. 2014; 11:291–307.
10. Campos LN, Guimarães MDC, Remien RH. Anxiety and depression symptoms as risk factors for nonadherence to antiretroviral therapy in Brazil. AIDS Behav. 2010;14(2):289–99.
11. Batavia AS, Secours R, Espinosa P, Jean Juste MA, Severe P, Pape JW, et al. Diagnosis of HIV-associated oral lesions in relation to early versus delayed antiretroviral therapy: results from the CIPRA HT001 trial. PLoS One. 2016; 11(3):e0150656. https://doi.org/10.1371/journal.pone.0150656.
12. X-Glick M, Berthold P, Danik J. Severe caries and the use of protease inhibitors. J Dent Res. 1998;77:77–84.
13. Y- Navazesh M, Mulligan R, Barrón Y, Redford M, Greenspan D, Alves M, Phelan J. A 4-year longitudinal evaluation of xerostomia and salivary gland hypofunction in the women's interagency HIV study participants. Oral Surg Oral Med Oral Pathol Oral Radiol Endod. 2003;95:693–8.
14. Z- Bretz WA, Flaitz C, Moretti A, Corby P, Schneider LG, Nichols CM. Medication usage and dental caries outcome-related variables in HIV/AIDS patients. AIDS Patient Care STDs. 2000;14:549–54.
15. Lins L, Farias É, Brites-Alves C, Torres A, Netto EM, Brites C. Increased expression of CD38 and HLADR in HIV-infected patients with oral lesion. J Med Virol. 2017; 89(10):1782–7. https://doi.org/10.1002/jmv.24852. Epub 2017 Jun 15
16. w- Mohamed N, Saddki N, Yusoff A, Jelani MA. Association among oral symptoms, oral health-related quality of life, and health-related quality of life in a sample of adults living with HIV/AIDS in Malaysia. BMC Oral Health. 2017;17:119. Published online 2017 Aug 22. https://doi.org/10. 1186/s12903-017-0409-y.
17. Ware JE. SF-36 health survey update. Spine. 2000;25:3130–9.
18. World Health Organization. Oral health surveys basic methods. 4th ed. Geneva: WHO; 1997.
19. Leroy E, Eaton KA, Savage A. Methodological issues in epidemiological studies of periodontitis - how can it be improved? BMC Oral Health. 2010;10:8.
20. Landis JR, Koch GG. The measurement of observer agreement for categorical data. Biometrics. 1977;33(1):159–74.
21. Krasse B. Caries risk: a practical guide for assessment and control. Chicago, IL: Quintessence; 1985.
22. Okoro CA, Strine TW, Eke PI, Dhingra SS, Balluz LS. The association between depression and anxiety and use of oral health services and tooth loss. Community Dent Oral Epidemiol. 2012;40:134–44.
23. Liberali SA, Coates EA, Freeman AD, Logan RM, Jamieson L, Mejia G. Oral conditions and their social impact among HIV dental patients, 18 years on. Aust Dent J. 2013;58(1):18–25.

24. Santo AE, Tagliaferro EP, Ambrosano GM, Meneghim MC, Pereira AC. Dental status of Portuguese HIV+ patients and related variables: a multivariate analysis. Oral Dis. 2010;16(2):176–84.

25. Aleixo RQ, Scherma AP, Guimaraes G, Cortelli JR, Cortelli SC. DMFT index and oral mucosal lesions associated with HIV infection: crosssectional study in Porto Velho, Amazonian region - Brazil. Braz J Infect Dis. 2010;14(5):449–56.

26. Soares GB, Garbin CA, Moimaz SA, Garbin AJ. Oral health status of people living with HIV/AIDS attending a specialized service in Brazil. Spec Care Dentist. 2014;34(4):176–84.

27. Pinheiro A, Marcenes W, Zakrzewska JM, Robinson PG. Dental and oral lesions in HIV infected patients: a study in Brazil. Int Dent J. 2004;54(3):131–7.

28. Saravani S, Zehi TN, Kadeh H, Mir S. Dental Health Status of HIV-Positive Patients and Related Variables in Southeast Iran. Int J High Risk Behav Addict. 2016;5(2):e29149.

29. Schwendicke F, et al. Socioeconomic inequality and caries: a systematic review and meta-analysis. J Dent Res. 2015;94(1):10–8.

30. Khazaei S, Keshteli AH, Feizi A, Savabi O, Adibi P. Epidemiology and risk factors of tooth loss among Iranian adults: findings from a large community-based study. Biomed Res Int. 2013;2013:786462.

31. Jaquet A, et al. Antiretroviral treatment and quality of life in Africans living with HIV: 12-month follow-up in Burkina Faso. J Int AIDS Soc. 2013;16:18867.

32. Fleming CA, Christiansen D, Nunes D, Heeren T, Thornton D, Horsburgh CR, Koziel MJ, Graham C, Craven DE. Health-related quality of life of patients with HIV disease: impact of hepatitis C coinfection. Clin Infect Dis. 2004;38:572–8.

28

A new tooth brushing approach supported by an innovative hybrid toothbrush-compared reduction of dental plaque after a single use versus an oscillating-rotating powered toothbrush

D. Klonowicz[1], M. Czerwinska[1], A. Sirvent[2] and J-Ph. Gatignol[3*]

Abstract

Background: An innovative hybrid toothbrush was designed functioning either in manual mode, in powered mode (sonic) or in combined mode (manual and powered). The primary aim of this study was to evaluate and compare the clinical efficacy of this first hybrid toothbrush (*Elgydium Clinic/Inava Hybrid*) used in combined mode to a marketed oscillating-rotating powered toothbrush (*Oral-B Vitality*) in the reduction of dental plaque after a single use. The secondary aims were to evaluate the tolerance and acceptability of each device.

Methods: It was a randomized, examiner-blind, single-center study performed on two parallel groups: hybrid toothbrush ($n = 33$) versus oscillating-rotating toothbrush (n = 33). A brushing exercise was conducted for two minutes on subjects presenting a "Silness and Löe Plaque Index" (PI) between 1.0 and 2.0 and a "Modified Gingival Index" between 1.0 and 2.0. They were not to have ever used an electric toothbrush. To assess the device effect after brushing, a paired t-test was applied on the change outcome (After-Before brushing). An unpaired t-test was used to compare the efficacy of both devices. A global tolerance assessment of each powered toothbrush was done on all the subjects. The number and percentage of reactions related to each toothbrush was collected and the final tolerance assessment was estimated.

Results: After a single use, the hybrid toothbrush used in combined mode presented a global anti-plaque efficacy characterized by a significant decrease of the global PI of 45% on average ($p < 0.0001$; paired t-test). It was as effective as the oscillating rotating toothbrush in plaque removal ($p > 0.05$; unpaired t-test). The global tolerance of both toothbrushes was judged as "Good" and they were equally appreciated by the users.

Conclusion: The results of this one-time use trial demonstrate the efficacy of the hybrid toothbrush used in combined mode for plaque removal. The hybrid toothbrush design allows each user to adapt tooth brushing to his preference (manual / sonic / combined), his skills or his mouth condition. We hypothesize that such an individualized approach can favor long term compliance with oral health recommendations and improve global oral wellness.

Keywords: Powered toothbrush, Sonic toothbrush, Oscillating-rotating toothbrush, Dental plaque, Manual toothbrush, Hybrid toothbrush

* Correspondence: jean.philippe.gatignol@pierre-fabre.com
[3]Innovation Unit Consumer HealthCare, 17 avenue Jean Moulin, 81106 Castres Cedex, France
Full list of author information is available at the end of the article

Background

Oral health is one of the major concerns of dental health care professionals [1]. Most of periodontal diseases (halitosis, gingivitis, periodontitis, gum abscesses, peri-implant mucositis, etc.) are bacteria-dependent, through biofilm formation and dental plaque accumulation [2]. Promotion of regular oral hygiene can contribute to the maintenance of a functional dentition throughout life [3]. Current available approaches to control bacterial plaque development can be categorized as either mechanical (toothbrushes, floss, interdental brushes, chewing sugar-free gums) or chemotherapeutical (toothpastes, mouthwashes, gels) [4]. In Western industrialized countries, the toothbrush is widely accepted as a simple, affordable and effective device to remove plaque in a shorter time [5, 6]. To date, dental professionals recommend brushing teeth twice a day for two minutes [7, 8]. However, a wide diversity in brushing methods does exist depending on the position and motion of the brush. There appears to be no consensus on the ideal technique neither for the general population nor for people of different ages or with particular dental conditions [9]. No method is satisfactory when considering interdental cleanliness. Tooth brushing is able to clean the buccal, lingual and occlusal tooth surfaces but the proximal and interdental areas are often stayed untouched [10] or roughly cleaned [11]. Furthermore, tooth brushing efficacy for plaque removal relies on several parameters: motivation and skills of the subject, the use of a brush that fits the mouth allowing it to reach all areas, as well as proper oral hygiene education with instructions on movement, duration and frequency of brushing [12]. As an example, the two-minute recommendation for brushing time is hardly ever reached in behavioral studies. Most people spend between 30 and 60 s brushing their teeth [13, 14], while plaque removal efficacy is known to be time-dependent [15–17].

Powered toothbrush was conceived in the 1950s with a view to improve and facilitate oral hygiene. It was designed to target patients with limited motor skills as well as orthodontic patients, who have difficulties in keeping their teeth hygienic and healthy [18]. Geriatric patients with impaired manual skills can also benefit from powered toothbrushes [19]. Since the 1980s, powered toothbrushes have rapidly developed to become an established alternative to manual tooth brushing [20, 21]. Tremendous work has been done in order to improved toothbrush design, head and bristles. Several modes of action can be found on the market (oscillation-rotation, side-to-side sonic action, counter oscillation, circular, ultrasonic, ionic) but two technologies are dominating: oscillation-rotation and sonic. With the former, a small round brush head rotates in one direction and then the other, with the latter, a traditional brush head moves laterally form side to side with a high vibrational speed (mean frequency range 250 Hz, i.e.

30,000 brush-strokes-per-minute). This latter agitates the fluids present in the mouth (water, saliva) to the degree that they are able to disrupt dental plaque colonies even beyond where the bristles of the brush actually touch [22–24]. This fluid-dynamics cleaning action, although considered as a secondary cleaning effect, is characteristic of sonic toothbrushes.

A new generation of toothbrush called hybrid toothbrush has been recently developed. Hybrid toothbrush means that it can be used either in manual mode (motor off), in powered mode (sonic) or in combined mode (manual gesture associated to sonic vibrations). These various modes allow the user to adapt tooth brushing to his desire or his mouth condition. However, the use of combined mode corresponds to a new way of brushing. Indeed, usual recommendations for sonic tooth brushing imply minimal hand movements. In this case, hybrid toothbrush could be used by applying slight pressure by slowly moving the brush head with a light circular motion.

The primary aim of this study was to evaluate and compare the clinical efficacy of the first hybrid toothbrush (*Elgydium Clinic/Inava Hybrid*) using combined mode to a marketed oscillating-rotating powered toothbrush (*Oral-B Vitality*) in the reduction of dental plaque after a single use. The secondary aims of the study were to evaluate the tolerance and acceptability of each device.

Methods

Experiment

The experiment was a randomized, examiner-blind, single-center study performed on parallel group. It took place at Dermscan Poland (Gdansk, Poland). In Poland, an electric toothbrush is considered to be a domestic electric apparatus. Conducting a clinical study with such devices does not require any approval by an ethics committee. However, the study was conducted in compliance with Good Clinical Practices and in accordance with the "Declaration of Helsinki." Written informed consents for participation in the clinical study were obtained for all participants.

Subjects

The planned number of subjects to be analyzed was 30 minimum per group. In order to participate in the study, subjects had to be aged between 18 to 70 years old, to present at least 20 natural teeth, without implants, prosthesis or dental braces on the studied teeth. To qualify for the study, subjects had to present a "Silness and Löe Plaque Index" between 1.0 and 2.0 and a "Modified Gingival Index" between 1.0 and 2.0. They were not to have ever used an electric toothbrush. Subjects having undergone surgery, chemical or physical treatment in the mouth in the last 3 months as well as subjects using preventive dental medications, antibiotics and/or steroids for 1 week before the study were excluded. Written informed consents for participation in the clinical study of its result were obtained for all participants before the beginning of the study.

Tested toothbrushes

> Hybrid toothbrush (*Elgydium Clinic/Inava Hybrid–* Pierre Fabre Oral Care): this toothbrush looks like a manual toothbrush with a traditional oval brush head shape associated to sonic technology (Fig. 1). It weights around 1.59 oz. The toothbrush neck is thin and flexible. The bristles have a conical design (18/100 at the basis and 1/100 at the tip) which increase softness. They are made of Tinex® fibers with rounded ends, offering high flexibility for a non-traumatic brushing of gums and enamel. The brushing technology can be chosen among three modes: manual, sonic or combined (manual and sonic). The sonic mode uses vibration technology; the brush head makes side-by-side movements and produces up to 28,000 strokes per minute for an effective plaque removal.

The instructions for use given to the subjects were the following (combined mode):

1. *Wet the toothbrush (brush bristles) and apply a small amount of toothpaste.*
2. *Place the brush bristles in contact with the tooth with a 45 ° inclination to the gums.*
3. *Turn the toothbrush on once in the mouth to activate the sonic mode.*
4. *Apply slight pressure by slowly moving the brush head with a light circular motion.*
5. *Keep an inclination (45 °) and constant contact with the teeth during brushing.*
6. *Be sure to clean all surfaces of your teeth; do not forget your tongue.*
7. *Brushing time: two minutes.*

> Oscillating-rotating toothbrush (Oral-B Vitality 2D Sensitive Clean - Procter & Gamble): this rechargeable electric toothbrush possesses a small circular brush head, with soft and highly flexible bristles convenient for sensitive gums (Fig. 2). It weights approximately 5.29 oz. This toothbrush uses rotation-oscillation action (=rotary technology); the brush head spins in a motion and makes 16 degree movements. It performs 7600 oscillations per minute. The instructions for use given to the subjects were the following:

1. *Wet brush head and apply a small amount of toothpaste. To avoid splashing, guide the brush head to your teeth before switching on the appliance.*
2. *Guide the brush head slowly from tooth to tooth, spending a few seconds on each tooth surface. Brush the gums as well as the teeth, first the outside, then the inside, finally the chewing surfaces. Do not press too hard or scrub. Do not forget to brush your tongue.*

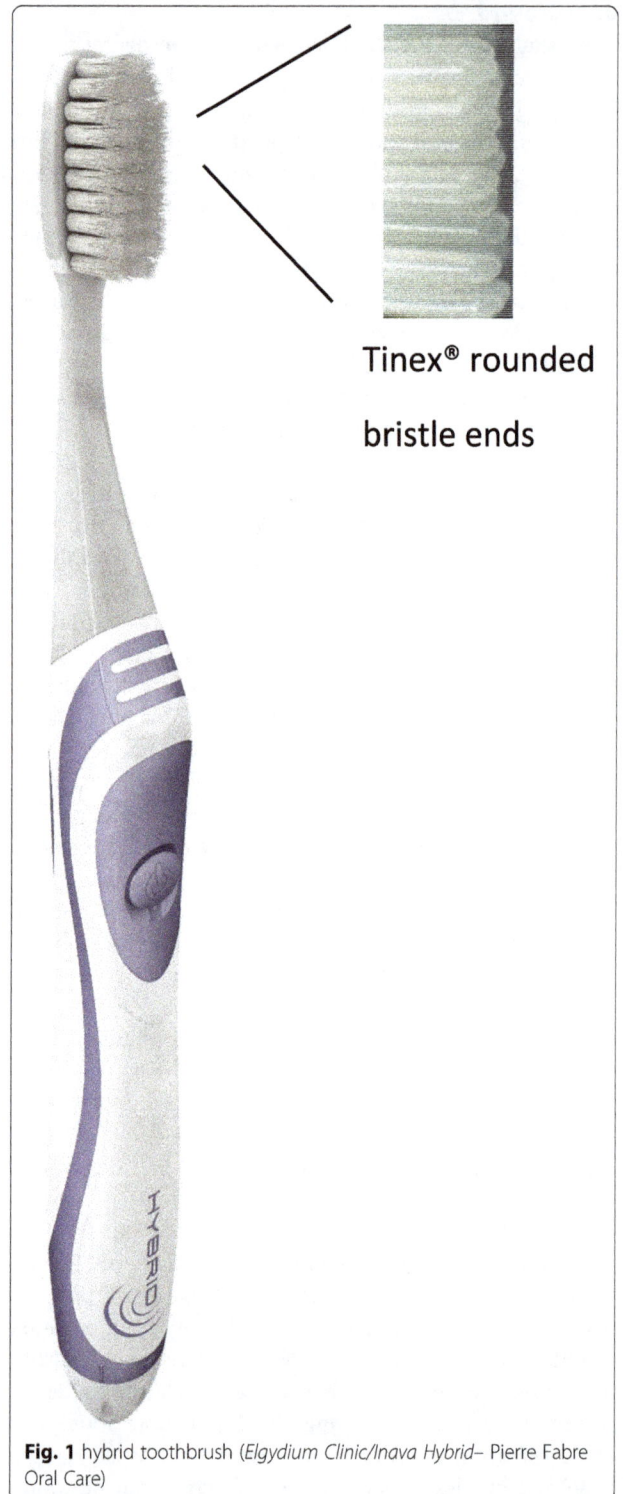

Tinex® rounded bristle ends

Fig. 1 hybrid toothbrush (*Elgydium Clinic/Inava Hybrid–* Pierre Fabre Oral Care)

3. *Brushing time: two minutes.*

Trial schedule

On the day of the study, the subjects came to the laboratory after refraining from all oral hygiene procedures for 24 h and without eating, drinking and smoking for the

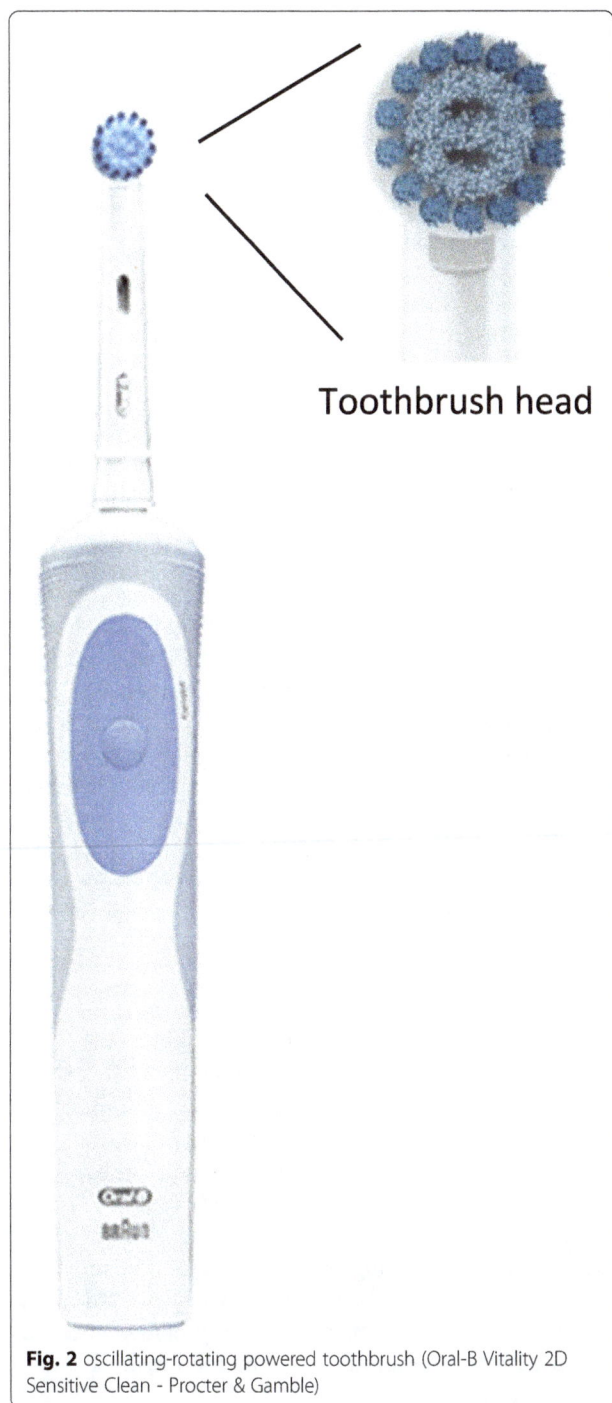

Fig. 2 oscillating-rotating powered toothbrush (Oral-B Vitality 2D Sensitive Clean - Procter & Gamble)

last 4 hours before the visit. The subjects read, signed and dated the information sheet (instructions on the product use and restrictions related to the study) and informed consent forms in duplicate. After a verification of the inclusion and non-inclusion criteria, the dentist performed a clinical examination of the state of the oral cavity. Only the subjects with a" Silness and Löe Plaque Index" (PI) score between 1.0 and 2.0 and "Modified Gingival Index "(MGI) score between 1.0 and 2.0 were

included in the study. After randomization, each participant received instructions on how to use the assigned toothbrush device. The same toothpaste was provided to all the subjects. A single brushing with the studied product (hybrid toothbrush) or the comparative product (oscillating-rotating device) was performed for exactly 2 minutes under supervision to ensure compliance with the manufacturer's usage instructions. Immediately after brushing, another clinical examination of the state of the oral cavity was performed by the dentist and another PI scoring was done. Possible adverse reactions were noted. For this post-brushing evaluation, the dentist was blinded as to the device used. The participants completed a self-assessment questionnaire of the products' acceptability after the first use.

Evaluation tools

> "Silness and Löe Plaque Index" (PI) [25]: this assessment is based on recording, on all natural teeth, the thickness of the plaque at the gingival margin rather than its coronal extent on the tooth surface area. The scoring system goes from 0 to 3 (**0**_no plaque / **1**_deposit of invisible plaque but can be removed by a curette / **2**_deposit of plaque covering $^1/_3$ of the cervical / **3**_deposit of plaque in abundance (more than $^1/_3$ of the cervical)]. The index for the subject was obtained by summing the indexes for all surfaces (lingual and labial) of natural teeth and dividing by the number of surfaces examined. Variations (before brushing - after brushing) were calculated and statistics were performed to determine the significance of any variation. The device was considered effective if it induced a significant decrease in the score of the plaque.

> "Modified Gingival Index" (MGI) devised by Lobene et al. [26]: gum status was evaluated using a score ranging between 0 to 4 (**0**_absence of inflammation/ **1**_mild inflammation or with slight changes in color and texture but not in all portions of gingival marginal or papillary / **2**_mild inflammation, such as the preceding criteria, in all portions of gingival marginal or papillary / **3**_moderate, bright surface inflammation, erythema, oedema $^{and}/_{or}$ hypertrophy of gingival marginal or papillary / **4**_severe inflammation: erythema, oedema $^{and}/_{or}$ marginal gingival hypertrophy of the unit or spontaneous bleeding, papillary, congestion or ulceration). The MGI was scored for selected teeth (12, 16, 24, 36, 32 and 44). The scores of the four areas (buccal/lingual/mesial/distal) of the tooth were summed and divided by four to give the MGI for the tooth. For each subject, the MGI was obtained by adding the values of each tooth and dividing by the number of teeth assessed.

> Tolerance assessment: before and after the first brushing, an examination of the subject's oral cavity was performed by the dentist to assess, either on soft tissues

(gums, tongue, lips, palate) or hard tissues (teeth), the following signs:

- clinical signs: ulceration, desquamation, dyschromia, erythema, bleeding, papules, edema, cheilitis or other on soft tissues; dyschromia, tooth decay or other on hard tissues.
- functional signs: pruritus, stinging, pain, burning sensation, change in the quantity of saliva, oral dysesthesia, taste perversion, sensation of discomfort or other on soft tissues; dyschromia or other on hard tissues.

For each sign, the intensity was scored as: **0**_none / **1**_very mild / **2**_mild/ **3**_moderate.

A global tolerance assessment of each powered toothbrush was done on all the subjects who used the device at least once. The number and percentage of reactions related to each toothbrush was collected and the final tolerance assessment was estimated either as: Excellent (no functional nor physical signs related to the study) product observed or reported by the subjects) / Very good / Good / Moderate / Bad.

Statistics

The raw variations (Δ) of the different studied parameters were calculated according to the following formulas:

$$\Delta = (PI_{t1} - PI_{t0}).$$

with: PI: Silness and Löe Plaque Index; t0: before brushing; t1: after brushing.

The descriptive statistics for quantitative data were computed for each time point, for each surface (lingual and labial) as well as for the change between (t1-t0).

To assess the effectiveness of the device after brushing, a paired t-test was applied on the change outcome (t1-t0). The normality assumption was checked with a Shapiro-Wilk test ($\alpha = 0.01$). The type I error probability (α) was set at 5% in bilateral mode. The software used was Microsoft Excel® 2010 and SAS® v9.2.

Results

A total of 66 subjects participated in the study (33 per group). The baseline demographics of the randomized subjects are given in Table 1.

Evaluation of plaque removal efficacy

Mean values of PI scores before and after a single brushing with either powered toothbrush are presented in Table 2.

Under these study conditions, after a single use, the hybrid toothbrush presented a global anti-plaque efficacy characterized by a significant decrease of the global PI of 45% on average ($p < 0,0001$; paired t-test); this effect was observed in 100% of subjects. The oscillating-rotating toothbrush used under the same conditions showed a similar efficacy: reduction of global PI of 43% on average ($p < 0.0001$; paired t-test); effect observed in 100% of subjects.

For each tooth brushing technique, removal of plaque was more effective on the labial side than on the lingual side (mean reduction of PI of 53% versus 37% respectively for the hybrid toothbrush and 52% versus 34% for the oscillating-rotating device). However, whatever the side and the device, the decrease of plaque index was statistically significant and observed on the totality of the participants.

The comparison of methods showed that the hybrid toothbrush (manual and sonic combination) was as effective as the oscillating rotating one in plaque removal after a single use ($p > 0.05$; unpaired t-test).

Global tolerance assessment

> With the hybrid toothbrush, 15 subjects (45%) presented reactions with causality assessment "likely or very likely." The most common reaction was bleeding (12 subjects, with very mild or mild intensity).

> With the oscillating-rotating powered toothbrush, 14 (42%) subjects presented reactions with causality assessment "likely or very likely." For 13 out of 14 participants, the reaction was bleeding with very mild or mild intensity.

However, no subject was withdrawn of the study due to theses reactions. Subjects neither modified methods of brushing nor temporally stopped the brushing due to the reactions.

Table 1 Baseline demographics of randomized subjects

		Hybrid ($n = 33$ subjects)	Oscillating-rotating ($n = 33$ subjects)
Age (years)	Mean (±SEM)	27.5 (±5.6)	30.2 (±7.4)
	Range	18–42	19–55
Gender	Male	14	6
	Female	19	27
LSPI	Mean (±SEM)	1.2 (±0.0)	1.2 (±0.0)
MGI	Mean (±SEM)	1.3 (±0.0)	1.2 (±0.0)

Table 2 evolution of mean PI after a single brushing for the hybrid and oscillating-rotating powered toothbrushes; comparison of devices' efficacy

PI	Device	Variation Δ (t1-t0) (mean ± SEM)	Δ%	Significance (paired t-test)	% of subjects with a positive effect
Global score	Hybrid	−0.5 ± 0.0	−45%	p < 0.0001	100%
	Oscillating-rotating	−0.5 ± 0.0	−43%	p < 0.0001	100%
	Comparison	0.0 ± 0.2		p = 0.5474	(unpaired t-test)
Labial side	Hybrid	−0.6 ± 0.0	−53%	p < 0.0001	100%
	Oscillating-rotating	−0.6 ± 0.0	−52%	p < 0.0001	100%
	Comparison	0.0 ± 0.2		p = 0.9273	(unpaired t-test)
Lingual side	Hybrid	−0.5 ± 0.0	−37%	p < 0.0001	100%
	Oscillating-rotating	−0.4 ± 0.0	−34%	p < 0.0001	100%
	Comparison	−0.05 ± 0.2		p = 0.3022	(unpaired t-test)

According to the investigator, bleeding reactions could be due not only to the toothbrushes (bristles), but also to the fact that the participants used this type of toothbrush (powered) for the very first time. As the teeth brushing was done under supervision, the subjects could have brushed too intensively... Considering this, the dentist judged the global tolerance of both powered toothbrushes as "Good."

Global appreciation of the powered toothbrushes
The participants completed a subjective evaluation questionnaire after their first use. A summary of the answers is presented in Figs. 3 and 4.

> The hybrid toothbrush was appreciated by the majority of the subjects for its characteristics; its intensity of vibration was just about right for 91% of the participants. The new hybrid sonic toothbrush was judged better than the usual manual one for 87% of the subjects.

> The oscillating-rotating toothbrush was also liked by the majority of the subjects; its intensity of vibration was considered just about right for 94% of the participants.

90% of the subjects rated the marketed oscillating-rotating toothbrush better than their usual manual one.

Discussion
The maintenance of periodontal health requires supragingival dental plaque removal. Tooth brushing is a key element in mechanical plaque control [6]. Several randomized, controlled clinical trials recognized a superiority of powered over manual toothbrushes in removing dental plaque [19, 20]. Without distinction on the type of powered toothbrushes used, an overall benefit of 11% reduction in plaque was shown at one to 3 months and 21% at longer than 3 months [19]. With regards to gingivitis, a 6% reduction was shown at one to 3 months and an 11% over the long term. In 2010, different power toothbrush technologies were compared for plaque and gingivitis control [27]. The authors concluded that, over a period of four to 12 weeks, brushes with a rotating-oscillating action appeared more effective than sonic ones for plaque and gingivitis reduction. However, they noticed that the difference

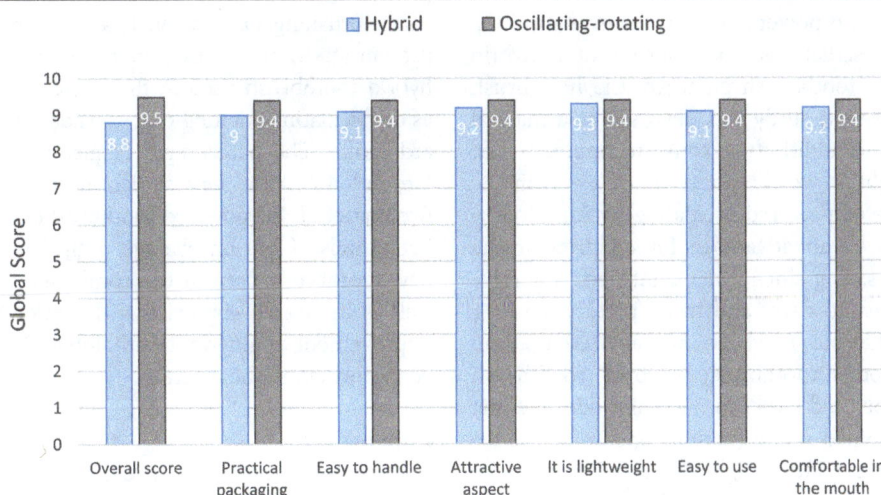

Fig. 3 mean global appreciation of the hybrid and the oscillating-rotating powered toothbrushes. Overall score was scored on a scale ranging from 0 (really dislike) to 10 (really like). Affirmations were scored on a scale ranging from 0 (totally disagree) to 10 (totally agree)

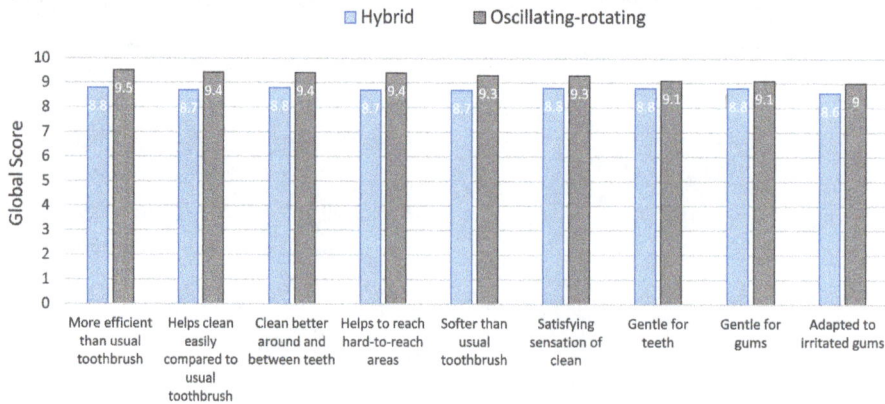

Fig. 4 mean global appreciation of the hybrid and the oscillating-rotating powered toothbrushes. Affirmations were scored on a scale ranging from 0 (totally disagree) to 10 (totally agree)

was small and its clinical importance, unclear. A recent review on the efficacy of powered toothbrushes following a single-use test highlighted the contribution of several factors to the observed efficacy on dental plaque: the power supply (rechargeable or replaceable battery), the mode of action, the brushing duration as well as the type of instructions [28]. The magnitude of the outcome was also highly dependent on the index scale used to score plaque for the evaluation.

These conflicting results may have contributed to the resistance of a portion of the population to becoming powered toothbrush users. Some consumers stay attached to their manual brushing experience, favor a traditional brush head characteristic and the ability to brush several teeth at once. Modifying oral hygiene habits is difficult to achieve and maintain over time [29]. Moreover, some of the powered toothbrush users sometimes return to their manual brush, either because of a vacation period, dead battery or hybrid usage (for example, manual tooth brushing in the morning and powered one in the evening) [30]. Based on these observations, the concept of a hybrid (manual and sonic) toothbrush emerged: the new brush evaluated in the present study was designed as a manual toothbrush with the addition of sonic technology. The final product is light (it weights three times less than the comparative marketed powered oscillating-rotating toothbrush), which can be an advantage for children or the elderly. It is space-saving since it does not need any electrical base. It is easy to carry and has a battery life of 1 month. The brush head needs to be replaced every 3 months, like any other toothbrush. "Hybrid" toothbrush means that it can be used either in manual mode, in sonic mode or in a combined mode (manual and sonic). Since the brush bristles are made of highly flexible Tinex® fibers, conically designed and rounded ended, a non-traumatic brushing of gums and enamel can be performed. Such bristles suit particularly well to sulcular tooth brushing. In

this technique, the brush is positioned at about 45 degrees to the tooth and the tooth brush bristles are pushed into the sulcus [31]. The brush is then moved back and forth and removed by a downward and outward movement in the top arch. The toothbrush is moved to another tooth and the process is repeated. People presenting gum sensitivity can benefit from this gentle brush. In the manual mode, the user can keep his familiar brushing technique; in the sonic mode, the "non-contact" brushing linked to fluid dynamics completes the soft mechanical scrubbing. Sonic toothbrushes used in combination with a fluoride toothpaste demonstrate significantly less interproximal plaque and deliver significantly higher concentration of fluoride in that plaque, compared to manual or oscillating-rotating toothbrushes [32]. A standardized in vitro test -performed on a phantom tooth model cleaned by a robot proved that the hybrid toothbrush (combined mode) eliminates ten times more plaque in the approximal spaces compared to a conventional ADA manual toothbrush (internal data). Brushing exercise such as the one reported in the present study, proved that the plaque removal ability of the hybrid toothbrush used in the combined mode is as good as an oscillating-rotating one, considered as the gold standard mode. The percentages of plaque reduction obtained (around 45%) are very similar to the one estimated by Rosema et al. for powered toothbrushes following a brushing exercise (46% on average) [28]. The tolerance of the new toothbrush used in the combined mode was good as well as its overall appreciation. In order to investigate the improvement of gingival health, longer term studies should be performed in the future.

Conclusion

The results of this one-time use trial demonstrate that the hybrid toothbrush (used in the combined mode) is as good as a marketed oscillating-rotating toothbrush for plaque removal. The hybrid technology -offering the choice between either the traditional manual brushing technique, the sonic mode or the combined mode- allows each user to adapt tooth brushing to his desire, his skills or his mouth condition. We hypothesize that such an individualized approach can favor long term compliance with oral health recommendations and improve global oral wellness [33].

Abbreviations
ADA: American Dental Association; MGI: Modified Gingival Index; PI: Silness and Löe Plaque Index

Acknowledgements
Not applicable

Funding
Funding for this study was provided by Pierre Fabre Oral Care for the design of the study, collection, analysis, and interpretation of data as well as in writing the manuscript.

Authors' contributions
DK and MC drew up the study protocol in collaboration with JPG. DK and MC performed the clinical evaluations. AS wrote the article. DK, MC and JPG proofread the article. All the authors approved the final version of the article.

Competing interests
Dr. Gatignol is employee ofInnovation Unit Consumer HealthCare - Institut de Recherche Pierre Fabre
Dr. Klonowicz and Dr. Czerwinska received funding from Dermscan Poland for their collaboration to the study.
Dermscan Poland and Laboratoire Dermscan (A. Sirvent) are part of the Dermscan Group, a CRO that received funding from Pierre Fabre Oral Care to conduct the study.
Elgydium Clinic/Inava Hybrid toothbrush is marketed by Pierre Fabre Oral Care.

Author details
[1]Dermscan Poland, Ul. Kruczkowskiego 12, 80-288 Gdansk, Poland.
[2]Laboratoire Dermscan, 114 Bd du 11 novembre 1918, 69100 Villeurbanne, France. [3]Innovation Unit Consumer HealthCare, 17 avenue Jean Moulin, 81106 Castres Cedex, France.

References
1. Van Der Weijden FA, Slot DE. Oral hygiene in the prevention of periodontal diseases: the evidence. Periodontol. 2011;55:104–23.
2. Baehni PC, Takeuchi Y. Anti-plaque agents in the prevention of biofilm-associated oral diseases. Oral Dis. 2003;9(suppl1):23–9.
3. Claydon N. Current concepts in toothbrushing and interdental cleaning. Periodontol 2000. 2008;48:10–22.
4. Choo A, Delac D, Brearley Messer L. Oral hygiene measures and promotion: review and considerations. Aust Dent J. 2001;46:166–73.
5. Löe H. Oral hygiene in the prevention of caries and periodontal disease. Int Dent J. 2000;50:129–39.
6. Grover D, Malhotra R, Kaushal S, Kaur G. Toothbrush – a key mechanical plaque control. Ind J Oral Sci. 2012;3:62–8.
7. American Dental Association. Available: http://www.mouthhealthy.org/en/az-topics/b/brushing-your-teeth (accessed on October 10, 2016).
8. UFSBD. Available: http://www.ufsbd.fr/espace-grand-public/votre-sante-bucco-dentaire/recommandations-hygiene-bucco-dentaire (accessed on October 10, 2016).
9. Wainwright J, Sheiham A. An analysis of methods of toothbrushing recommended by dental associations, toothpastes and toothbrush companies and in dental texts. Br Dent J. 2014;217:E5.
10. Kinane DF. The role of interdental cleaning in effective plaque control: need for interdental cleaning in primary and secondary prevention. In: Lang NP, Attström R, Löe H, editors. Proceedings of the European workshop on mechanical plaque removal. Berlin: quintessence, publishing co.; 1998. p. 156–68.
11. Mastroberardino S, Grazia Cagetti M, Cocco F, Campus G, Pizzocri J, Strohmenger L. Vertical brushing versus horizontal brushing: a randomized split-mouth clinical trial. Quintessence Int. 2014;45:653–61.
12. Frandsen A. Mechanical oral hygiene practices. In: Löe H, Kleinman DV, editors. Dental plaque control measures and oral hygiene practices. Oxford-Washington DC: IRL Press; 1986. p. 93–116.
13. MacGregor I, Rugg-Gunn A. A survey of toothbrushing sequence in children and young adults. J Periodontal Res. 1979;14:225–30.
14. Van der Weijden FA, Timmerman MF, Nijboer A, et al. A comparative study of electric tooth- brushes for the effectiveness of plaque removal in relation to toothbrushing duration. J Clin Periodontol. 1993;20:476–81.
15. Honkala E, Nyyssonen V, Knuuttila M, Markkanen H. Effectiveness of children's habitual toothbrushing. J Clin Periodontol. 1986;13:81–5.
16. Van der Weijden FA, Timmerman MF, Danser MM, et al. Approximal brush head used on a powered toothbrush. J Clin Periodontol. 2005;32:317–22.
17. Gallagher A, Sowinski J, Bowman J, et al. The effect of brushing time and dentifirice on dental plaque removal *in vivo*. J Dent Hyg. 2009;83:111–6.
18. Manhold J. 2015. About us: Inventor, Philippe-G. Woog, Ph.D. [Online]. BROXO. Available: http://eu.broxo.com/about-us/inventor (Accessed October 10, 2015).
19. Verma S, Bhat KM. Acceptability of powered toothbrushes for ederly individuals. J Public Health Dent. 2004;64:115–7.
20. Yaacob M, Worthington HV, Deacon SA, et al. Powered versus manual tooth brushing for oral health (review). Cochrane Database Syst Rev. 2014;6:art n° CD002281.
21. Van der Weijden FA, Slot DE. Efficacy of homecare regimens for mechanical plaque removal in managing gingivitis: a meta review. J Clin Periodontol. 2015;42(Suppl16):S77–91.
22. Stanford CM, Srikantha R, Wu CD. Efficacy of the Sonicare toothbrush fluid dynamic action on removal of human supragingival plaque. J Clin Dent. 1997;8(1 Spec n°):10–4.
23. Hope CK, Wilson M. Effects of dynamic fluid activity from an electric toothbrush on in vitro oral biofilms. J Clin Periodontol. 2003;30:624–9.
24. Schmidt JC, Zaugg C, Weiger R, Walter C. Brushing without brushing? A review of the efficacy of powered toothbrushes in noncontact biofilm removal. Clin Oral Investig. 2013;17:687–709.
25. Löe H. The gingival index, the plaque index and the retention index systems. J Periodontol. 1967;38:610–6.
26. Lobene RR, Weatherford T, Ross NM, et al. A modified gingival index for use in clinical trials. Clin Prev Dent. 1986;8:3–6.
27. Deacon SA, Glenny AM, Deery C, et al. Different powered toothbrushes for plaque control and gingival health. Cochrane Database Syst Rev. 2010;12:CD004971.
28. Rosema NAM, Slot D, Van Palenstein Helderman WH, et al. The efficacy of powered toothbrushes following a brushing exercise: a systematic review. Int J Dent Hyg. 2016;14:29–41.
29. Inglehart M, Tedesco LA. Behavioral research related to oral hygiene practices: a new century model of oral health promotion. Periodontol 2000. 1995;8:15–23.
30. Rosema NAM, Adam R, Grender JM, et al. Gingival abrasion and recession in the manual and oscillating-rotating power brush users. Int J Dent Hyg. 2014;12:257–66.
31. European Federation of Periodontology Available: http://weblink2.consult-pro.com/user/BkojAog7yFCwPkwyV1ZnLQ (Accessed on November 4, 2016).
32. Sjörgren K, Lundberg AB, Birkhed D, et al. Interproximal plaque mass and fluoride retention after brushing and flossing a comparative study of powered toothbrushing, manual toothbrushing and flossing. Oral Health Prev Dent. 2004;2:119–24.
33. Mariotti A, Hefti AF. Defining periodontal health. BMC Oral Health. 2015; 15(suppl1):S6.

Evaluation of the relationship between maxillary posterior teeth and the maxillary sinus floor using cone-beam computed tomography

Yechen Gu[1,2,3], Chao Sun[2,4], Daming Wu[2,4,5]* ⓘ, Qingping Zhu[2,3]*, Diya Leng[2,4,5] and Yang Zhou[2,4,5]

Abstract

Background: Maxillary posterior teeth have close anatomical proximity to the maxillary sinus floor (MSF), and the race, gender, age, side and presence/absence of adjacent teeth may influence the mean distances between the root apices and the MSF. This study aimed to evaluate both the relationship between the maxillary posterior teeth and MSF, and the influence of adjacent teeth loss on the distance between the maxillary posterior roots and MSF.

Methods: Cone-beam computed tomography images were collected from 1011 Chinese patients. The relationship between the maxillary posterior teeth and the MSF was divided into three types: Type OS (the root apex extending below/outside the MSF), Type CO (the root apex contacting with the MSF), Type IS (the root apex extending above/inside the MSF). The minimum vertical distances between the maxillary posterior roots apices and the MSF were recorded. The correlations of the distances with gender and age were analyzed. The distances between the maxillary posterior root apices and the MSF with different types of adjacent teeth loss was evaluated.

Results: Type OS was the most common relationship of all posterior root apices ($P<0.05$). Type IS was highest in the palatal roots (PRs) of the maxillary first molars (MFMs) and the mesiobuccal roots (MBRs) of the maxillary second molars (MSMs) (24.8% and 21.6%) ($P<0.05$). The frequency of Type IS decreased with age except the premolar roots and PRs of the MSMs ($P<0.05$). The MBRs of the MSMs had the lowest distances to the MSF (0.8 ± 2.5 mm), followed by the distobuccal roots of the MSMs (1.3 ± 2.7 mm) and the PRs of the MFMs (1.4 ± 3.4 mm) ($P<0.05$). Age was an important influencing factor to the mean distances while gender had little effects. The distance between the maxillary second premolar root apices and the MSF decreased with the absence of adjacent teeth ($P<0.05$).

Conclusions: The maxillary molars showed greater proximity to the MSF than premolars. Age had significant impacts on the relationship between maxillary posterior roots and MSF. The absence of maxillary first molars will influence the proximity of maxillary second premolar root apices to MSF.

Keywords: Cone-beam computed tomography, Maxillary posterior teeth, Maxillary sinus floor, Root apices

* Correspondence: wdming@njmu.edu.cn; zhuqpp@163.com
[2]Jiangsu Key Laboratory of Oral Diseases, the Affiliated Stomatological Hospital of Nanjing Medical University, 136 Hanzhong Road, Nanjing 210029, People's Republic of China
Full list of author information is available at the end of the article

Background

The maxillary sinus (MS) is an important anatomic structure beside the nasal cavity and close to the root apices of maxillary posterior teeth. The maxillary sinus floor (MSF) is formed by the alveolar process of the maxilla and situated 5 mm inferior to the nasal floor at approximately 20 years old [1]. The inferior wall of sinus is lined with Schneiderian membrane which is changeable during the development of relevant disease [2]. Previous studies indicated that the volume of MS pneumatization is not a permanent state but a metabolic process, increasing at about 12 years old and reaching the lowest point at about 20 years old with the complete eruption of the maxillary third molars [3, 4]. In addition, the MS pneumatization can be affected by the extraction of the maxillary posterior teeth, especially several adjacent teeth, teeth with apices intruded into the sinus and maxillary second molars [1, 5, 6].

Due to the close anatomical proximity of the root apices of maxillary posterior teeth to the MSF, teeth infections may spread into the MS through periapical tissues and cause odontogenic maxillary sinusitis, which account for 10%~ 12% of all sinusitis [7]. The periapical and marginal lesion of roots close to or extending into the MSF could cause inflammatory changing of sinus mucosal lining and result in maxillary sinusitis in the end [8]. The infection can also intrude into the sinus via bone marrow, blood vessels and lymphatics. Mehra and Murad reported that when there is a close proximity of root apices of teeth with necrotic pulp and the MSF, the MS can also be influenced [9]. If clinical operation errors occur during root canal treatment, the root canal shaping instruments, flushing fluid and filling materials can extrude to the MS subsequently. In addition, a perforation of MSF can occur and result in oroantral fistula during tooth extraction, and a pathological change of MS can also occur for the improper implant therapy [10]. All these reasons can result in various complications, such as odontogenic maxillary sinusitis, endo-antral syndrome and traumatic alterations, which are complex problems for dentists and otolaryngologists [7, 11].

Periapical and panoramic radiographies are conventional imaging techniques used for treatment planning and evaluating the close relationship of the root apices and the MSF. However, they can only provide two-dimensional (2D) images, causing superposition and magnification of anatomic structures impending proper diagnosis. During periapical surgery, the 2D radiographies cannot determine the risk of perforation of MSF [12]. In past 20 years, cone-beam computed tomography (CBCT) has gradually got into the public eyes. As a three-dimensional (3D) imaging technique, CBCT has important significances in clinical diagnosis

and planning process, contributing to the establishment of effective therapeutic protocols [13]. When compared with conventional CT, CBCT works with lower radiation, higher resolution and shorter scanning time [14]. CBCT can provide high-quality 3D images of oral and maxillofacial regions and evaluate the relationship between the maxillary root apices and MS clearly.

Previous studies evaluated the proximity of the maxillary posterior teeth to the MSF. For example, Jung et al. [15] reported that the mesiobuccal roots (MBRs) of the maxillary second molars (MSMs) were closest to the MSF in Korean people, but they did not analyze the correlations of the distances with gender and age. Von Arx et al. [16] evaluated the distances between maxillary premolar roots and the MSF in Switzerland population, and found that gender, age, side, and presence/absence of premolars failed to influence significantly the mean distances between premolar roots and the MS. Kilic et al. [17] and OK et al. [18] evaluated the relationship between the maxillary posterior teeth root tips and the MSF in Turkey population respectively, both of them found that there were no significant statistical differences between the right and left side measurements, but them had different conclusions in the relationships between males and females. In addition, OK et al. [18] also found that the relationship between the posterior teeth and the MSF differed according to the age decade interval. However, few studies have investigated the relationship between the root apices of maxillary posterior teeth and the MSF in Chinese population, and whether the gender, age, side and presence/absence of adjacent teeth influence the mean distances between the root apices and the MSF also unclear. Therefore,the aim of this study was to evaluate the anatomic proximity of the maxillary posterior roots apices to MSF in Chinese population according to age, gender and side. In addition, the distances between the root apices of maxillary posterior teeth and the MSF with different situation of adjacent teeth loss were also evaluated.

Methods

CBCT images collections

This study was approved by the Ethical Committee Department, the Affiliated Stomatological Hospital of Nanjing Medical University (PJ2015–047-001), and the written informed consent was obtained from the patients. High-quality CBCT images were randomly collected from the Department of Radiology, the Affiliated Stomatological Hospital of Nanjing Medical University from May 2017 to October 2017.

The reasons for CBCT scanning include dental implants, endodontic treatment, treatment planning before orthodontics and diagnosis of facial trauma. The CBCT images showed the maxillary premolars, molars and MSF clearly. The exclusion criteria for the CBCT images were as following: (1) Maxillary premolars or molars with caries, unformed apices, root resorption or fractures. (2) Maxillary premolars or molars with root canal fillings, posts or coronal restorations. (3) The presence of periapical or periradicular lesions, or MS diseases. (4) Patients have been experienced orthodontic treatment, or experienced traumatic injury which disturbing the normal anatomy of MS.

CBCT images of 1745 maxillary first premolars (MFPs), 1663 maxillary second premolars (MSPs), 1331 maxillary first molars (MFMs) and 1360 MSMs from 1011 individuals (476 males and 535 females) were selected. The age of these patients was ranged from 18 to 85 years, with mean age of 47.7 ± 15.6 years. The patients were divided into 3 groups: 18–40 years group, 41–60 years group and ≥ 61 years group.

CBCT images evaluations

CBCT images were obtained using a CBCT scanner (NewTom VG, QR srl., Verona, Italy) with the following parameters:110kVp, 3.6–4.8 mA, a voxel size of 0.2 mm and a field of view of 12×8 cm or 15×15 cm. The as-low-as-reasonably achievable principle was strictly followed, exposing patients to the least amount of radiation while still obtaining the most useful information for a proper diagnosis. All images were acquired by an experienced radiologist according to the manufacturer's instructions.

To ensure the reliability of the values, two endodontists calibrated their interpretations by reviewing 20 CBCT images of MSF and maxillary posterior teeth selected before the experimental reading. The intra and inter-examiner reliability were assessed by Cohen's kappa statistical analysis. They assessed the CBCT images with NNT4.6 software (QR srl., Verona, Italy) simultaneously. The software reorientation was performed parallel to the occlusal surface before measuring in reconstruction. The contrast and brightness of the images could be adjusted using the software to ensure optimal visualization. The vertical relationship between the maxillary posterior root apices and the MSF were evaluated in CBCT sagittal and coronal planes simultaneously (Fig. 1): (1) Type OS: the root apex extending below/outside the MSF; (2) Type CO: the root apex contacting with the MSF; (3) Type IS: the root apex extending above/inside the MSF.

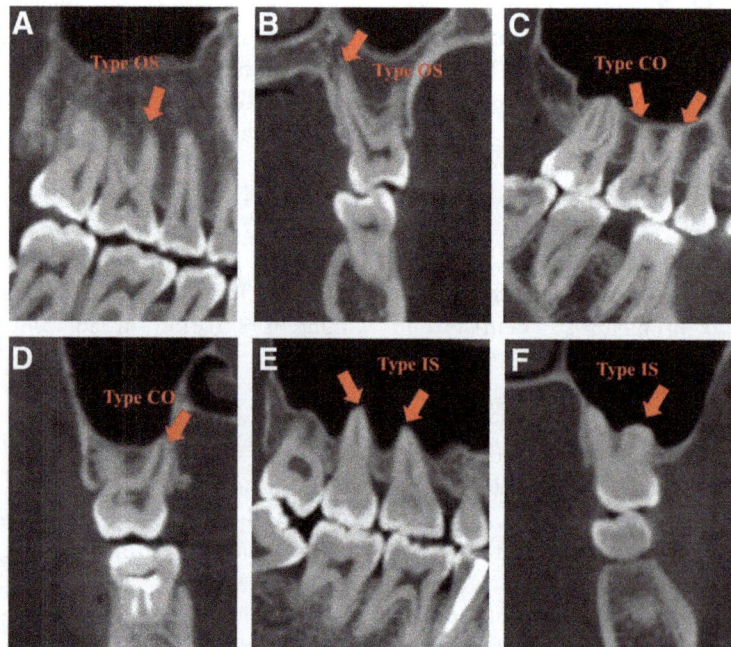

Fig. 1 CBCT images of three vertical relationships between maxillary posterior teeth and MSFs in sagittal (**a**, **c** and **e**) and coronal planes (**b**, **d** and **f**). **a** Type OS: MBR of a right MFM; **b** Type OS: PR of a left MFM; **c** Type CO: MBR and DBR of a right MFM; **d** Type CO: PR of a right MSM; **e** Type IS: PRs of right maxillary molars; **f** Type IS: MBR of a left MSM

The vertical distance of the maxillary posterior root apices to the MSF was measured according to previous studies [19]. Briefly, the vertical distance between the root apices of each maxillary posterior tooth and the closest border of the MSF was measured in serial sagittal and coronal planes with a slice thickness of 0.2 mm. The shortest distance was recorded. A negative value was recorded if the root apex intruded into the MSF. Only one value was recorded if the roots were fused (Fig. 2). The correlations of the vertical relationship and distance with age and gender were analyzed.

In order to evaluated the changes in the distances of root apices of maxillary posterior teeth to MSF in right and left side with different situation of adjacent teeth loss, the CBCT images of the patients who experienced one side tooth extraction more than 6 months were assessed. Then the vertical distance of the side that with tooth extraction were compared with the other side that without tooth extraction.

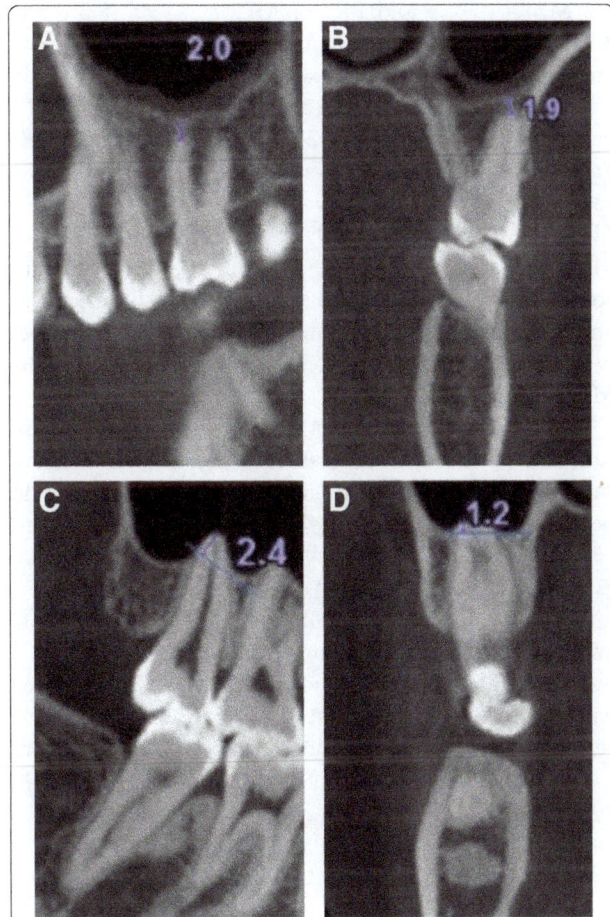

Fig. 2 The shortest distances between the root apices and the MSFs were measured. **a** CBCT sagittal plane, positive value; **b** CBCT coronal plane, positive value; **c** CBCT sagittal plane, negative value; **d** CBCT coronal plane, negative value

Statistical analysis

The statistical analysis was performed using the SPSS 22.0 (IBM Corp., Armonk, NY, USA) at a significance level of $P<0.05$. The association between the distance measurements and the patient's age, gender and side were assessed using the chi-square test and the Kruskal-Wallis test. The Wilcoxon test was used to analyze the influence of adjacent teeth loss.

Results

The kappa values for the intra-examiner agreements of each examiner were 0.923 and 0.933, respectively. Regarding inter-examiner agreement, the kappa values were 0.898 and 0.877 for the first and second assessments, respectively. There was a good intra-examiner and inter-examiner agreement.

The vertical relationship between the maxillary posterior root apices and the MSF

The distribution of the relationship between maxillary posterior root apices and the MSF were shown in Tables 1 and 2. Type OS was the most common relationship of all root apices to the MSF, and it was the highest in the MFPs ($P<0.05$). Type IS was highest in the palatal roots (PRs) of the MFMs and the MBRs of the MSMs (24.8% and 21.6%). The frequency of Type IS decreased with age except the premolar roots and PRs of the MSMs ($P<0.05$) .

There were no significant differences between males and females in the occurrences of Type IS in all posterior roots ($P>0.05$). There were no significant differences between two sides as well ($P>0.05$).

The distances between the maxillary posterior root apices and the MSF

There was no significant differences between right and left side maxillary posterior root apices of the distances ($P>0.05$).

The MFPs had the largest distances, while the MBRs of the MSMs had the lowest distances for both males and females, followed by the distobuccal roots (DBRs) of the maxillary second molars and the PRs of the maxillary first molars ($P<0.05$). There were no significant

Table 1 Distribution of the relationship between maxillary premolars root apices and the MSFs by age (%)

Age	MFPs			MSPs		
	Type OS	Type CO	Type IS	Type OS	Type CO	Type IS
18-40y	85.2	10.8	4	52	32.3	15.7
41-60y	95	5	0	71	25.8	3.2
>60y	97.5	2.5	0	81.7	13.9	4.4

Table 2 Distribution of the relationship between maxillary molars root apices and the MSFs by age (%)

Age	MBR			DBR			PR		
	Type OS	Type CO	Type IS	Type OS	Type CO	Type IS	Type OS	Type CO	Type IS
MFMs 18-40y	41.5	36.8	21.7	40.4	37.9	21.7	37.7	25.7	36.6
MFMs 41-60y	61.5	30.7	7.8	62.3	31.7	6.0	52.8	30.1	17.1
MFMs >60y	74.6	22.6	2.8	76.0	21.2	2.8	63.2	27.6	9.2
MSMs 18-40y	29.5	35.1	35.4	36.8	39.0	24.2	44.2	35.7	20.1
MSMs 41-60y	48.7	40.4	10.9	60.0	31.6	8.4	65.7	28.2	6.1
MSMs >60y	54.0	37.4	8.6	66.7	26.5	6.8	66.7	25.2	8.1

differences in the mean distance between males and females ($P>0.05$) (Table 3).

The distances between the root apices and the MSF increase with age in all roots of posterior teeth and there were significant differences among groups ($P<0.05$) (Table 4).

The distance between the root apices and the MSF influenced by loss of adjacent teeth

The distance between root apices of the MSPs and the MSF was significantly shorter with loss of adjacent teeth (Tables 5 and 6).

Discussion

The close anatomic distance between the maxillary posterior root apices and the MSF result in various complications during disease development and dental treatment process. In present study, the proximity of the maxillary posterior root apices to the MSF in a native Chinese population was studied. The results showed that the Type OS (the root apex extending below/outside the MSF) was observed in 91.9% of MFPs, which is consistent with previous studies [17, 20, 21], indicating that the roots of MFPs have little relationship with the MSF. For MSPs, the frequencies of Type IS (the root apex extending above/inside the MSF) were observed a few times as many as the MFPs and the Type OS accounted for 66.0%, which showed that the relationship of the MSPs is relatively close to the MSF. There were no significant differences between the left and right premolars, which is also in agreement with the findings of Kilic et al. [17] and OK et al. [18]. For

maxillary molars, the Type IS was observed more frequently in the PRs of the MFMs (24.8%) and the MBRs of the MSMs (21.6%), indicating that dentists should pay more attentions to the two roots during the dental treatment, because the perforation of MSF in the areas is more likely to occur. However, Pagin et al. [20] reported that the root protrusions (Type IS) in Brazilian population were 3.2%, 1.8% and 5.5% for MBRs, DBRs and PRs of MFMs, 12.9%, 8.3% and 4.1% for MBRs, DBRs and PRs of the MSMs. Jung and Cho [15] reported that the root protrusions in Korean population were 32.5% and 30.1% for MBRs and DBRs of MFMs, and 36.7% and 34.3% for MBRs and DBRs of MSMs. OK et al. [18] reported that the root protrusions in Turkey population were 34.2% for MBRs of MFMs and 30.9% for MBRs and DBRs of MSMs. These results were different with the present study. Possible explanation is that ethnic difference is an important factor to influence the relationship between the maxillary posterior root apices and the MSF.

The MS pneumatization varied with age [1, 3]. Kalender et al. [22] reported that the lateral recess of the MS is more likely to interpose between roots in people aged 18–54 years compared to those aged 55 years and older in Turkish population. Tian et al. [21] investigated the mean distances between posterior root apices and the MSF in Chinese population, and they found that the mean distances to the MFS increased and the frequencies of Type IS decreased with age. Considering that the Type IS was closely related to the development of odontogenic maxillary

Table 3 The shortest vertical distances between the maxillary posterior root apices and the MSFs according to sex ($\bar{x} \pm SD$, mm)

	MFPs	MSPs	MFMs			MSMs			P
			MBR	DBR	PR	MBR	DBR	PR	
Male	6.0 ± 4.4	2.5 ± 3.6	1.9 ± 3.3	1.8 ± 3.1	1.3 ± 3.2	0.7 ± 2.4	1.2 ± 2.6	1.8 ± 3.0	
Female	5.8 ± 4.4	2.6 ± 3.6	2.0 ± 3.4	1.9 ± 3.3	1.5 ± 3.5	0.8 ± 2.7	1.4 ± 2.8	2.2 ± 3.4	>.05
Total	5.9 ± 4.4	2.5 ± 3.6	1.9 ± 3.3	1.9 ± 3.1	1.4 ± 3.4	0.8 ± 2.5	1.3 ± 2.7	2.0 ± 3.2	

Table 4 The shortest vertical distances between the maxillary posterior root apices and the MSFs according to age ($\bar{x} \pm$ SD, mm)

Age	MFPs	MSPs	MFMs			MSMs			P
			MBR	DBR	PR	MBR	DBR	PR	
18-40y	4.9 ± 3.9	1.7 ± 3.0	1.2 ± 2.9	1.2 ± 2.8	0.8 ± 3.1	0.2 ± 2.3	0.8 ± 2.4	1.3 ± 2.7	.00*
41-60y	6.8 ± 4.3	3.4 ± 3.8	2.6 ± 3.3	2.6 ± 3.2	2.1 ± 3.5	1.5 ± 2.7	2.1 ± 3.0	2.8 ± 3.5	
≥61y	8.3 ± 4.6	4.6 ± 4.0	3.8 ± 3.9	3.7 ± 3.8	3.0 ± 3.9	2.2 ± 3.2	2.9 ± 3.4	3.5 ± 3.9	

*The distances between the root apices and the MSFs increased with age and there were significant differences among the groups

sinusitis, so the present experiment focused on the Type IS proportion in Chinese population. The results showed that the frequency of Type IS decreased with age for all maxillary posterior roots. Therefore, age is the important factor to influence the relationship between the maxillary posterior root apices and the MSF.

The results of this study showed that the root apices of MFPs had the maximum distance to the MSF (5.9 ± 4.4 mm), which were consistent with the previous reports in Turkey and Brazilian populations [17, 19], indicating that the inadequate endodontic treatments of the MFPs make less impacts on the condition of the MS mucosa when compared with the maxillary molars because of a closer anatomic relationship between maxillary molars and the sinus floor [23]. It was interest to find that the MBRs of MSMs had the minimum distance to the MSF (0.8 ± 2.5 mm), which was in agreement with the previous studies using CBCT technology in Romania and Chinese populations [21, 24]. However, Yoshimine et al. [25] reported that the PRs of the MFMs had the shortest distance to the MSF (1.67 ± 2.36 mm) in Japanese population. Kilic et al. [17] and Kwak et al. [26] found that the shortest distance was observed in DBRs of the MFMs (2.74 ± 3.23 mm and 0.25 ± 2.17 mm, respectively) in Korean and Turkey populations. Ethnic and different measurement methods may influence the distances between the maxillary posterior root apices and the MSF. In this study, the distances between all roots and the MSF increased with age, indicating that younger people had more probability to have odontogenic maxillary sinusitis caused

by iatrogenic factors. However, the proportion of periodontitis and periapical periodontitis is also higher among the elderly, so it is not possible to infer that the incidence of odontogenic maxillary sinusitis in the elderly is lower than the young people.

Tooth extraction can influence the location of the MSF [1]. von Arx et al. [16] measured the distances of the MFPs with or without the presence of MSPs and found the distances tended to be greater with the presence of MSPs, but the results didn't have significant differences. In this study, the changes of vertical relationship between the maxillary posterior root apices and the MSF after the extraction of adjacent teeth were evaluated using the self-control study. The results showed that when the MFMs or the MFPs was absent, the distances between the roots of the MSPs and the MSF decreased significantly, while other roots had no significant effect. Compared with premolars, MFMs were closer to the MSF and had relatively more obvious impact on the reconstruction of the MSFs. Therefore, it can be inferred that the loss of the MFMs may lead to a forward expansion to the maxillary sinus and influence the distances of MSPs to the MSF.

Conclusions

With the limitations of this study, it may be concluded that the MBRs of MSMs appeared to be the closest to the MSF. The frequency of root apices extending outside the MSF increased with age, while the frequency of the root apices extending inside or contacting with the MSF decreased with age. The absence of the MFMs could influence the proximity of the MSPs roots to the MSF.

Table 5 Comparison of the vertical distances of root apices of maxillary premolars with/without adjacent teeth ($\bar{x} \pm$ SD, mm)

	BR/PR	P
MFPs A	4.7 ± 3.6	.31
MFPs P	5.0 ± 3.9	
MSPs A	2.6 ± 2.6	.01*
MSPs P	1.9 ± 2.3	

A/P Absence/Presence of adjacent teeth
* There were significant differences in 2 PM with or without absence of adjacent teeth

Table 6 Comparison of the vertical distances of root apices of the maxillary molars with/without adjacent teeth ($\bar{x} \pm$ SD, mm)

	MBR	DBR	PR	P
MFMs A	2.6 ± 2.3	1.8 ± 2.2	1.5 ± 2.4	.41
MFMs P	2.0 ± 2.4	2.0 ± 2.8	1.8 ± 2.9	
MSMs A	0.7 ± 1.2	1.1 ± 1.4	1.6 ± 1.9	.66
MSMs P	0.8 ± 1.5	1.4 ± 1.5	1.9 ± 2.2	

A/P Absence/Presence of adjacent teeth

Abbreviations
2D: Two-dimensional; 3D: Three-dimensional; CBCT: Cone-beam computed tomography; DBRs: Distobuccal roots; MBRs: Mesiobuccal roots; MFMs: Maxillary first molars; MFPs: Maxillary first premolars; MS: Maxillary sinus; MSF: Maxillary sinus floor; MSMs: Maxillary second molars; MSPs: Maxillary second premolars; PRs: Palatal roots

Funding
This work was supported by a Project Funded by the Priority Academic Program Development of Jiangsu Higher Education Institutions (PAPD2014–37), the Natural Science Foundation of Jiangsu Province (BK20151560), the Cadre health care research of Jiangsu Province (BJ15031), the Scientific Research of Jiangsu Provincial Commission of Health and Family Planning (H2017050).

Authors' contributions
All authors made substantial contributions to the present study. YG and CS contributed to acquisition of data, data analysis, writing the paper. DL and YZ contributed to CBCT images evaluation and data analysis. DW and QZ contributed to the study design, interpretation of the results, writing the paper, supervision. All authors have read and approved the final manuscript.

Competing interests
The authors declare that they have no competing interests.

Author details
[1]Department of Endodontics, Stomatological Hospital Affiliated to Soochow University, Suzhou Stomatological Hospital, Suzhou, Jiangsu, People's Republic of China. [2]Jiangsu Key Laboratory of Oral Diseases, the Affiliated Stomatological Hospital of Nanjing Medical University, 136 Hanzhong Road, Nanjing 210029, People's Republic of China. [3]Department of Oral Special Consultation, the Affiliated Stomatological Hospital of Nanjing Medical University, 136 Hanzhong Road, Nanjing 210029, People's Republic of China. [4]Department of Radiology, the Affiliated Stomatological Hospital of Nanjing Medical University, 136 Hanzhong Road, Nanjing 210029, People's Republic of China. [5]Department of Endodontics, the Affiliated Stomatological Hospital of Nanjing Medical University, 136 Hanzhong Road, Nanjing 210029, People's Republic of China.

References
1. Sharan A, Madjar D. Maxillary sinus pneumatization following extractions: a radiographic study. Int J Oral Maxillofac Implants. 2008;23:48–56.
2. Lu Y, Liu Z, Zhang L, Zhou X, Zheng Q, Duan X, et al. Associations between maxillary sinus mucosal thickening and apical periodontitis using cone-beam computed tomography scanning: a retrospective study. J Endod. 2012;38:1069–74.
3. Alfaraje L. Surgical and radiologic anatomy for oral implantology. U.S: Quintessence; 2013.
4. Asaumi R, Sato I, Miwa Y, Imura K, Sunohara M, Kawai T, et al. Understanding the formation of maxillary sinus in Japanese human foetuses using cone beam CT. Surg Radiol Anat. 2010;32:745–51.
5. Jung YH, Nah KS, Cho BH. Maxillary sinus pneumatization after maxillary molar extraction assessed with cone beam computed tomography. Korean J Oral Maxillofac Radiol. 2009;39:109–13.
6. Wehrbein H, Diedrich P. Progressive pneumatization of the basal maxillary sinus after extraction and space closure. Fortschr Kieferorthop. 1992;53:77–83.
7. Ariji Y, Obayashi N, Goto M, Izumi M, Naitoh M, Kurita K, et al. Roots of the maxillary first and second molars in horizontal relation to alveolar cortical plates and maxillary sinus: computed tomography assessment for infection spread. Clin Oral Investig. 2006;10:35–41.
8. Maloney P, Jeong D. Maxillary sinusitis of odontogenic origin. Curr Allergy Asthma Rep. 2009;9:238–43.
9. Mehra P, Murad H. Maxillary sinus disease of odontogenic origin. Otolaryngol Clin N Am. 2004;37:347–64.
10. Doud Galli SK, Lebowitz RA, Giacchi RJ, Glickman R, Jacobs JB. Chronic sinusitis complicating sinus lift surgery. Am J Rhinol. 2001;15:181–6.
11. Watzek G, Bernhart T, Ulm C. Complications of sinus perforations and their management in endodontics. Dent Clin N Am. 1997;41:563–83.
12. Oberli K, Bornstein MM, von Arx T. Periapical surgery and the maxillary sinus: radiographic parameters for clinical outcome. Oral Surg Oral Med Oral Pathol Oral Radiol Endod. 2007;103:848–53.
13. Estrela C, Bueno MR, Leles CR, Azevedo B, Azevedo JR. Accuracy of cone beam computed tomography and panoramic and periapical radiography for detection of apical periodontitis. J Endod. 2008;34:273–9.
14. Ludlow JB, Ivanovic M. Comparative dosimetry of dental CBCT devices and 64-slice CT for oral and maxillofacial radiology. Oral Surg Oral Med Oral Pathol Oral Radiol Endod. 2008;106:106–14.
15. Jung YH, Cho BH. Assessment of the relationship between the maxillary molars and adjacent structures using cone beam computed tomography. Imaging Sci Dent. 2012;42:219–24.
16. von Arx T, Fodich I, Bornstein MM. Proximity of premolar roots to maxillary sinus: a radiographic survey using cone-beam computed tomography. J Endod. 2014;40:1541–8.
17. Kilic C, Kamburoglu K, Yuksel SP, Ozen T. An assessment of the relationship between the maxillary sinus floor and the maxillary posterior teeth root tips using dental cone-beam computerized tomography. Eur J Dent. 2010;4:462–7.
18. Ok E, Güngör E, Colak M, Altunsoy M, Nur BG, Ağlarci OS. Evaluation of the relationship between the maxillary posterior teeth and the sinus floor using cone-beam computed tomography. Surg Radiol Anat. 2014;36:907–14.
19. Estrela C, Nunes CA, Guedes OA, Alencar AH, Estrela CR, Sliva RG, et al. Study of anatomical relationship between posterior teeth and maxillary sinus floor in a subpopulation of the Brazilian central region using cone-beam computed tomography - part 2. Braz Dent J. 2016;27:9–15.
20. Pagin O, Centurion BS, Rubira-Bullen IR, Alvares Capelozza AL. Maxillary sinus and posterior teeth: accessing close relationship by cone-beam computed tomographic ccanning in a Brazilian population. J Endod. 2013;39:748–51.
21. Tian XM, Qian L, Xin XZ, Wei B, Gong Y. An analysis of the proximity of maxillary posterior teeth to the maxillary sinus using cone-beam computed tomography. J Endod. 2016;42:371–7.
22. Kalender A, Aksoy U, Basmaci F, Orhan K, Orhan AI. Cone-beam computed tomography analysis of the vestibular surgical pathway to the palatine root of the maxillary first molar. Eur J Dent. 2013;7:35–40.
23. Nascimento EH, Pontual ML, Pontual AA, Freitas DQ, Perez DE, Ramosperez FM. Association between odontogenic conditions and maxillary sinus disease: a study using cone-beam computed tomography. J Endod. 2016;42:1509–15.
24. Georgescu CE, Rusu MC, Sandulescu M, Enache AM, Didilescu AC. Quantitative and qualitative bone analysis in the maxillary lateral region. Surg Radiol Anat. 2012;34:551–8.
25. Yoshimine S, Nishihara K, Nozoe E, Yoshimine M, Nakamura N. Topographic analysis of maxillary premolars and molars and maxillary sinus using cone beam computed tomography. Implant Dent. 2012;21:528–35.
26. Kwak HH, Park HD, Yoon HR, Kang MK, Koh KS, Kim HJ. Topographic anatomy of the inferior wall of the maxillary sinus in Koreans. Int J Oral Maxillofac Surg. 2004;33:382–8.

Income and wealth as correlates of socioeconomic disparity in dentist visits among adults aged 20 years and over in the United States, 2011–2014

Alexander Kailembo[1]*(iD), Carlos Quiñonez[2], Gabriela V. Lopez Mitnik[1], Jane A. Weintraub[3], Jennifer Stewart Williams[4,5], Raman Preet[4], Timothy Iafolla[1] and Bruce A. Dye[1]

Abstract

Background: Most studies in the United States (US) have used income and education as socioeconomic indicators but there is limited information on other indicators, such as wealth. We aimed to assess how two socioeconomic status measures, income and wealth, compare as correlates of socioeconomic disparity in dentist visits among adults in the US.

Methods: Data from the National Health and Nutrition Examination Survey (NHANES) 2011–2014 were used to calculate self-reported dental visit prevalence for adults aged 20 years and over living in the US. Prevalence ratios using Poisson regressions were conducted separately with income and wealth as independent variables. The dependent variable was not having a dentist visit in the past 12 months. Covariates included sociodemographic factors and untreated dental caries. Parsimonious models, including only statistically significant ($p < 0.05$) covariates, were derived. The Akaike Information Criterion (AIC) measured the relative statistical quality of the income and wealth models. Analyses were additionally stratified by race/ethnicity in response to statistically significant interactions.

Results: The prevalence of not having a dentist visit in the past 12 months among adults aged 20 years and over was 39%. Prevalence was highest in the poorest (58%) and lowest wealth (57%) groups. In the parsimonious models, adults in the poorest and lowest wealth groups were close to twice as likely to not have a dentist visit (RR 1.69; 95%CI: 1.51–1.90) and (RR 1.68; 95%CI: 1.52–1.85) respectively. In the income model the risk of not having a dentist visit were 16% higher in the age group 20–44 years compared with the 65+ year age group (RR 1.16; 95%CI: 1.04–1.30) but age was not statistically significant in the wealth model. The AIC scores were lower (better) for the income model. After stratifying by race/ethnicity, age remained a significant indicator for dentist visits for non-Hispanic whites, blacks, and Asians whereas age was not associated with dentist visits in the wealth model.

Conclusions: Income and wealth are both indicators of socioeconomic disparities in dentist visits in the US, but both do not have the same impact in some populations in the US.

Keywords: Disparities, Inequalities, Socioeconomic position, Income, Wealth, Dental utilization, Dental visits

* Correspondence: alexkailembo@gmail.com
[1]National Institutes of Health, National Institute of Dental and Craniofacial Research, Bethesda, USA
Full list of author information is available at the end of the article

Background

Despite general improvements in oral health status due to advancement in social and living conditions, oral diseases remain among the most prevalent human diseases globally and a major public health problem. The 2015 Global Burden of Disease Study estimated that oral conditions (untreated dental caries, chronic periodontitis, and edentulism) ranked among the top ten health conditions, affecting 3.5 billion people worldwide [1]. The profile of oral diseases is not homogeneous between or within countries; the burden is substantially higher among poorer and disadvantaged populations in both high- and low-income countries, including the United States (US) [2–4]. In the US, people of lower socioeconomic position have a higher burden of oral diseases compared with those who are socioeconomically better off, and these disparities also apply to issues of access to oral health services. A study among US adults reported that people living in poverty and those with the least education had fewer dentist visits compared with more affluent and educated individuals [5].

Having a dentist visit in the past 12 months is one of the 17 Healthy People (HP) 2020 oral health objectives in the US [6]. The HP 2020 initiative contains health promotion and disease prevention national goals and objectives set by the US Department of Health and Human Services (HHS) for improving the health of all Americans. There are 12 Leading Health Indicators in HP 2020, and oral health is represented by the objective "to increase the proportion of children, adolescents, and adults who used the oral health care system in the past year." Utilizing dental care in the past 12 months is correlated to higher levels of dental health satisfaction and overall quality of life [7]. Furthermore, differences in access to dental care still exist and a major reason for not having a dentist visit is financial circumstances [8]. For example, dental care utilization in the past 12 months among poor adults in the US was around 20% compared to approximately 50% among high income adults in 2014 [9].

Most studies in the US have used income [10, 11] and education [5, 12] as socioeconomic indicators to assess the association between lower socioeconomic position and lower rates of dentist visits, but there is limited information on other socioeconomic indicators, such as wealth, which measures accumulated assets rather than income alone. Yet there are arguments that health studies should include wealth as a socioeconomic indicator [13]. The wealth index has been widely used as a proxy of socioeconomic position in studies conducted in low- and middle-income settings. Based on methodology developed by Filmer and Pritchett [14], the index combines data on durable assets (car, refrigerator, and television), housing characteristics (dwelling floor and roof material), and access to services (drinking water source and electricity supply) and uses Principal Component Analysis to generate weights for household

assets [14, 15]. However, in the US setting, where most households have durable assets and access to electricity and water supplies, it may be more appropriate to measure wealth differently, by combining income and assets such as cars, homes, savings, and stocks.

Even though income and wealth are positively correlated, they measure different things. For example, older adults may have little income but may have accumulated substantial wealth, through a combination of a lifetime of work and/or inheritance from ancestors. Recent immigrants and racial minorities, even those with high incomes, may be less likely to have significant familial or inherited wealth [16]. Income and occupation status among retired people lose their significance as measures of socioeconomic position and wealth becomes more important [17, 18]. Another example of the difference between income and wealth has been shown in studies using home ownership as a measure of wealth. Home owners may have more income to spend on health care than non-home owners because non-home owners still have to make rent payments [19]. Most recently, wealth rather than income was reported to be more sensitive as an indicator of socioeconomic disparity in health-related outcomes [13]. However, the best choice of socioeconomic measure will depend upon the purpose of the analysis and the policy context.

The purpose of this study is to improve understanding of income and wealth as correlates of socioeconomic disparity in dentist visits among adults in the US so that policy makers may be better informed about targeting interventions to improve access to dental care. The objective is to assess how two socioeconomic status measures, income and wealth, compare as correlates of socioeconomic disparity in dentist visits among adults in the US.

Methods
Data source

Data from the 2011–2014 National Health and Nutrition Examination Survey (NHANES) were used for this study. NHANES is a cross-sectional survey conducted by the National Center for Health Statistics (NCHS) of the Centers for Disease Control and Prevention (CDC) that uses a stratified, multistage sampling design to obtain a representative probability sample of non-institutionalized, civilian population of all ages in the US. NHANES data are used to assess the health, nutritional status and health behaviors of the eligible population using self-reported responses, standardized physical examinations and laboratory tests. The NHANES protocol was developed and reviewed to be in compliance with the HHS Policy for Protection of Human Research Subjects (45 CFR part 46). The protocol was approved by the NCHS Research Ethical Review Board and underwent annual review. Sample persons were informed of the survey process and their rights as a participant by interviewers and by written materials. Written informed consent was freely obtained from each individual participant. Only de-identified observations were used and presented in aggregated summary form. The current study combined the 2011–2012 and 2013–2014 NHANES cycles to derive a study sample covering the 2011–2014 period. Data from both cycles were collected via in-home interviews, with health examinations and laboratory tests conducted in mobile examination centers (MEC). Data for this analysis were obtained from responses to the home interviews and results from the dental examinations. The home interviews used a structured questionnaire that assessed demographic and socioeconomic characteristics and various health-related issues, including oral health. The dental examinations were conducted by trained dentists in the MEC on all eligible participants aged 1 year and older. The 2011–2012 and 2013–2014 NHANES data sets followed the same protocols and are in the public domain, analyzed using only de-identified observations and presented in aggregated summary form. Further details on NHANES survey sample design are provided elsewhere [20].

Study population

The available data set of the 2011–2014 NHANES comprised 19,931 participants of all ages. From this study population, 8602 participants who were younger than 20 years were excluded. Additionally, all participants aged 20 years and over with no dental examination information (422) and those with missing observations (1661) were excluded. A complete flowchart of participants is available in Additional file 1.

Published response rates were 73% and 70% respectively for the interview and examination samples in the 2011–2012 cycle and 71% and 69% respectively for the 2013–2014 cycle [21, 22]. To increase the precision of estimates, NHANES oversamples some population subgroups. For NHANES 2011–2014, the primary change was the addition of an oversample of Asian persons. Oversampling was also carried out for Hispanic, non-Hispanic black, low-income white persons, and older white adults aged 80 years and over [20]. Sampling weights used in this data analysis are provided in the data files which are in public domain.

Variables

The outcome was derived from the question "About how long has it been since you last visited a dentist?" Participants who responded "6 months or less" or "more than 6 months but not more than 12 months" were defined as having a dentist visit in the past 12 months. Participants who responded "more than 12 months" or "never have been" were classified as not having a dentist visit in the past 12 months.

The income variable was based on the poverty income ratio (PIR) calculated by dividing family income to the poverty level threshold specific to family size and survey year. The PIR followed the HHS federal poverty guidelines (FPG) which are issued each year, in the Federal Register, for determining financial eligibility for certain federal programs such as Head Start, Supplemental Nutrition Assistance Program (SNAP) and the National School Lunch Programs. Additional information can be located at http://aspe.hhs.gov/poverty/11poverty.shtml. Ratios below 1.00 indicate that family income is below the official definition of poverty and ratios of 1.00 or greater indicate family income at or above the poverty level. Income was categorized into four PIR groups [23]: PIR greater or equal to 3.00 (high income); PIR greater or equal to 2.00 and less than 3.00 (middle income); PIR greater or equal to 1.00 and less than 2.00 (near poor); and PIR less than 1.00 (poor).

The wealth variable was constructed using a combination of family monthly income and home ownership variables. We chose to use wealth as a socioeconomic variable in addition to income because some authors have argued that income in combination with assets such as housing is a better indicator of health than income alone [24]. Wealth was categorized into three groups – high, middle and low wealth groups. High wealth corresponds to participants in households with more than $2900 USD of monthly income and who are home owners. Middle wealth corresponds to participants with either more than $2900 USD of monthly income and who are non-home owners or are home owners with less than $2900 USD of monthly income. Low wealth corresponds to participants in households with less than $2900 USD of monthly income and who are non-home owners. The choice of $2900 USD cut-off point was influenced by NHANES data reporting. The monthly income variable made available to the public is not presented as a continuous variable but rather as a range value in dollars. For example, $0 - $399 coded as 1, $400 - $799 coded as 2, $800 - $1249 coded as 3 etc. Therefore, our final binary categorization ensured participants' income is as close to the US median value as possible and are equally divided.

Other variables used in the analyses were chosen based on Andersen's behavioral model of health service use [25]. Predisposing factors included sex, age, race/ethnicity, country of birth, marital status, education, and smoking status. Age was categorized as 20–44 years, 45–64 years, and 65 years and over. Race/ethnicity was recoded as non-Hispanic white, Hispanic, non-Hispanic black, and non-Hispanic Asian. Country of birth was dichotomized as born in the US or born in another country. Marital status was recoded as married or cohabiting, widowed or separated, and never married. Educational attainment was classified as having more than 12 years, 12 years, and less than 12 years of school. Smoking status was categorized as current, former, and never smokers. Job status was an enabling factor being expressed as having a job versus not having a job. Need factors were self-rated oral health and the presence of untreated caries. Self-rated oral health was based on the question "Overall, how would you rate the health of your teeth and gums?" Participants were defined as satisfied if they responded excellent, very good or good, and not satisfied if they responded fair or poor. Presence of untreated dental caries (yes/no) was derived from the NHANES clinical dental examination.

Statistical analysis

Only records with complete data on all study variables were analyzed. The analyses were carried out using STATA 13 software (StataCorp, 2013). Sample weights and survey design variables were used to account for unequal probability of participant selection, nonresponse, and sampling error. Absolute numbers, weighted percentages, and standard errors (SE) were estimated to assess the prevalence of not having a dentist visit in the past 12 months. Differences between percentages were calculated by using two-sided t-tests at the $\alpha = 0.05$ level following recommended NHANES analytical and tutorial guidelines. Because education is associated with income and wealth in some populations, we assessed for collinearity between income and wealth with education and found weak correlation: 0.39 (income) and 0.25 (wealth).

Unadjusted (univariable) and parsimonious Poisson regression models were derived separately for income and wealth using generalized linear models with long link and Poisson distribution. The models described associations between income, wealth, socio-demographic factors, health behaviors and need factors and not having a dentist visit. The Poisson regression models were first adjusted for age, sex, race/ethnicity, country of birth, marital status, education, smoking status, job status, self-rated oral health and presence of untreated caries. The criterion for inclusion in the parsimonious models was $p < 0.05$ in the full adjusted models. Associations are presented as prevalence ratios (RRs) with 95% confidence intervals (CIs). The income and wealth models were compared using the Akaike Information Criterion (AIC) as a means of model selection. The AIC estimates the relative information lost when a given model is used to approximate reality. It selects the better model given a set of available data. A preferred model is the one with a minimum AIC valuee [26, 27]. Due to significant interactions by race/ethnicity, the results in the parsimonious models were stratified by race/ethnicity.

Results

The study sample of adults aged 20 years and over in the US was 9246. The weighted prevalence of selected demographic and socioeconomic characteristics are presented in Table 1. Almost half of the adults were aged 20–44 years and about 18% were 65 years and over. The proportion of females to males was just above 50%. Just over two-thirds of the adults were non-Hispanic white (69%), approximately 12% were non-Hispanic black and 5% were non-Hispanic Asian. Almost two-thirds of adults had more than 12 years of education (64%), while only 15% had less than 12 years of education. Almost half of the adults aged 20 years and over lived in high income households, whereas 17% lived in poor households (below the federal poverty level). Almost half (48%) were in the high wealth group while 22% belonged to the low wealth group.

Table 1 also shows the prevalence of not having a dentist visit in the past 12 months among adults aged 20 years and over by sociodemographic characteristics. The overall prevalence was 39%, with a significant difference between participants who did or did not have a dentist visit. This difference held true for all groups except for the non-Hispanic Asian and middle income groups. An income gradient was observed whereby participants in the poorest group had the highest prevalence (58%) and those in the highest income group had the lowest prevalence (24%) of not having a dentist visit. A wealth gradient was also observed. The prevalence was highest in the lowest wealth group (57%) and lowest in the highest wealth group (25%). Not having a dentist visit was more prevalent among adults aged 20–44 years, males, Hispanics, those with the least education, current smokers, those who reported poor oral health, and those with the presence of untreated dental caries.

The income and wealth regression models are presented in Table 2. In the univariable model, adults in the poor (RR = 2.44 95% CI 2.17–2.73) and low wealth (RR = 2.30 95% CI 2.05–2.58) groups were over two times more likely to not have a dentist visit in the past 12 months compared with those with high income and high wealth. Participants aged 20–44 years were 24% (RR = 1.24 95% CI 1.10–1.38) more likely to not have a dentist visit compared with those aged 65 years and over. However, there were no differences between adults aged 45–64 years and those 65 years and over. For adults aged 20 and above in the US, the following factors were associated with not having a dental visit in the past 12 months: being male; Hispanic; non-Hispanic black; born outside the US; widowed or separated; never married; least educated; a current smoker; not satisfied with oral health; having no job; and with untreated dental caries.

In the parsimonious income model, adults in the poor group were close to twice as likely to not have a dentist visit (RR = 1.69; 95% CI: 1.51–1.90) and those aged 20–44 years were 16% more likely to not have a dentist visit than those aged 65 years and over (RR = 1.16; 95% CI: 1.04–1.30). In the parsimonious wealth model, adults in the low wealth group were close to

Table 1 Prevalence of not having a dentist visit in the past 12 months among adults aged 20 years and over, NHANES, 2011–2014[d]

Characteristic		Total study participants n (%)[a]	Participants not having dentist visit n[b]	% (SE)[c]
	Total	9246	4171	38.8 (1.3)
Age groups	20–44 years	4057 (45.7)	1942	42.9 (1.7)[*]
	45–64 years	3149 (36.5)	1340	35.6 (1.7)[*]
	65+ years	2040 (17.8)	889	34.7 (1.7)[*]
Sex	Female	4792 (52.1)	1985	36.1 (1.5)[*]
	Male	4454 (47.8)	2186	41.7 (1.5)[*]
Race/ethnicity	Non-Hispanic White	3938 (69.1)	1604	34.0 (1.4)[*]
	Hispanic	1931 (14.1)	1011	53.9 (2.2)[*]
	Non-Hispanic Black	2190 (11.6)	1093	49.2 (1.8)[*]
	Non-Hispanic Asian	1187 (5.2)	463	38.3 (2.1)
Country of birth	Born in the United States	6598 (83.3)	2941	37.3 (1.4)[*]
	Born in other countries	2648 (16.7)	1230	46.2 (1.7)[*]
Marital status	Married/cohabiting	5348 (62.1)	2226	35.0 (1.5)[*]
	Widowed/separated	2059 (18.8)	1047	46.6 (1.7)[*]
	Never married	1839 (19.1)	898	43.4 (1.6)[*]
Education	More than 12 years	5234 (64.4)	1884	30.9 (1.2)[*]
	12 years	1995 (20.5)	1034	47.4 (1.6)[*]
	Less than 12 years	2017 (15.1)	1253	60.6 (1.9)[*]
Income	High income	3415 (48.2)	905	23.8 (1.3)[*]
	Middle income	1222 (14.1)	556	41.9 (2.5)
	Near poor	2412 (21.0)	1379	55.9 (1.5)[*]
	Poor	2197 (16.7)	1331	58.0 (2.1)[*]
Wealth	High	3441 (47.6)	1002	24.8 (1.3)[*]
	Middle	3088 (30.1)	1547	47.3 (1.7)[*]
	Low	2717 (22.3)	1622	57.1 (1.6)[*]
Job status	With a job	5068 (61.9)	2167	37.7 (1.4)[*]
	Without a job	4178 (38.1)	2004	40.5 (1.5)[*]
Smoking status	Never smoker	5230 (56.4)	2121	34.6 (1.8)[*]
	Former smoker	2148 (24.0)	949	36.1 (1.5)[*]
	Current smoker	1868 (19.6)	1101	54.3 (1.5)[*]
Self-rated oral health status	Satisfied	6231 (72.7)	2335	31.1 (1.4)[*]
	Not satisfied	3015 (27.3)	1836	59.3 (1.5)[*]
Untreated dental caries	No	6579 (75.4)	2528	32.0 (1.3)[*]
	Yes	2667 (24.6)	1643	59.5 (1.7)[*]
Dentist visit in the past 12 months	Yes	5075 (61.2)		
	No	4171 (38.8)		

[*] $p < 0.05$ (t-statistic)
[a] n (%) Number and weighted percent of entire study participants
[b] n Number of respondents not having a dentist visit in the past 12 months
[c] %(SE) Weighted percent and Standard Error of participants not having a dentist visit in the past 12 months
[d] Data source – National Health and Nutrition Examination Survey (NHANES), 2011–2014

twice as likely to not have a dentist visit compared with those in the high wealth group (RR = 1.68; 95% CI: 1.52–1.85) and unlike the income model, there were no significant differences within age subgroups in the multivariable wealth model. This result shows that age and income were independently associated with not having dentist visits but the age association attenuated to non-significance in the presence of wealth.

Table 2 Income, wealth and other factors associated with not having a dentist visit in the past 12 months among adults aged 20 years and over in the United States[d]

		Unadjusted Model RR (CI)	Pars Income Model[a] RR (CI)	Pars Wealth Model[b] RR (CI)
Age groups	20–44 years	**1.24 (1.10–1.38)**	**1.16 (1.04–1.30)**	ns
	45–64 years	1.03 (0.93–1.13)	1.02 (0.94–1.12)	ns
	65+ years[c]	1.00	1.00	
Sex	Female[c]	1.00	1.00	1.00
	Male	**1.15 (1.07–1.24)**	**1.14 (1.06–1.22)**	**1.13 (1.05–1.21)**
Race/ethnicity	Non-Hispanic White[c]	1.00	1.00	1.00
	Total Hispanics	**1.58 (1.42–1.77)**	**1.16 (1.07–1.25)**	**1.20 (1.10–1.76)**
	Non-Hispanic Black	**1.45 (1.31–1.60)**	**1.12 (1.05–1.20)**	**1.12 (1.04–1.21)**
	Non-Hispanic Asian	1.13 (0.97–1.30)	**1.22 (1.09–1.37)**	**1.20 (1.07–1.35)**
Country of birth	Born in the United States[c]	1.00		
	Born in other countries	**1.24 (1.14–1.35)**	ns	ns
Marital status	Married/cohabiting[c]	1.00	1.00	1.00
	Widowed/separated	**1.33 (1.22–1.45)**	**1.16 (1.09–1.24)**	**1.09 (1.03–1.16)**
	Never married	**1.24 (1.14–1.35)**	1.02 (0.95–1.09)	1.00 (0.94–1.08)
Education	More than 12 years[c]	1.00	1.00	1.00
	12 years	**1.54 (1.42–1.66)**	**1.17 (1.09–1.25)**	**1.23 (1.15–1.32)**
	Less than 12 years	**1.96 (1.79–2.14)**	**1.26 (1.16–1.36)**	**1.33 (1.25–1.42)**
Job status	With a job[c]	1.00		
	Without a job	**1.07 (1.01–1.14)**	ns	ns
Smoking status	Never smoker[c]	1.00	1.00	1.00
	Former smoker	1.04 (0.94–1.16)	1.05 (0.95–1.15)	1.00 (0.90–1.10)
	Current smoker	**1.57 (1.40–1.76)**	**1.18 (1.08–1.29)**	**1.17 (1.07–1.27)**
Self-rated oral health status	Satisfied[c]	1.00	1.00	1.00
	Not satisfied	**3.22 (2.73–3.80)**	**1.35 (1.24–1.47)**	**1.37 (1.26–1.48)**
Untreated dental caries	No[c]	1.00	1.00	1.00
	Yes	**1.86 (1.72–2.01)**	**1.30 (1.21–1.39)**	**1.32 (1.23–1.41)**
Income	High[c]	1.00	1.00	n/a
	Middle	**1.76 (1.57–2.00)**	**1.48 (1.31–1.67)**	n/a
	Near poor	**2.35 (2.07–2.66)**	**1.80 (1.58–2.05)**	n/a
	Poor	**2.44 (2.17–2.73)**	**1.69 (1.51–1.90)**	n/a
Wealth	High[c]	1.00	n/a	1.00
	Middle	**1.90 (1.74–2.08)**	n/a	**1.57 (1.44–1.71)**
	Low	**2.30 (2.05–2.58)**	n/a	**1.68 (1.52–1.85)**

RR Prevalence ratios using Poisson regression models, *CI* 95% Confidence Intervals, *n/a* Not Applicable, *ns* Not Significant
[a] Parsimonious income model excluding country of birth and job status variables
[b] Parsimonious wealth model excluding age, country of birth and job status variables
[c] Reference Category
[d] Data source – National Health and Nutrition Examination Survey (NHANES), 2011–2014
All bolded entries are statistcally significant

The effect of being in either the Total Hispanic or Non-Hispanic Black group attenuated from the unadjusted to the parsimonious income and wealth models. This means that relative to being in the Non-Hispanic White group, the likelihood of those in either the Total Hispanic or Non-Hispanic Black group having had no dentist visits decreased in the presence of other socio-demographic factors. In contrast, there was positive attenuation for the Asian group, relative to the Non-Hispanic White group, for both the income and wealth models. The parsimonious models showed increased and significant associations between being in the

Asian group and having no dentist visits which suggests possible offsetting sociodemographic effects in the unadjusted models. Overall, the risk indicators in both models were: being male; Hispanic; non-Hispanic black; widowed or separated; least educated; a current smoker; not satisfied with oral health; and having untreated caries. The income and wealth models were compared using the AIC. The AIC values for the parsimonious income and wealth models were 10,829 and 10,895 respectively. These results indicate that the income models are marginally better than the wealth models (the smaller the AIC value, the better the model).

The analyses were stratified by race/ethnicity because of significant interactions. Figure 1 uses the parsimonious models to summarize the association (RRs). The figure presents income, wealth and other factors as binary variables to compare between the highest and lowest groups. In the income and wealth models, the poor and the low wealth respondents were more likely to not have a dentist visit in all four race/ethnic groups compared to the least poor and the high wealth groups. In the income model, age was a significant factor. Compared to participants aged 65 years and over, the non-Hispanic white and non-Hispanic Asian adults aged 20–44 years were more

likely to not have a dentist visit, while the same association was not significant among non-Hispanic black and Hispanics. In the wealth model, age was not a significant factor in all race/ethnic groups.

Discussion

This study is the first to describe both income and wealth as correlates of socioeconomic disparity in dentist visits among adults using NHANES data. Important differences were observed (especially in age groups) when each measurement was used. Age was not significant for wealth but significant for income. There were also significant interactions by race/ethnicity for income and wealth.

The overall prevalence of not having a dentist visit in the past 12 months among adults aged 20 years and over was 39%. This prevalence is consistent with other findings. For example, a report released in 2016 by the National Center for Health Statistics (NCHS) presented the proportion of adults aged 18 years and over without a dentist visit in 2014 at 38% [28]. However, studies using the Medical Expenditure Panel Survey (MEPS) data have reported higher percentages: 65% of adults aged 18–64 years did not see a dentist in 2013 [29]. Study design, sampling frame, reference periods, lead-in statements, question

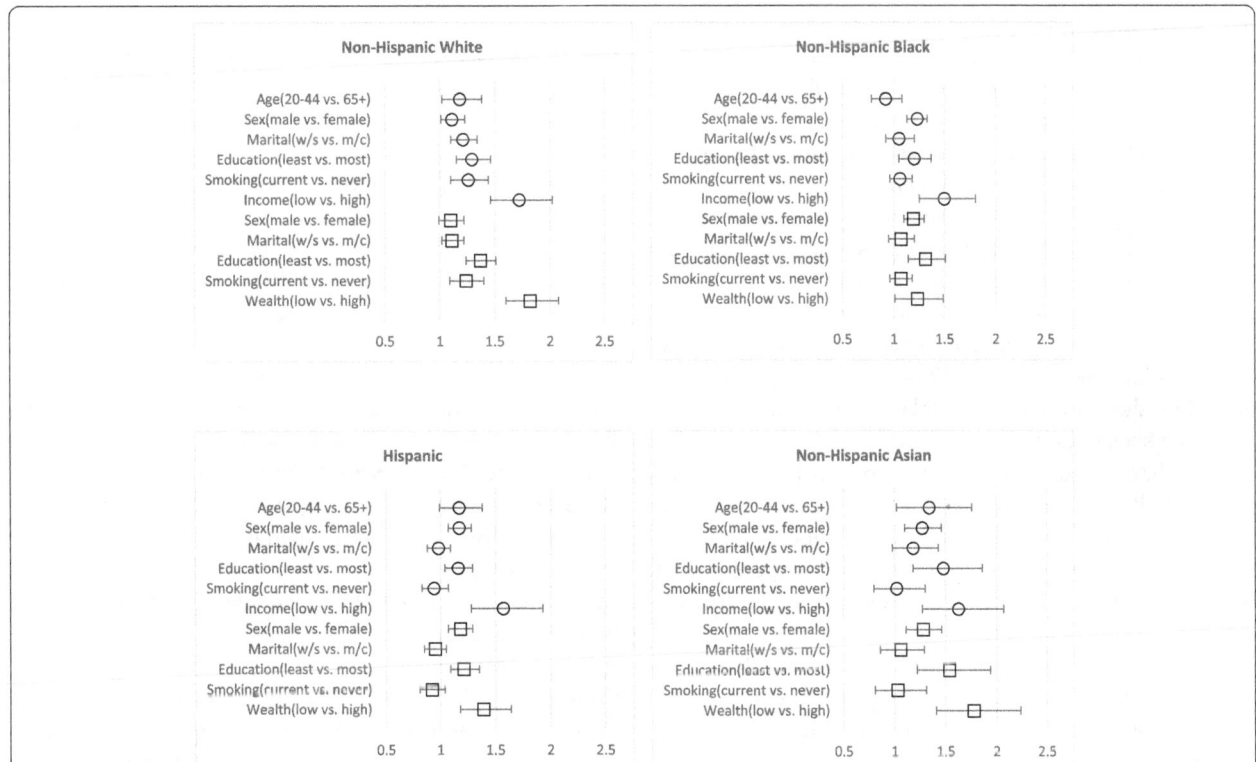

Fig. 1 Income, wealth and other factors associated with not having a dentist visit in the past 12 months stratified by race/ethnicity among adults aged 20 years and over in the United States[+]. Each race/ethnicity plot contains two parsimonious multivariable regression models. Income represented by a circle (o). Wealth represented by a square (□). Measure of associations are prevalence ratios using Poisson regression models. Significant associations ($p < 0.05$) are those greater the one (in the figure) and do not cross the one line in the x-axis. Marital status – widowed/divorced/separated vs. married/cohabiting. [+] Data source – National Health and Nutrition Examination Survey (NHANES), 2011–2014

wording, and social desirability bias are some of the reasons for these different estimates [12].

Despite differences in these overall estimates of dentist visits, demographic and socioeconomic indicators such as sex, race/ethnicity and socioeconomic position have shown consistent associations across national US surveys. For example, persons in lower socioeconomic positions (commonly measured via income status and education) were significantly more likely than those in higher socioeconomic positions to not have a dentist visit in the past 12 months, as were non-Hispanic blacks; Hispanics were significantly more likely than non-Hispanic whites [12]. Similar findings were found in our study where participants in lower socioeconomic positions (measured by income status and wealth) were consistently more likely than those in higher socioeconomic positions to not have a dentist visit in the past 12 months. Other studies have also shown the same pattern in different contexts. A study among adults aged 50 years and over in 14 European countries reported higher rates of dental services utilization among the high-income group compared with the low-income group [30]. Income and education have also been reported as factors in not seeking oral health services in many other global contexts [31, 32].

Explanations for observed socioeconomic disparities have been put forward in the literature. The Commission on Social Determinants of Health (CSDH) produced a landmark report on the impact of social determinants of health (via unfair economic arrangements and poor social policies and programs) on the unequal distribution of health experiences, where health and illness invariably follow a social gradient [33]. Bartley [34] has also reviewed the four theories proposed to lie behind inequality in health and access to health care, namely behavioral, psychosocial, material, and life-course approaches [34]. Importantly, even well-defined material and neo-material resources (income, living conditions) and health behaviors (smoking, diet) do not fully explain health inequality, let alone the social gradient, which may be much more difficult to characterize. The persistent health inequality observed at all levels of the social gradient may be explained by the psychosocial model and the concept of buffering resources such as social capital, social support, social relations, social participation, and self-efficacy. Whatever the case, health inequalities are affected by a complex interaction of these pathways during a person's life-course depending on the context and the population [34].

Our study shows that both income and wealth have strong associations with dentist visits, similar to findings in previous studies. For example, a study among US adults aged 51 years and older in 2008 showed the separate effects of income and wealth on dental utilization [35]. Likewise, a recent study among Japanese adults aged 50 to 75 years showed that both wealth-related and income-related

inequalities in dental care use existed, with greater impact shown by wealth [36]. Our findings also show that results differ when measurements of income or wealth are used. For instance, age was significant in the income model but was not significant in the wealth model. Possible explanations for the observed differences may be that wealth reflects net accumulation of advantage and disadvantage over the life course while income reflects the direct and immediate impacts of a lack of resources. Moreover, without adjusting for wealth, participants aged 20–44 years were more significantly likely to not have a dentist visit but after adjusting for wealth and other sociodemographic factors the association was not significant. One possible explanation is that there are other cultural factors impacting on dental utilization.

There are some limitations. This is a cross-sectional study and causation cannot be inferred. We show that income and wealth are associated with dental visits. Furthermore, the study analyzed self-reported data, which might be subject to information and social desirability biases. For example, while respondents may report poor oral health, they could be misclassified based on clinical examination, or respondents might be more prone to provide socially acceptable responses or unable to correctly recall an event or to accurately evaluate their caries severity. Our outcome variable – not having a dentist visit in the past 12 months – may also capture a heterogeneous group of people who had various reasons for their answers to the question "about how long is it since you last visited a dentist?" Some people may have poor oral health because they had not visited the dentist in the past two or 3 years, whereas others may not have visited the dentist in the past 4 years, but have good oral health. We acknowledge that the outcome variable is not comprehensive but we are confident of its relevance, given that in the Healthy People 2020 objectives, one of the oral health objectives (OH-7) is to increase the proportion of children, adolescents, and adults who used the oral health care system in the past 12 months [6].

This is the first study of its kind to analyze wealth as a socioeconomic variable using NHANES data. We used two indicators - monthly family income and home ownership - to construct a wealth variable. Nevertheless, the results of our study should be interpreted with caution because capturing an individual's wealth is a complex undertaking. One common method of measuring wealth is using Principal Component Analysis to generate weights indicative of household wealth. For this method to work, it requires gathering large amounts of information from respondents, such as ownership of material goods, savings, consumption of goods and services, etc. Unfortunately, due to data limitations we were not able to derive a wealth index using this method, but we think our approach may open doors for future surveys to incorporate more questions regarding household assets to create a wealth index that can give more precise measures of economic well-being. Lastly, we are unable to account for the role of environmental and psychosocial factors such as social capital, social support, geo-locality (urban/rural residence), as well as dental insurance and out of pocket payments. Studies have shown the impact of these determinants in oral health services utilization [37–39] but unfortunately, information on such factors was not collected in the NHANES.

Conclusion

In the US, adults in lower socioeconomic positions (low wealth or income) are less likely to have annual dentist visits yet the socioeconomic patterning varies by age, race/ethnicity and other factors. This study showed that income may be a better measure of socioeconomic disparity than wealth, although wealth may well be a more suitable socioeconomic measure in older adult populations. There is clearly a need for further research into ways of more precisely measuring socioeconomic disparities in dentist visits in the US. Importantly, these findings strengthen the call to action regarding policy based on socioeconomic inequalities in oral health.

Abbreviations

AIC: Akaike Information Criterion; CI: 95% Confidence Interval; CSDH: Commission on Social Determinants of Health; ERB: Ethical Review Board; HHS: US Department of Health and Human Services; HP: Healthy people; MEC: Mobile Examination Centers; MEPS: Medical Expenditure Panel Survey; NCHS: National Center for Health Statistics; NHANES: National Health and Nutrition Examination Survey; ORs: Odds Ratios; PIR: Poverty Income Ratio; SE: Standard Errors; US: United States

Acknowledgements

We are grateful to the participants of NHANES 2011-2012 and 2013-2014 cycles and to the CDC/NCHS for making the NHANES dataset publicly available. Support for the NHANES study was provided by the Federal Government of the United States. We are also grateful to the feedback received from our reviewers.

Funding

AK was a dental public health resident at NIDCR in the United States for the year 2016–2017. The remaining authors involved in this study did not receive any funding.

Authors' contributions

AK conceived the study, developed the first draft and undertook the statistical analyses. BD participated in the conception of the manuscript, data analysis and writing the first draft. GM assisted with statistical analysis. CQ, JW, JSW, RP, TI, GM, and BD checked the analyses, provided critical inputs and advised at all stages of the manuscript. All authors approved the final draft. The authors thank the reviewers for their important feedback and commentary.

Competing interests

The authors declare that they have no competing interests.

Author details

[1]National Institutes of Health, National Institute of Dental and Craniofacial Research, Bethesda, USA. [2]University of Toronto, Toronto, Canada. [3]University of North Carolina, Chapel Hill, USA. [4]Umeå University, Umea, Sweden. [5]Research Centre for Generational Health and Ageing, University of Newcastle, Callaghan, Australia.

References

1. GBD 2015 DALYs and HALE Collaborators. Global, regional, and national disability-adjusted life-years (DALYs) for 315 diseases and injuries and healthy life expectancy (HALE), 1990–2015: a systematic analysis for the Global Burden of Disease Study 2015. Lancet (London, England). 2016; 388:1603–58.
2. Hosseinpoor AR, Itani L, Petersen PE. Socio-economic inequality in oral healthcare coverage: results from the world health survey. J Dent Res. 2012; 91:275–81.
3. Watt RG. Social determinants of oral health inequalities: implications for action. Community Dent Oral Epidemiol. 2012;40(Suppl 2):44–8.
4. Sheiham A, Alexander D, Cohen L, et al. Global oral health inequalities: task group--implementation and delivery of oral health strategies. Adv Dent Res. 2011;23:259–67.
5. Sabbah W, Tsakos G, Sheiham A, Watt RG. The role of health-related behaviors in the socioeconomic disparities in oral health. Soc Sci Med. 2009;68:298–303.
6. Healthy People 2020. 2010. (https://www.healthypeople.gov/. Accessed 6/5/2017).
7. U.S. Department of Health and Human Services. Oral health in America: A report of the surgeon General. Rockville: U.S. Department of Health and Human Services, National Institute of Dental and Craniofacial Research, National Institutes of Health; 2000.
8. Locker D, Maggirias J, Quinonez C. Income, dental insurance coverage, and financial barriers to dental care among Canadian adults. J Public Health Dent. 2011;71:327–34.
9. Nasseh K, Vujicic M. Dental care utilization steady among working-age adults and children, up slightly among the elderly. Illinois: Health Policy Institute Research Brief American Dental Association; 2016.
10. Nasseh K, Vujicic M. Dental care utilization rate continues to increase among children, holds steady among working-age adults and the elderly. Illinois: Health Policy Institute Research Brief American Dental Association; 2015. p. 2001–10.
11. Wall TP, Vujicic M, Nasseh K. Recent trends in the utilization of dental care in the United States. J Dent Educ. 2012;76:1020–7.
12. Macek MD, Manski RJ, Vargas CM, Moeller J. Comparing oral health care utilization estimates in the United States across three nationally representative surveys. Health Serv Res. 2002;37:499–521.
13. Pollack CE, Chideya S, Cubbin C, Williams B, Dekker M, Braveman P. Should health studies measure wealth? A systematic review. Am J Prev Med. 2007; 33:250–64.
14. Filmer D, Pritchett LH. Estimating wealth effects without expenditure data—or tears: an application to educational enrollments in states of India*. Demography. 2001;38:115–32.
15. Howe LD, Galobardes B, Matijasevich A, et al. Measuring socio-economic position for epidemiological studies in low- and middle-income countries: a methods of measurement in epidemiology paper. Int J Epidemiol. 2012;41:871–86.
16. Pew Research Center. "On Views of Race and Inequality, Blacks and Whites are Worlds Apart."2016.
17. Duncan GJ, Daly MC, McDonough P, Williams DR. Optimal indicators of socioeconomic status for Health Research. Am J Public Health. 2002;92: 1151–7.
18. Van Ourti T. Socio-economic inequality in ill-health amongst the elderly. Should one use current or permanent income? J Health Econ. 2003;22:219–41.
19. Costa-Font J. Housing assets and the socio-economic determinants of health and disability in old age. Health Place. 2008;14:478–91.
20. Johnson CL, Dohrmann SM, Burt VL, Mohadjer LK. National health and nutrition examination survey: sample design, 2011–2014. Vital and health statistics Series 2, Data evaluation and methods research; 2014. p. 1–33.
21. Response rates for NHANES 2011–2012 by Age and Gender. 2012. (https://www.cdc.gov/nchs/data/nhanes/response_rates_cps/rrt1112.pdf. Accessed 12/9/2016).
22. Response rates for NHANES 2013–2014 by Age and Gender. 2014. (https://www.cdc.gov/nchs/data/nhanes/response_rates_cps/2013_2014_response_rates.pdf. Accessed 12/9/2016).

23. Keppel KG, Pearcy JN, Klein RJ. Measuring progress in healthy people 2010, Healthy People 2010 statistical notes: from the Centers for Disease Control and Prevention/National Center for Health Statistics; 2004. p. 1–16.
24. Galobardes B, Shaw M, Lawlor DA, Lynch JW, Davey Smith G. Indicators of socioeconomic position (part 2). J Epidemiol Community Health. 2006;60:95–101.
25. Andersen RM. Revisiting the behavioral model and access to medical care: does it matter? J Health Soc Behav. 1995;36:1–10.
26. Hu S. Akaike Information Criterion: North Carolina State university. Raleigh: Center for Research in scientific computation; 2012.
27. Lumley T, Scott A. AIC and BIC for modeling with complex survey data. J Survey Stat Methodology. 2015;3:1–18.
28. National Center for Health S. Health, United States. Health, United States, 2015: with special feature on racial and ethnic health disparities. Hyattsville: National Center for Health Statistics (US); 2016.
29. Nasseh K, Vujicic M. Dental care utilization rate highest ever among children, continues to decline among working-age adults. Health Policy Institute Research Brief. Illinois: American Dental Association; 2014.
30. Listl S. Income-related inequalities in dental service utilization by Europeans aged 50+. J Dent Res. 2011;90:717–23.
31. Petersen PE, Kjoller M, Christensen LB, Krustrup U. Changing dentate status of adults, use of dental health services, and achievement of national dental health goals in Denmark by the year 2000. J Public Health Dent. 2004;64:127–35.
32. Molarius A, Engstrom S, Flink H, Simonsson B, Tegelberg A. Socioeconomic differences in self-rated oral health and dental care utilisation after the dental care reform in 2008 in Sweden. BMC Oral Health. 2014;14:134.
33. Marmot M, Friel S, Bell R, Houweling TA, Taylor S. Closing the gap in a generation: health equity through action on the social determinants of health. Lancet. 2008;372:1661–9.
34. Bartley M. Health inequality: an introduction to concepts, theories and methods. Cambridge: Wiley; 2016.
35. Manski RJ, Moeller JF, Chen H, St Clair PA, Schimmel J, Pepper JV. Wealth effect and dental care utilization in the United States. J Public Health Dent. 2012;72:179–89.
36. Murakami K, Hashimoto H. Wealth-related versus income-related inequalities in dental care use under universal public coverage: a panel data analysis of the Japanese study of aging and retirement. BMC Public Health. 2016;16:24.
37. Hendryx MS, Ahern MM, Lovrich NP, McCurdy AH. Access to health care and community social capital. Health Serv Res. 2002;37:85–101.
38. Vargas CM, Dye BA, Hayes K. Oral health care utilization by US rural residents, National Health Interview Survey 1999. J Public Health Dent. 2003;63:150–7.
39. Yu ZJ, Elyasi M, Amin M. Associations among dental insurance, dental visits, and unmet needs of US children. J Am Dent Assoc. 2017;148:92–9.

What factors are associated with dental general anaesthetics for Australian children and what are the policy implications? A qualitative study

John Rogers[1]* , Clare Delany[1], Clive Wright[2], Kaye Roberts-Thomson[3] and Mike Morgan[1]

Abstract

Background: Dental general anaesthetics undertaken on young children are amongst the most common of all potentially preventable hospitalisations of children in Australia. They are costly for families and the community and entail some risk. The aim of the study was to explore the views of stakeholders about factors associated with children's dental general anaesthetics in Victoria, Australia and to identify policy implications.

Methods: Interviews with stakeholders were used to develop a framework of factors. Interview data were subject to qualitative analysis, informed by Interpretative Phenomenological Analysis.

Results: Eight themes that encompassed 30 main factors were identified through focused discussions with 16 stakeholders. While the safety of dental general anaesthetics has improved and mortality rates are low, side effects are common. Push factors for children's dental general anaesthetics include a perceived greater 'child-focus'; preferred models of care; low oral health literacy; parent guilt; convenience; and some dentists reluctance to treat high needs children in the clinic. Factors that may decrease the prevalence of dental general anaesthetics include: prevention of dental caries; using alternative approaches; an appropriate workforce mix; enhancing oral health literacy; and development of guidelines.

Conclusion: The prevalence of hospitalisation of children to treat dental caries is increasing. Many factors influence the prevalence of paediatric dental general anaesthetics - relating to the child, parent, oral health professional, financial impact, health risk, and accessibility to facilities. There are quality of care and convenience benefits but also high costs and possible health risks. Family, workforce and health system factors have been identified that could decrease the prevalence of paediatric dental general anaesthetics.

Keywords: Dental caries, Children, Dental general anaesthetics, Potentially preventable dental hospitalisations

Background

Dental general anaesthetics (DGAs) undertaken in hospitals or day procedure centres on young children are amongst the most common of all hospitalisations of children in Australia. Of the 130,792 DGAs in 2013–14, 20,607 were 0–9 year-olds hospitalised for potentially preventable reasons [1]. The number of Potentially Preventable Dental Hospitalisations (PPDHs) in this age group has been increasing. Between 2013-14 and 2015–

16 there was a 17% increase to 4891 in Victoria, making PPDHs the highest of all Potentially Preventable Hospitalisations (PPHs) and double the rate for asthma admissions [2]. These PPHs are admissions for conditions where hospitalisation is considered to have been avoidable if timely and adequate non-hospital care had been provided [1] or if the condition had been prevented in the first place. In 2015–16 the principal diagnosis for over 90% of PPDHs in children was dental caries [3], meaning that almost all DGAs were PPDHs. Just over half of children's PPDHs (53%) were conducted in public hospitals in Victoria in 2015–16 [4].

* Correspondence: jgrogers@unimelb.edu.au
[1]University of Melbourne, Melbourne, Victoria, Australia
Full list of author information is available at the end of the article

Reducing PPHs is an objective in health care reform with the aim of improving patients' outcomes, reducing pressure on hospitals and enhancing health system efficiency and cost effectiveness [5]. PPDHs are one of 11 PPHs that are included in the National Healthcare Agreement [6] between the Australian Government and the state and territory governments as a performance indicator [7]. Reducing the rates of PPDHs is a key strategy in the Australian National Oral Health Plan 2015–2024 [8].

The most recently published guidelines for indications for DGA for children and adolescents have been developed by the American Academy of Pediatric Dentistry [9]. Indications are proposed for: patients who cannot cooperate due to lack of psychological or emotional maturity and/or mental, physical or medical disability; patients for whom local anaesthesia is ineffective because of acute infection, anatomic variations, or allergy; the extremely uncooperative, fearful, anxious or uncommunicative child or adolescent; those requiring significant surgical procedures; patients for whom the use of general anaesthesia may protect the developing psyche and/ or reduce medical risk; and patients requiring immediate, comprehensive oral/dental care [9]. Higher quality dental care can often be provided in a DGA because it is easier to manage saliva and the tongue in the more controlled environment. A systematic review of 20 studies from 14 countries concluded that dental care under a GA improves the overall quality of life of children with high levels of parental satisfaction [10].

Concerns about DGAs for children include the family and health system costs and mortality and morbidity risks. The average cost of a DGA for under 15 year-olds in Western Australia has been estimated at $2039 and $5234 when indirect costs are added [11]. Richardson and Richardson estimated that the cost of the 50,000 PPDHs in Australia in 2008–09 was $233 million, an average cost of $4660 [12]. There is little information published on the morbidity and mortality impacts of DGAs in Australia. The overall GA mortality rate in children was estimated to be 1:150,000 in 2005 [13]. Knapp and colleagues systematic review quoted above found that some quality of life sub scales worsened after a DGA [10]. Qualitative research has also found that some children report that they were scared during the DGA process [14] while parents have reported being shocked at the amount of blood and the behavioural state of their child [15].

There may be variations in views among Oral Health Professionals (OHPs) about indications for conducting DGAs in children. DGA guidelines from the United Kingdom indicate that the majority of dental services for children can be carried out using either local anaesthesia or local anaesthesia with conscious sedation, and that patient/carer preferences are a condition that rarely justifies

a GA [16]. United Kingdom guidelines for people living with learning disabilities state that a DGA for people with a disability should be the '*last choice of treatment*' [17]. In the Australia context, Alcaino and colleagues have noted that '*although most children will cope with dentistry in the normal setting, many more may benefit from delivery of extensive dentistry in one session under GA*' [13]. In the Australian public dental system there have been indications that children who are considered difficult to treat in the dental chair are referred for a DGA without consideration of alternative care [18]. The most recent Australian DGA guidelines for children were developed by the Australasian Academy of Paediatric Dentistry in 2002 and published in 2005 [19]. There are no standard Australian policy guidelines for referral for publicly funded DGAs.

The literature that has examined factors which influence dental hospitalisation of children is generally descriptive and is predominantly derived from cross sectional studies which limit the ability to ascribe causality. Few studies have measured the strengths of associations or controlled for potentially confounding factors. Information is available on DGA frequency [1, 20], individual characteristics of those who have a DGA [11, 21, 22], and the impact of environmental factors such as access to water fluoridation and primary dental care [23]. However, little is known about the factors that drive the decisions of OHPs when they encounter a child in their clinic including how they make decisions about the most appropriate treatment for a particular dental problem. There are also few references in the literature to DGA mortality in Australia or the access to operating theatres.

The decision to perform a DGA is potentially influenced by the perspectives and clinical reasoning of the individual oral health professional and more broadly by drivers within the health and education systems. Identifying these factors, including how they intersect, is necessary for the development of strategies to reduce the rates of PPDHs as called for in the Australian National Oral Health Plan 2015–2024 [8].

Therefore the aim of this study was to explore the views of stakeholders in the public dental health system about factors associated with children's DGAs and to identify policy implications. The main research question was 'What is the perception of OHPs and Hospital Admission Decision Makers (HADMs) about factors associated with the frequency of DGAs among children in Victoria, Australia?'

Methods

The research design was qualitative drawing from interpretivism [24] and phenomenology [25]. These methodologies are appropriate when the research aims to understand people's interpretations, perceptions, perspectives and experiences of a particular situation (or phenomenon). These research paradigms acknowledge that people experience and understand the same 'objective reality' in very different ways, which then shapes their decision making [26].

A two stage process was used to collect data. The first stage involved interviewing OHPs and HDAMs working in the public sector to identify factors which might influence decisions to perform a DGA for a child. These data were analysed and a framework of factors influencing DGAs developed.

The framework was then used in stage two of data collection. Paediatric dentists were interviewed using the framework to encourage these participants to reflect on their own decisions and the influences they had encountered. Paediatric dentists undertake the majority of DGAs in Victoria. Participants either agreed or disagreed with the identified factors and added their perspective. In-depth interviews were also held with HDAMs to explore factors relating to health system policy and practice of dental hospitalisation in Victoria.

Stage one discussions took place between the chief investigator (JR) and 11 OHPs and two HDAMS. Discussions were held between August 2012 and May 2014 and lasted from 30 to 90 min. Notes were taken and discussed with the participants. Memos or 'notes to self' on emerging categories and ideas were written during the discussions. Thematic analysis was undertaken [26] and the framework developed. Participants were purposefully selected [27] on the basis of their experience and expertise related to DGAs in Victoria particularly in the public sector. The OHPs included four paediatric dentists, two dentists, two dental therapists, and three dental public health specialists as listed in Table 1. Both HDAMs were senior public hospital executives. All of the stakeholders who were approached agreed to participate.

In the stage two data collection, in-depth interviews were conducted with three of the paediatric dentists and three HADMs. The HADMs included two Department of Health policy makers and a senior public hospital executive as shown in Table 1. All participants were purposefully selected on the basis of positions they hold in the public sector provision of dental general anaesthesia in Victoria. The paediatric dentists also had private

practice experience. The framework and research questions are presented in the Results.

The in-depth interviews were conducted by the chief investigator (JR) from May 2014 to June 2015. Participants were provided with a plain language statement about the research and signed consent forms. Open-ended questions were used to allow the participants to add their interpretation and understanding of what they thought was important. The semi-structured nature of the discussions encouraged participants to respond more freely than a structured interview format [24]. Interviews generally ran from 60 to 90 min. Comprehensive notes were taken during the interviews. These notes were compiled and provided to the participants to check their accuracy.

Analytical plan for data

Interview data from both stages were subject to qualitative analysis, informed by Interpretative Phenomenological Analysis (IPA) [28]. Analysis of data within the IPA approach is flexible but with general procedures that define the approach and ensure its rigor. Procedures followed in stage one were: JR reading and re-reading the notes of discussions with OHPs and HDAMs to identify the matters or themes that were raised by participants; annotating notes with the themes that arose; reviewing the memos written during the interviewing process to support an understanding of the concepts within the data; and clustering participant themes. Notes and themes were then reviewed by MM and CW and consensus reached on main and subordinate themes.

A framework was developed using the identified themes of factors associated with DGAs in children. The framework was then used in stage two. Notes of the interviews were compiled as for the discussions with the OHPs and HDAMs and as mentioned, provided to the participants to check their accuracy. Verbatim quotes were checked in this way. Themes were then written up using selected participant statements with interpretative commentary. These steps were followed by preparing a discussion of identified themes against what is presently known in the literature

Table 1 Study participants

	Number	Years of experience related to DGAs (average)
Preliminary discussions		
Oral health professionals (OHPs) – 4 paediatric dentists, 2 dentists, 2 dental therapists and 3 dental public health specialists.	11	28 years
Hospital admission decision maker (HADMs)	2	
In-depth interviews		
Paediatric dentists	3	23 years
HADMs	3	

and reflection on the research to identify policy implications and further areas for research.

Results

Discussions were held with 11 OHPs and two HDAMs to develop the framework. While the sample was only a relatively small proportion of the dental and hospital policy professionals in Victoria, the most influential people associated with dental hospitalisation in the public sector were included. The average years of relevant experience was 28 years, as shown in Table 1.

A thematic analysis of the discussions identified eight key themes that encompassed 30 main factors that the participants considered are relevant to understanding the frequency of dental hospitalisation of children in Victoria (Table 2). Themes (T) were: T1, criteria for DGAs; T2, child factors; T3, dental provider factors; T4, parent factors; T5, risk; T6, financial impact; T7, access to general anaesthetic facilities; and T8, treatment provided. Theme 3, dental provider factors, comprised the sub themes of paediatric dentist factors, general dentist factors, and dental therapist factors.

Questions for the in-depth semi structured interviews in stage two of the data collection were based on the framework and are presented in Table 3. The questions were different for the paediatric dentists and HADMs to reflect these groups different roles in relation to DGAs. The in-depth interviews confirmed that the themes in the framework were relevant. Further detail emerged from these interviews.

Theme 1 criteria for DGAs

All participants noted that it was preferable to prevent dental caries rather than have to treat it. While all participants indicated that a DGA was required for higher quality outcomes for young children with extensive or complex dental treatment needs and/or behavioural issues, there were variations in views about the appropriate threshold. A commonly mentioned indicator from paediatric dentists was if the child required treatment in all four quadrants of the mouth. It was noted that some operators have a lower DGA threshold such as when a child will not tolerate the placement of rubber dam. Several OHPs spoke of peers in the public and private

Table 2 Framework of themes and factors associated with Dental General Anaesthetics (DGAs) in children in Victoria

Themes	Main associated factors
1. Criteria for DGAs	• Importance of preventing dental caries • Variation in views about appropriate threshold for paediatric DGAs • Perceived increase in dental caries prevalence and dental care needs • Change in attitude by OHPs to DGAs • Limitation of existing guidelines
2. Child factors	• Greater emphasis on children's attitude toward dental treatment • Possible change in behavioural management techniques
3. Dental provider factors	
3.1. Paediatric dentist factors	• Quality of care • Case selection for DGAs
3.2. General dentist factors	• Reluctance to treat young children • Changes in general dental practice • Limited alternatives to DGAs
3.3. Dental therapist factors	• Increased employment in private practice • Role as primary oral health care workers
4. Parent factors	• Convenience of DGAs • Parenting styles • Oral health literacy • Guilt • Cultural variations
5. Risk	• Improved safety of DGAs • Mortality • Morbidity
6. Financial impact	• Private sector DGA cost • Public sector DGA cost
7. Access to general anaesthetic facilities	• Economic efficiencies • Dental provider issues • Department of Health policy factors • Rural hospital issues.
8. Treatment provided and follow-up after a DGA	• Emergency and elective DGAs • Appropriate dental treatment under DGAs • Follow up prevention appointments

Table 3 Interview questions

Questions for paediatric dentists
'What do you consider to be the key factors related to DGAs in Victorian children?'
Prompts:
- Criteria for DGAs
- OHP factors
- Parent and child factors
- Indications for DGAs
- Access to DGA facilities
- DGA costs
- DGA risks.

Questions for Hospital admission decision makers (HADMs)
- 'What is the current policy, associated guidelines and practice related to access to hospital theatres for DGA?'
- 'Have the current policy/guidelines/practice changed?'
Prompts:
- Funding changes
- Any difference in factors for metropolitan and rural hospitals.
- Influence of waiting lists.

sector who tended to use DGA as a 'first resort' or as the 'default choice'.

Four of the five paediatric dentists believed that there had been an increase in dental caries prevalence in Victorian children since 2000 with a consequent increase in dental treatment needs. None of these participants had readily available data to quantify this perceived change.

Four paediatric dentists spoke of the change in attitudes toward DGAs by general and paediatric dentists.

'Twenty years ago, treating a young child under GA was generally seen as a failure by clinicians to manage care in the dental clinic. Fewer hold this view now'. (Paediatric dentist)

No published Australian guidelines on criteria for DGAs were acknowledged as best practice by any of the participants.

'The Australasian Academy of Paediatric Dentistry published guidelines in 2005 but there have not been any updates'. (Paediatric dentist)

Participants working in the public system noted that there were no standard Australian policy guidelines for referral for publicly-funded DGAs.

'It would be fantastic to establish a national group to agree on guidelines that can be accepted at a national level'. (Paediatric dentist)

Theme 2 child factors

There was agreement that there is a greater emphasis on the child's attitude toward dental treatment compared to 30 years ago. The child is now more likely to be asked than told what they want or need.

Behavioural management techniques used in dentistry appear to have changed.

'There is now less acceptance by children, parents and dental providers of 'chasing the child' and 'rough and tumble' in the dental chair'. (Paediatric dentist)

A paediatric dentist with experience working in a children's hospital noted that there has been a general increase in 'child focus' across all health disciplines.

'The accepted best practice is 'do not stress the child'. (Paediatric dentist)

A 'pain free' policy has led to a shift to use general anaesthesia in the hospital for procedures previously undertaken under local anaesthesia. For example, short general anaesthesia is now used in medical procedures such as lumbar punctures in order to be kinder ('less stressful') to the child. Nitrous oxide (relative analgesia) sedation is also now in widespread use in hospital medical clinics and its use has also increased in the hospital dental clinics.

Theme 3 dental provider factors
Paediatric dentist factors

The two main areas relating to paediatric dentists identified by participants were quality of care and case selection for DGAs. Case selection responses have been included under Theme 1 Criteria for DGAs.

Four of the five paediatric dentists indicated that a DGA can be the preferred model of care.

'Higher quality treatment is possible, especially for preschool children'. (Paediatric dentist)

'It can be more predictable with less complications'. (Paediatric dentist)

'A DGA for a child can be a preferred model of care for a quality outcome and ability to manage all treatment'. (Paediatric dentist)

These informants considered that treatment under a DGA can be less haphazard and provide the most efficient outcome. Dental treatment completed in a one-hour DGA session could require four to six appointments in a dental clinic. It was noted that the quality of care possible also depends on the length of the GA session.

Two of the paediatric dentists stated that undertaking a DGA does not necessarily allow higher quality care to be provided, nor does it improve the chances of being able to provide subsequent care to children in a dental clinic. It was noted that under a GA it is difficult to obtain an x-ray and it may not be possible to check the occlusion. In addition, quality can be compromised because of mouth rather than nasal intubation. It was reported that many anaesthetists do not like using nasal intubation. A paediatric dentist referred to research about DGAs and their impact on a child's attitude to future dental care.

'DGAs don't necessarily reduce the anxiety a child may have about receiving dental treatment in a dental clinic in the future'. (Paediatric dentist).

General dentist factors

All of the clinician participants (the paediatric dentists, general dentists, and dental therapists) considered that general dentists may be reluctant to treat young children due to a lack of confidence because they may not have had the necessary training or experience. A general view was that there was not sufficient practical experience during basic dental degree training. For example, a paediatric dentist noted that dental students may not have the opportunity to give a block local anaesthetic to a child, or learn about alternative sedation techniques to DGAs such as using relative analgesia.

It was reported that there can be a shortage of appropriate patients for dental students to be able to develop their behavioural management and clinical skills. Many children who attend student clinics do not require care beyond examinations and the placement of fissure sealants. It was also noted that training in relative analgesia and also intravenous sedation is limited in Victoria.

'It is a tragic loss of opportunity that there is no course of training in intravenous sedation available in Victoria'. 'There is a desperate need for a wider range of options than avoidance of treatment or full general anaesthesia'. (Dentist)

Three participants raised an issue about perception of the professional status of dentists.

'If a general dentist is having difficulty managing the dental care of a child, he or she may refer the child to a paediatric dentist in order to save face with parents'. (Dentist)

Participants mentioned changes in general dental practice that have affected DGA rates such as more referral options with increased numbers of registered paediatric dentists and less acceptance by children, parents and

dental providers of 'rough and tumble' in the dental chair.

Dental therapist factors

The dental therapist participants, in common with other OHPs as mentioned under T1, indicated that it was preferable to prevent dental caries rather than treat it and that DGAs were required in certain circumstances. Several participants noted that more private practices are employing dental therapists who manage most of the dental care for children. Participants involved in education or service delivery noted that oral health and dental therapist training focuses on managing the general clinical care of children and that they were efficient and effective primary oral health care workers.

The dental therapist participants spoke of cases where they were asked to provide a second opinion after parents had been told by another OHP that their child would require a DGA. In these cases the dental therapists reported that they were able to manage the child in the dental chair. Therapists acknowledged that paediatric dentists had advanced skills and would refer children to them if the treatment required was outside a therapists scope of practice.

Theme 4 parent factors

While parents were not interviewed, most study participants commented on parent factors that affected the frequency of DGAs. Comments were made about convenience, parenting styles, oral health literacy, guilt, and cultural variations.

Participants noted that some parents consider a DGA to be convenient because treatment can be completed in one session, rather than three or more visits to a dental clinic. This reduces the time needed for parents to take time off work in addition to potentially there being less expense for childcare for other children.

'A DGA is attractive to parents who are time-poor and asset-rich'. (Paediatric dentist)

Some respondents framed parents' requests as an example of 'permissive' parenting styles compared to 'authoritative' or 'authoritarian' styles, which may have led to an increase in DGAs as parents were less likely to insist on their child 'behaving in the dental chair'.

Comments were made about the wide variation in oral health literacy among parents. Several participants mentioned that parents accessing private care for their child generally had higher oral health literacy, but some were influenced by anti-fluoride articles they had accessed on the internet. These parents were more likely to use herbal toothpastes that do not have the dental caries prevention impact of fluoride toothpastes. Three paediatric dentists also mentioned the variation in the perceived importance of primary teeth to parents.

> *'Some parents do not value primary teeth'.* (Paediatric dentist).

Some parents were not aware of the impact of diet on oral health. Others were, but considered it too difficult to change feeding habits and a DGA was the price they were prepared to pay.

Several paediatric and general dentists noted that parents can become defensive when issues of diet are raised, possibly because of feelings of guilt that their child had dental caries.

> *'Some parents feel guilty that their child has dental caries'.* (Paediatric dentist)

Several paediatric dentists noted that more parents are asking that white fillings rather than silver crowns are used to cap decayed molar teeth because these parents are concerned that visible dental work was a sign of parental neglect. A general dentist commented that there may be occasions when an OHP could 'trade on' parental guilt when discussing the need for a DGA.

Several OHPs noted that some parents are reluctant for their children to have care under a DGA. Cultural variations in parental attitudes toward DGAs were raised.

> *'There are cultural variations, for example some parents with Asian backgrounds are more concerned about the risks of a DGA'.* (Paediatric dentist).

Theme 5 risk

When paediatric dentists mentioned risk, they indicated that the safety of a DGA had improved with new anaesthetic drugs and better monitoring. The newer anaesthetic agents have fewer side effects. With better monitoring, problems are detected earlier when intervention can occur. Nausea was noted by some paediatric dentists as a still common side effect.

Paediatric dentists noted that DGA-linked child deaths were rare in Australia. The fatalities mentioned were limited to the death of a young child in Broken Hill in 1998 and a fatality in a Brisbane dental clinic more than 20 years ago. Both deaths were associated with the children's underlying medical problems.

Theme 6 financial impact

Participants mentioned costs to the family and to the health system. Paediatric dentists reported that costs ranged from $2500 to $8000 in the private sector, with most admissions costing between $3500 and $5000.

> *'In the private sector there are three direct cost components to a DGA: the anaesthetist's fee, clinician's fee and facility bed fee'.* (Dentist).

Participants noted that costs are predominantly 'out of pocket', with Medicare reimbursement only available for part of the anaesthetist fee.

> *'Private insurance rebates may cover only about half of the DGA costs'.* (Dentist).

Hospital administrators advised that the national Independent Hospital Pricing Authority determined through a survey of public hospitals that the average cost for the most common DGA (dental extractions and restorations) was $3029 in public hospitals in 2012–13 [29]. These direct costs do not include indirect costs such as childcare for other children and loss of income from taking time off work.

Theme 7 access to DGA facilities

Four issues concerning access to operating theatres were identified from participants' responses: economic efficiencies, dental provider issues, Department of Health and Human Services policy, and rural hospital issues.

Several participants who had worked in the private hospital system noted that general dental treatment of children was perceived as less economically viable for a facility than extraction of wisdom teeth, the placement of grommets, or the removal of tonsils and adenoids.

> *'Whereas a dental clinician may see three to five children in a three-hour session, a maxillofacial surgeon could extract the wisdom teeth of six patients, grommets could be placed in the ears of six children, or 10–15 cataract operations could be performed'.* (Paediatric dentist).

Participants with experience in the public system commented that a DGA can be a lower priority than a general anaesthetic for procedures that are monitored for waiting times by the Department of Health and Human Services and publically reported. Using the limited theatre resources for DGAs means that less time is available for procedures for which waiting times are reported publicly. Respondents commented that in busy hospitals there was a pressure on access to operating theatres.

> *'There is never enough theatre time'. 'If it is not counted (for waiting list reporting) it does not count'.* (Hospital admission decision maker)

Paediatric dentists noted that access to operating theatres was more difficult in the public system compared to the private system. However, they did note that some paediatric dentists and general dentists complained about poor access to private facilities for DGAs. Both an experienced general dentist and a hospital manager said that clinicians who appreciated that private hospitals and day procedure centres need to make a profit, and arranged their cases and length of treatment accordingly, appeared to have little problem accessing theatres.

The impact on DGA rates of hospital admission policy changes was raised by HDAMs. An example was a change in policy by the then Victorian Department of Health in 2011. Patients who attended emergency departments could not be recorded as an admission if they were admitted directly to a public hospital bed. A HDAM noted that total public hospital admissions decreased in 2012–13 compared to 2011–12, but then increased again in 2013–14 as hospitals established different arrangements for this group.

Two HDAMs indicated that there may be fewer barriers to DGAs in smaller rural hospitals, compared to larger metropolitan facilities. This is because small rural hospitals in Victoria are globally funded, not casemix funded, and have fewer medical specialty services competing for theatre time. It was noted that rural hospitals can have a regular general anaesthetic session for local dentists, that is, a 'dental list' every week or month. Where this occurs, there is some pressure on dentists to use these sessions and not risk losing them which may reduce access for providing timely DGA care for high needs cases.

Theme 8 treatment provided and follow-up after a DGA

Paediatric dentists explained that emergency DGA cases, where a child has an infected tooth causing a swollen face, can take less than 15 min in theatre because only the teeth that are causing pain or infection and grossly decayed teeth are extracted. Non-emergency sessions are generally longer and more comprehensive treatment is provided.

The need to provide appropriate dental treatment under DGA was mentioned by most paediatric dentists. Paediatric dentists spoke of the need for 'aggressive treatment' to reduce the prevalence of repeat DGAs. Most interviewees indicated the need to discuss oral hygiene and diet with the family after their child's DGA to reduce the likelihood of repeat DGAs for the child or their siblings.

Discussion

This research has explored the views of OHPs and HADMs about factors associated with the frequency of DGAs among children. The in-depth interviews with paediatric dentists and HDAMs confirmed that the themes in the framework developed from initial focused

discussions with participants were relevant. A wide range of factors were identified. These can be organised into 'push' factors for DGAs and potential factors to decrease DGA rates.

Push factors for children's DGAs

It is evident that approaches to the dental hospitalisation of children have been changing as a result of societal, technical and dental provider influences. Seven factors were identified that may increase DGA prevalence: a perceived greater 'child-focus' with emphasis on not stressing the child; a perceived increase in dental caries in children; DGAs as a preferred model of care; parents low health literacy; parent guilt; convenience for parents; and some dentists reluctance to treat children because they have not had the training and/or experience. These factors will be discussed before addressing the identified factors that are likely to decrease DGA prevalence.

The impact of a perceived greater 'child-focus' on the frequency of DGAs is difficult to quantify. Several participants noted that there had become a greater emphasis in 'not stressing the child' which was possibly associated with more permissive rather than 'authoritative' or 'authoritarian' parenting styles. There was a general view amongst OHPs that there is now less acceptance by parents, children and OHPs of 'rough and tumble' in the dental chair. It was noted by a paediatric dentist that this approach was in keeping with a more pain free policy that has been adopted in general health care.

Four of the five paediatric dentists stated that they considered that children's dental caries rates and consequently dental treatment needs had increased in Victoria since 2000. High dental treatment needs have been shown to be a key driver of DGAs [30]. There is a lack of population data on trends in children's oral health in Australia to test this perception. The results of the only two child population oral health surveys that have been conducted in Australia indicate that dental caries rates in 5–6 year olds have remained similar between 1987 and 88 and 2014–16, with significant reductions in rates in 12 year-olds [31]. However the children accessing paediatric dentists would more likely be high risk children and not representative of the general population.

Jamieson and Roberts-Thomson have suggested that one possible reason for the increased rate of dental hospitalisation of Australian children between 1997 and 98 and 2003–2004 was the increased number of paediatric dentists, *'whose preferred modality for treatment may be a general anaesthetic'* [20]. A more recent shift by Australian paediatric dentists towards the use of DGAs may have occurred. As raised earlier, Alcaino and colleagues noted in 2013 that *'although most children will cope with dentistry in the normal setting, many may benefit from delivery of extensive dentistry in one session under GA'.* [13]. Cameron, who wrote the corresponding section on GA in the 2008 edition of this reference book, suggested that the need for a DGA is the clinician's last solution to treating a child's dental problem [32]. Cameron noted that *'In most instances, a caring attitude in association with a period of familiarisation will allow the child to be treated conservatively'* and that *'If, after seeing the child several times, the clinician feels the child needs dental work, but is unmanageable, a general anaesthetic should be considered'.* These comments are more in keeping with UK guidelines [16, 17] but are not included in the 2013 edition of the reference book [13].

Dental hospitalisation is to some extent what investigators of medical practice variation call 'preference-sensitive' [33]. Variation may reflect differences in patient or clinician preferences or cost. A 2013 review by the Australian Commission on Safety and Quality in Health Care (ACSQHC) into medical practice variation noted that information asymmetry in health care can be an issue, and that patient preferences can be driven by clinicians. This phenomenon is referred to as 'supplier-induced demand' [33]. The other driver of medical care variation identified in the ACSQHC report was 'supply-sensitive care' – when more resources, equipment and workforce are available, the more they will be used [33].

These workforce supply factors and information asymmetry between OHPs and parents may be relevant to DGA rates in Victoria. The low oral health literacy levels of some parents were noted by OHP participants as well as the possibility of OHPs using parental guilt that their child has dental caries when discussing the need for a DGA. Also the latest examination of supply and demand in the Australian oral health workforce concluded that there was generally an excess supply of dentists, a shortage of dental therapists, and *'no current perceived shortage'* of paediatric dentists in the private sector in the metropolitan areas with a likely excess of paediatric dentists in the near future except in the public sector and rural and remote areas [34]. The number of registered paediatric dentists in Victoria has increased from four in 1995 to 41 in 2018 [35]. While several participants noted cases where they may have been an element of preference and/or supply sensitive demand in Victoria, the extent of such demand pressures is difficult to quantify and is worthy of further research with larger sample sizes and interviews with paediatric dentists working in the private sector.

Several of the participants mentioned that DGA is convenient for parents because treatment can be completed in one session, rather than three or more visits to a dental clinic. It was noted that DGA can be attractive to parents who are time-poor and asset-rich. Patient/practitioner convenience is considered a contraindication for DGA in the 2017 American APD guidelines for

DGA [9]. This area is not considered in the Australasian APD 2005 guidelines for children's DGA. Whether there is a need for new guidelines in Australia will be discussed under policy implications of the study.

All of the OHP participants considered that general dentists may be reluctant to treat young children due to a lack of confidence because they may not have had the necessary training or experience. A general view was that there was not sufficient practical experience during basic dental degree training. Participants also mentioned changes in general dental practice that may have affected DGA rates such as more referral options with increased numbers of registered paediatric dentists and less acceptance by children, parents and dental providers of 'rough and tumble' in the dental chair.

Potential factors to decrease DGA rates

Factors that were identified that are likely to decrease DGA prevalence included: the prevention of dental caries which is the major 'cause' of DGAs in children; use of alternatives to DGAs; an appropriate workforce mix; enhancing the oral health literacy of parents; and development and use of evidence-informed guidelines for DGAs. These factors will be reviewed and policy implications considered before discussing the impact of DGAs on health and costs, strengths and limitations of the study, and what further research is required.

All participants agreed that it was preferable to prevent dental caries rather than have to treat it. Primarily this requires addressing the social determinants, that is the 'upstream', 'causes of causes', such as the political and economic drivers [36]. Addressing sugar consumption is fundamental because sugar is the major proximal cause of dental caries [37]. Other interventions include extending community water fluoridation [38] and using other health professionals such as child health nurses for screening and referral for dental care [39].

Alternatives to DGAs that participants raised included enhanced child management techniques and use of sedation. A recent pragmatic randomised control trial in Western Australia using dental therapists compared use of atraumatic restorative treatment procedures with the standard care approach for preschool children with dental caries [40]. At 12 months follow up, there was a 45% lower rate of referral for specialist care in the intervention group. These children also reported lower levels of dental fear.

The Dental Board of Australia requires dental practitioners to undertake a training course before they are endorsed to provide intravenous sedation. As noted by a participant, the only Australian course is in Sydney, New South Wales. Just seven Victorian dental practitioners were endorsed in 2018 compared to 49 dental practitioners in New South Wales [41]. There is a need to understand the barriers faced by Victorian practitioners to becoming endorsed. It is likely that training and cost of equipment are key issues.

Several participants commented that a workforce mix is required that provides effective and efficient oral health care to meet community needs. The use of dental and oral health therapists as the primary health care workers with dentists and paediatric specialists available for work outside therapists scope of practice was considered ideal.

Enhancing the oral health literacy of parents would help to address the information asymmetry that exists between them and OHPs and allow for fully informed consent about options to DGA. Poor understanding of the importance of primary teeth and the preventive impact of fluoride were reported by interviewees. A concerning trend was the observed increase in the use of herbal toothpaste rather than fluoride toothpaste.

In relation to DGA guidelines, while all dental clinicians interviewed indicated that a DGA was required for children with high dental treatment needs and/or behavioural issues, views about thresholds varied. Some saw a DGA as the last resort, while others had a lower threshold for hospitalisation. Recently developed clinical guidelines for the Victorian public dental sector support a move away from DGA being the first resort for children for whom dental treatment in a dental chair is not considered possible. A dedicated prevention services appointment is mandated before a DGA service is offered. Recall systems must be implemented for children who do have a DGA [42]. These guidelines also outline what are the most appropriate and long lasting treatment options for a DGA. However the guidelines do not address indications for DGA, and as noted by several participants, there are no standard Australian policy guidelines for referral for publicly funded DGA.

Several paediatric dentists considered that the 2005 Australasian APD guidelines required updating. These guidelines are mostly similar to the 2017 American APD guidelines. A key difference is that there are two additional contraindications for DGA in the latter guidelines: a very young patient with minimal dental needs that can be addressed through therapeutic interventions, and patient/practitioner convenience. New Australian guidelines would need to take into account an enhanced child focus in health care generally, increased DGA safety, treatment shifts, and parent demand.

Health impacts

Participants considered that the health risks of DGAs were low. Paediatric dentist participants noted that deaths under DGA were rare. Two child deaths under DGA in Australia over the last 20 were discussed. Both deaths were associated with the children's underlying medical

problems. A third child death was raised by one of the participants after the study was completed but no publically available details were found. Child DGA mortality appears to be rare in Australia and lower than the 1:150,000 rate for child GA mortality identified in 2005 [13].

Paediatric dentists indicated that the safety of DGAs had improved with new anaesthetic drugs and better monitoring, a finding supported by an international review of DGAs [43]. Newer anaesthetic agents have fewer side effects and improved monitoring allows problems to be detected earlier when intervention can occur. However nausea was noted by some paediatric dentists as a still common side effect of DGA and could be distressing for the child and parents.

Possible adverse impacts of general anaesthesia on young children's neuro-development is an active area of research [44]. The United States Food and Drug Administration issued a warning in 2016, updated in 2017, that exposure to anaesthetic and sedative drugs for more than 3 h may cause adverse effects on young children's developing brain [45]. Children's DGAs however rarely last longer than half this time [44, 46]. Nelson and Xu in a review of research into the neurological effects of sedation and DGA in children concluded that it is likely to be many years before it is possible to determine the impact on learning and behaviour with confidence [47]. Further research on the side effects of DGAs is required.

Costs

Based on the conservative assumption that public and private DGAs average $3029 [29], the estimated direct DGA costs for dental Diagnostic Related Groups would have been $571.8 million in Australia in 2013–14. These costs do not include indirect costs such as childcare for other children and loss of income from taking time off work.

Strengths and limitations

The strength of the qualitative research approach employed in the study was that a detailed exploration of the contributing factors impacting on DGAs was possible. A more comprehensive understanding of decision making contexts related to DGAs was obtained, particularly for factors that are difficult to quantify. Open ended questions allowed participants to describe their perceptions about DGAs. Interviews with HDAMs allowed a deeper understanding of the policy nuances that impact on DGA rates. While the sample was small and targeted, it allowed a set of perspectives on DGAs to be compiled that have not been explored in depth in the literature.

A limitation of the study was that participants worked predominantly in the public sector and although many had also experience in private settings, paediatric dentists working predominantly in the private sector were not interviewed. The key focus for policy and practice implications is therefore in the public sector. Another limitation was that interviews were not audio recorded. While this approach risked loss of data, it was possible to create a more collegial tone between the researcher and participants interviewed, facilitating in-depth discussion about sensitive issues. The principal investigator took notes which were compiled and provided to the participants to check accuracy.

Research required

The research identified the complex nature of decision making around dental hospitalisation for children at the OHP and parent level. Decisions whether children should receive dental treatment under GA can be complex and raise diagnostic conundrums. The interests of the child, parent and dental provider may align or differ. Issues in the social processes between these participants include power relations, information asymmetry, parental guilt, professional prestige, and commercial pressures. Further research with a medical sociology lens that includes interviewing parents and children would deepen understanding of the complexities related to decision making for DGAs. More research is also required on cost benefit analysis of DGA and alternatives, health and cost impacts, education and workforce issues, and access to operating theatres in the public and private systems. Interviews with private paediatric dentists are required to identify their perspectives on DGAs.

Policy implications

Policy implications of the study include: expanding courses to train OHPs in alternatives to DGAs; follow up with the family after a DGA to discuss oral hygiene and diet to reduce the likelihood of repeat DGAs for the child or their siblings; address oral health workforce imbalances; enhance families oral health literacy particularly related to the prevention of dental disease and alternatives to DGAs; enhance initiatives to prevent dental caries, the proximal 'cause' of most DGAs in children; and develop Australian DGA guidelines.

Conclusion

The prevalence of hospitalisation of children to treat dental caries is increasing. Many factors influence the prevalence of paediatric dental general anaesthetics – relating to the child, parent, oral health professional, financial impact, health risk, and accessibility to facilities. There are quality of care and convenience benefits but also high costs and possible health risks. Family, workforce and health system factors have been identified that could decrease the prevalence of paediatric dental general anaesthetics.

Abbreviations
DGAs: Dental general anaesthetics; HADMs: Hospital admission decision makers; OHPs: Oral health professionals; PPDHs: Potentially preventable dental hospitalisations

Acknowledgements
JR thanks the Oral Health CRC and his Advisory Committee members for support to conduct his PhD - Professor Ivan Darby (chair), Professor Geoffrey McColl, Associate Professor Andrea de Silva, and his three supervisors (MM, FACW and KRT) who have co-authored this article.

Funding
Not applicable.

Authors' contributions
JR conducted the study as part of his PhD thesis with the Oral Health Collaborative Research Centre (CRC), Melbourne Dental School, The University of Melbourne, Victoria, Australia. CD, MM, FACW, and KRT provided assistance with study design, data analysis and critical revision of the manuscript. All authors read and approved the final manuscript.

Competing interests
The authors declare that they have no competing interests.

Author details
[1]University of Melbourne, Melbourne, Victoria, Australia. [2]University of Sydney, Sydney, New South Wales, Australia. [3]University of Adelaide, Adelaide, South Australia, Australia.

References
1. Chrisopoulos S, Harford JE, Ellershaw A. Oral health and dental care in Australia: key facts and figures 2015. Canberra: Australian Institute of Health and Welfare; 2016.
2. Victorian Health Intelligence Information Surveillance System (VHIIS). https://hns.dhs.vic.gov.au/3netapps/vhisspublicsite/ViewContent.aspx?TopicID=1. Accessed 11 Nov 2017.
3. Rogers J. Dental hospitalisation of children. Australian and New Zealand Journal of Dental and Oral Health Therapy. 2017;6(1):1,4–5.
4. Department of Health and Human Services (DHHS). Victorian admitted episode dataset (VAED). Melbourne: Department of Health and Human Services (DHHS); 2017.
5. Katterl R, Anikeeva O, Butler C, Brown L, Smith B, Bywood P. Potentially avoidable hospitalisations in Australia: causes for hospitalisations and primary health care interventions. Adelaide: Primary Health Care Research & Information Service; 2012.
6. Burnham R, Bhandari R, Bridle C. Changes in admission rates for spreading odontogenic infection resulting from changes in government policy about the dental schedule and remunerations. Br J Oral Maxillofac Surg. 2011; 49(1):26–8.
7. AIHW. National Healthcare Agreement: P1 18-selected potentially preventable hospitalisations, 2015. Australian Institute of Health and Welfare: Canberra; 2015.
8. Australian Government. Healthy mouths healthy lives:Australia's National Oral Health Plan 2015-2014. Adelaide: Council of Australian Governments (COAG) Health Council; 2015.
9. American Academy of Pediatric Dentistry. Behavior guidance for the pediatric dental patient. Pediatr Dent. 2017;39(6):246–59.
10. Knapp R, Gilchrist F, Rodd HD, Marshman Z. Change in children's oral health-related quality of life following dental treatment under general anaesthesia for the management of dental caries: a systematic review. Int J Paediatr Dent. 2017;27(4):302–12.

11. Alsharif AT, Kruger E, Tennant M. Dental hospitalization trends in Western Australian children under the age of 15 years: a decade of population-based study. Int J Paediatr Dent. 2015;25(1):35–42.

12. Richardson BJ, Richardson JR. End the decay: the cost of poor dental health and what should be done about it. Melbourne: Brotherhood of St. Laurence; 2011.

13. Alcaino EA, McDonald J, Cooper MG, Malhi S. Pharmacological behaviour management. In: Cameron AC, Widmer RP, editors. Handbook of Pediatric Dentistry. 4th ed. Mosby: Elsevier; 2013. p. 25–46.

14. Rodd H, Hall M, Deery C, Gilchrist F, Gibson BJ, Marshman Z. 'I felt weird and wobbly.' child-reported impacts associated with a dental general anaesthetic. Br Dent J. 2014;216(8):E17.

15. Goodwin M, Sanders C, Pretty IA. A study of the provision of hospital based dental general anaesthetic services for children in the northwest of England: part 1-a comparison of service delivery between six hospitals. BMC Oral Health. 2015;15:50.

16. Davies C, Harrison M, Roberts G. UK national clinical guidelines in paediatric dentistry: guideline for the use of general anaesthesia (GA) in paediatric dentistry. London: Royal College of Surgeons of England; 2008.

17. Royal College of Surgeons of England: Clinical guidelines and integrated care pathways for the oral health care of people with learning disabilities. Faculty of Dental Surgery, the Royal College of Surgeons of England, British Society for Disability and Oral Health 2012.

18. Dental Health Services Victoria. Avoiding anaesthesia: Treating kids at the chair. https://www.dhsv.org.au/news/news-stories/general-news-stories/2015-news/avoiding-anaesthesia-treating-kids-at-the-chair. Accessed 11 Nov 2017.

19. Australasian Academy of Paediatric Dentistry. Standards of care. Australia: Australasian Academy of Paediatric Dentistry; 2005.

20. Jamieson LM, Roberts-Thomson KF. Dental general anaesthetic trends among Australian children. BMC Oral Health. 2006;6:16.

21. Schroth RJ, Quinonez C, Shwart L, Wagar B. Treating early childhood caries under general anesthesia: a National Review of Canadian data. J Can Dent Assoc. 2016;82:20.

22. Kruger E, Tennant M. Potentially preventable hospital separations related to oral health: a 10-year analysis. Aust Dent J. 2015;60(2):205–11.

23. Rogers JG, Adams GG, Wright FAC, Roberts-Thomson K, Morgan MV. Reducing potentially preventable hospitalizations of young children: A community level analysis. JDR Clinical & Translational Research. 2018; 3(3)272-8.

24. Cresswell J. Qualitative inquiry and research design: choosing among five approaches. London: Sage publications; 2013.

25. Greenfield BH, Jensen GM. Understanding the lived experiences of patients: application of a phenomenological approach to ethics. Phys Ther. 2010; 90(8):1185–97.

26. Rice P, Ezzy D. Qualitative research methods. A health focus. Oxford: Oxford University Press; 1999.

27. Palys T. Purposive Sampling. In: Given L, editor. The Sage Enclyclopedia of Qualitative Research Methods. Thousand Oaks: Sage Publications; 2008.

28. Braun V, Clarke V. Successful qualitative research: a practical guide for beginners. London: Sage; 2013.

29. Independent Hospital Pricing Authority. National Hospital Cost Data Collection (NHCDC) Australian Public Hospitals Cost Report 2012–12, Round 17. Canberra: Commonwealth of Australia; 2015.

30. Ramdaw A, Hosey MT, Bernabe E. Factors associated with use of general anaesthesia for dental procedures among British children. Br Dent J. 2017; 223(5):339–45.

31. Do LG, Luzzi L, Ha D.H, Roberts-Thomson K.F., Chrisopoulos S, Armfield J.M. and Spencer A.J. : Trends in child oral health in Australia. In: Oral health of Australian children - The National Child Oral Health Study 2012–14. Do LG, Spencer AJ. Adelaide: University of Adelaide Press; 2016: 288–297.

32. Cameron AC. In: Cameron AC, Widmer RP, editors. Handbook of Pediatric Dentistry. 3rd ed. Mosby: Elsevier; 2008.

33. Australian Commission on Safety and Quality in Health Care (ACSQHC). Medical Practice Variation: Background Paper. Sydney: ACSQHC; 2013.

34. Health Workforce Australia. Australia's Future Health Workforce - Oral Health - Detailed report. Canberra: Department of Health, Australian Government; 2014.

35. Dental Board of Australia. Statistics. Registrant Data 2018. Dental specialists 2018. http://www.dentalboard.gov.au/About-the-Board/Statistics.aspx. Accessed 24 Apr 2018.

36. Watt RG, Heilmann A, Listl S, Peres MA. London charter on oral health inequalities. J Dent Res. 2016;95(3):245–7.

37. Sheiham A, James W. Diet and dental caries the pivotal role of free sugars reemphasized. J Dent Res. 2015;94(10):1341–7.

38. National Health and Medical Research Council (NHMRC). Information Paper – Water fluoridation: dental and other human health outcomes. Canberra: NHMRC; 2017.

39. Rogers JG. Evidence-based oral health promotion resource. Melbourne: Victorian Department of Health; 2011.

40. Arrow P, Klobas E. Minimum intervention dentistry approach to managing early childhood caries: a randomized control trial. Community Dent Oral Epidemiol. 2015;43(6):511–20.

41. Dental Board of Australia. Statistics. 2018. Endorsements 2018. http://www.dentalboard.gov.au/About-the-Board/Statistics.aspx. Accessed 24 Apr 2018.

42. Dental Health Services Victoria (DHSV). Treatment planning for children managed under dental general anaesthesia. In: Clinical Guideline 18 - Version, vol. 3. Melbourne: DHSV; 2017. p. 1–5.

43. Farsi N, Ba'akdah R, Boker A, Almushayt A. Postoperative complications of pediatric dental general anaesthesia procedure provided in Jeddah hospitals, Saudi Arabia. BMC Oral Health. 2009;9:6.

44. Davidson AJ, Disma N, de Graaff JC, Withington DE, Dorris L, Bell G, Stargatt R, Bellinger DC, Schuster T, Arnup SJ, et al. Neurodevelopmental outcome at 2 years of age after general anaesthesia and awake-regional anaesthesia in infancy (GAS): an international multicentre, randomised controlled trial. Lancet. 2016;387(10015):239–50.

45. US Food and Drug Administration. FDA drug safety communication: FDA review results in new warnings about using general anesthetics and sedation drugs in young children and pregnant women. 2016 https://www.fda.gov/Drugs/DrugSafety/ucm532356.htm. Accessed 24 Apr 2018. Update issued 2017. FDA Drug Safety Communication: FDA approves label changes for use of general anesthetic and sedation drugs in young children. https://www.fda.gov/Drugs/DrugSafety/ucm554634.htm. Accessed 24 Apr 2018.

46. Andropoulos DB, Greene MF. Anesthesia and developing brains - implications of the FDA warning. N Engl J Med. 2017;376(10):905–7.

47. Nelson TM, Xu Z. Pediatric dental sedation: challenges and opportunities. Clin Cosmet Investig Dent. 2015;7:97–106.

Permissions

The contributors of this book come from diverse backgrounds, making this book a truly international effort. This book will bring forth new frontiers with its revolutionizing research information and detailed analysis of the nascent developments around the world.

We would like to thank all the contributing authors for lending their expertise to make the book truly unique. They have played a crucial role in the development of this book. Without their invaluable contributions this book wouldn't have been possible. They have made vital efforts to compile up to date information on the varied aspects of this subject to make this book a valuable addition to the collection of many professionals and students.

This book was conceptualized with the vision of imparting up-to-date information and advanced data in this field. To ensure the same, a matchless editorial board was set up. Every individual on the board went through rigorous rounds of assessment to prove their worth. After which they invested a large part of their time researching and compiling the most relevant data for our readers.

The editorial board has been involved in producing this book since its inception. They have spent rigorous hours researching and exploring the diverse topics which have resulted in the successful publishing of this book. They have passed on their knowledge of decades through this book. To expedite this challenging task, the publisher supported the team at every step. A small team of assistant editors was also appointed to further simplify the editing procedure and attain best results for the readers.

Apart from the editorial board, the designing team has also invested a significant amount of their time in understanding the subject and creating the most relevant covers. They scrutinized every image to scout for the most suitable representation of the subject and create an appropriate cover for the book.

The publishing team has been an ardent support to the editorial, designing and production team. Their endless efforts to recruit the best for this project, has resulted in the accomplishment of this book. They are a veteran in the field of academics and their pool of knowledge is as vast as their experience in printing. Their expertise and guidance has proved useful at every step. Their uncompromising quality standards have made this book an exceptional effort. Their encouragement from time to time has been an inspiration for everyone.

The publisher and the editorial board hope that this book will prove to be a valuable piece of knowledge for researchers, students, practitioners and scholars across the globe.

List of Contributors

Ryota Nomura, Yuko Ogaya, Saaya Matayoshi, Yumiko Morita and Kazuhiko Nakano
Department of Pediatric Dentistry, Division of Oral Infection and Disease Control, Osaka University Graduate School of Dentistry, 1-8 Yamada-oka, Suita, Osaka 565-0871, Japan

Yaqi Deng, Yannan Sun and Tianmin Xu
Department of Orthodontics, Peking University School and Hospital of Stomatology, Beijing 100081, People's Republic of China

Thankam Thyvalikakath
Dental Informatics Core, Department of Cariology, Operative Dentistry and Dental Public Health, Indiana University School of Dentistry, Research Scientist, Center for Biomedical Informatics, Regenstrief Institute, Inc, 1050 Wishard Boulevard, R2206, Indianapolis, IN 46202, USA

Mei Song
Microbicide Trials Network, Magee-Womens Research Institute, 204 Craft Avenue, Pittsburgh, PA 15213, USA

Titus Schleyer
Center for Biomedical Informatics, Regenstrief Institute, Inc. Indiana University School of Medicine, 1101 West Tenth Street, Indianapolis, IN 46202, USA

Amal Elamin and Malin Garemo
Department of Health Sciences, College of Natural and Health Sciences, Zayed University, Abu-Dhabi, United Arab Emirates

Andrew Gardner
School of Molecular Sciences, University of Western Australia, Crawley, Perth, WA 6009, Australia

Zhi Cui, Ping Yan and Han Jiang
The State Key Laboratory Breeding Base of Basic Science of Stomatology (Hubei-MOST) and Key Laboratory of Oral Biomedicine Ministry of Education, School and Hospital of Stomatology, Wuhan University, Luoyu Road, Wuhan City 237, China

Zhao Wei
Department of Dentistry, Second Hospital of Baoding, 338 Dongfeng West Road, Baoding, China

Minquan Du
Department of Prevention Dentistry School and Hospital of Stomatology, Wuhan University, 237 Luoyu Road, Wuhan, China

Se-Hwan Jung
Department of Preventive Dentistry, College of Dentistry, Gangneung-Wonju University, 120 Gangneungdaehag-ro, Gangneung City, Gangwon Province 25457, South Korea

Myoung-Hee Kim
Center for Health Equity Research, People's Health Institute, 36 Sadangro 13-gil, 2nd floor, Dongjak-gu, Seoul 07004, South Korea

Jae-In Ryu
Department of Preventive and Social Dentistry, College of Dentistry, Kyung Hee University, 26 Kyungheedae-ro, Dongdaemun-gu, Seoul 02447, South Korea

Shalini Nayee, Charlotte Klass and Jennifer E. Gallagher
King's College London Dental Institute, Population and Patient Health Division, Denmark Hill, London SE5 9RS, UK

Gail Findlay
Institute for Health and Human Development, University of East London Stratford Campus, Water Lane, London E12 4LZ, UK

Falk Schwendicke and Karim Elhennawy
Department of Operative and Preventive Dentistry, Charité –Universitätsmedizin Berlin, Aßmannshauser Str. 4-6, 14197 Berlin, Germany

Osama El Shahawy and Reham Maher
Department of Pediatric Dentistry, Cairo University, Giza, Egypt
Department of Pediatric Dentistry, Cairo University, 11 el Saraya Street, Manial, Cairo, Egypt

Thais Gimenez and Fausto M. Mendes
Department of Pediatric Dentistry, School of Dentistry, University of São Paulo, Av. Lineu Prestes, São Paulo 2227, Brazil

Brian H. Willis
Institute of Applied Health Research, University of Birmingham, Edgbaston, Birmingham B15 2TT, UK

Giuliana Bontà
Department of Biomedical, Surgical and Dental Sciences, University of Milan, Via Beldiletto 1, 20142 Milan, Italy

Maria Grazia Cagetti and Laura Strohmenger
Department of Biomedical, Surgical and Dental Sciences, University of Milan, Via Beldiletto 1, 20142 Milan, Italy
WHO Collaboration Centre for Epidemiology and Community Dentistry, Via Beldiletto 1, 20142 Milan, Italy

Fabio Cocco and Guglielmo Campus
WHO Collaboration Centre for Epidemiology and Community Dentistry, Via Beldiletto 1, 20142 Milan, Italy
Department of Surgery, Microsurgery and Medicine Sciences, School of Dentistry University of Sassari, Viale San Pietro, 43 Sassari, Italy

Peter Lingstrom
Department of Cariology, Institute of Odontology, The Sahlgrenska Academy, University of Gothenburg, Medicinaregatan 12 A-G, P.O. Box 450, 405 30 Gothenburg, Sweden

Lingli Wu
Department of Dentistry, Key Laboratory of Oral Diseases of Gansu Province, Northwest University for Nationalities, Lanzhou, China

Xiaoli Gao
Dental Public Health, Faculty of Dentistry, The University of Hong Kong, 3rd Floor, Prince Philip Dental Hospital, 34 Hospital Road, Sai Ying Pun, Hong Kong

Juliana de Aguiar Grossi, Renata Nunes Cabral and Soraya Coelho Leal
Faculdade de Ciências da Saúde, Universidade de Brasília, Campus Universitário Darcy Ribeiro, Asa Norte, Brasília, DF 70910-900, Brazil

Ana Paula Dias Ribeiro
Faculdade de Ciências da Saúde, Universidade de Brasília, Campus Universitário Darcy Ribeiro, Asa Norte, Brasília, DF 70910-900, Brazil
Department of Restorative Dental Sciences, College of Dentistry, University of Florida, 1395 Center Dr, Gainesville, FL 32610-0415, USA

Katarzyna Grocholewicz and Joanna Janiszewska-Olszowska
Department of Interdisciplinary Dentistry, Pomeranian Medical University in Szczecin, Al. Powstancow Wlkp. 72, 70-111 Szczecin, Poland

Magda Aniko-Włodarczyk, Olga Preuss and Grzegorz Trybek
Department of Oral Surgery, Pomeranian Medical University in Szczecin, Szczecin, Poland

Ewa Sobolewska
Department of Dental Prosthetics, Pomeranian Medical University in Szczecin, Szczecin, Poland

Mariusz Lipski
Department of Preclinical Conservative Dentistry and Preclinical Endodontics, Pomeranian Medical University in Szczecin, Szczecin, Poland

Kari Elisabeth Dahl and Giovanna Calogiuri
Department of Public Health, Faculty of Social and Health Sciences, Inland Norway University of Applied Sciences, Hamarveien 112, 2418 Elverum, Norway

Birgitta Jönsson
The Public Dental Health Service. Competence Centre of Northern Norway (TkNN), Tromsø, Norway
Institute of Odontology, Department of Periodontology, The Sahlgrenska Academy, University of Gothenburg, Gothenburg, Sweden

Gunnar Dahlén, Haidar Hassan, Susanne Blomqvist and Anette Carlén
Department of Oral Microbiology and Immunology, Institute of Odontology, Sahlgrenska Academy, University of Gothenburg, Box 450, SE 40530 Gothenburg, Sweden

Jin Ah Kim
College of Nursing Science, Kyung Hee University, Seoul, Korea

Hayon Michelle Choi
Graduate School of Public Health, Seoul National University, Seoul, Korea

Yunhee Seo
Graduate School of Public Health, Ajou University, Suwon, Korea

Dae Ryong Kang
Center of Biomedical Data Science / Institute of Genomic Cohort, Wonju College of Medicine, Yonsei University, 20 Ilsan-ro, Wonju, Gangwon-do 26426, Korea

Borany Tort, Youn-Hee Choi, Yun-Sook Jung and Keun-Bae Song
Department of Preventive Dentistry, School of Dentistry, Kyungpook National University, 2177 Dalgubeol-daero, Jung-gu, Daegu 700-412, Republic of Korea

Eun-Kyong Kim
Department of Dental Hygiene, College of Science and Technology, Kyungpook National University, 386 Gajangdong, Sangju 742-711, Republic of Korea

Mina Ha
Department of Preventive Medicine, Dankook University College of Medicine, 119, Dandae-ro, Dongnam-gu, Cheonan-si, Chungnam 330-714, Republic of Korea

Young-Eun Lee
Department of Dental Hygiene, Daegu Health College, 15 Youngsong-Ro, Buk-Gu, Daegu 702-722, Republic of Korea

Teddy Nagaddya, Florence Nakaggwa, Mary Gorrethy N-Mboowa, Peter Kirabira and John Charles Okiria
Clarke International University (CIU) formerly International Health Sciences University (IHSU), Plot 4686, St. Barnabas Road Kisugu-Namuwongo, , Kampala, Uganda

Fiona Atim
Clarke International University (CIU) formerly International Health Sciences University (IHSU), Plot 4686, St. Barnabas Road Kisugu-Namuwongo, Kampala, Uganda
St. Lawrence University, Kampala, Uganda

Kirstine Juhl Thuesen and Dorte Haubek
Section for Pediatric Dentistry, Department of Dentistry and Oral Health, Health, Aarhus University, Vennelyst Boulevard 9, 8000 Aarhus C, Denmark

Hans Gjørup
Center for Oral Health in Rare Diseases, Department of Maxillofacial Surgery, Aarhus University Hospital, Noerrebrogade 44, 8000 Aarhus C, Denmark

Jannie Dahl Hald Torben Harsløf and Bente Langdahl
Department of Endocrinology and Internal Medicine, Aarhus University Hospital, Tage-Hansens Gade 2, Aarhus, Denmark

Malene Schmidt
Aarhus Municipal Dental Service, Groendalsvej 2, 8000 Aarhus C, Denmark

Rosalia Leonardi and Simone Muraglie
Department of Orthodontics, Policlinico Universitario "Vittorio Emanuele", University of Catania, Catania, Italy

Salvatore Crimi
Department of Maxillofacial Surgery Policlinico G Martino, University of Messina, Messina, Italy

Marco Pirroni
Private practice, Bologna, Italy

Giuseppe Musumeci
Department of Biomedical and Biotechnological Sciences, Human Anatomy and Histology Section, School of Medicine, University of Catania, Catania, Italy

Rosario Perrotta
Department of Plastic Surgery, Director of the Master'sDegree in Plastic Surgery, University of Catania, Catania, Italy

U. Wide J.Hagman, H. Werner and M.Hakeberg
Department of Behavioral and Community Dentistry, Institute of Odontology, The Sahlgrenska Academy, University of Gothenburg, SE-40530 Gothenburg, Sweden

Hey Chiann Wong, Yuxuan and Ooi Shaju Jacob Pulikkotil
School of Dentistry, International Medical University, Kuala Lumpur, Malaysia

Cho Naing
Institute for Research, Development and Innovation (IRDI), International Medical University, 5700 Kuala Lumpur, Malaysia
Division of Tropical Heath and Medicine, James Cook University, Townsville, Australia

Hye-Kyung Lee and Joo-Cheol Park
Departments of Oral Histology-Developmental Biology and Dental Research Institute, School of Dentistry, Seoul National University, 101 Daehagro, Chongro-gu, Seoul 110-749, South Korea.

Soo Jin Kim
Office of Biostatistics, Institute of Medical Sciences, Ajou University School of Medicine, Suwon, South Korea

Young Ho Kim
Department of Orthodontics, Institute of Oral Health Science, Ajou University School of Medicine, Suwon, South Korea

Youngkyung Ko
Department of Periodontics, College of Medicine, Seoul St Mary's Hospital, The Catholic University of Korea, Seoul, South Korea

Suk Ji
Department of Periodontics, Institute of Oral Health Science, Ajou University School of Medicine, 164, World cup-ro, Yeongtong-gu, Suwon, South Korea

Kylie Gwynne, Norma Binge and Anthony Blinkhorn
Poche Centre for Indigenous Health, University of Sydney, Room 223 Edward Ford Building, Sydney, New South Wales, Australia

Yvonne Dimitropoulos and Michelle Irving
Poche Centre for Indigenous Health, University of Sydney, Room 223 Edward Ford Building, Sydney, New South Wales, Australia
University of Sydney School of Dentistry, Mons Road, Westmead, Sydney, NSW 2145, Australia

Alexander Holden
University of Sydney School of Dentistry, Mons Road, Westmead, Sydney, NSW 2145, Australia

Magandhree Naidoo and Shenuka Singh
School of Health Sciences, Discipline of Dentistry, University of KwaZulu-Natal, Westville Campus, South Africa

Paula R. Blasi, Melissa L. Anderson, Jennifer Nelson and Jennifer B. McClure
Kaiser Permanente Washington Health Research Institute, 1730 Minor Ave, Suite 1600, Seattle, WA 98101, USA

Chloe Krakauer
Department of Biostatistics, University of Washington, F-600, Health Sciences Building 1705 NE Pacific Street, Seattle, WA 98195, USA

Terry Bush
Optum Center for Wellbeing Research, 999 3rd Ave., Suite 2000, Seattle, Washington 98104, USA

Sheryl L. Catz
Betty Irene Moore School of Nursing, University of California-Davis, 2450 48th Street, Suite 2600, Sacramento, CA 95817, USA

Magdalena Sulewska and Ewa Duraj
Department of Periodontal and Oral Mucosa Diseases, Medical University of Białystok, ul. Waszyngtona 13, 15-269 Białystok, Poland

Beata Bugała-Musiatowicz
Dental Practice, ul. Żeromskiego 1A/1U, 15-349 Białystok, Poland

Emilia Waszkiewicz-Sewastianik and Jan K. Pietruski
Dental Practice, ul. Waszyngtona 1/34, 15-269 Białystok, Poland.

Małgorzata Pietruska
Department of Periodontal and Oral Mucosa Diseases, Medical University of Białystok, ul. Waszyngtona 13, 15-269 Białystok, Poland
Dental Practice, ul. Waszyngtona 1/34, 15-269 Białystok, Poland

Robert Milewski
Department of Statistics and Medical Informatics, Medical University of Białystok, ul. Szpitalna 37, 15-295 Białystok, Poland

Eugeniusz Sajewicz
Department of Biocybernetics and Biomedical Ingeenering, Białystok University of Technology, ul. Wiejska 45c, 15-351 Białystok, Poland

Vinicius da Costa Vieira and Liliane Lins
School of Medicine, Federal University of Bahia, Praça XV de Novembro, Largo do Terreiro de Jesus s/n, Salvador, Bahia CEP 400260-10, Brazil

Viviane Almeida Sarmento
School of Dentstry, Federal University of Bahia, Salvador, Bahia, Brazil

Eduardo Martins Netto and Carlos Brites
Research Laboratory of Infectious Diseases, Edgard Santos Federal University Hospital, Salvador, Bahia, Brazil

D. Klonowicz and M. Czerwinska
Dermscan Poland, Ul. Kruczkowskiego 12, 80-288 Gdansk, Poland

A. Sirvent
Laboratoire Dermscan, 114 Bd du 11 novembre 1918, 69100 Villeurbanne, France

J-Ph. Gatignol
Innovation Unit Consumer HealthCare, 17 avenue Jean Moulin, 81106 Castres Cedex, France

Yechen Gu
Department of Endodontics, Stomatological Hospital Affiliated to Soochow University, Suzhou Stomatological Hospital, Suzhou, Jiangsu, People's Republic of China
Jiangsu Key Laboratory of Oral Diseases, the Affiliated Stomatological Hospital of Nanjing Medical University, 136 Hanzhong Road, Nanjing 210029, People's Republic of China
Department of Oral Special Consultation, the Affiliated Stomatological Hospital of Nanjing Medical University, 136 Hanzhong Road, Nanjing 210029, People's Republic of China

Qingping Zhu
Jiangsu Key Laboratory of Oral Diseases, the Affiliated Stomatological Hospital of Nanjing Medical University, 136 Hanzhong Road, Nanjing 210029, People's Republic of China
Department of Oral Special Consultation, the Affiliated Stomatological Hospital of Nanjing Medical University, 136 Hanzhong Road, Nanjing 210029, People's Republic of China

Chao Sun
Jiangsu Key Laboratory of Oral Diseases, the Affiliated Stomatological Hospital of Nanjing Medical University, 136 Hanzhong Road, Nanjing 210029, People's Republic of China

Department of Radiology, the Affiliated Stomatological Hospital of Nanjing Medical University, 136 Hanzhong Road, Nanjing 210029, People's Republic of China

Daming Wu, Diya Leng and Yang Zhou
Jiangsu Key Laboratory of Oral Diseases, the Affiliated Stomatological Hospital of Nanjing Medical University, 136 Hanzhong Road, Nanjing 210029, People's Republic of China
Department of Radiology, the Affiliated Stomatological Hospital of Nanjing Medical University, 136 Hanzhong Road, Nanjing 210029, People's Republic of China
Department of Endodontics, the Affiliated Stomatological Hospital of Nanjing Medical University, 136 Hanzhong Road, Nanjing 210029, People's Republic of China

Alexander Kailembo, Gabriela V. Lopez Mitnik, Timothy Iafolla and Bruce A. Dye
National Institutes of Health, National Institute of Dental and Craniofacial Research, Bethesda, USA

Carlos Quiñonez
University of Toronto, Toronto, Canada

Jane A. Weintraub
University of North Carolina, Chapel Hill, USA

Raman Preet
Umeå University, Umea, Sweden

Jennifer Stewart Williams
Umeå University, Umea, Sweden
Research Centre for Generational Health and Ageing, University of Newcastle, Callaghan, Australia

John Rogers, Clare Delany and Mike Morgan
University of Melbourne, Melbourne, Victoria, Australia

Clive Wright
University of Sydney, Sydney, New South Wales, Australia

Kaye Roberts-Thomson
University of Adelaide, Adelaide, South Australia, Australia

Index

A

Acceptance and Commitment Therapy, 164, 170-171

Actinomyces Naeslundii, 119, 121, 125

Antiretroviral Therapy, 227-228, 232

Atraumatic Restorative Treatment, 96-97, 102, 267

Autism Spectrum Disorder, 165, 197-198, 201-205

B

Blood Lead Level, 133, 135-139

C

Campylobacter Ureolyticus,, 120

Canine Bud Extraction, 140-142, 145-146

Cariogram, 76-85

Cognitive Behaviour Therapy, 164-165, 171

Cone Beam Computed Tomography, 10, 13, 22-23, 48, 162, 248

Corah Dental Anxiety Scale, 86, 93

Corticotomy-assisted Orthodontic Treatment, 218-219, 225

D

Dental Caries, 5-7, 34-41, 50-54, 56-58, 75-76, 78, 84, 97, 102, 117-118, 126-127, 129-132, 134, 137-139, 164-166, 168, 170, 194-197, 227, 232, 249-250, 259, 269-270

Dental Caries Susceptibility, 76, 78

Dental Fear and Anxiety, 86, 89-90, 93-94

Dental General Anaesthetics, 259, 262, 269

Dentinogenesis Imperfecta (DI), 148

Diagnostic Meta-analyses, 67-68

Diarrhea, 140-141, 144-145

Disparities, 41, 56, 89, 207, 216, 249-250, 256-258

Dmft, 34-40, 76, 78-80, 82, 84, 122, 124, 127, 131, 134, 137-138, 191, 196-203, 227-233

E

Edentulousness, 112, 118

Evidence-based Dentistry, 31, 67

F

Fluoride Toothpaste, 190, 192-193, 195-196, 268

G

Gingival Crevicular Fluid, 120, 125, 181-183, 189

Gingival Index, 41, 133-135, 137, 139, 197, 199, 201, 234-235, 237, 241

Gingival Inflammation, 197, 199, 201, 203

Gingivitis, 124, 133, 136, 138, 165, 170, 228-229, 235, 239, 241

Glass Ionomer, 96-97, 100, 102

H

H. Felis, 2-3

H. Pylori, 1-8, 120, 122-124

Haemophilus Parainfluenzae, 119-121

Hscl-25, 111, 113-118

Human Dental Fibroblast Cells, 1-2, 8

Hybrid Toothbrush, 234-241

I

Il10-1082 A > G, 172-173, 175

Inflamed Pulp, 1-8

J

Junctional Epithelium, 182, 188-189

L

Lactobacilli, 77, 83

Lymphoma, 227-228

M

Malocclusion, 11, 14-15, 19-20, 23, 218-219

Mandibular Anterior Teeth, 10

Mandibular Cortical Index, 103-106, 108-110

Manual Toothbrush, 234, 236, 240

Maxillary Central Incisors, 10, 18-19, 21-22

Maxillary Lateral Incisors, 10, 18-19, 22, 163

Maxillary Posterior Teeth, 242-245, 248

Maxillary Sinus Floor, 242, 248

Missing Teeth, 36-37, 40, 81, 118, 163, 227, 229, 231

Molar Incisor Hypomineralization, 96, 102

N

Nested Pcr Method, 1-3, 5, 8

O

Odds Ratios, 52, 114, 116, 126, 129, 133-134, 138, 257

Odontogenic Ameloblast-associated Protein, 182, 188-189

Oral Bacteria, 2, 119-120, 123

Oral Hygiene Practices, 34-35, 41, 191, 193, 204, 241

Orthodontics, 10-15, 20, 23, 43, 155, 162, 188, 218-219, 223-226, 244

Oscillating-rotating Toothbrush, 234, 236, 239-240

Osteogenesis Imperfecta (OI), 148

Osteoporosis, 103-105, 107-110

P

Palatally Displaced Canine, 155, 161-163

Panoramic Radiograph, 11, 103-106, 109-110, 149

Periodontal Disease, 24-27, 29, 31, 33, 112, 117, 122, 125, 138, 171, 179-181, 183, 189, 204, 219, 228-230, 241

Phalanx Iii, 103-105

Plaque Index, 34, 36, 41, 133-135, 137-139, 183, 185, 188, 197, 199, 201, 203, 218-221, 225, 234, 237-238, 241

Powered Toothbrush, 234-235, 237-238, 240-241

Psychological Intervention, 164-166, 168, 170

Q

Quantitative Ultrasound, 103-104, 109

R

Radiomorphometric Indices, 103, 109

Rapid Urease Test, 119-120, 124-125

Root Apices, 242-247

Root Resorption, 10-14, 16-17, 19-23, 219

S

Self-efficacy, 206-217, 256

Sonic Toothbrush, 234, 239

Staphylococcus Epidermidis, 119-121

Streptococcus Salivarius,, 120

Supragingival Dental Plaque, 119

Surface-to-surface Matching, 155, 157, 162

Syphilis, 227-228

T

Transverse Maxillary Deficiency, 218

V

Visual and Radiographic Caries Detection, 67-68

W

Waveone, 42-43, 47-49

www.ingramcontent.com/pod-product-compliance
Lightning Source LLC
Chambersburg PA
CBHW061314190326

41458CB00011B/3806

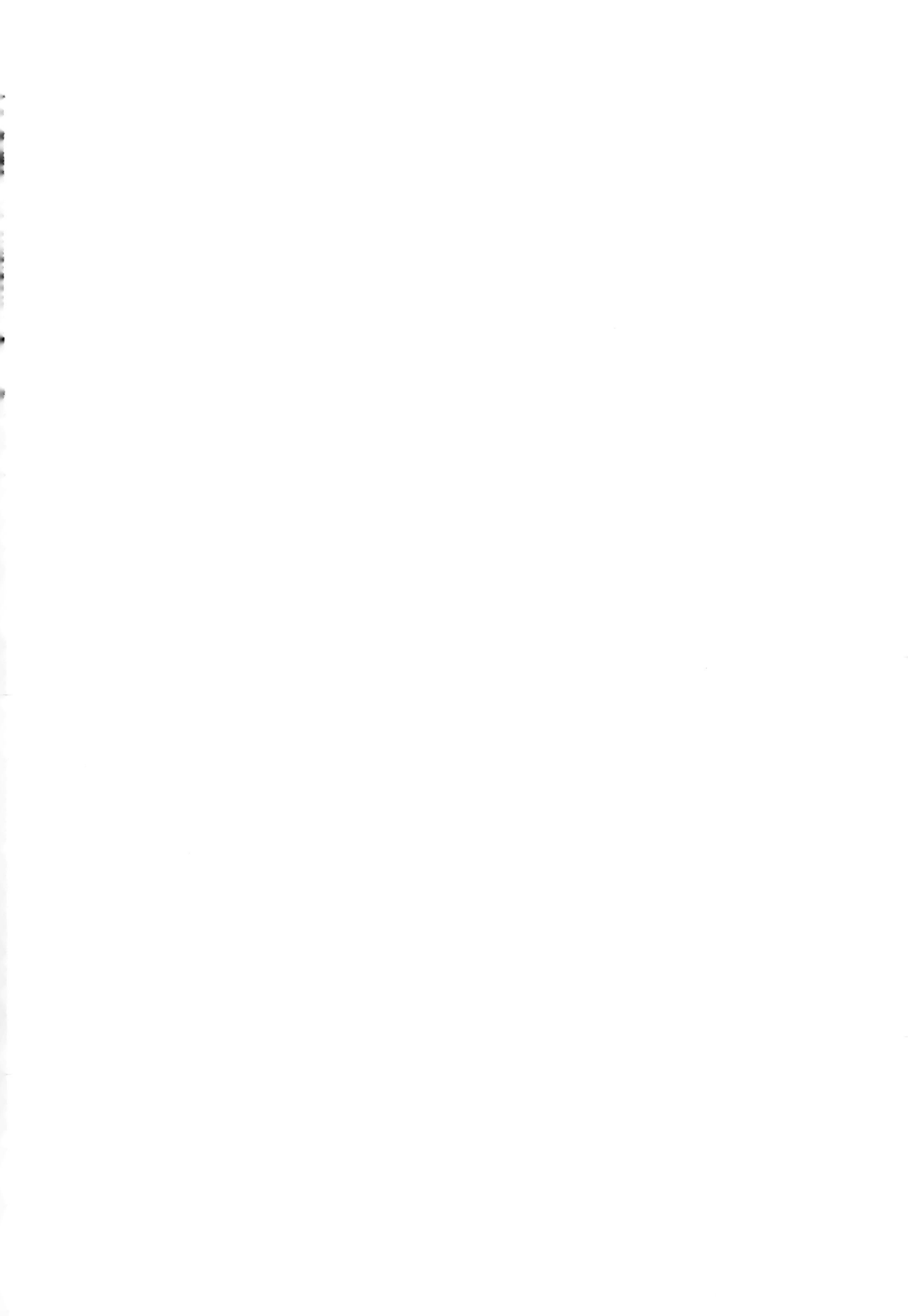